RENEWALS 458-4574
DATE DUE

OCT 1 8			
NOV 1 0			
MAR 2 9			
APR 1 3			
APR 2 8			
DEC 1 2			
ILL 830812		MAY 0 7 2000	
		NO RENEWALS	
JUL 0 8			
OCT 0 2			
		MAR 2 5	
APR 0 9			
GAYLORD			PRINTED IN U.S.A

Trauma and Memory

TRAUMA AND MEMORY

Clinical and Legal Controversies

Edited by

PAUL S. APPELBAUM, M.D.
A. F. Zeleznik Professor of Psychiatry
Chairman, Department of Psychiatry
University of Massachusetts Medical Center

LISA A. UYEHARA, M.D.
Assistant Professor of Psychiatry,
Tufts University School of Medicine
Private Practice of Psychiatry and Psychoanalysis

MARK R. ELIN, PH.D
Assistant Professor,
Tufts University School of Medicine,
Department of Psychiatry,
Division of Neuropsychology,
Baystate Medical Center

New York   Oxford
OXFORD UNIVERSITY PRESS
1997

Oxford University Press

Oxford   New York
Athens   Auckland   Bangkok   Bogota
Bombay   Buenos Aires   Calcutta   Cape Town
Dar es Salaam   Delhi   Florence   Hong Kong   Istanbul
Karachi   Kuala Lumpur   Madras   Madrid
Melbourne   Mexico City   Nairobi   Paris
Singapore   Taipei   Tokyo   Toronto

and associated companies in
Berlin   Ibadan

Library of Congress Cataloging-in-Publication Data
Trauma and memory : clinical and legal controversies /
edited by Paul S. Appelbaum, Lisa A. Uyehara, Mark R. Elin.
p.   cm.   Includes bibliographical references and index.
ISBN 0–19–510065–4
1. Adult child abuse victims—Psychology.
2. Recovered memory.
3. Psychic trauma.
4. Autobiographical memory.
5. False memory syndrome.
I. Appelbaum, Paul S.   II. Uyehara, Lisa A.   III. Elin, Mark R.
[DNLM: 1. Stress Disorders, Post-Traumatic.   2. Memory.
3. Repression.   4. Child Abuse.
WM 170 T7772 1997]
RC569.5.C55T734   1997   616.85′82239—dc20
DNLM/DLC   for Library of Congress   96–27699

9 8 7 6 5 4 3 2 1

Printed in the United States of America
on acid-free paper

Contents

Contributing Authors, ix

Introduction, xiii

I The Controversy Over the Delayed Recall of Traumatic Memories

1. Some People Recover Memories of Childhood Trauma That Never Really Happened, 3
   Ira E. Hyman, Jr. and Elizabeth F. Loftus

2. The Argument for the Reality of Delayed Recall of Trauma, 25
   Richard P. Kluft

II Current Concepts of Memory

3. Neuroanatomical Correlates of the Effects of Stress on Memory: Relevance to the Validity of Memories of Childhood Abuse, 61
   J. Douglas Bremner, Steven M. Southwick, and Dennis S. Charney

4. Inaccuracy and Inaccessibility in Memory Retrieval: Contributions from Cognitive Psychology and Neuropsychology, 93
   Wilma Koutstaal and Daniel L. Schacter

5. Psychoanalysis, Memory, and Trauma, 138
   Robert M. Galatzer-Levy

6. The Nature and Development of Children's Event Memory, 158
   Michelle D. Leichtman, Stephen J. Ceci, and Marjorie B. Morse

7. An Integrative Developmental Model for Trauma and Memory, 188
   Mark R. Elin

III   The Memory of Trauma

8. Memory and Posttraumatic Stress Disorder, 225
    Julia A. Golier, Rachel Yehuda, and Steven M. Southwick

9. Traumatic Memories, 243
    Bessell A. van der Kolk

10. Continuous Memory, Amnesia, and Delayed Recall of Childhood Trauma:
    A Clinical Typology, 261
    Mary R. Harvey and Judith L. Herman

11. Traumatic Experiences: The Early Organization of Memory in School-Age
    Children and Adolescents, 272
    Robert S. Pynoos, Alan M. Steinberg, and Lisa Aronson

Part IV   Trauma and Memory: Evaluation and Treatment

12. Psychoanalysis, Reconstruction, and the Recovery of Memory, 293
    Howard B. Levine

13. Psychodynamic Therapy for Patients with Early Childhood Trauma, 316
    Julia A. Matthews and James A. Chu

14. Hypnosis and Hypnotherapy, 344
    Fred H. Frankel and Nicholas A. Covino

15. Cognitive Therapy of Dissociative Identity Disorder, 360
    Colin A. Ross

16. Memories of Trauma in the Treatment of Children, 378
    Maria C. Sauzier

17. Diagnosis, Pathogenesis, and Memories of Childhood Abuse, 394
    Lisa A. Uyehara

V   The Trauma Debate and the Legal System

18. Legal Rights of Trauma Victims, 425
    Wendy J. Murphy

19. For Whom Does the Bell Toll? Repressed Memory and Challenges for the Law—
    Getting Beyond the Statute of Limitations, 445
    Rose R. Zoltek-Jick

20. Ethical and Clinical Risk Management Principles in Recovered Memory Cases:
    Maintaining Therapist Neutrality, 477
    Robert I. Simon and Thomas G. Gutheil

21. Child Victims in the Legal System, 496
    Diane H. Schetky

VI   Reflections on Trauma and Memory

22. Reflections on Trauma and Memory, 511
    Paul S. Appelbaum

    Index, 529

Contributing Authors

PAUL S. APPELBAUM, M.D.
A.F. Zeleznik Professor of Psychiatry,
Chairman, Department of Psychiatry,
University of Massachusetts Medical Center,
   Worcester, MA

LISA ARONSON, PH.D.
Director of Evaluations, Trauma Psychiatry
   Program,
Department of Psychiatry and Biobehavioral
   Sciences,
University of California at Los Angeles

J. DOUGLAS BREMNER, M.D.
Assistant Professor of Psychiatry and
Fellow in Diagnostic Radiology/Nuclear
   Medicine
Yale University School of Medicine
Research Psychiatrist,
VA Connecticut and National Center for
   PTSD

STEPHEN J. CECI, PH.D.
The Helen L. Carr Professor of Develop-
   mental Psychology,
Cornell University

DENNIS S. CHARNEY, M.D.
Professor of Psychiatry and Associate Chair
   for Research,
Yale University School of Medicine
Chief of Psychiatry,
VA Connecticut and National Center for
   PTSD

JAMES A. CHU, M.D.
Assistant Professor of Psychiatry
Harvard Medical School
Clinical Director,
Dissociative Disorders & Trauma Program
McLean Hospital, Belmont, MA

NICHOLAS A. COVINO, PSY.D.
Assistant Professor of Psychology,
Harvard Medical School
Director, Psychology Division,
Beth Israel Hospital, Boston, MA

MARK R. ELIN, PH.D.
Assistant Professor, Tufts University School
   of Medicine,
Department of Psychiatry, Division of
   Neuropsychology
Baystate Medical Center, Springfield, MA

FRED H. FRANKEL, M.B. CH.B., D.P.M.
Professor of Psychiatry,
Harvard Medical School
Psychiatrist-in-Chief,
Beth Israel Hospital, Boston, MA

ROBERT M. GALATZER-LEVY, M.D.
Lecturer in Psychiatry,
University of Chicago
Training and Supervising Analyst,
Chicago Institute for Psychoanalysis

JULIA A. GOLIER, M.D.
Department of Psychiatry
Yale University

THOMAS G. GUTHEIL, M.D.
Professor of Psychiatry,
Harvard Medical School
Co-director, Program in Psychiatry
   and the Law,
Massachusetts Mental Health Center,
   Boston, MA

MARY R. HARVEY, PH.D.
Director of Victims of Violence Program,
   Cambridge Hospital
Assistant Clinical Professor of Psychology in
   the Department of Psychiatry, Harvard
   Medical School

JUDITH L. HERMAN, M.D.
Director of Training at Victims of Violence
  Program, Cambridge Hospital
Associate Clinical Professor of Psychiatry,
  Harvard Medical School

IRA E. HYMAN, JR., PH.D.
Associate Professor of Psychology,
Western Washington University

RICHARD P. KLUFT, M.D.
Clinical Professor of Psychiatry
Temple University School of Medicine
Director, Dissociative Disorders Program
The Institute of Pennsylvania Hospital,
  Philadelphia, PA

WILMA KOUTSTAAL, PH.D.
Post-Doctoral Researcher, Department of
  Psychology,
Harvard University

JOHN H. KRYSTAL, M.D.
Associate Professor of Psychiatry,
Yale University School of Medicine
Director of Clinical Research
VA Connecticut and National Center for
  PTSD

MICHELLE D. LEICHTMAN, PH.D.
Assistant Professor of Psychology
Harvard University

HOWARD B. LEVINE, M.D.
Faculty, Boston Psychoanalytic Institute
Faculty, Massachusetts Institute for
  Psychoanalysis
Private Practice, Brookline, MA

ELIZABETH F. LOFTUS, PH.D.
Professor of Psychology,
University of Washington

JULIA A. MATTHEWS PH.D., M.D.
Assistant Professor of Psychiatry,
University of Massachusetts Medical School
Attending Psychiatrist, Adult Mental Health
  Unit,
University of Massachusetts Medical Center,
  Worcester, MA

MARJORIE B. MORSE, M.A., J.D.
Department of Psychology
Harvard University

WENDY J. MURPHY, ESQ.
Of Counsel, Law Firm of Brody, Hardoon,
  Perkins, and Kesten
Boston, MA

ROBERT S. PYNOOS, M.D., M.P.H.
Professor of Psychiatry and
Director, Trauma Psychiatry Program,
Department of Psychiatry and Biobehavioral
  Sciences,
University of California at Los Angeles

COLIN A. ROSS, M.D.
Associate Clinical Professor of Psychiatry,
Southwestern Medical Center, Dallas, Texas
Medical Director,
The Colin A. Ross Institute for
  Psychological Trauma,
Richardson, Texas

MARIA C. SAUZIER, M.D.
Faculty, Harvard Medical School,
The Cambridge Hospital

DANIEL L. SCHACTER, PH.D.
Professor of Psychology,
Harvard University

DIANE H. SCHETKY, M.D.
Associate Clinical Professor of Psychiatry,
University of Vermont College of Medicine
  (at Maine Medical Center)
Private Practice, Rockport, ME

ROBERT I. SIMON, M.D.
Clinical Professor of Psychiatry and
Director, Program in Psychiatry and Law,
Georgetown University School of Medicine,
  Washington, DC

STEVEN M. SOUTHWICK, M.D.
Associate Professor of Psychiatry,
Yale University School of Medicine
Director of PTSD Program,
VA Connecticut and National Center
  For PTSD

ALAN M. STEINBERG, PH.D.
Research Health Scientist, Trauma
  Psychiatry Program,
Department of Psychiatry and Biobehavioral
  Sciences,
University of California at Los Angeles

LISA A. UYEHARA, M.D.
Private practice of psychoanalysis and
  psychiatry.
Assistant Professor of Psychiatry,
Tufts University Medical School

BESSEL A. VAN DER KOLK, M.D.
Professor of Psychiatry,
Boston University
Clinical Director, Trauma Center,
Human Resources Institute, Brookline, MA

RACHEL YEHUDA, PH.D.
Associate Professor of Psychiatry,
Mt. Sinai School of Medicine
Director of Trauma Studies,
Bronx VA Medical Center

ROSE R. ZOLTEK-JICK, LL.B, LL.M
Associate Professor of Law,
Northeastern University School of Law

Introduction

Rarely in our world of subspecialized knowledge have disparate disciplines been so joined in the cauldron of public debate as by the controversy over trauma and memory. Psychology, psychiatry, neuroscience, and law each have struggled to understand and respond to the perplexities that attend the recollection of memories of traumatic events. This book presents the contributions of these various fields with the aim of shedding light on the theoretical and practical aspects of trauma and its impact on memory.

The heart of the controversy lies in the question that has captured headlines, generated television documentaries, and sparked debates among professionals and laypeople alike: can persons who have been severely traumatized—especially by sexual abuse in childhood—endure prolonged periods during which they fail to remember the traumatic episodes, only later to recover accurate memories of the events? Critical issues of science, psychotherapy, and law turn on the answer to this question. Before considering some of these issues, it may be worthwhile to reflect on how the relationship between trauma and memory rose to prominence in public discourse.

Abuse of children burst onto the social agenda in the 1960s and 1970s, as researchers began to document the stunning rates of physical abuse to which children were subjected. In the wake of these accounts, other investigators reported an equally horrifying incidence of sexual abuse of children, usually, though not invariably, girls. The short-term consequences of sexual abuse—anxiety, depression, and behavioral problems among them—were documented first. Other evidence soon pointed to the conclusion that long-term effects were common as well. Links between childhood sexual abuse and some of the most difficult adult psychiatric disorders, including depression, eating disorders, and borderline personality disorder, were suggested by patients' accounts of their early experiences.

Some patients who related histories of abuse, however, had not always recollected these events. A number had recovered their memories prior to entering treatment, while others developed them in the course of therapy. Given the highly charged nature of their recollections, which often implicated family members in acts of sexual abuse, and the enormous consequences they held for those involved, controversy soon erupted over the legitimacy of the memories. Were they veridical, or had they been induced by the popular media or the suggestive techniques of therapists themselves? Was it possible for people to forget traumatic events that nevertheless caused them great psychic distress, only to remember them years later? Or had we entered a world of fantasy, a latter day version of the witch trials of Salem?

The debate implicated major theoretical and practical issues in every field that it touched. From the perspective of neuroscience, if memories can be recovered accurately years or even decades after the events they record, the brain must have mechanisms for retaining memories out of consciousness and permitting their retrieval. What are those mechanisms, and how do they function at the level of neural systems and cells? Are only some memories—specifically those of traumatic events—susceptible to being put aside in this way, or does this represent a more general means of dealing with memory? If the former, how does the brain distinguish between traumatic and non-traumatic memories? When memories do return, are they always accurate? If they are sometimes inaccurate, what variables influence the degree to which they deviate from fidelity to the actual occurences?

These questions of neuroscience have profound implications for the practice of psychotherapy, so much of which is devoted to the treatment of persons plagued by events that occured in the distant past. Clinicians now debate whether accurate memories of patients' personal histories can be retrieved in the consulting room. Moreover, the technical necessity for veridical recollection is also in dispute: some theorists argue that assisting patients to arrive at a coherent belief system regarding their past is more important than establishing the accuracy of their memories, while others disagree.

Where clinicians stand on the relationship between remembering and successful treatment shapes their approach to the role of memory in therapy. Some psychotherapists encourage recollections, especially of trauma, often using special techniques derived for this purpose. Others believe that doing so raises an unacceptable risk that inaccurate memories will result, which can distort the course of therapy and have untold consequences for patients' lives. Cautious practitioners urge that patients be warned that even memories they have long held or retrieved spontaneously may be inaccurate. Meanwhile, worries grow about the effect of such practices on the therapeutic relationship, as clinicians ponder the consequences of overtly expressing skepticism about their patients' accounts.

Trauma is inherently about harm, and harm in our society usually calls for a remedy. Little surprise, then, that the courts have played so prominent a role in the trauma and memory debate. Indeed, the courts—in some cases more so than the scientific literature—have become the battleground on which opposing theories of memory and its vicissitudes have struggled for ascendance. Highly publicized criminal cases have turned on memories of witnesses that were lost to consciousness for decades. Victims of sexual abuse, seeking delayed recompense, have brought their alleged abusers into court up to scores of years after the traumas were inflicted, their claims based on newly recovered recollections. Therapists, too, have found themselves the targets of suits by patients who believe ''memories'' of abuse were negligently implanted in the course of therapy, or by patients' family members who now find themselves accused—falsely, they argue—of having perpetrated abuse.

What constitutes a just outcome of such cases seems to have evoked different intuitions among many observers. Courts and legislatures have created, and then in some cases set aside, special mechanisms for granting access to civil remedies for victims who claim to have lost the ability to retrieve their memories for long periods of time. The proper bounds of suits against therapists, including whether family members should have standing to seek redress, are a matter of active contention. Whether child witnesses, who are often alleged victims of abuse, deserve special protections as they testify has been considered by courts at every level up to the U.S. Supreme Court, and no one is persuaded that the issue is settled.

These are some of the questions with which this volume is concerned. Unlike books that focus only on the scientific or clinical aspects of this area, we have sought to provide a bridge for researchers, clinicians, and policymakers from their own area of expertise to the other fields of knowledge that impact this controversy. In doing so, we have recruited many of the leading experts in diverse disciplines. No effort has been made to restrain controversy. Our contributors take different views on unsettled issues of science, therapy, and policy. By maximizing the perspectives presented, we hope to offer readers the chance to reach their own conclusions on these contentious issues.

Part I of the book begins with presentations on the core of the controversy: the question of whether memories of trauma can be repressed. To understand the issues raised by this debate, we turn in Part II to recent advances in understanding relevant aspects of memory, from neurobiological, cognitive, psychoanalytic, and developmental perspectives. Moving from the basic science of memory to more clinical concerns, Part III addresses memories of trauma per se: how they are manifest in both adults and children, and how they may differ from nontraumatic recollections. Part IV focuses on the concerns of clinicians with regard to the treatment of patients with memories of trauma, including contributions from psychoanalysis, psychodynamic psychotherapy, hypnotherapy, cognitive behavioral therapy, and eclectic approaches. In Part V we consider the ways in which these debates over science and clinical technique have spilled over into the courts and some of the implications for social policy towards victims of trauma. Finally, we close in Part VI with an attempt to integrate the responses to the controversies detailed in the earlier chapters, and to reflect on the broader impact of the trauma and memory debate.

Trauma and memory is the proverbial moving target. New data appear continuously, innovative theories are proposed, new treatments are developed. No volume can fully anticipate what the future will bring. It is our hope, however, that the chapters in this book will serve readers as a framework of knowledge into which they can integrate the information that will appear in years to come. If we have provided that intellectual scaffolding, we will have accomplished our aim.

I

THE CONTROVERSY OVER DELAYED RECALL OF TRAUMATIC MEMORIES

1

Some People Recover Memories of Childhood Trauma That Never Really Happened

IRA E. HYMAN, JR.
ELIZABETH F. LOFTUS

A woman in her late 20s enters therapy for problems that she is currently experiencing, perhaps an eating disorder, depression, or relationship difficulties. Early in therapy, the therapist asks the woman if she was ever sexually abused and the woman answers that she was not. The woman honestly believes that she was never abused. Over time, the therapist keeps returning to the issue of child abuse. The therapist tells the woman that her problems indicate severe childhood trauma and that the woman cannot expect to improve until she remembers the childhood trauma. The woman starts to think more about sex abuse, she reads about abuse in popular books, and she eventually has nightmares about sex abuse. Finally she recovers a memory of sexual abuse that happened when she was young. She begins to participate in group therapy for adults recovering from child sexual abuse and she uncovers more memories of childhood sexual abuse. In this situation, the woman may be recovering memories of abuse that actually occurred or she may be creating memories in response to the demands of the therapy situation. This is not the story of one individual, but rather the story of many individuals (both men and women, but predominantly women).

Child abuse is a horrible crime. Abuse is damaging to the child and may result in severe long-term consequences. Many adults remember their abuse (or at least part of their abuse) and these memories may be the source of psychological distress. When clients present abuse memories as part of their adult problems, they may desperately need help in addressing those memories.[1] Talking about memories of traumatic experiences may enable people to deal with the trauma and move on in their lives.[2] In therapy, clients may rewrite the past into a version that allows future growth; they may create new narrative truths for their lives.[3,4]

Other individuals who have experienced the trauma of childhood abuse forget about it. Whether this forgetting involves normal memory mechanisms or whether it is due to "repression" or some other abnormal memory mechanism is unclear.[5–8] Nonetheless, many writers have pursued a Freudian thread and have argued that forgotten traumas lie buried in the unconscious and continue to affect emotions, thoughts, and behaviors. Before the adult problems can be improved, the repressed memories must be recovered and addressed. Several techniques have been suggested as possible aids in memory recovery, including guided imagery, journaling, support groups, hypnosis, sodium amytal interviewing, visiting old home sites, viewing old photos, dream interpretation, and free association.[9–18] These techniques are sometimes used by individuals who have read self-help books;[10,14] sometimes they are employed by therapists during therapy not generally focused on memory recovery, and sometimes as part of therapy aimed at memory recovery. If such techniques accurately result in the recovery of childhood trauma memories and if memory recovery is necessary for the cure of psychological problems, then these memory recovery techniques might be justified.

Unfortunately, memory recovery techniques may result in the creation of false childhood memories. If a client creates memories of childhood abuse, then concern for the original problem that caused the person to seek therapy may be swept aside during the deluge of interest in the memories of childhood abuse. If clients create false memories of childhood abuse, they may find that other problems come with the newly found memories. Since traumatic memories can cause psychological distress, many individuals experience deep pain, regardless of the truth content of the memories. If the person acts on the memories by accusing family members or bringing litigation, this invariably leads to devastation within the larger family. Numerous detailed case histories documenting such devastation have recently been published.[19–21]

In this chapter we demonstrate that adults can be led to create false childhood memories. Because of this basic truth about memory, we argue that therapy focused on the recovery of unremembered childhood trauma runs the risk of creating false memories of childhood sexual abuse. If a person recovers memories of child sexual abuse through therapy, it is impossible to discern, without corroborating evidence, whether the person has recovered a true memory that had previously been unavailable or has created a false memory in response to the suggestions and demands of therapy. Given the difficulty in distinguishing true from false memories, and given the lack of evidence for repression, as well as for the necessity of memory recovery in the healing process, we contend that therapy focused on memory recovery does not provide enough documented benefits to justify the risk of false memory creation.

Evidence for False Childhood Memories

Human memory is fallible, and one common source of such errors is the introduction of additional information after an event occurs. For example, in traditional studies of eyewitness memory, people are first presented with an event (occasionally, a staged event but more commonly, a videotape or a series of slides). At some point after the event, some participants in the study are provided incorrect information about the event. If, for instance, they viewed a series of slides concerning a car accident in which one car went past a stop sign, the misleading post-event information may suggest the car passed a yield sign. Control participants are given either no additional information or correct post-event information about the event. When later asked if they remember seeing whether the car passed a stop sign or a yield sign, many people who were given misleading information claim that they saw a yield sign. In other words, they demonstrate that the misinformation has become part of the memory for the original event. The effect of misleading post-event information is robust and easily replicated, although the precise explanation for the memory errors is hotly contested.[22–29]

But what does the change of a stop sign to a yield sign have to do with memories of child abuse? We can argue that suggestions of abuse can be accepted as part of one's memory for childhood, much as the suggestions of a yield sign are accepted as part of one's memory for a viewed traffic accident. But as others have suggested, such a generalization appears to be a rather large leap.[30–32] In the typical eyewitness memory experiment, uninvolved college students are trying to recall the details of an event recently observed. With respect to false suggestions of childhood sexual abuse, people are trying to recall personally involving, emotionally arousing events that happened to them during their childhood. Details versus a whole event, mundane experiment versus emotionally arousing event, uninvolved observer versus involved participant—these are all differences that could conceivably make the introduction of errors more difficult. Certainly these differences limit the ability to make generalizations between eyewitness memory studies and suggestions of false childhood sexual abuse, unless we can demonstrate that memory errors work in a fashion similar for those involving whole, emotional, self-involving events.

We have been working independently for the last few years to find an experimental paradigm for the creation of false childhood memories.[33–37] Our original intention was to find out if people create false childhood memories. Once memory creation was demonstrated, we turned our attention to factors that contribute to and hinder memory creation.

Lost in a Mall

Loftus[19,38] described several cases in which people created false memories of being lost. A 14-year-old adolescent named Chris was one such case. For 5 days Chris was given written versions of several events that had happened when he was young and was asked to write about any additional information that he remembered each day. The events were generated by Chris's older brother Jim, and three events were things that had really happened. One event, however, was something that did not happen: the description claimed that Chris had been lost in a specific shopping mall at age 5 and that he was rescued by an elderly man. Over the course of 5 days, Chris supplied additional information about being lost (such as his emotional response, what the man looked like, and his mother's response). When he was asked to rate the clarity of all of his memories, the false event of being lost was given his second-highest rating. In addition, when he was told that one of the events was false, Chris actually selected a true event as the false event. This is the creation of a whole, emotional, self-involving event—a clear demonstration that people can come to believe that a suggested false event happened and that they can describe the event as a persoanl memory.

Loftus and Pickrell[37] extended these findings by using the same basic procedure with more participants. Twenty-four participants were asked about three true events from their childhood and about one false event. As with the demonstration using Chris, the false event was being lost at a specific place at age 5. The false event was constructed with the aid of the family member who had provided the true events. This family member made sure that the details (such as location and who was there) were consistent with things that could have occurred and that the event had not happened. The participants first responded to the events in writing and then were interviewed about the events twice within the next month. Of the 24 participants, 7 indicated in their written response that they remembered the false event. Six (25%) continued to remember the false event in both interviews. Loftus and Pickrell found that participants recalled about 70% of the true events and that people did not recall any additional true events throughout the interviews. They also found that people rated their memories of the true events as being more clear than their memories of the false event.

The work of Loftus and her colleagues demonstrates that people create false childhood memories in response to false events presented in a leading experimental context. Nonetheless, it can be argued that the work, while more generalizable than traditional eyewitness memory studies, is of limited value in its application to possible false memories of child abuse. The primary limitation is the nature of the suggested event. Getting lost, at least for brief moments, is a common childhood experience. In addition, many people have heard stories of being lost. Thus people have a script for being lost and it may be relatively easy for them to construct memories of being lost on a particular occasion. Convincing people of other false events, however, may be substantially more difficult.

Punch Bowls at Weddings

Hyman, Husband, and Billings[34] used a similar methodology but employed a variety of false events. In both studies, they mailed a questionnaire about childhood events to the parents of college students (the parents were asked about events in typical categories of activities for middle-class American families). Based on the parent responses, the students were asked to remember a series of childhood experiences assumed to be true. They were also asked to remember one experimenter-created false event. The students thought their goal was to accurately recall the events and that their memories would be compared to the information supplied by their parents. They were interviewed two to three times within 1 week and told that they could expect to remember more after continuing to think about the events.

In the first study, Hyman et al. used two false events: an overnight hospitalization for a high fever and possible ear infection, and a birthday party with pizza and a visit by a clown. Each student was asked about one of the false events and told that it occurred at age 5. (Although both hospitalizations and birthdays were categories supplied to parents, neither an overnight hospital visit for an ear infection nor a party with a clown was reported by any of the parents.) The students were interviewed twice and asked about all events in both interviews. Both true and false events were first cued with an event title (e.g., hospitalization) and an age. If the student could not recall the event or started to describe an event that did not match the parent (or false) event, the interviewer provided additional cues of location, people involved, and one or two activities.

In the first interview, the 20 students recalled 62 of the 74 true events (all students were asked about two to five true events). In the second interview, they recalled an additional three true events (perhaps a recovery of information in response to repeated questioning). For false events, no student described the false event as a memory in the first interview, but in the second interview, 4 of 20 (20%) incorporated the false information and constructed an event description.

Although Hyman et al.'s second study was similar to the first, there were a few changes. Three different false events were used (again each participant was asked about only one). The first false event was running around at the wedding reception of a family friend, bumping into the table holding the punch bowl, and spilling punch on the parents of the bride. The second false event was grocery shopping with a parent when the store's fire-extinguisher sprinkler system activated, forcing them to evacuate the store. The third false event was being left in the car in a parking lot and releasing the brake, which caused the car to roll into something. In addition to using different events, Hyman et al. also began the interviews by cueing with the full list of cues in the first interview and only the title and age in subsequent interviews. Instead of two interviews as in the earlier study, there were three interviews spaced 1 day apart (Monday, Wednesday, Friday, for example). Finally, the suggested age of the false event was varied (2, 6, or 10).

As with the first study, the true events were well recalled in the first interview (182 of 205, or 89%) and more events were recalled in subsequent interviews (195 of 205, or 95% in interview three). In the first interview, no student provided a memory for the false event, but by the third interview, 13 of the 56 (23%) students constructed a false memory in response to the false event. Hyman et al. noted that 6 memories were clear false memories, 5 were partial false memories, and 2 were clear descriptions of images but the students were unsure that the images were memories. Neither the false event (wedding, store, car) nor the suggested age (2, 6, 10) affected the rate of false memory creation. These studies show that the event used may not matter; people create memories of being lost, being hospitalized, and turning over punch bowls.

Hyman et al. also provided a tentative insight into the process of memory creation. Since no students created false memories in the first interview, it was possible to look at how the students responded to the false events in the first interviews and see if that predicted memory creation by the end of the study. In the first experiment, all of the students who created memories had discussed self-knowledge related to the false event in the first interview. For example, one student who created a memory of hospitalization talked about visits to the doctor for ear infections. A student who created a memory of a birthday party with a clown and pizza described a birthday party at McDonalds and, in the second interview, described having pizza at McDonalds and claimed that a clown appeared at the party. Based on these observations from the first study, in the second experiment Hyman et al. classified the students based on whether they supplied some related self-knowledge in the first two interviews. They found that those students who did so were more likely to create false memories by the third interview. Thus, the students appeared to construct a memory by using the suggested false event and related self-knowledge.

Hyman and his colleagues have replicated memory creation in two additional studies and have begun to investigate factors related to memory creation.[33,35] Hyman and Billings[33] correlated memory creation with four measures of cognitive/personality differences: the Dissociative Experiences Scale (DES),[39] the Creative Imagination Scale (CIS),[40] the Tellegen Absorption Scale (TAS),[41] and the Marlowe-Crowne Social Desirability Scale (SDS).[42] They found that both the DES ($r = .48$) and the CIS ($r = .36$) were significantly correlated to memory creation, thus indicating that individual differences contribute to memory creation. The DES is a measure of the tendency to have experiences that disrupt the normal integration of consciousness and personality. The correlation of the DES with memory creation indicates that people exhibiting a high frequency of dissociative experiences may be likely to create memories and perhaps to create personalities. Hyman and Billings argued that such findings should contribute to the ongoing dialogue concerning the causes of dissociative identity disorders. The CIS is a measure of both imagery vividness and hypnotizability. Both factors have been found to be related to memory errors in traditional eyewitness memory studies.[43,44]

By using the same basic methodology as Hyman et al., Hyman and Pentland,[35] investigated the role of guided imagery in memory creation. They asked students to imagine the childhood events that they could not remember (both true and false events) and then to describe these images. They found that around 40% of these guided imagery participants created false memories, while approximately 15% of a control group that simply thought about the nonremembered events created memories.

In addition to these studies that focused on memory creation in teenagers, college students, and adults, other researchers have shown that children will also create whole, self-involving, emotional events. By using a methodology similar to that of Hyman et al., Ceci and his colleagues found that more than a third of the preschool students they studied created false memories over the course of numerous interviews (sometimes up to 12) in which they were repeatedly asked about both true and false events.[45,46] In this research, preschoolers were led to believe that when they were younger, they had fallen off their tricycle and had to get stitches in their leg, or even more unusual, that they had gotten their hand caught in a mousetrap and had to go to the hospital to get it removed. Specifically, 17% of the 3–4-year-old subjects remembered the tricycle accident during the first suggestive interview, but after approximately 10 weeks of repeated interviewing, the figure rose to 31%.[46] As for the hand in the mousetrap, of all subjects (ages 3–6) interviewed, 34% falsely assented to this event during the first session, and the same percentage did so at the seventh session.

Taken together, the studies on false memory creation show that it is indeed possible to implant a false memory—in adults as well as in children. In some of the studies the participants begin by denying that they remember the fictitious events, but over time they increasingly assent to them. In other studies the percentage of participants who embrace the false event stayed constant across interviews. While we do not fully understand when the rate of belief rises, the results are clear in showing that people can be led to remember experiencing some highly unusual events.

The Processes Involved in Memory Creation

Several factors present in the basic methodology presented above probably contribute to false memory creation. First, we think the social demands are important. Participants are expected to remember past events and are told that they will remember more of them. Participants are presented with the false events by reliable sources—the experimenter and a family member. In addition, once the participant starts to remember an event, there is social encouragement (in the form of both nonverbal and verbal behaviors) to continue remembering it. This all contributes to a demanding social context. The importance of social demands for cognitive processes has often been demonstrated[47] and has also been shown to influence the acceptance of false information into memory of an event.[48–52]

Once a person begins to acquiesce to the social demands, they do not simply accept the false events as described. Instead, those who create memories first think of the false event in terms of their self-knowledge.[33,34] When first asked about turning over a punch bowl at a wedding reception, some college students will talk about at whose wedding it could have been, where it could have happened, if they would have done such a thing, what their parents' likely response might have been, and other related knowledge. When these students later think about the false event, they also bring to mind related self-knowledge. These individuals then construct a memory that includes both the false event and some accurate self-knowledge. Memory construction has been demonstrated in material ranging from word lists[53] to short stories,[54] and it has often been found in memory for autobiographical events.[55,56]

Finally, a person must confront the constructed memory in the subsequent interviews and decide if this is something remembered, something imagined, or something known from other sources.[57] Generally, people do not carefully monitor whether an image that comes to mind is a memory; typically, they accept these as memories. Sometimes people engage in more careful reality monitoring. Several aspects of the interview situations we have described, however, can make these reality monitoring decisions more difficult. The repetition of the false information across several interviews may lead to some confusion in monitoring the source of information.[58] Clearer mental images are generally thought by people to be indicative of memory accuracy,[59,60] and thus clear mental images due to individual differences[33] or experimental manipulation[35] may increase errors in reality monitoring. In addition, if the created memory contains both true and false information, a person may be biased by the true information when deciding if the constructed event is real.

Thus the creation of false childhood memories depends on the pressure of social demands, the constructive nature of remembering, and the difficulty in reality monitoring in these situations. As more and more research on the creation of false childhood memories is conducted, it is becoming increasingly evident that there is a continuity between the lab studies of memory errors and these studies of false childhood memories. That is, the two sets of research overlap in terms of the factors that predict or are correlated with memory errors. This observation increases our confidence in generalizing from one setting to another. Put another way, we expect to find that relevant factors explored in laboratory studies of memory errors will also be relevant to the creation of childhood memories.

Application to Therapy

If people can be led by suggestion to remember false childhood experiences, does this mean that people will also create false memories of child abuse in therapy? This is the critical question with which we opened: Is it likely that the woman who recovers memories after several leading therapy sessions actually has created false memories? Several differences between the experiments described and therapy contexts still limit our ability to generalize. At the very least is the nature of the event. In the studies of false childhood memories, single episodes of emotional, but not overly traumatic, events have been suggested. Sexual or other abuse may be harder to suggest. In addition, recovered abuse memories often involve multiple events and it may be more difficult to suggest a series of events. Ceci, Loftus, Leichtman, and Bruck[46] found that although children were willing to accept positive and negative emotional false events, they were less likely to accept the negative emotional events. Work with adults has not directly addressed whether this aspect of the false event (i.e., its positive or negative quality) matters. (For example, would adults be as likely to believe that they lost a $10 bill in a parking lot as they would to believe that they had found a $10 bill?) Nonetheless, a variety of false memories have been created in different research projects, thus indicating that false memory creation can be accomplished—even for rather negative experiences.

Another difference between the experimental and therapeutic contexts that may limit generalization between the two is the manner in which the false event is suggested. In the experimental context, participants are directly informed that the false event occurred. Although some individuals dispute this claim (arguing that the parent must have confused again which kid did what), most accept the accuracy of the parent's report. The suggestion of abuse in therapy is much more probabilistic: the client is informed that she or he has characteristics indicative of possible repressed memories of child sexual abuse.[10,14] Of course, suggestions based on probability can also be made very forcefully, as exhibited in Bass and Davis's work: "So far, no one we've talked to thought she might have been abused, and then later discovered that she hadn't been. The progression always goes the other way, from suspicion to confirmation. If you think you were abused and your life shows the symptoms, then you were"[10] (p. 22). Such writing includes little to indicate that the suggestion is only a possibility and that the symptoms do not clearly discriminate those who were abused from those who weren't. We both have heard stories from former clients of therapists that some therapists make similar suggestions in therapy. Clients with a variety of problems have often been told that their problems are generally related to child sexual abuse and then asked if anything like that ever happened to them.

Although there are limits to the generalizability of the current research, there are also limits to how much closer research can come to suggestions of abuse. For obvious ethical reasons, researchers cannot explicitly suggest to a participant that she or he was traumatically abused. But given the success that researchers have had with suggestions of single events, and sometimes rather unpleasant ones at that, we are learning something about the basic mechanisms by which such false memories can be implanted. Although repeated events, and highly traumatic events, may be more difficult to suggest successfully, there is no a priori reason to believe that people will not create such memories as well. In fact, as we demonstrate later, real world examples have shown us that such memories have indeed been created in the minds of numerous individuals with the involvement of certain questionable therapeutic procedures. These observations, in part, convince us that there are features of some therapy contexts that are more powerful than those of experimental contexts, and thus, false memory creation is more likely in the therapy settings where these features are present.

At times, therapy focuses on the recovery of unavailable memories, and many authors have offered suggestions for memory recovery techniques.[9-18] Lindsay and Read[61] referred to such therapy as *Memory Recovery Therapy* (MRT) and noted that several memory recovery techniques may contribute to false memory creation. Techniques that increase the demand to recover memories of abuse, that encourage constructive memory processes, and that discourage careful reality monitoring most likely will increase the chance of false memory creation. Some techniques undoubtedly contribute to memory creation through more than one mental mechanism.

Demand to Remember in Therapy

The demands in therapy contexts can be very high. Authority increases the probability of accepting suggestions,[49–52] and the therapist is a powerful authority figure. The therapist is an expert and a person who cares about the client. If this person suggests abuse, the client will assume that there must be a reason for the suggestion. Often these reasons are couched in the language of science and presented as facts. The reasons may include erroneous indications of relationships between current features and child abuse, and personal impressions of the prevalence of repressed memories.

The therapist may present the recovery of memories as critical in the overall healing process—this would lead clients to be more motivated rememberers/creators than the participants in research projects. Participating in group therapy in which others describe memories of child abuse also contributes to the demands of therapy. Several studies have shown that individuals conform to majorities.[47,48] In addition, the repeated suggestions of abuse probably contribute to the feeling on the part of clients that recovering such memories is important. Overall, the demands to remember events in therapy, particularly if therapy extends for any length of time, can be much higher than the demands to remember events in a short-term psychology experiment.

In her description of the Memory Recovery Therapy that she experienced, Laura Pasley[62] described her desire to remember as being very strong. The desire depended on her therapist's emphasis on the need to remember, the approval she obtained from her therapist, the need to be a part of the group in group discussions of sexual abuse, and her own desire to improve. When the social forces and personal motivations combine, particularly over long periods of time, the demand to remember events may lead to the creation of memories.

Memory Construction in Therapy

Other aspects of therapy may contribute to false memory creation by encouraging memory integration and construction. Hyman and his colleagues[33,34] have found that students who integrate false events with self-knowledge are more likely to create false memories. If therapists suggest child abuse to a client who does not have such memories, they may also suggest activities that encourage memory construction. Suggestions to look at old photographs, visit childhood homes, and talk about other childhood experiences may encourage the integration of suggestions of child abuse with self-knowledge. Questions about who would have been the perpetrator directly ask a client to integrate the abuse with self-knowledge. Similarly, interpretations of dreams as being informative about abuse also directly integrate self-knowledge and abuse. When the client returns later to contemplate the possibility of abuse, the client may well construct a memory based on the suggestions of abuse and on previously accessed self-knowledge.

Claridge,[11] for example, described encouraging clients to reconstruct memories as a means to recover memories. First she helped clients to identify current situations that made them feel uncomfortable. She then asked the clients to generate traumatic childhood scenes that were related to the current situations. With these "memory fragments" she helped the clients construct a childhood and childhood traumas that made sense of current concerns. While it is not clear that a process that explicitly involves clients in memory construction aids in memory recovery, it will increase the incidence of false memories.

Reality Monitoring in Therapy

Therapy may also contribute to false memory creation by discouraging careful reality monitoring. Other less obvious methods may also be employed. For example, a therapist may display interest when a client describes a memory but little interest when a client discusses his or her doubts about the memory. Fredrickson[14] directly addressed such issues early in her book by telling clients to put aside doubts and to accept returning images and thoughts as memories. Later in her book she revisited the issue of whether the memories are real. She does not, however, emphasize the importance of corroborating evidence; she actually discounts it by noting that such evidence is hard to find and it doesn't always convince a client when it appears. Instead, she emphasizes the authenticity of the memory itself: the fit with adult problems, the depth of pain, the amount of details. She notes that *disbelief* is an indication of the authenticity! Essentially, she tells her readers to accept their memories—especially if they are hard to believe. In this fashion, a therapist can discourage careful reality monitoring and actually turn reality monitoring against itself.

Some memory recovery techniques, such as hypnosis and the use of "truth" drugs, may create false memories by increasing the demand to remember events, encouraging memory integration and construction, and decreasing careful reality monitoring. Guided imagery techniques for memory recovery may also influence all three processes. Imagery techniques often include high demands on clients to remember events. First, imagery treatments force a client to participate; the therapist requires the description of an image. In addition, the client will be informed that the techniques will help in memory recovery. The formation of mental images is likely a constructive process based on suggestions and past knowledge (for example, picturing oneself in a scene of abuse and trying to imagine who is the abuser). In addition, once a clear image is formed, this influences reality-monitoring decisions; people generally think that more vivid memories are more accurate.[59]

Memory Recovery Therapy

Do therapists actually engage in Memory Recovery Therapy? Probably few therapists use all of the above practices and few clients have probably experienced all of these questionable techniques. In that sense, there is no type of therapy that is called Memory Recovery Therapy and, as far as we know, no schools that teach something called Memory Recovery Therapy. Nonetheless, the use of some of these techniques aimed at recovering memories may be fairly commonplace. Certainly the number of publications (both popular and academic) suggesting some of these techniques emphasizes the general acceptance of therapy aimed at memory recovery.[9–18] In addition, Poole, Lindsay, Memon, and Bull[63] recently surveyed active clinical psychologists—all with doctoral level training. Poole et al. found that nearly three-quarters of the clinical psychologists had used some memory recovery techniques at least occasionally to aid clients in recovering memories of child sexual abuse and that a few of the therapists tended to use these techniques frequently. Yapko's[64,65] surveys also indicate widespread belief among therapists in the prevelance of repression and in the usefulness of memory recovery techniques. Others[30] have suggested that the use of memory recovery techniques may be an even greater problem with less well-trained therapists. In general, it appears that therapy aimed at the recovery of childhood abuse memories is more common than many individuals wish to believe.

If such therapy is common, and assuming that these techniques can lead to memory creation rather than genuine memory recovery, then the creation of false childhood memories may be a societal problem of sizable magnitude.[61] False memory creation is a problem created in large measure by how therapy is conducted. For that reason, we think it is a problem that all psychologists, both clinical and cognitive, should unite to solve.

Bizarre Recovered Memories

Most of our discussion has been directed toward memories of childhood sexual abuse recovered via suggestive therapy techniques. We also want to briefly address more unusual recovered memories, which, for the sake of nomenclature, we will refer to as "bizarre." These include memories of the first few years of life, satanic ritual abuse (SRA), past lives, and alien abductions. For a variety of reasons, we argue that such memories should be viewed with a strong dose of skepticism. There is little reliable evidence that people can recall events from before age 2,[66,67] no cogent evidence for memories of repeated SRA that are repressed and de-repressed,[68] and, as far as we know, no evidence for reincarnation or alien abduction. Thus it is unlikely that people can accurately recover memories of these bizarre occurrences. The explanation for these bizarre memories, however, creates problems for all participants in the recovered memory debate. They provide problems for those who argue for the general accuracy of virtually all recovered memories, and they provide a different set of problems for those (like ourselves) who argue that some recovered memories may be false.

Problems Viewing Bizarre Recovered Memories as Accurate

For those who would argue that recovered memories are generally accurate, these bizarre recovered memories stretch one's credibility. Simply put, these memories are too strange to be true. For example, the memories of the Ingram family, as reported by Wright,[69,70] are certainly hard to believe. Many family members recovered memories of repeated SRA that occurred over many years, including activities that should have left scars on the survivors, places where bones and others remains should have been buried, ritual abortions that should have left physiological evidence, sacrifices, and participation by many well-known members of the community that would have been hard to hide. The tales told by Wright are hard to believe; but that in itself is not a compelling reason to discredit the stories of the Ingram family. In addition, some members of the family, particularly the father, Paul Ingram, now claim that the memories were false. But denials by an individual accused of abuse and who once pleaded guilty to the abuse are not convincing (even though he experienced incredibly leading and demanding interviews by friends and the family minister). There was, however, a lack of corroborating evidence. In the Ingram case there is no physical evidence of the scars, pregnancies, abortions, sacrifices, or participation by others. This is a compelling reason to doubt the stories.

In addition, cases of bizarre recovered memories often violate well-known principles of memory. People do not remember much from early childhood and generally nothing from the first few years of life—a phenomenon referred to as *childhood amnesia*. Although Freud[71] discussed childhood amnesia in the language of repression, modern scholars focus more on cognitive, developmental, and biological explanations.[66,67] Whatever the contributions of cognition, development, and biology might be, we do not expect people to recover memories from the first few years of life.

Another problem concerns what we know to be true about repeated events that occur in our lives. People develop scripts (or schemata) for frequently recurring events and, although they may lose some specifics, the general pattern of these events is retained.[72–74] Thus, we expect people to have better memory of the gist of repeated events, not to forget them completely.[6,68,75] Terr,[76] however, argued that repeated traumatic events would be more likely to be repressed, although little supporting evidence was provided. For these reasons, many of the bizarre recovered memories violate all that we know about the workings of human memory, and are worthy of being viewed with skepticism.

Problems with Viewing Bizarre Recovered Memories as False Memories

Bizarre recovered memories also present a difficult case for those who would argue that some recovered memories, and particularly these unusual recovered memories, are false. Although these memories are too strange to be true, they are also too strange to be created. We are often asked when we talk about false memories why and how someone could create something like these bizarre memories or like the Ingram family's memories (the family mentioned earlier in which many individuals recovered memories of abuse and SRA). In some measure, this is a problem for our view that false memories are constructed from external suggestions and some personal knowledge. The personal knowledge of SRA and alien abduction must be minimal for those who have not experienced SRA and alien abduction.

One way to account for these unusual memories is to clarify the meaning of related self-knowledge. Although we have argued that connections are made to personal memories, this is not the only form of self-knowledge that people possess. Connections made to self-attitudes (such as what or who a person likes and dislikes) may be sufficient for memory creation. In addition, although we have focused on the self-related aspect of the knowledge, it may be that simply developing connections to any knowledge (such as having heard or read similar stories) is sufficient. At this point we don't know how personal the additional knowledge needs to be or if connections to self-knowledge are necessary for memory creation or if such connections merely make memory creation more likely.

Another way to view unusual recovered memories is that these memories may be more likely to be accepted wholesale in the face of strong social demands and/or the willingness of the individual to accept the reality of the suggestions. This may have been the case for Paul Ingram who, in the course of very demanding interviews,[69,70] came to believe the stories of SRA that his daughters told. Ofshe reported that during his interview with Ingram, he suggested a false event and found that Ingram agreed that the event probably happened, formed an image of the event, prayed about the event, and later accepted the image as a memory.[68] In this case, there was little apparent connection made to other information about Paul Ingram's life, but the social demands were intense and Paul Ingram appeared very willing to accept the reality of the suggested event.

Another explanation for some of the bizarre memories is that these memories are dreams and images that are accepted as memories. The dreams or images could come from something happening in a person's life, like reading and talking about abuse, or could be an unusual dream that felt unexplained, such as feeling immobilized. The individual may then interpret the dreams or images as memories of abuse that happened or memories of alien forces. This may be due to lenient reality-monitoring strategies used by some individuals. These lenient strategies, or the willingness to see the dreams and images as real, may reflect individual differences, or suggestions from a therapist.

Perhaps the memories are constructed gradually, beginning with viewing innocent contacts (kisses and hugs by a father) as unwanted abuse, expanding to created memories of sexual contact, and gradually constructing memories of SRA (this appears to be a possible explanation for the recovered memories of Paul Ingram's daughters[69,70]). In such cases, there may be a real memory at the core of the bizarre memory. The individual may constantly reconstruct that memory to meet the demands of a therapy situation in which the person is expected to recover more memories. These additional memories are often expected to be worse, since they have remained hidden and since the person has not improved after recovering the previous memories. In Laura Pasley's description of her experiences during Memory Recovery Therapy, she noted that her memories were created over time and that they gradually became more unusual.

These bizarre memories would, assumedly, be more difficult to create, requiring more social demand over longer periods of time, more constructive work, or greatly diminished reality-monitoring strategies. Nonetheless, we think a view that such memories are false is more plausible than the view that they are accurate. Thus we suggest that the more bizarre the memories, the more they should be viewed with skepticism.

Faulty Arguments Based on Unusual Recovered Memories

One additional concern we have with these bizarre memories is that they can lead to two erroneous forms of argument. Proponents of the view that these memories are accurate sometimes argue—erroneously—that their view must be correct because their opponents cannot disprove the existence of aliens or reincarnation. In these situations, the simplest course is to not accept concepts without evidence if the data can be explained in some simpler fashion. The burden of proof should rest not with the doubters of aliens to disprove the existence of aliens (an impossible task as it turns out), but rather with the proponents of aliens to produce some reliable evidence for their existence. This same argument applies for the documentation that someone can completely repress memories of SRA and then accurately recover those memories.

For those who argue that bizarre memories are false, one risk is the temptation to make a faulty generalization to all recovered memories. We have heard people argue that since the more bizarre recovered memories are false (e.g., memories from the period following one's conception in the fallopian tubes, of sexual encounters with aliens, of having been Cleopatra), then all other memories recovered with similar techniques are also false. The logic is obviously faulty, as one set of memories could be false while the other is not. Although some dogs have spots, it does not follow that all dogs have spots. Put another way, the truth of recovered memories of sexual abuse does not depend on the truth of recovered memories of alien abduction.

CONCLUSION

As a way of concluding, we advocate a serious consideration of the risks of therapy aimed at the recovery of memories of childhood sexual abuse. To better appreciate our argument, it is helpful to understand the attraction of therapy aimed at recovering memories—an idea based on hand-me-down Freudian thinking.[71,77–79] In simple form, the Freudian notion has a few key ideas. An adult has problems because of some unresolved childhood problem (which for Freud is a failure to deal with a conflict, and for many modern writers it is the remains of a traumatic experience). The unresolved issues or experiences are repressed, which means they are hidden from conscious thought but are nonetheless able to influence thought, emotions, and behaviors. If treatment focuses on simply curing the visible problems, then the unconscious, repressed ideas will remain and be expressed in some new problem. The only method of curing is first to face the repressed material that is hidden in the unconscious.

This old concept of treatment is particularly troubling to us because the basic assumptions are poorly supported. First there is little evidence for repression.[6,38,79] People can forget events for a number of years and later remember the events. A handful of studies have found that adults claim to have recovered memories of child sexual abuse after having not thought about the abuse for a period of time.[15,80,81] But repression is not the only mechanism that explains forgetting and remembering; for example, others have argued for the importance of encoding specificity.[5,6,82] In addition, there is evidence that people can forget sexual abuse,[8] but there is little evidence that the rate of forgetting is higher than that for other types of events, and there is no need whatsoever to assume repression as a mechanism in any of these cases.[7] Trying to disprove repression is a bit like trying to disprove UFOs—a nearly impossible task. In some measure, the best we can do is show that forgetting and remembering can be explained more easily in terms of normal memory processes. But given that the notion of repression has been around for nearly 100 years, hasn't there been time enough for investigators to produce some solid evidence for its existence as a mechanism underlying the forgetting and subsequent remembering of experiences?

Even if solid evidence for repression were to be found one day, we would still need evidence that the recovery of memories is necessary for treatment or even helpful in achieving a cure for a client's problems. As Lindsay and Read[83] recently noted, there is no evidence that treatment aimed at memory recovery is effective compared with control groups of any sort. Case studies are not convincing, due to a lack of pre- and post-therapy measures, a failure to report the number of cases attempted, and the lack of meaningful comparison treatments. Thus the benefits of therapy aimed at recovering memories of childhood sexual abuse have not been clearly demonstrated.

We want to point out that it is possible to remember some experience that one has not thought of in many years. Anyone who doubts that long-forgotten memories can be recalled need only visit an old family home site not visited in years, flip through an old photo album, or attend a high school reunion. Memories may come flooding back, and sometimes verification can be produced. Moreover, discussions in therapy may provide cues that bring to mind previously forgotten events. In such situations, memories may return with little or no prompting by a therapist. This does not mean that the memories were repressed, or dissociated, or whatever fancy term one wants to use. A simpler explanation is that the memories simply responded to an effective retrieval cue. We have also argued elsewhere[6] that some of the techniques used in Memory Recovery Therapy may very well lead to the recovery of true memories. Techniques that provide additional retrieval cues (types of events, suggestions to visit old home sites, a supportive environment for remembering), for example, can result in recovery of memories. In fact, in some of the research previously reviewed, people remembered more of the true events with repeated interviews.[33–35]

The problem is that the very same techniques can and do result in the creation of false childhood memories. To make matters worse, it is very difficult to tell the difference between the recovered true memories and the created false memories. In one study, people's reported confidence in their memories was essentially equal for recovered true memories and created false memories.[33] Confidence in the recovered true and the created false memories was lower than confidence in always-remembered true memories, but it was higher than confidence in unrecalled true memories. Moreover, several studies have shown that when participants are asked to choose which event was the false event, those participants who created false memories often experienced difficulty in correctly identifying the false event.[34,38] After analyzing dozens of recovered true memories and created false memories, it is clear that there is little about the content of the memories that distinguishes the two categories. (One reason for some of the difficulty may be that some of recovered true memories actually may be creations like the false memories; the participants may have created a memory to match the information supplied. Were this the case, we would expect no differences between the recovered true memories and the created false memories.[33]) Thus, if a person is asked about childhood sexual abuse, does not recall such events, and participates in therapy with memory recovery as a goal, they may recover a true memory and they may create a false memory. Without corroborating evidence, discriminating true from false memories will be virtually impossible.[61]

Therapists need to weigh the possible benefits of recovering true memories against the risk of creating false memories. The benefits of recovering memories have not yet been adequately demonstrated. Memory creation is clearly possible and the consequences of memory creation can be lethal both for the individual who creates memories and for the people who are falsely accused in the wake of those memories. To appreciate how the risks associated with memory recovery therapy might exceed the possible benefits, consider the dilemma faced by a physician in this hypothetical analogy. Suppose this physician is considering prescribing a brand new drug for cancer. The drug, if given to patients who definitely have cancer, might help them. But if given to patients who do not have cancer, the drug has a good chance of causing cancer. If the physician could not give a test in advance to determine whether the patient had cancer, should she prescribe the drug?

We have focused on the possibility of memory creation for several reasons: (1) this is a problem caused by risky therapy practices; (2) the practices are based on certain mistaken or unsupported notions about how human memory works; and (3) we are psychologists who specialize in the study of memory. But the debate about recovered memory has many implications for our society, the most significant of which concern reports of genuine child abuse. If reports of abuse become widely discounted and discredited due to questionable practices and uncritical acceptance of all claims, no matter how dubious, the important progress made in the last 20 to 30 years will be undermined. Any retreat from that progress is one more tragic consequence of the uncritical hunt for missing memories that goes awry and ends up creating false memories. True victims may become lost in the surge of emphasis on false memories of child abuse. One outcome of working together to decrease therapy-caused creation of child abuse memories is that we can then focus our energies where they should be: on preventing real abuse from happening in the first place and, when we fail, on helping the genuine victims heal and punishing the genuine violators sternly.

References

1. Harvey MR, Herman JL: Amnesia, partial amnesia, and delayed recall among survivors of childhood trauma. Consciousness Cogn 1994; 3:295–306.
2. Harber KD, Pennebaker JW: Overcoming traumatic memories. *In* S-A Christianson (Ed.), The Handbook of Emotion and Memory: Research and Theory. Hillsdale, NJ: Erlbaum, 1992, pp. 359–387.
3. Cohler BJ: Memory recovery and the use of the past: a commentary on Lindsay and Read from psychoanalytic perspectives. Appl Cogn Psychol 1994; 8:365–378.
4. Spence DP: Narrative Truth and Historical Truth: Meaning and Interpretation in Psychoanalysis. New York: Norton, 1982.
5. Bower GH: Awareness, the unconscious, and repression: an experimental psychologist's perspective. *In* JL Singer (Ed.), Repression and Dissociation: Implications for Personality, Psychopathology, and Health. Chicago: The University of Chicago Press, 1990, pp. 209–231.
6. Hyman IE Jr, Loftus EF: Memory: modern conceptions of the vicissitudes of early childhood memories. *In* DA Halperin (Ed.), False Memory Syndrome: Therapeutic and Forensic Perspectives. Washington, DC: American Psychiatric Press, in press.
7. Loftus EF, Garry M, Feldman J: Forgetting sexual trauma: What does it mean when 38% forget? J Consult Clin Psychol 1994; 62:1177–1181.

8. Williams LM: Recall of childhood trauma: A prospective study of women's memories of child sexual abuse. J Consult Clin Psychol 1994; 62:1167–1176.

9. Alpert JL: Retrospective treatment of incest victims: Suggested analytic attitudes. Psychoanal Rev 1991; 78:425–435.

10. Bass E, Davis L: The Courage to Heal: A Guide for Women Survivors of Child Sexual Abuse. New York: Harper & Row, 1988.

11. Claridge K: Reconstructing memories of abuse: A theory-based approach. Psychotherapy 1992; 29:243–252.

12. Courtois CA: Theory, sequencing, and strategy in treating adult survivors. New Dir Ment Health Serv 1991, Fall; 51:47–60.

13. Edwards DJA: Cognitive therapy and the restructuring of early memories through guided imagery. J Cogn Psychotherapy: Int Q 1990; 4:33–50.

14. Fredrickson R: Repressed Memories: A Journey to Recovery from Sexual Abuse. New York: Simon & Schuster, 1992.

15. Herman JL, Schatzow E: Recovery and verification of memories of childhood sexual trauma. Psychoanal Psychol 1987; 4:1–14.

16. Maltz W: Adult survivors of incest: how to help them overcome the trauma. Med Aspects Hum Sex 1990; December: 42–47.

17. Olio KA: Memory retrieval in the treatment of adult survivors of sexual abuse. Trans Anal J 1989; 19:93–100.

18. Roland CB: Exploring childhood memories with adult survivors of sexual abuse: concrete reconstruction and visualization techniques. J Ment Health Counseling 1993; 15:363–372.

19. Loftus EF, Ketcham, K: The Myth of Repressed Memories: False Memories and Allegations of Sexual Abuse. New York: St. Martin's Press, 1994.

20. Ofshe RJ, Watters, E: Making Monsters: False Memories, Psychotherapy, and Sexual Hysteria. New York: Charles Scribner's, 1994.

21. Pendergrast M: Victims of Memory: Incest Accusations and Shattered Lives. Hinesburg, VT: Upper Access, 1994.

22. Belli RF: Influences of misleading postevent information: misinformation interference and acceptance. J Exp Psychol Gen 1989; 118:72–85.

23. Lindsay DS: Misleading suggestions can impair eyewitnesses' ability to remember event details. J Exp Psychol Learn Mem Cogn 1990; 16:1077–1083.

24. Loftus EF: Eyewitness Testimony. Cambridge, MA: Harvard University Press, 1979.

25. Loftus EF: When a lie becomes memory's truth: memory distortion after exposure to misinformation. Curr Dir Psychol Sci 1992; 1:121–123.

26. Loftus EF, Donders K, Hoffman HG, Schooler JW: Creating new memories that are quickly accessed and confidently held. Mem Cogn 1989; 17:607–616.

27. McCloskey M, Zaragoza M: Misleading postevent information and memory for events: arguments and evidence against memory impairment hypothesis. J Exp Psychol Gen 1985; 114:3–18.

28. Tversky B, Tuchin M: A reconciliation of the evidence on eyewitness testimony: comments on McCloskey and Zaragoza. J Exp Psychol Gen 1989; 118:86–91.

29. Zaragoza MS, Lane SM: Source misattributions and the suggestibility of eyewitness memory. J Exp Psychol Learn Mem Cogn 1994; 20:934–945.

30. Berliner L, Williams LM: Memories of sexual abuse: a response to Lindsay and Read. Appl Cogn Psychol 1994; 8:379–387.

31. Olio KA: Truth in memory. Am Psychol 1994; 49:442–443.

32. Pezdek K: The illusion and illusory memory. Appl Cogn Psychol 1994; 8:339–350.

33. Hyman IE Jr, Billings FJ: Individual differences and the creation of false childhood memories. Memory, in press.
34. Hyman IE Jr, Husband TH, Billings JF: False memories of childhood experiences. Appl Cogn Psychol 1995; 9:181–197.
35. Hyman IE Jr, Pentland J: Guided imagery and the creation of false childhood memories. J Memory Lang 1995; 35:101–117.
36. Loftus EF, Coan D: The construction of childhood memories. *In* D. Peters (Ed.), The Child Witness in Context: Cognitive, Social and Legal Perspectives. New York: Kluwer, 1994.
37. Loftus EF, Pickrell JE: The formation of false memories. Psychiatr Ann 1996; 25:720–725.
38. Loftus EF: The reality of repressed memories. Am Psychol 1993; 48:518–537.
39. Bernstein EM, Putnam FW: Development, reliability, and validity of a dissociation scale. J Nerv Ment Dis 1986; 174:27–735.
40. Wilson SC, Barber TX: The creative imagination scale as a measure of hypnotic responsiveness: applications to experimental and clinical hypnosis. Am J Clin Hypn 1978; 20:235–249.
41. Tellegen A, Atkinson G: Openness to absorbing and self-altering experiences (''absorption''), a trait related to hypnotic susceptibility. J Abnorm Psychol 1974; 83:268–277.
42. Crowne DP, Marlowe D: A new scale of social desirability independent of psychopathology. J Consult Psychol 1960; 24:349–354.
43. Barnier AJ, McConkey KM: Reports of real and false memories: The relevance of hypnosis, hypnotizability, and context of memory test. J Abnorm Psychol 1992; 101:521–527.
44. Schooler JW, Loftus EF: Multiple mechanisms mediate individual differences in eyewitness accuracy and suggestibility. *In* JM Pucket, HW Reese (Eds.), Mechanisms of Everyday Cognition. Hillsdale, NJ: Erlbaum, 1993, pp. 177–203.
45. Ceci SJ, Huffman ML, Smith E, Loftus EF: Repeatedly thinking about non-events. Consciousness Cogn 1994; 3:388–407.
46. Ceci SJ, Loftus EF, Leichtman MD, Bruck M: The possible role of source misattributions in the creation of false beliefs among preschoolers. Int J Clin Exp Hypn 1994; 42:304–320.
47. Asch SE: Studies of independence and conformity: I. A minority of one against a unanimous majority. Psychol Monogr 1956; 70(9).
48. Betz AL, Skowronski JJ, Ostrom TM: Shared realities: social influence and episodic memory. Manuscript submitted for publication, 1993.
49. Ceci SJ, Ross DF, Toglia MP: Suggestibility of children's memory: psycholegal implications. J Exp Psychol Gen 1987; 116:38–49.
50. Chambers KL, Zaragoza M: The effect of source credibility and delay on eyewitness suggestibility. Poster presented at the 34th annual meeting of the Psychonomic Society, Washington, DC, November 1993.
51. Dodd DH, Bradshaw JM: Leading questions and memory: some pragmatic constraints. J Verbal Learn Verbal Mem 1980; 19:695–704.
52. Greene E, Flynn MS, Loftus EF: Inducing resistance to misleading information. J Verbal Learn Verbal Behav 1982; 21:207–219.
53. Roediger HL, McDermott KB: Creating false memories: remembering words not presented in lists. J Exp Psychol Learn Mem Cogn 1995; 21:803–814.
54. Bartlett FC: Remembering: A Study in Experimental and Social Psychology. Cambridge: Cambridge University Press, 1932.
55. Barclay CR, DeCooke PA: Ordinary everyday memories: some of the things of which selves are made. *In* U Neisser, E Winograd (Eds.), Remembering Reconsidered: Ecological and Traditional Approaches to the Study of Memory. Cambridge: Cambridge University Press, 1988, pp. 91–125.

56. Neisser U: John Dean's memory: a case study. *In* U Neisser (Ed.), Memory Observed: Remembering in Natural Contexts. San Francisco: Freeman, 1982, pp. 139–159.
57. Johnson MK, Hastroudi S, Lindsay DS: Source monitoring. Psychol Bull 1993; 114:3–28.
58. Zaragoza MS, Mitchell KF: Effect of repeated exposure to misleading suggestions on source misattribution errors. Paper presented at the 35th annual meeting of the Psychonomic Society, Washington, DC, November 1994.
59. Johnson MK, Foley MA, Suengas AG, Raye CL: Phenomenal characteristics of memories for perceived and imagined autobiographical events. J Exp Psychol Gen 1988; 117:371–376.
60. Rubin DC, Kozin M: Vivid memories. Cognition 1984; 16:81–95.
61. Lindsay DS, Read JD: Psychotherapy and memories of childhood sexual abuse: a cognitive perspective. Appl Cogn Psychol 1994; 8:281–338.
62. Pasley L: Misplaced trust: a first-person account of how my therapist created false memories. Skeptic 1994; 2(3):62–67.
63. Poole DA, Lindsay DS, Memon A, Bull R: Psychotherapy and the recovery of memories of childhood sexual abuse: U.S. and British practitioners' beliefs, practices, and experiences. J Consult Clin Psychol 1995; 63:426–437.
64. Yapko MD: Suggestibility and repressed memories of abuse: a survey of psychotherapists' beliefs. Am J Clin Hypn 1994; 36:163–171.
65. Yapko MD: Suggestions of Abuse: True and False Memories of Childhood Sexual Traumas. New York: Simon & Schuster, 1994.
66. Pillemer DB, White SH: Childhood events recalled by children and adults. *In* HW Reese (Ed.), Advances in Child Development and Behavior, Vol. 21. San Diego: Academic Press, 1989, pp. 297–340.
67. Usher JA, Neisser U: Childhood amnesia and the beginnings of memory for four early life events. J Exp Psychol Gen 1993; 122:155–165.
68. Ofshe RJ, Watters E: Making monsters. Society 1993; 30:4–16.
69. Wright L: Remembering Satan—Part I. The New Yorker 1993, May 17: 60–81.
70. Wright L: Remembering Satan—Part II. The New Yorker 1993, May 24: 54–76.
71. Freud S: Childhood memories and screen memories. *In* J Strachey (Ed. and Trans.), The Standard Edition of the Complete Psychological Works of Sigmund Freud, Vol. 6. London: Hogarth Press, 1974, pp. 43–52. (Original work published 1901)
72. Linton M: Transformations of memory in everyday life. *In* U Neisser (Ed.), Memory Observed: Remembering in Natural Contexts. San Francisco: Freeman, 1982, pp. 77–91.
73. Neisser U: Nested structure in autobiographical memory. *In* DC Rubin (Ed.), Autobiographical Memory. Cambridge: Cambridge University Press, 1986, pp. 71–80.
74. Nelson K: The ontogeny of memory for real events. *In* U Neisser, E Winograd (Eds.), Remembering Reconsidered: Ecological and Traditional Approaches to the Study of Memory. Cambridge: Cambridge University Press, 1988, pp. 244–276.
75. Goodman GS, Quas JA, Batterman-Faunce JM, Riddlesberger MM, Kuhn J: Predictors of accurate and inaccurate memories of traumatic events experienced in childhood. Consciousness Cogn 1994; 3:269–294.
76. Terr LC: Childhood traumas: an outline and overview. Am J Psychiatry 1991; 148:10–20.
77. Freud S: Repression. *In* J Strachey (Ed. and Trans.), The Standard Edition of the Complete Psychological Works of Sigmund Freud, Vol. 14. London: Hogarth Press, 1957, pp. 141–158. (Original work published 1915)
78. Erdelyi MH: Repression, reconstruction, and defense: history and integration of the psychoanalytic and experimental frameworks. *In* JL Singer (Ed.), Repression and Dissociation. Chicago: University of Chicago Press, 1990, pp. 1–32.

79. Holmes DS: The evidence for repression: an examination of sixty years of research. *In* JL Singer (Ed.), Repression and Dissociation. Chicago: University of Chicago Press, 1990, pp. 85–102.

80. Briere J, Conte J: Self-reported amnesia for abuse in adults molested as children. J Traumatic Stress 1993; 6:21–31.

81. Loftus EF, Polonsky S, Fullilove MT: Memories of childhood sexual abuse: remembering and repressing. Psychol Women Q 1994; 18:67–84.

82. Christianson S-A, Nilsson L-G: Hysterical amnesia: a case of aversively motivated isolation of memory. *In* T Archer, L-G Nilsson (Eds.), Aversion, Avoidance, and Anxiety: Perspectives on Aversively Motivated Behavior. Hillsdale, NJ: Lawrence Erlbaum Associates, 1989, pp. 289–310.

83. Lindsay DS, Read JD: "Memory Work" and recovered memories of childhood sexual abuse: scientific evidence and public, professional, and personal issues. Psychol Public Policy Law 1995; 1:846–908.

2

The Argument for the Reality of Delayed Recall of Trauma

RICHARD P. KLUFT

In any debate over the reality of recovered memory, it is useful to clarify the grounds of the debate, that is, to specify the issue that is being debated. If arguments are being proposed to the effect that there is no such thing as recovered memory, so that any apparently recovered memory can be discounted a priori, the premise of the debate can be formulated: resolved, that there is no demonstrable instance in which accurate, once unavailable memories have been recovered. I have avoided the use of the terms *recovered memory* and *repressed memory* in the resolution itself because these terms not only have become politicized, but the former term has no correlation to traditional clinical literature, and the latter represents an overgeneralized use of the term *repression*, which is only one of the processes by which the defensive exclusion of autobiographical experience from available and routinely retrievable memory may occur.

If the affirmative case is proven, then there is no such thing as a recovered memory. Should the negative prevail, such a phenomenon exists. The debate concerns whether there are demonstrable instances of the recovery of repressed, dissociated, or otherwise unavailable memory. Circumspect authorities would observe that since it is impossible to prove a negative, the debate can only be won by the affirmative side's discounting of any and all evidence that repressed and recovered memories exist. This is why vigorous attacks have been launched against virtually every article that appears to document this phenomenon, and efforts have been made to overextend implications that memory not only can be but will be distorted by various forms of suggestion and influence. Another consideration in this debate is that the affirmative side must make its case by advancing falsifiable arguments. Opinions cannot be stated as if they were facts. All recovered memories must be demonstrated to be false by objective data, and by unimpeachable corroborations of their falseness, not simply by allegations or statements of belief. Pope[1] has explored this dilemma very thoughtfully. That is, advancing lines of reasoning that cannot be tested, but permit the infinite, defensive rationalization of one's point of view from a lofty retreat remote from all threat of disconfirmation, falls short of scientific acceptability.

In this study, I will address a number of issues. I will not, however, offer a detailed review of the general clinical literature that speaks to the existence of recovered memory. I do not wish to add to the literature in which extrapolations from theories, general principles, or research of questionable relevance to clinical practice are employed to advance arguments about proper treatment of the traumatized. Instead, I will begin by presenting the type of clinical vignettes that make the recovery of previously unavailable memories a clinical fact, if not a research finding. I will then present findings from my recent clinical research on allegations of abuse made by patients with dissociative identity disorder. Finally, I will offer observations on a series of additional related topics.

Clinical Experiences Supporting the Recovery of Long-Unavailable Memories

For many years, in addition to conducting a psychiatric practice in Philadelphia, I had the privilege of treating patients in a small city surrounded by farmlands and semirural areas. During that period, that city's population base was stable, with relatively little mobility. For most of that time the area was underserved by mental health professionals and there was relatively little therapist-switching. I had the opportunity to observe the life cycles of many families over a period of 18 years. It was predominantly in this setting that I followed 210 patients with dissociative identity disorder (DID; formerly multiple personality disorder [MPD]) and was able to sketch out the natural history of this disorder.[1a] I came to know many patients and their families in a manner that I rarely experienced in my urban practice, and I remained in contact with them over a prolonged period of time. Often information that was unavailable during my patients' treatments came my way a decade later. In this setting I learned that many of the allegations of abuse that were made by my patients (whether always in conscious awareness or recovered in therapy) were in fact true, even allegations that were vehemently denied by their families at the time when I first treated the patients. I also learned that some of the accusations were lies, and that some were based on misperceptions or distorted recall. In 1984 I cautioned that the therapist "must remain aware . . . that material influenced by intrusive inquiry or iatrogenic dissociation may be subject to distortion. In a given patient, one may find episodes of photographic recall, confabulation, screen phenomena, confusion between dreams or fantasies and reality, irregular recollection, and willful misrepresentation. One awaits a goodness of fit among several forms of data, and often must be satisfied to remain uncertain."[2] I did not encounter instances in which false accusations were triggered in therapy, but I must acknowledge that the possibility exists.

Here I will focus on several examples of confirmed recovered memories. My files contain hundreds of such confirmations.

In the mid-1970s I was treating a female colleague who seemed unable to sort out her relationships with men. A bright and attractive woman, she had distanced herself from her alcoholic family only after winning her own battles with addiction. As her psycho-analytically oriented psychotherapy proceeded, which was supported by her participation in Alcoholics Anonymous, we both appreciated that she became unable to express herself whenever transference feelings toward me came under exploration. After several months of mutual confusion, we decided to use hypnosis to explore her block. She was an excellent hypnotic subject. While in trance she recovered memories of her first therapy, which was conducted by an addiction counselor. He had encouraged the development of an extremely positive transference and then exploited it to seduce her. Once out of trance she was mortified, but she steeled herself to report that, although she had completely forgotten that particular experience, she had reenacted the same pattern with the leader of a therapy group. She had not felt comfortable enough to admit her growing fears that the same might happen with me. Now her shutting down whenever she began to experience feelings toward me made sense to both of us. Her therapy continued to a successful conclusion, and her relationships with men became satisfactory to her.

A decade later, her former alcoholism counselor came to me for psychotherapy. After several sessions, he revealed what he considered the two worst things he had ever done. While an active alcoholic, he had molested his own daughter. When he became a recovering alcoholic and respected therapist, he had become infatuated with a beautiful young patient and had manipulated her idealization of him to seduce her. "You know her. You treated her. You must think I'm a real bastard." He spoke briefly about his relationship with my other patient, confirming her hypnotically retrieved account in detail. The next day, he left me a message which said that he was too embarrassed to return. He transferred to a therapist who had never known his victim.

In another case, two sisters, who were long estranged, were reunited after twenty years as they attended their dying mother. One sister, who was my patient, had always been aware of sexual abuse by her father and had recovered memories of abuse by a baby-sitter in the course of her therapy. She asked her sister if the sister had any knowledge of such an incident. Her sister not only recalled the event but supplied details that confirmed additional circumstances which my patient had recovered in the course of her treatment but which she had not yet shared with her sister. Each confirmed the other's recollection of father-daughter incest, with reference to several specific instances. Furthermore, their dying mother apologized to my patient for her harsh treatment of her, which my patient had recovered in psychotherapy but had doubted to be true.

Another example of confirmed recovered memories concerns a man who had served in Vietnam as a Marine who maintained in therapy that he and his unit had seen no combat over a particular period. However, also in therapy, he recovered memories of an attack on his base and of his killing several armed Vietnamese attackers. After recovering these memories, he disbelieved them. At a Washington, D.C. commemoration for Vietnam veterans he became irritated when a wartime buddy reminded him of his role in this firefight. He told the friend that he must be wrong, that he had never fired his weapon in combat. The man was shocked, and shook his head, uncomprehending. "You were a fuckin' hero, man!" The patient's military records reveal that his unit had indeed been in combat and had maintained a defensive perimeter around a supply base that was frequently under attack throughout the period during which the patient maintained that his unit had seen no action. For reasons unrelated to this account, this man had joined the Marines, hoping to be killed. He had repeatedly volunteered for hazardous duty in the effort to bring about his own death. Although he eagerly placed himself at risk, he was passionately opposed to taking another human life. Ultimately, he was able to confront the fact that despite his beliefs and apparent wish to die, when faced with a genuine life-and-death decision, he had methodically and efficiently dispatched several enemy combatants at close range, an act that was witnessed by his buddy. His repugnance and conflict over this action apparently drove it from his memory. It took months to work through his guilt over his having taken the lives of the Vietcong attackers.

A woman with multiple personality disorder underwent hypnosis to access personalities and to explore missing periods of time in her life. During her assessment and treatment, she had denied that she had ever been mistreated by a previous therapist. Fourteen months later, a personality that was contacted through hypnosis indicated that the patient's prior psychiatrist had exploited her sexually. Against my advice, she revealed this information to her prior psychiatrist. When he learned that his former patient was revealing his boundary violations, he telephoned me. He asked me to treat him, he admitted his indiscretions, and he insisted that since he was now my patient, I could not reveal what I knew, due to my duty of confidentiality! He was not pleased when I reminded him that I had never agreed to treat him, and that I was not disposed to accept the constraints he tried to impose. This case was one of several in which alleged therapist abuses, which were often not in patients' conscious awareness at the beginning of the patients' therapy with the author, were later confirmed.[3,4]

A married woman in her late 20s who had been adopted at birth came for a consultation to discuss the pluses and minuses of tracing her birth parents. Now the mother of two toddlers, she was increasingly curious about her own origins. After she located her birth parents, she returned to discuss her reactions. During this interview she spoke at length about the mental illness of her adoptive mother, who ultimately had been institutionalized as a paranoid schizophrenic. While discussing her adoptive mother's suspiciousness and unusual behavior (such as shooting a rifle at aircraft flying over the family farm), she dissociated into an alter personality and began to talk about a psychotic ritual of her mother's, a practice that was repeated over and over again. In it, her mother and she undressed. Her mother made her lie under a blanket on her abdomen and crawl out between her legs to be "born." Then her mother would express delight at her daughter's birth. When the patient switched back to her previous personality, she was amnestic for the above revelations. However, within minutes, she had a flashback of bizarre enematization experiences at her mother's hands.

She decided to enter treatment to explore these phenomena and to better understand herself. Much abuse material emerged under hypnosis. After the third hypnotic session the patient was sure that the recollections were inaccurate, but she appreciated that her long-standing depression was fading. We discussed how to approach the resolution of her uncertainly. Her adoptive parents were deceased. They had raised her on an isolated farm in a wooded rural area with no close neighbors. No close relatives of her parents were available as resources. I asked her to bring in any school and medical records, and any family materials or photo albums in her possession for us to review. I really had no hopes that anything would emerge, but wanted to leave no stone unturned. The next day she called me in tears. Not only had she found albums, she had found her mother's diaries, which described her mother's "experiments on the girl." They included detailed accounts of every abuse the patient had shared with me. Unable to tolerate having this material in her home, she presented me with a box of her mother's diaries and with yearly school pictures of herself, on the backs of which were written her mother's comments and planned experiments (i.e., abuses). When I asked her what she thought I should do with these materials, she paused thoughtfully and replied: "Someday you may find people don't believe child abuse happens, and that people can forget their abuse. If you ever need to prove it happens, you have this box." That conversation occurred in 1978. Upon an 18-year follow-up, she is integrated, symptom-free, and well. Several years after the conclusion of her therapy she went to graduate school in psychology. She currently is a practicing mental health professional.

A Pilot Study Exploring Validation of Recovered Memories of Childhood Abuse and Other Traumatic Experiences in Patients with Dissociative Identity Disorder

A series of 34 DID patients who were in treatment with the author during a 30 day period from mid-August through mid-September 1995 were the subjects of a pilot study meant to determine the feasibility of conducting a larger study on documenting and disconfirming the memories recovered by DID patients in psychotherapy (see Kluft[5]). I was interested both in the occasions in which documentation of abuses alleged by DID patients took place and in instances of definitive disconfirmation of such allegations. I excluded from this study patients seen for brief hospital care or assessment only during this period of time. Also excluded were patients seen for medication management alone, whose psychotherapy was being provided by a non-physician colleague. Furthermore, in order to be included in the study, patients had to have fulfilled DSM-IV criteria for DID while under my observation, even if they did not do so during the period of the study.

The charts of the remaining 34 DID patients were reviewed and instances of documented abuse were tabulated, along with the sources of the documentation. With three exceptions, all documentations occurred naturalistically and serendipitously, as in the context of therapy or in connection with obtaining prior records from professional or legal sources. One of these exceptions was when an MPD patient was about to bring charges against an alleged abuser and the author contrived a plan to assess the reliability of the allegations; they were disconfirmed. In the second exception, information suggested that the patient was in imminent danger if some materials retrieved under hypnosis were accurate. A strategy for confirmation or disconfirmation without disturbing the therapy was developed. The danger was confirmed and ultimately police intervention was required (for a description of this case, which was fictionalized to protect confidentiality, see Kluft[6]). The third exception concerned a hospitalized DID patient who returned from a pass for a holiday dinner and alleged that her father had sexually assaulted her. She was immediately assessed at a rape center, where no firm evidence of sexual assault was found, but it could not be ruled out. The patient herself tried to reconstruct her day by asking family members whom she perceived as nonabusive. She concluded that in fact she had never been alone with her father, so her account of that day had to be false. It remained possible, and was suspected by some involved in her care, that she was reacting to a flashback of a prior incestuous assault that was misperceived as contemporary reality.

Thirty-two of the 34 DID patients were female. All 34 would have satisfied DSM-IV[7] criteria for DID at the beginning of their treatment, but at the time of this study, several were integrated and many had ceased to manifest overt signs of DID. They had been in treatment with the author for an average of 5.5 years (range: 3 months to 19 years). This reflects the fact that DID patients with a good prognosis tend to get well relatively rapidly, whereas those with poorer prognoses tend to accumulate in the caseload of the dissociative disorders specialist.[8,9] Some patients were integrated and being seen for follow-up at infrequent intervals, but most were still quite dissociative and were seen from one to four times a week in active psychotherapy with the author.

Of the 34 patients, 19 (56%) were found to have instances of confirmed abuse. Data demonstrated that the longer a patient was known to me, the more likely it was that an incident of alleged abuse would be confirmed (Kluft, unpublished observations). There were very few confirmations among patients seen for less than a year. My data suggest that usually patients must be in an advanced state of recovery in order to pursue confirmation productively. Also, over time, more and more information is likely to become available from other sources who initially may distance themselves from the patient. Furthermore, as abusers die, become ill, or move away, other sources are likely to speak up.

As Table 2-1 indicates, several patients had multiple sources of confirmation; and

Table 2–1. Sources of Confirmation of Abuse Allegations for 19 DID Patients[a]

	Total	C	R
Confirmation by a sibling who witnessed abuse[b]	12	4	8
Confirmation by one parent of abuse by the other parent	5	3	2
Confession by abusive parent (deathbed or serious illness)	4	1	3
Confession of abusive parent (other circumstances)	3	1	2
Confirmation by police/court records	3	2	1
Confirmation to author by abusive therapist	2	1	1
Confirmation by a childhood neighbor of witnessed abuse	1		1
Confession by abusive sibling (during terminal illness)	1		1
Confession of abusive sibling (other circumstances)	1		1
Confirmation by relative (neither parent nor sib)	1		1
Confirmation by friend who witnessed and interrupted abuse attempt	1		1
TOTALS	34	12	22

[a]C = Always recalled; R = recovered in therapy.
[b]For three patients, sibs confirmed both C and R material; one report unclassified because the dissociative handling of the incident involved depersonalization and derealization, but not frank amnesia.

many times, sibling confirmation indicates that more than one sibling verified the patient's account. For example, one patient had eight siblings, all of whom confirmed the patient's abuse, and three of whom confirmed it directly to the author. For this patient, there were also confirmations by one parent of intrafamilial abuse and by police reports of extrafamilial abuse.

Sibling confirmation is not unusual in abuse situations, but often one sibling will confirm the abuse while another will deny it vociferously. In this study, sibling confirmation was tabulated only when all siblings other than the one making the allegation were in accord or acknowledged the plausibility of abuse. For example, for two patients, one sibling supported the allegations and another disputed it vigorously. I did not tabulate these allegations as confirmed. Had I done so, the number of confirmed cases would have increased by 5, to 71% of my series. I chose the more conservative road. I did not consider one sibling's statement that he or she had also been abused as a confirmation of the allegations made by the index patient. Sibling confirmation often was a function of the duration of therapy and the survival or death of the parents. Several siblings began by denying that the index patient had or could have been abused, but years later, they either recovered memories on their own or in treatment, or admitted that they had lied when they denied the index patient's abuse. In several families, some siblings denied anything that was amiss until at least one parent (usually the abuser) died. Only then would they confirm the abuse, since their relationships to the abusive parent would not be compromised. In the situation defying classification, the memory of abuse had been retained, but it was experienced as dreamlike and unreal, and had not been accorded credibility by the patient.

One parent's confirmation of another's abusiveness might be understood as emerging from the context of domestic discord, where allegations, false and otherwise, are common weapons. In this study, all five such confirmations were buttressed by abusers' confessions in four cases, and by sibling confirmation in the fifth. Most of these confirmations were made by mothers about their deceased or dying husbands; in the last instance, a patient confronted her mother about physical abuse in a family therapy session with the author. The mother admitted the actions in question, but she defended her physical abuse of her daughter on the grounds that her daughter was evil. She maintained that her daughter was possessed by the devil and that she needed to "beat the devil out of her." Her husband confirmed his wife's abusiveness, and shame-facedly, offered no justification for his passivity.

Confessions by abusers on their deathbeds or in the throes of terminal illness were made mostly by male members of the Roman Catholic faith, who literally feared going to hell unless they took appropriate preventive steps by confessing their sins and making amends. One father begged for his daughter's forgiveness; another apologized to his daughter's husband for the mess he had made of her life. A third father broke down in tears when his daughter said that regardless of whether he could admit what he did to her, she forgave him. When he recovered his composure, he admitted having abused her and her sisters, and offered the rationalization that he thought that she and her sisters were too young to be harmed by what he had done, especially since they seemed to have forgotten it. Another confessor, an abusive mother, offered no rationale for her disclosure, but appeared to have been moved by the patient's efforts to tend to her during her terminal illness. She tried to straighten out their relationship before she died. An abusive older brother dying of cancer (also of the Roman Catholic faith) apologized to his sister for abusing her. He offered to talk to me, but died before this could be arranged. The three other confessions that were not made on deathbeds were made by mothers who had been physically but not sexually abusive. Two were made in the presence of the author. One confession made directly to a patient appears to have occurred in the context of the mother's recovery work in a 12-step program.

Two boundary-violating therapists confessed their abuse of their patients directly to the author. One patient encountered previous neighbors when she returned to her old neighborhood in an effort to make peace with her past. In this case a neighbor admitted with guilt and shame that she and other neighbors had known of the abuse, but had not known what to do in an era before child abuse was discussed openly. In one unusual instance, a patient returned to her parents' home on an errand with a friend. The patient entered the house first, upon which her father dropped his pants and insisted on sexual favors. The patient "spaced out." When her friend, whose presence was not anticipated by the parents, walked through the door a few moments later, the friend witnessed, and later described to the author, finding the patient's father with his trousers and underwear around his ankles, trying to force the patient to perform a sexual act. The patient was amnestic for this event for several weeks.

Most of the patients made many allegations that could neither be proven nor disproven with the available data, and some made allegations that were not very likely to be accurate. For example, 13 patients (38%) at one time alleged that they had suffered satanic ritual abuse. One such allegation was disproven (see below). None reported alien abductions, prior lives, or similar phenomena. One patient alleged that she was the victim of military mind control experiments. Her father had been involved in military intelligence, but this in and of itself is no confirmation. His career may or may not have been connected to a set of factual occurrences, but in any case, it may have served as the nidus of a confabulation or fantasy that was mistaken as reality.

Only three of the 34 patients (9%) had instances of disconfirmation of an instance of alleged abuse. Disconfirmation required evidence that disproved the allegation in question: it was not a mere tally argument to the effect that it was not credible. Recanting was not considered disconfirmation, because it has no more or no less credibility than an initial allegation, and it usually occurs under circumstances of profound interpersonal pressure. This pressure has many features of interrogatory suggestibility, which is known to cause false statements frequently (discussed clearly in Brown[10,11]). Disavowal by an alleged abuser was no more considered proven disconfirmation than was mere allegation considered confirmation of abuse.

An example of a disconfirmed allegation is that of a woman who came to a session with numerous wounds on her chest and breasts in shapes suggestive of satanic symbolism. She alleged that she had been accosted by a man she remembered from her participation in a satanic cult. She also alleged that she had been taken to a secluded location, brutally raped, and cut by this man, who, she said, had threatened to come after her and kill her if she did not return to the cult by the next satanic ''holiday.'' The patient refused gynecologic assessment, but agreed to have her wounds assessed and treated. I asked a board-certified forensic pathologist to join the surgeon who evaluated and treated the wounds. The forensic pathologist determined to a degree of medical certainty that the wounds were self-inflicted. When gently confronted, the patient decompensated, became suicidal, and was hospitalized. Over a period of time, it was possible to reconstruct a plausible scenario of what had occurred. After she had decided against filing charges and the use of hypnosis would not compromise her credibility as a witness, hypnosis was used to explore her experience. While in trance, she recalled coming to a certain location and beginning to have a flashback. It appeared that she perceived the vivid imagery of the flashback as if it were external reality, and that one of her cult-identified alters had both raped the body with a blunt object and inflicted the chest and breast wounds. The patient was helped to become co-conscious while this cult-identified alter retold its story. This allowed her to better appreciate her circumstances. It remains uncertain whether the man she had accused initially had abused her in the past and had been a member of the cult to which she had belonged. As unlikely as such allegations may seem, they are not disproven or beyond the realm of possibility. They are members of a class of allegations about which there is considerable doubt, and for which there is minimal confirmatory evidence.[12,13]

In a second instance of disconfirmed allegation, a DID patient of mine was admitted to another facility after a suicide attempt. For administrative reasons, she remained there for her hospital care. There she was exposed to therapies in which there was uncensored discussion of ritual abuse experiences. Upon discharge, she returned to me with elaborate memories of ritual abuse. She had come to believe that she had been abused in a cult in California during a particular period of time. Unique factors in her case made it possible to demonstrate by school records that the patient had been in Pennsylvania during the time in question, and that there were no other times in her life when she might have had the purported exposures and experiences.

Confronted with this, the patient admitted that she had been puzzled that her memories so clearly paralleled those of another patient in her therapy group. She herself raised the possibility of contagion. Over the subsequent years it became apparent that the patient had become murderously angry at me because of the circumstances that necessitated her being treated elsewhere. Talk about satanism and the suggestion by peers that she might have suffered cult abuse provided her with a ready displacement for her rage at me and for her perception of me as cruel and deliberately abusive to her. She had returned to me completely out of contact with her rage at me, but she was determined to bring her satanic abusers to justice. Needless to say, chaotic negative transferences dominated her therapy for some time after she repudiated the cult memories.

The third instance of disconfirmed allegation, which was noted briefly above, involved an allegation of an incestuous rape at a family gathering. The patient was sent to a specialized forensic unit, where no findings consistent with the allegation were reported, and family members sympathetic to the patient convincingly demonstrated to her that there had been no occasion during which she was alone with her father that day. This is a situation in which incest had been alleged on many occasions, but had not been confirmed. Her experience may have been a flashback or fantasy that was misperceived as reality, a fabrication, or a manifestation of related phenomena.

It may be thought that the patients who made disconfirmed reports of abuse should be considered as without credibility. However, of these 3 patients, the second and third patients had confirmed instances of abuse. The second patient had confirmation of incest with her father by her father's confession, her mother's admission, and the testimony of three sisters, all of whom were incest victims and one of whom bore a child by her father. Her brother confessed to incest as well. She had confirmation of both recovered memories of abuse and of those that were always available. The third patient had made accusations of sexual exploitation against a teacher, who was convicted and jailed for his offenses. This is a very pragmatic demonstration that neither the truth nor falsity of one allegation can be used to determine the truth or falsity of another.

Of the 19 DID patients who had made allegations that were confirmed, 10 of the 19, or 53%, had always retained conscious awareness of the abuses that were later confirmed, and they had reported these abuses in some manner or other within the first few interviews. However, 13 of 19, or 68%, obtained documentation during the course of their treatment of abusive events that they had not recalled prior to treatment. Four patients (21%) received confirmation of incidents or situations that they had always recalled, as well as confirmation of events and circumstances that were recovered during the course of therapy. That some abuse incidents may be recalled while others are not was noted by Williams,[14,15] who found that patients who may have forgotten the abuses documented in medical records might offer accounts of additional abuse experiences that were retained in available memory.

It is of interest that in all cases but two, the first discovery of all of these incidents in therapy occurred in connection with the use of hypnosis. One later confirmed memory emerged while a patient was discussing dynamic material; another memory was recovered while a patient was receiving eye movement desensitization reprocessing (EMDR)[16] treatment for a traumatic scenario which the patient had always remembered. In one case, in which an incest allegation was confirmed by both parents, the material was first uncovered under hypnosis after 8 years of treatment and after complete and total denial under initial hypnotic exploration.

In contradiction to positions taken by numerous proponents of the extreme false memory perspective, these findings seem to indicate that memory of genuine trauma can be absent from awareness for protracted periods of time and then recovered, and that genuine trauma can be documented in the childhood and adulthood of many adults with DID. Furthermore, these findings cast doubt on the argument that materials emerging from hypnotic exploration should be discounted in a peremptory manner. It seems that there are indeed many systems and/or forms of memory, and that they may have very different characteristics. Treating memory as a unitary phenomenon that can be discussed in glib generalizations is a dangerous oversimplification.

It might be argued that the documented incidents represent the only true abuses that were endured, forgotten, and recovered; i.e., the majority of allegations made by DID patients and others that recover abuse recollections are false. It might also be argued that the documented incidents represent only the tip of the iceberg of the sum total of true abuses that are endured, forgotten, and recovered; i.e., most allegations of abuse made by DID patients and others who recover such memories are accurate. There is no evidence for either extreme stance. The memories that were either confirmed or disconfirmed represent a fraction of all of the memories reported and recovered in these patients' treatment. The percentage of all allegations of childhood and adult abuse and the percentage of such allegations made on the basis of recovered memories that are accurate and inaccurate are currently unknown. To play on the catch-phrase of *The X-Files* (a currently popular television program in which there is a conspiracy to deny the existence of many widely doubted phenomena) with regard to recovered memories, ''the truth is *not* out there.'' Since all extreme, polarized statements about the accuracy of recovered memories must be made on the basis of discounting solid evidence that speaks to the contrary point of view,[5,17–19] they call into question the scholarship, integrity, and motivation of those who make them. Statements denying the possibility of the recovery of accurate, previously unavailable memories, and statements insisting that one can be confident of the recovery of such memories, are both grossly irresponsible.

Let us examine some of the further implications of the findings of this study. Recovered memories have been confirmed, but it is crucial to appreciate that this confirmation was often of a certain class of behaviors rather than a validation of the precise details that were recovered in therapy. It remains possible that the detail of what is recalled lacks accuracy because the patient's accurate memory is for the central details of a trauma; therefore, perhaps the original details never were in memory, have decayed, or have been contaminated in the course of their registration, retention, retrieval, and reporting. It is also possible that those details which are recalled are the result of a process of reconstruction, which is an aspect of narrative purpose. These details constitute an unwitting artifact of the act of remembering and reporting, much as secondary revision occurs in the process of recounting a dream to a psychoanalyst.

Pragmatically, what this means is that confirmations did not invariably contain all the details of the patient's own account. Often the confirmation was of a class of events rather than of specific events. That is, a patient's sister might recall coming upon their father in sex acts with the patient, but the sister rapidly turned away and could say no more than "He was naked, on top of you." However, on some occasions the confirmation was of specific events in great detail, or even much more detailed than the patient's own accounts, which were incomplete and fragmentary (see van der Kolk and Fisler[20]). A patient described driving her bicycle down a hill into a tree in an attempt to kill herself. She had only the vaguest and most fragmentary recollection of this event. However, an older brother had witnessed this episode and was able to recount it to me in great detail. The patient had been hospitalized for her injuries. Hospital records confirm both the accident and the extent of her injuries, but do not address her intent.

I have not attempted to develop categories with regard to the degree of detail of patients' memories because the data were not collected in a manner that would allow me to make orderly comparisons. Furthermore, the data had been prepared over 10 years without any awareness of the factors that might be useful in this study of memory. For example, when a psychiatrist admitted "sexual contacts" with a patient, I did not attempt to press to see if the patient's recollections were confirmed in detail, although it is possible that the psychiatrist might have been able to do so. However, it is possible to state that in this study, instances of detailed abuse scenarios that were confirmed in detail, detailed scenarios that were confirmed in a general way, vague scenarios that were confirmed in a vague manner, and vague scenarios that were confirmed in great detail were all encountered. This suggest to me that traumatic memory may not be a uniform phenomenon but consist of detailed recollections, vague recollections, fragmentary recollections and implicit memories inferred from symptoms, reenactments, and somatic memories[20] (and unconscious flashbacks[21]).

Interestingly, as this chapter was being revised, Pope and Hudson[22] proposed two criteria and two "rule-outs" for demonstrating the repression of traumatic memories. The two criteria are as follows. "First, an investigator must exhibit cases where it can be established *that the traumatic events actually occurred"*[22] (p. 716; italics in the original). They indicate that while legitimate trauma may be covert and unwitnessed, such uncorroborated events cannot be considered as constituting scientific proof in the case in question. "Second, one must establish that the individual actually developed amnesia for the events" (*ibid*). One must rule out normal childhood amnesia and amnesia that is due to organic causes. The authors do not explain how these can be ruled out if the amnesia is reversed.

In addition, Pope and Hudson ask that investigators rule out amnesia that may be alleged to achieve secondary gain for the patient. Under secondary gain, they include patients' failure to disclose because of embarrassment or "some psychological or legal advantage from professing amnesia" (*ibid*). Furthermore, they request that one exclude amnesia that is due to normal forgetfulness. They conclude: "Thus, a satisfactory demonstration of repression must show cases of noncontrived amnesia among neurologically intact individuals over the age of 6 who experienced events sufficiently traumatic that no one would be expected to simply forget them" (*ibid*).

Nearly all of the cases in this paper fulfill these criteria. The events that are under discussion are those which were confirmed (Table 2-1) or disconfirmed. None of the confirmed memories were from the first 6 years of life, nor were any of the patients in this series 6 years of age or younger. It is impossible to say that some did not suffer head injury, because many had been beaten badly on many occasions. However, no retrieved and confirmed memory had to do with a situation in which head trauma played a role. Only one patient in this series had confirmed neurological disease, and she did not have a recovered memory confirmed. However, an allegation of hers was demonstrated to be false. A second patient had been knocked unconscious when she threw herself in front of a vehicle in a suicide attempt. Even prior to that, she suffered nonepileptic seizures with three negative neurological work-ups, including normal electroencephalograms and CAT scans. She had both confirmed and disconfirmed memories of trauma.

With regard to secondary gain, the argument always exists that the secondary gain sought by these patients was their remaining in treatment and getting my sustained attention. It is my impression that this indeed was a factor in three cases. The remaining patients, however, seemed very motivated to complete their treatment as soon as possible. It is worth noting, in light of the nasty spirit of discussion that all too often pervades this field, that there are some gratifications inherent to being in compassionate and caring treatment. Trauma patients, and DID patients in particular, can become very attached to their therapists. However, one cannot infer from attachment, or even from regressive dependency, that the amnesia is being used in the service of secondary gain. There are egregious exceptions to this generalization, which occur when the therapist is preoccupied with the issue of trauma to the point of differentially reinforcing such reports, or when the therapist provides undue gratification or encourages regressive dependency. However, that the therapy of a traumatized patient focuses on trauma is no more proof of the therapist's exerting a distorting impact than is a treatment of a person with depression which focuses on affective issues. None of the patients in this series were involved in current legal proceedings. One had made charges against an extra-familial abuser which had led to this person's conviction and imprisonment, but this was 3 years before her treatment began.

All patients suffered considerable shame and used the shame scripts described by Nathanson.[23] However, their shame was not in connection with their abuse experiences as historical events. Instead, it centered on their perceptions of their own reactions and roles in these scenarios. For example, one woman, whose incest was confirmed by her father's confession and by her mother's corroboration as a witness, had rediscovered her incest experiences through hypnosis. However, it took another 6 years before she acknowledged that she felt very aroused by the incest and enjoyed much of it in spite of herself, and that she learned that if she responded to her father's advances by being more sexually aggressive than he was himself, she could avoid being beaten or threatened into submission.

This study demonstrates that the phenomenon of recovered memory is a clinical reality and that research formulations which bypass this class of observations are contriving to neglect a legitimate set of findings. Scientific formulations that disregard facts are suspect. Freud's obituary of Charcot states this eloquently (although I realize that referring to the words of Charcot in this context is somewhat analogous to quoting Polonius in Shakespeare's *Hamlet* on integrity and honesty):

> Charcot, indeed, never tired of defending the rights of purely clinical work, which consists of seeing and ordering things, against the encroachments of theoretical medicine. On one occasion there was a small group of us, all students from abroad, who, brought up on German academic physiology, were trying his patience with our doubts about his clinical innovations. "But that can't be true," one of us objected, "it contradicts the Young-Helmholtz theory." He did not reply, "So much the worse for your theory, clinical facts come first" or words to that effect; but he did say something which made a great impression on us: "La theorie, c'est bon, mais ca n'empeche pas d'exister. . . . [Theory is good, but it doesn't prevent things from existing]"[24] (p. 13).

I will close this section of my remarks by reminding the reader that this is not the first report of the credibility of accounts made by patients with DID, although it is the first to explicitly link specific memories to corroboration, as opposed to demonstrating that such patients have indeed suffered abuse. Bliss[25] found that some allegations made by 8 of 9 DID patients could be documented to some extent. Coons and Milstein[26] found that 85% of their 20 DID patients had experienced confirmable abuse. More recently, Hornstein and Putnam[27] found that 95.3% of their series of dissociative children and adolescents had experienced corroborated abuse, a finding that is comparable to the 95% corroboration rate found by Coons[28] in a similar group of patients. However, these studies did not address the confirmation of recovered memories, only the legitimacy of representing that DID and similar forms of DDNOS (dissociative disorder not otherwise specified) have genuine traumatic antecedents.

Hypnosis and the Recovery of Memory: A Paradigm of the Impact of Interpersonal Influence

It has become fashionable to attack the credibility of material that is recovered in hypnosis. Even experts who firmly believe that it is possible for memories of trauma to become unavailable and then be recovered often decry hypnosis as a concession to the critics of their basic point of view. Therefore, it is useful to discuss the issue of hypnosis, because as a rule, its discussion in the more recent literature has been lacking in depth and thoughtfulness. Welcome exceptions are an excellent review by Brown[10] and a monograph produced by the American Society of Clinical Hypnosis.[29]

Furthermore, I would ask the reader to study this section on hypnosis as a set of observations on interpersonal influence and persuasion in general, of which hypnosis may be seen as an exemplar or a paradigm. The overall subject of interpersonal influence and persuasion is too enormous to address in this context. Today's patient lives in a stimulus-dense environment with regard to trauma. It is difficult if not impossible to avoid a subject that is so much a part of our culture and concerns at the close of the twentieth century.

Hypnosis is discussed as if it were a uniform clinical intervention with a predictable, distorting effect. This is far from the truth. Defining hypnosis is a scholar's nightmare. Some describe it in terms of the phenomena associated with it. Others use the paradigm of the differential distribution of attention, with hypnosis involving focused concentration in some directions and consequent inattention to others. State and trait variables and concepts play a role in many theories, while contextual factors play a role in others. A major debate concerns whether hypnosis is defined as an altered state or in terms of social psychological variables. Many attempt to define hypnosis by its antecedents (i.e., the presence of an induction ceremony), while others regard hypnosis as a phenomenon that may occur spontaneously, by autohypnosis, or by its deliberate induction (heterohypnosis). The interested reader is referred to an excellent discussion by Lynn and Rhue of available theories.[30]

Not only is it difficult to define hypnosis, but there is also a consensus among scholars that hypnosis is a facilitator of treatment rather than a treatment in and of itself.[31,32] For example, hypnosis in the service of directive treatment will catalyze a very different set of interventions than it would in a permissive expressive form of psychotherapy. It is easy to erroneously attribute to hypnosis the characteristics of the treatment it facilitates.

As an illustration of this principle, let us imagine three scenarios in which hypnosis is used to explore a period of time for which a patient has amnesia and during which the therapist suspects abuse might have occurred. In the first instance, the patient, in trance, is requested to return to the time in question and is asked questions such as: "Were you being hurt?" "You see someone. Is it your father?" "Is he wearing any clothes?" Such an approach is very provocative and suggestive, and might lead the patient toward confabulation. In the second circumstance, the patient, in trance, is requested to return to the time in question and is asked questions such as: "What do you observe?" "Can you identify the person you noticed?" "Does anything more strike your attention?" Such an approach is very open ended and permissive, and is realtively unlikely to promote confabulation. In a third situation, the clinician is working with a patient who expects to find a memory of abuse on the basis of already known traumata, a hypothesis of a friend or relative, something encountered in the media or professional reading, the tenor of the therapy to date, or a recent dream. Under these circumstances even the most circumspect approach will run the risk of uncovering a potentially inaccurate set of findings that are contaminated far in advance of the intervention's occurrence.

Furthermore, the capacity to respond to hypnotic interventions and suggestions is far from uniform. Not only are there many different degrees of hypnotizability, but within each there is a diversity of hypnotic talents. That is, two subjects with the same degree of hypnotizability may not have the same type of responses to a given stimulus (e.g., the capacity to hallucinate visually or ablate painful sensations). Therefore, one patient may respond to suggestions or requests to manifest phenomena that another patient cannot demonstrate, and vice versa. I have seen instances in which the assumption was made that a patient had had visual hallucinations of abuse in response to a therapist's suggestive inquiries under hypnosis and had mistaken them for historical reality, when objective testing demonstrated that the patient lacked the capacity to respond to suggestions by having visual hallucinations.

In addition, the subject is further complicated by the fact that hypnotic phenomena do not require the formal induction of trance in order to occur. Spontaneous trance and self-induced or autohypnotic trance phenomena can occur in any setting, so that the hypnotic responsiveness of a susceptible individual is not simply or invariably linked to the intervention of the person who is said to have induced a state of hypnosis.

The central point is that the term *hypnosis,* when applied to a diverse array of therapies offered to a variety of individuals, encompasses a very wide and complex domain of phenomena and responses. General statements about hypnosis and its impacts must be regarded with caution. More often than not, when it is alleged that hypnosis has thus and so an effect, the truth is that hypnosis may have such an effect, but that such an effect is not inevitable. Often what is attributed to hypnosis is due to other factors in the treatment situation[33] or in the scientific experiment.[34] McConkey demonstrated that given a patient's hypnotizability and the demand characteristics of an experimental situation, the formal induction of hypnosis did not increase the likelihood that memory distortion would occur or be increased.[34]

Because hypnosis is thought to have the potential to generate pseudomemories and can have the effect of making the subject very sure that what has been experienced is actual ("concretization") its use in court is problematic.[35–39] In legal situations, it is problematic to use an intervention that may adversely affect an individual's ability to be a credible witness, or to run the risk that someone may suffer adverse consequences on the basis of a faulty report. It is unfortunate that a press toward disambiguation often characterizes legal rulings on hypnosis, and that many authorities press for the adoption of forensic restrictions and practices in the clinical use of hypnosis.

This results in a frequent dilemma. What is possible is described as if it were probable, and what is now (inaccurately) assumed to be probable is further inflated and assumed to be true. On this basis, expert testimony may be offered or scientific articles written. Extreme and atypical practices that illustrate the actualization of the possible become the paradigms to which opponents of the possibility of the recovery of actual memories refer (see Loftus and Ketcham,[40] and Ofshe and Watters[41]). The outlying case becomes represented as a typical instance and is played up by irresponsible media and by colleagues with particular axes to grind.

A more careful reading of the hypnosis literature[10,11,34] reveals that of three factors traditionally associated with hypnotic memory distortion—expectations/demand characteristics, hypnotizability, and the induction of hypnosis—the actual induction of hypnosis does not contribute to the degree of error in patients' reports. That is, what is traditionally ascribed to the use of hypnosis is in fact due to the trait of hypnotizability and its impact in nonhypnotic situations, and the expectations and social influences brought to bear on the patients. The salient factors involve the application of techniques of interpersonal influence to potentially suggestible subjects. In short, the use of hypnosis is accorded both a potency and an impact that reside elsewhere and that play a role in nonhypnotic situations as well. Therefore, much of what is said about hypnosis and memory in the literature that is skeptical of the possibility of the recovery of memory with hypnosis is based on questionable assumptions or on older allegations that should be modified in light of more recent findings.

This may help the reader to appreciate why—despite the widespread current tendency to make global condemnations that discredit the clinical use of hypnosis in uncovering material—it is not incomprehensible that hypnosis, used gently and without the exertion of undue influence and suggestions, was associated with the majority of the accurate recoveries of memories in this series. Hypnosis was not involved with the confabulated and discredited memories. Whereas the recovery of accurate memories with hypnosis has been demonstrated, it is my feeling that if the number of disproven incidents were higher, they might have included instances in which hypnotically retrieved materials were disproven. It is important for the reader to appreciate that the types of questionable practices often assumed to be associated with hypnosis in the polarized atmosphere of the false memory debate did not play a part in these therapies. They are not typical of the practice of experts in the treatment of trauma.

In sum, caricatured and oversimplified generalizations about the dangers of hypnosis discredit the usefulness of this venerable clinical tool in the treatment of the traumatized. This is a very dangerous situation, because in addition to patients with dissociative identity disorder,[42] many patients with chronic and severe posttraumatic stress disorder are also highly hypnotizable.[43,44] As noted above, even in the absence of formal hypnosis (heterohypnosis) following a ceremony of induction, autohypnosis and spontaneous trance phenomena will be encountered in these patient populations. Many dissociative and posttraumatic symptoms respond well to therapies facilitated by hypnosis. Hypnosis is often a most useful modality with which to facilitate their restructuring and resolution.[45–48] It would be a shame to throw the baby out with the bathwater by unduly restricting the use of hypnosis in traumatized populations.

This having been said, the use of hypnosis should be avoided in all circumstances in which the patient is, anticipates, or may be involved in forensic proceedings, unless it has been determined that its use will not be detrimental to the patient and/or the case. This decision should not be made by the clinician alone, but with the advice of a legal professional safeguarding the patient's interests who is familiar with the particular case and the relevant regulations in the appropriate jurisdiction. When a determination is made to use hypnosis to retrieve materials that may be used in forensic proceedings, forensic guidelines should be used.[29,37,38]

The Dilemma of Dissociation in the Repressed Memory Debate

It is unfortunate that one aspect of the oversimplification of the debate over the possibility of recovering memories has been the lumping together, under a common heading, of many defensive processes and cognitive operations that remove material and affect from conscious awareness. Although a strong case can be made for collapsing the differences among terms because of their muddled connotations, their histories of being used interchangeably, and the uncertainty of whether some distinctions reflect theories (often changed or discredited over time) rather than tangible reality,[49] a strong argument can be made that the differences between repression and dissociation are considerable and quite salient in the current context.

Repression comes to us from the tradition of Freudian psychoanalysis. It involves the defensive exclusion of content from conscious representation because of its unacceptable nature. Our concepts of repression stem from an hydraulic metaphor.[50] Most of what is repressed is related to unacceptable drives and their derivative wishes, and it never has achieved conscious representation. Additional repressed material consists of material that was conscious, but has been removed from consciousness because it is unacceptable and/or intolerable. With regard to formerly conscious material, such repressed material is removed from awareness after having been conscious, that is, ex post facto. Anxiety is often the remaining conscious residue of repression.

Dissociation comes to us from the tradition of Janet and his colleagues. Although originally it was associated with the failure of the mind to retain cohesion due to a lowered supply of mental energy or ''cerebral glue,'' modern concepts of dissociation are guided by the neodissociation theories of Hilgard[51] and current cognitive psychology. Dissociation is a special form of consciousness in which events that normally would be connected with one another are divided from one another.[50] Yet the very information that has been excluded often makes its presence known in symptomatic manifestations of many varieties. As Spiegel observes, dissociation also has the capacity to serve as "a defense not only against warded-off memories, fears, and wishes, but against trauma while it is occurring. . . . The essence of trauma is physical helplessness, the loss of control over one's body and environment at a time when pain and damage are being threatened or inflicted. One's will and desire is overridden by another's brutality, by accident, or by nature's indifference. When physical control is lost, mental control becomes paramount"[48] (pp. 261–262).

Dissociation involves the segregation of some sets of information from others in a relatively rule-bound manner.[52] Its metaphors are drawn from cognitive studies and information-processing models. For example, Spiegel[52a] has used the computational model of parallel distributed processing from the work of Rumelhart and McClelland[53] to describe a variety of processors working on stored information simultaneously. Kluft[54] has drawn on psychoanalytic sources to derive an understanding of dissociation as the study of "the elsewhere thought known," arguing to counter Freud's[55] insistence that it is impossible for the mind to possess a second conscious state of which the owner is unaware. Not only has dissociation of all sorts been historically associated with trauma,[56] but recent studies[57–59] have demonstrated that dissociative responses occur quite commonly in documented trauma (such as exposure to earthquakes, firestorms, shootings, etc.) in nonpatient populations.

In my understanding, when material is repressed, it enters a state of storage in which it may come into contact with and be influenced by a wide variety of other mental content, and when repressed material is recovered it may be subject to considerable distortion in the process. Furthermore, the very nature of what is repressed may be highly imbued with wishes, fears, and fantasies which are experienced as having an interpersonal and object-related dimension involving significant others. Hence, it is fertile ground for the generation of fantasy-imbued pseudomemories.

Conversely, what is dissociated may be held in relative isolation and may always remain a known entity within some of the parallel distributed processes and the structures that serve them. In this model, what is recovered from such a storage situation has not necessarily been distorted, contaminated, or imbued with fantasies. If such material leaks into a second process that is associated with comonplace consciousness, it may do so either eruptively or in a piecemeal and gradual manner. If, on the other hand, it is accessed more directly by techniques such as hypnosis or EMDR (eye movement desensitization and reprocessing),[16] it is conceivable that the dissociated material will behave more as if it were material that was always in full consciousness. On the basis of the research that has been discussed above, I have come to the opinion that material that is truly repressed is far more subject to contamination than memory that is directly accessed from a parallel distributed processing system, and that material from dissociated processing systems that leaks or breaks through occupies an intermediate likelihood of being distorted. If this were a sufficient conceptualization, it would turn the tables on the current wisdom which holds that hypnotically retrieved information is more problematic. Unfortunately, although this formulation holds up in the study noted above, it is without general applicability. As I noted in 1984, the same populations in which such clear recall can occasionally be documented are vulnerable to mistaking phenomena with different origins as autobiographic history. This may be related to the relative ease with which most patients who dissociate can mistake what they experience visually for what has in fact befallen them. (See Belli and Loftus[60] for a useful source-monitoring perspective on the recovery of inaccurate memories.) We are left with what we had from the start: no memory that cannot be externally corroborated is useful for any purpose other than in the service of therapy.

Therefore, we have evidence that dissociation is a defense and reaction associated with trauma, and we must entertain the possibility that what is dissociated may have been conscious in a manner of speaking all along, and may conceivably be retrieved without much distortion in some cases. Furthermore, the recovery of memory is a dissociation paradigm rather than a repression paradigm in many cases, and there is a considerable body of research literature to the effect that what has been dissociated from consciousness can be recovered. Erdelyi observes: "Formally, the recovery paradigm is realized when a second test of memory contains stimulus information not accessible in an earlier test, as in hypermnesia and reminiscence. It may be concluded from such a situation that the information was originally unconscious—dissociated from consciousness."[61]

In summarizing the literature, Erdelyi concludes: "Despite some past controversies[62] (see also M. H. Erdelyi, unpublished observations, 1994), the phenomenon of reminiscence (recovery of items in later trials that were not accessible on earlier ones) and hypermnesia (overall increase of memory from an earlier test to a later test) have become undisputed[62–64] (see also M. H. Erdelyi, unpublished observations, 1994). Such accessible increments, as Ballard[65] reluctantly acknowledged in his monograph, logically imply the existence of unconscious contents, for the recovered material has to come from somewhere. Hypermnesia and reminiscence effects are not only reliable, but powerful."[61]

Although I would prefer a reconciliation between the languages of Spiegel and Erdelyi so that they would not be viewed as discussing different phenomena, it is clear that both clinically and in the laboratory, the recovery of once unavailable material is commonplace rather than nonexistent. The furor over repression and the trendy term that is more buzz word than scientific concept, "robust repression,"[40] has distracted us from an appropriate focus on the importance of dissociation in such matters. Despite the confusion that surrounds the meaning and the domain of the term,[66] dissociation seems to be a demonstrable and readily researchable phenomenon.

Before leaving this section, I want to reflect briefly on the striking absence of cogent discussions of psychogenic amnesia, or dissociative amnesia in DSM-IV[7] or in the current literature. There has been such a strong focus on memories of child abuse (especially childhood sexual abuse) in the recovered memory debate that there has been a considerable neglect of the fact that amnesia is a venerable clinical phenomenon, and that people block out their perceptions and experiences of traumas other than abuse. This happened, for instance, to the marine in combat I alluded to above; and combat-related amnestic syndromes are well documented in the literature.[56] Not infrequently these patients were treated with hypnosis or drug-facilitated interviews. One of my first amnesia cases involved a woman's blocking out of the industrial accident that crushed and nearly amputated her index finger. Under hypnosis, she recalled and abreacted the incident, the reality of which was undeniable and the recovered details of which were confirmed independently by witnesses. Let us thus bear in mind that when we step back from the fury of the current turmoil, we find overlooked clinical and research literature that can offer valuable insights.

Reflections on the Current Literature

Della Femina, Yeager, and Lewis[67] demonstrated that often individuals with docu-mented histories of abuse withhold acknowledging their abuse, even when confronted. Herman and Schatzow[68] found that 64% of their 53 incest victim patients had some degree of amnesia and 28% had severe amnesia for their sexual abuse experiences, and over 70% of the total series had some corroboration for their allegations of abuse. This is a pioneering contribution, weakened somewhat by the less than stringent criteria for assessing corroboration. Linda Meyer Williams[14,15] found that 38% of women with documented childhood sexual abuse had forgotten the documented episode, and an-other 10% had forgotten the abuse at some time earlier but recalled it again at the time of the study. Briere and Conte[69] found that 59% of 450 subjects who had endured forced sexual experiences had forgotten the abuse for a period of time. Factors associ-ated with reversible amnesia were abuse at an earlier age, repetitive abuse, threats of death for making revelations, associated physical injuries, and mistreatment by more than one abuser. Loftus, Polonsky, and Fullilove[70] discovered that 19% of 100 women in substance abuse treatment had had delayed memories of having been sexually abused during their childhoods. The authors speculated that perhaps more had been abused but had not yet recovered their memories. The senior author's reversal on this issue[71] in the heat of the false memory debate is interesting to contemplate, and may represent the application of motivated skepticism to her own work. Cameron[72] studied 60 women over 6 years, of whom 42% had complete amnesia for childhood abuse and 23% had only partial memory for their abuse. Roesler and Wind[73] found that 28% of 228 survivors of childhood sexual abuse had repressed memories of their abuse. Feldman-Summers and Pope[74] found that 23.9% of a surveyed population of American psy-chologists reported having experienced childhood abuse. Approximately 40% of these reported a period of forgetting the abuse in whole or in part. Approximately half of those who reported forgetting the abuse also reported corroboration of their abuse allegation, a percentage close to that reported in my research presented above. Forgetting the abuse was related to its severity, and the most frequent factor associated with remembering it was being in therapy. Burgess et al.[75] prospectively followed 19 children who were sexually abused in day care settings. Sixteen percent had totally forgotten their documented abuse, and 26% had partially forgotten it. Finally, Albach and her colleagues[76] studied a Dutch sample of 97 sexually abused women in comparison with a control group of 65 control subjects. They found that amnesia for a traumatic event was very rare in the control group (1%), but common (35%) in the traumatized group. In this study, memories of abuse generally returned not in therapy, but spontaneously, triggered by abuse-related stimuli.

Most of these studies can be criticized because the abuse allegations were not corroborated and/or because the corroboration of allegations was attested to by the patients alone. However, cases of corroborated abuse with recovery of abuse memories were documented. As a whole, however, these studies demonstrate that patients who have suffered childhood abuse will frequently forget their experiences of abuse, and that the recovery of these memories may occur both in and outside of therapy. Furthermore, these findings indicate that a recovered memory of abuse may actually refer to an historical event rather than to a fantasy, despite arguments to the contrary (e.g., Frankel[77]). Consequently, a circumspect reading of the literature suggests that a recovered memory should no more be peremptorily discounted than immediately endorsed. The slow and steady process of therapy rather than simplistic confrontation schemes is the appropriate forum for the slow and circumspect study of all such materials.

Perspectives on Discrediting the Possible Recovery of Repressed Memory

Limitations of space preclude the possibility of my making a detailed critique of the arguments against the possibility of the recovery of repressed or otherwise unavailable memory. However, I will comment briefly on a small number of the issues that have been raised in that connection.

Often the argument is made that there are no data to sustain the notion of repression, so that any material alleged to have been repressed and then recovered is a priori suspect. Concepts such as repression and the unconscious mind have proven very elusive subjects of study in the experimental setting. Many laboratory models that have been advanced are far from convincing as paradigms.

The work of Holmes[78] is frequently cited in arguments opposing the existence of repression. It is of historical note that this work appears in an important book[79] containing 18 contributions, 17 of which come to different conclusions than that of Holmes. In this publication, Holmes demonstrates that several experimental constructs of repression were subject to plausible alternative explanations. Unfortunately, he uses motivated skepticism[80] adroitly. His dismissal of the possible relevance of criticism of his paradigms and his disregard of anecdotal clinical information is glib and cavalier.

In his 1970 study he tested the hypothesis that the recall of experiences is determined by the intensity of affect associated with the experiences at the time of recall; that the intensity of the affect associated with given experiences declines over time; and that the affect associated with displeasure will decline more rapidly than that associated with pleasant experiences. He had college students keep a diary of their pleasant and unpleasant experiences for a week. They were to score each experience for pleasantness and unpleasantness on a nine-point scale. A week later they were asked unexpectedly to write down the experiences from their diary cards and to score them again. The results indicated that unpleasant experiences showed greater declines than did pleasant ones and were less likely to be recalled. Holmes concluded that recall of unpleasant experiences was due to reduced affective intensity rather than to repression. He speculated that intensity was reduced because unpleasant experiences, such as failing a French test, were found not to matter that much, or remediative actions could alter the nature of the experience. He also proposed that, with further thought, the attitudes toward the events might become more positive, and therefore the intensity of the negativity would be reduced.

I would like to raise the possibility that the nature of the phenomena that Holmes studied is somewhat different from the materials encountered by clinicians working with traumatized populations. An incestuous experience or a gang-rape might be more traumatic than failing a French test. I do not quarrel with Dr. Holmes' experiment per se, but I do think that trauma-related problems of memory may be managed in a different manner and that this different manner may involve repression and dissociation. I do not think his experimental universe was sufficiently diverse to support his conclusions. Although I consider Holmes's work thought-provoking and ingenious, I seriously doubt that his arguments against the possibility of the recovery of memories[81] deal with the phenomena in question.

When we turn to the famous lost-in-the-mall scenario (see Chapter 1) of Elizabeth Loftus, who is often regarded as a very influential participant in the debate over recovered memory, we encounter another family of difficulties. In her study, 5 young subjects, ''all friends and relatives of our research group''[82,83] were taken through a reflection on early life experiences, most of which were accurate, but one of which— the experimentally suggested one—was not. The subjects were led by siblings and others to believe that they had been lost in a mall, when this had not occurred. Not only was it possible to cause the subjects to report this, but they often confabulated additional details as their stories took on lives of their own. On this basis she argued that it is possible for therapists to implant false memories that will be elaborated further and regarded as credible.[82,83]

I wonder about the generalizability of this experiment, and am troubled by its ethics. Young children were exposed to deliberately mendacious behavior by their siblings and concerned others, and were then told they were duped. I question whether the possible deleterious long-term effects on the relationship of those involved is acceptable. I wonder about the appropriateness of the strategy of teaching children to become involved in systematic deception. I also wonder about the message conveyed about authority figures and the nature of truth that is given to the young subjects. Were I on a human subjects review committee, I would not have passed on this one. When Dr. Loftus has been asked about this, she dismisses such concerns by stating there have been no adverse effects. She offers as proof that when the children understood what had occurred, some of her own subjects took to doing similar deceptions with their friends.[83] To me this is chilling. Perhaps these subjects are only engaging in a benign attempt to achieve mastery, but I would like to raise the possibility that adult authority figures have taught them to think that truth is a malleable commodity that can be distorted at one's convenience or whimsy. These children may be demonstrating the mechanism of identification with the aggressor, a severely pathological defensive adaptation.

I also think the design leaves much to be desired, because it does not narrow the variables in a manner that allows the results to mean anything. It becomes a Rorschach to confirm one's bias. We see a study not of memory but of social persuasion. Whether the implantation of the so-called memory by an older sibling who says he was there as an eye-witness and who has a powerful affective relationship with and position of authority over the child mirrors the position of the therapist is questionable. The therapist was not a first-hand witness to a patient's past, and the therapist is not lying, or trying consciously to systematically direct the patient's perception of the truth, or using techniques verging on the interrogatory. In addition, children are accustomed to the idea of getting lost.[84] It is a normal fear, it is the plot of innumerable fairy tales, and it is the subject of myriad maternal warnings. Children likely have a preexisting schema in mind with regard to getting lost, which can be tapped readily by suggestion because it is already present.[84] With regard to incest, however, the incest fantasies described as universal by Freud are not traumatic in nature, like the ones reported by incest victims. We cannot assume that there is a schema for abrupt anal or oral rape, for example, that is lying dormant and ready to be brought to immediate fruition by a therapist who asks a bland question about whether the patient has had any unwanted sexual experiences.

As a study on social persuasion, however, the lost-in-the-mall scenario demonstrates that when a family has a story about how an event happened, it may drive out the autobiographical memory of those involved. This need not be an instance in which a child is convinced that an event has occurred when it has not. It could just as easily explain how a child is persuaded that an event that did occur has not occurred, a possibility Loftus herself has acknowledged.[83] It is a curious irony that in 1983, a syndrome was described in which the family conspires to deny the reality of a traumatic event, and finally the victim endorses the alternate reality. This, of course, is the child sexual abuse accommodation syndrome, which was explored by Roland Summit—one of the experts frequently attacked by those who believe that recovered memories of childhood sexual abuse should be discredited. Loftus's lost-in-the-mall scenario offers confirmation of Summit's earlier observations: a family determined to distort a child's sense of reality has a good chance of achieving its objectives.

It is possible that insights gained from Loftus's lost-in-the-mall scenario and Summit's child sexual abuse accommodation syndrome may cast some light on a phenomenon that is of great interest in the current false memory controversy. Retractors are individuals who at one time believed that they were abused, but who have come to believe that their memories of abuse are inaccurate. Some retractors change their minds in the context of strong interpersonal pressures that have features in common with those exerted upon individuals in the lost-in-the mall scenario and the child sexual abuse accommodation syndrome. Could it be that retractors rather than therapy patients demonstrate the forces that Dr. Loftus has studied? This could prove an interesting subject for future research.

Another aspect of the Loftus research that has received little attention is that only a small minority of the subjects who received misdirection cues took the indicated misdirections. Most did not. This research might be cited as evidence that most persons, even those subjected to an intense campaign to distort their memories and induce confabulations, will reject such suggestions.

Since the reader of this chapter may have heard many an attack on the gullibility and ineptitude of clinicians by speakers representing themselves as guardians of science, it may be useful to consider an analysis from the perspective of a clinician who worries that the perfect can be the enemy of the good, and that taking too literally the warnings of researchers can destroy the capacity to render good therapy.

The progress of science is a parade of paradigms[85] that strut their arrogant hour upon the stage, expressing themselves in allegories called experiments, depreciating, belittling, and berating everything the paradigm of choice does not embrace. Paradigms collapse by virtue of their exclusion of or failure to address data they had deemed unimportant within the worldview of that particular paradigm. In the language of Greek tragedy, every paradigm has a tragic flaw, overstates its applicability (overweening pride), and is humiliated by fate (retribution).

By disregarding information, paradigms embrace the same mechanisms that we find in the more familiar processes of dissociation, repression, denial, splitting, and even more primitive mechanisms. Perhaps the excesses of such uses of science so fascinate me as a clinician because it helps me to appreciate that laboratory science that is unanchored in common sense is a primitive character disorder verging on decompensation into psychosis, a term that indicates that there is a major failure to appreciate reality. We mock the mad scientist in a grade-B movie and enjoy his or her downfall precisely because, like an incestuous Greek king or a Shakespearean regicide, the order of the universe is destroyed by his or her arrogance and false attempts to impose his or her self-deceived facsimile of natural order upon reality, and his or her defeat is necessary in order to preserve the true order of the world. It follows that the attempt to conform clinical practice rigidly to scientific findings is doomed to defeat, because it will introduce borderline and/or psychotic features into the thinking of the clinician.

Additional Remarks on the Recollection and the Nonrecollection of Trauma

Terr[86] describes types of trauma that are of a single blow and recalled clearly, and types that are repetitive and may be dissociated to a greater or lesser extent. Her primary example for the recall of single-blow trauma is her example of the children of Chow-chilla, who were kidnapped and buried in a trailer. A common example of repetitive trauma is incest. While I have commented on aspects of this theory elsewhere,[87] my focus here is that the example for recalled trauma is a collective group experience and the example for the less well–recalled trauma is a private one. Perhaps what occurs in a group context, with fellow sufferers who share and discuss the experience, is more difficult to abolish completely from memory than that which is faced in solitude and about which communication may be forbidden or limited. Perhaps in the middle of globally recalled traumata there are islands of amnesia that may be reversed at a later date.

Not infrequently, those who maintain that trauma is not forgotten illustrate their argument that no one who has suffered through a war or endured the Holocaust has forgotten their experience. I am not sure that such a global statement is accurate, but I am confident that it is at the least, very incomplete. It has long been appreciated that the more combat and bombardment soldiers endure, the more they demonstrate distur-bances of memory.[88] They do not forget that they were combatants, but they may not recall their entire combat experience (as in the story of the marine cited above). Likewise, among the Holocaust survivors I have interviewed, I have not encountered any who did not recall being caught up in the Holocaust, but I have spoken to many who, despite the inextinguishable recollection of unspeakable horrors, had considerable gaps in their autobiographical memories of their personal ordeals.

A sensitive reading requires us to take a very close look at the allegation that people do not forget real trauma. It is far too global an allegation, and begs a good many questions. For example, is it not possible that a traumatized person can forget some, but not all of a trauma, or some incidents, but not all instances, of traumatization? If this is the case, is it not possible that some memories that might arise in treatment or elsewhere could be brought to awareness once again (i.e., recovered) memory? In other words, is it not possible that we may find amnesia in the middle of memory, and vice versa? Often the most strong statements of one polarized point of view contain the essence of the opposite position within them.

Elizabeth Loftus, Ph.D., is a brilliant researcher and scholar. She has described her own experiences of abuse and reflected upon her incomplete recollection of it. Her words are captured in a deposition cited by Whitfield.[89] She both denies she repressed the memory of the abuse, and speaks of her uncertainty about the number of occur-rences, and of her memory having taken and destroyed her recollections of her abuser. In the same account we find both recollection and the absence of recollection. This might be understood as either confusing, or expectable. As Whitfield notes, trauma dissociates and confuses memory, and trying to block traumata out with guilt, shame, and/or threats of harm can drive its mental representation out of awareness.

Loftus's experience can be understood as capturing the essence of the intimately intertwined nature of both the memory and the banishing from memory of traumatization. Rather than polarized opposites, they may be understood by analogy with the intrusive and numbing aspects of the posttraumatic response. While there are some instances in which clear and striking memory is retained, and some in which its abolition is virtually complete, more often, the two processes proceed side by side. An example of this may be that often only the central aspect of a traumatic event is recalled. The details may neither be registered not retrieved.

Conclusions

To return to where we began, if the debate over the possibility of the delayed recall of disremembered trauma could be phrased, "resolved, that there has never been one instance in which repressed memories of genuine trauma have been recovered," we could all go home at this point. Such instances have been demonstrated. Although it is difficult to demonstrate such phenomena in laboratory situations or in the adversarial atmosphere of the courtroom, in the setting of the psychotherapist's office, the documentation of the recovery of what has been forgotten is a clinical commonplace. Furthermore, what has been forgotten tends to exert an influence from behind the scenes (as in the first example, of a patient's having unwittingly repeated her trauma in a new setting and having protected against the repetition of such a scenario with the author without consciously appreciating why she was doing this). This suggests that when material is unavailable to declarative autobiographical memory, it may nonetheless inform the mind in a more indirect or implicit fashion, which suggests a plurality of memory systems at work (see Spiegel and Scheflin,[19] van der Kolk and Fisler,[20] and Maldonado and Spiegel[47]).

Both relatively accurate and relatively inaccurate recollections are familiar visitors to the consulting room of the clinician and the laboratory of the scientific investigator. Every experiment that demonstrates the potential unreliability of memory implicitly relies on the accuracy of human memory to allow its subjects to follow the experimenter's instructions. That contemporary mental health scientists find themselves in the midst of an impassioned debate over the delayed recall of trauma is unfortunate in the extreme, because virtually all perspectives have something of importance to contribute, but they have been stretched beyond the bounds of credibility by the most extreme among their proponents.

Human memory is an extremely complex phenomenon. It appears to comprise several systems for the registration, retention, and recovery of information and experience; these several systems have diverse neuroanatomical and neurophysiologic substrates. There is no a priori reason to assume or assert that all forms of memory will handle a given stimulus in a similar manner. Therefore, global statements about the nature and function of memory are likely to prove premature. An already intricate situation is further confused when the very nature of what is to be remembered and recalled is itself complex, confusing, ambiguous, and overwhelming, and the mind that must perceive it, receive it, store it, and make it available once again is involved in a process of ongoing change and development.

However, many scholars have rushed to cleave the Gordian knot of memory and simplify our understanding of its vicissitudes with the sword of premature closure. They propose particular visions of how memory works and how it may be betrayed, promote often draconian reforms in the practice of psychotherapy, and offer frequently scathing and trenchant criticisms of those who do not share their points of view. This rush toward disambiguation has been embraced by the media, and by many within the professions who either find their arguments convincing, or look to them to provide guidance in these troubling, confused, and litigious times.

Depending on one's perspective, this situation is alarming, amusing, or both. I find it alarming, but choose to reflect momentarily on some of its amusing aspects. Those who maintain that all or most recovered memories are false have promoted to positions of ascribed and self-proclaimed expertise individuals with minimal direct experience in the treatment of the traumatized or in researching the consequences of trauma. Most of these individuals put forth as experts have made their contributions in other areas of study. They extrapolate paradigms and findings from these areas to the study of trauma and memory for traumatic experiences. They do so without having proven that their proceeding in this manner has ecological validity. By claiming to be more scientific, they purport to seize what they understand or represent to be the intellectual high ground. The problem that might appear to be difficult to address, their relative amateur status in the trauma field, is solved by its implicitly being decreed a virtue. This has been accomplished by depreciating and disparaging those who work with trauma and who might be understood to know something about traumatized populations. With a clever turn of phrase and a sophistry or two, the work of those who actually deal with trauma and its consequences is discounted as flawed and dismissed, and therefore need not be reckoned with. With similar maneuvers, those who treat and study trauma themselves are mocked and derided, and are alleged to create the circumstances and conditions that they treat.

The result is the enshrinement of persons as experts on trauma whose acquaintance with the realities of work in the trauma field is vicarious and limited. Those who have never treated a trauma victim are accorded credibility when they advise clinicians how to proceed and how not to proceed, although their advice is more consistent with their research and/or politics than any proven efficacy or effectiveness. Whitfield[89] has described this as the "false expert syndrome." In view of the lucrative nature of being such an expert these days, I would suggest that an alternative title might be the "false expensive expert syndrome," referred to by the acronym "FEES."

Whereas an infectious disease specialist would not be faulted if all of his patients suffered infectious diseases, and an oncologist would not be faulted if all of his patients suffered malignancies, that the trauma specialist's practice is replete with patients complaining of trauma is held to be prima facie evidence that something is very much amiss. Alone among specialists, the fact that their practices are full of patients whose complaints match their expertise is not seen as a tribute to their competence and reputation, and/or a consequence of their referral patterns, but an indictment of their manner of practicing their profession. Since the veracity of much of what they treat is doubted, they are accused of creating iatrogenic conditions and false memories in epidemic numbers. I myself am frequently accused of diagnosing every patient I see as having DID. However, of the 34 patients in the study cited above, only 3 came to me without a trauma history and/or a dissociative disorder diagnosed or suspected by another clinician. Two of the three patients approached me for the treatment of self-diagnosed dissociative disorders, and the third identified herself as an incest victim. This last patient was the only one for whom I was the first to raise the issue of a dissociative disorder diagnosis. Therefore, I have had minimal opportunity to earn the reputation accorded me by those who do not know my work.

Therefore, many of the critics of those who maintain that memories of trauma may be removed and then returned to conscious awareness are unburdened with the need to address trauma on an ongoing basis and unfettered with the implications of clinical observations (which they give themselves permission to dismiss as anecdotal). They feel free to pontificate in a manner that sounds plausible if all contradictory information is dismissed, but which appears fatuous to the person who refuses to oversimplify by discarding a priori information associated with an opposing point of view. Many pundits who promote the false memory perspective remind me of the song, ''I'm an Old Cowhand.'' Perhaps the reader will remember the lyrics, which include, ''I'm an old cowhand, from the Rio Grande. . . . I'm a cowboy who never saw a cow, never roped a steer 'cause I don't know how. . . . Yippeeiokayay!''

Those who steadfastly maintain the alternative polarized position have comparable grounds for self-reproach. However, they have not made as many extreme statements in recent years. It is unclear to me whether they are a wiser group, or whether they have been saved from making fools of themselves, because the media has so lionized those who promote the false memory point of view, that they have had relatively few opportunities to do so.

References

1. Pope KS: Memory, abuse, and science: questioning claims about the false memory epidemic. Am Psychol 1996; 51:957–974.
1a. Kluft RP: The natural history of multiple personality disorder. *In* RP Kluft (Ed.), Childhood Antecedents of Multiple Personality. Washington, DC: American Psychiatric Press, 1985, pp. 197–238.

2. Kluft RP: Treatment of multiple personality disorders. Psychiatr Clin North Am 1984; 7:121–134a.
3. Kluft RP: Dissociation and subsequent vulnerability: a preliminary study. Dissociation 1990; 3:167–173.
4. Kluft RP: Incest and subsequent revictimization: the case of therapist-patient sexual exploitation, with a description of the sitting duck syndrome. *In* RP Kluft (Ed.), Incest-related Syndromes of Adult Psychopathology. Washington, DC: American Psychiatric Press, 1990, pp. 263–287.
5. Kluft RP: The confirmation and disconfirmation of memories of abuse in dissociative identify disorder patients: a naturalistic clinic study. Dissociation 1995; 8:253–258.
6. Kluft RP: In harm's way. *In* S Kahn, E Fromm (Eds.), Changes in the Therapist: A Casebook. (in preparation).
7. American Psychiatric Association: Diagnostic and Statistical Manual of Mental Disorders (4th ed). Washington, DC: American Psychiatric Association, 1994.
8. Kluft RP: Treatment trajectories in multiple personality disorder. Dissociation 1994; 7:63–76.
9. Kluft RP: Clinical observations on the use of the CSDS Dimensions of Therapeutic Movement Instrument (DTMI). Dissociation 1994; 7:272–283.
10. Brown D: Pseudomemories, the standard of science, and the standard of care in trauma treatment. Am J Clin Hypn 1995; 37:1–24.
11. Brown D: Sources of suggestion and their applicability to psychotherapy. *In* JL Alpert (Ed.), Sexual Abuse Recalled: Treating Trauma in the Era of the Recovered Memory Debate. Northvale, NJ: Aronson, 1995, pp. 61–100.
12. Fraser GA: The Phenomenon of Ritualistic Abuse. Washington, DC: American Psychiatric Press, 1997.
13. Ross CA: Satanic Ritual Abuse: Principles of Treatment. Toronto: University of Toronto Press, 1995.
14. Williams LM: Adult memories of childhood abuse: preliminary findings from a longitudinal study. The Advisor 1992; 5:19–20.
15. Williams LM: Recall of childhood trauma: a prospective study of women's memories of child sexual abuse. J Consult Clin Psychol 1994; 62:1167–1176.
16. Shapiro F: Movement Desensitization and Reprocessing: Basic Principles, Protocols, and Procedures. New York: Guilford, 1995.
17. Nash MR: Memory distortion and sexual trauma: the problem of false negatives and false positives. Int J Clin Exp Hypn 1994; 42:346–362.
18. Schooler JW: Seeking the core: the issues and evidence surrounding recovered accounts of sexual trauma. Consciousness Cogn 1994; 3:452–469.
19. Spiegel D, Scheflin AW: Dissociated or fabricatred: psychiatric aspects of repressed memory in criminal and civil cases. Int J Clin Exp Hypn 1994; 42:411–432.
20. van der Kolk BA, Fisler R: Dissociation and the fragmentary nature of traumatic memories: overview and exploratory study. J Traumatic Stress 1995; 8:505–525.
21. Blank AS: The unconscious flashback to the war in Viet Nam veterans: clinical mystery, legal defense, and community problem. *In* SM Sonnenberg, AS Blank, JA Talbott (Eds.), The Trauma of War. Washington, DC: American Psychiatric Press, 1985, pp. 293–308.
22. Pope HG, Hudson JI: Can individuals "repress" memories of childhood abuse? An examination of the evidence. Psychiatr Ann 1995; 25:715–719.
23. Nathanson DL: Shame and Pride. New York: Norton, 1992.
24. Freud S: Charcot. *In* J Strachey (Ed. and Trans.), The Standard Edition of the Complete

Psychological Works of Sigmund Freud, Vol. 3. London: Hogarth Press, 1962 (Original work published in 1912).

25. Bliss EL: Spontaneous self-hypnosis in multiple personality disorder. Psychiatr Clin North Am 1984; 7:135–148.
26. Coons PM, Milstein V: Psychosexual disturbances in multiple personality: characteristics, etiology, and treatment. J Clin Psychiatry 1986; 47:106–110.
27. Hornstein NL, Putnam FW: Clinical phenomenology of child and adolescent multiple personality disorder. J Am Acad Child Adolesc Psychiatry 1992; 31:1055–1077.
28. Coons PM: Confirmation of childhood abuse in childhood and adolescent cases of multiple personality disorder and dissociative disorder not otherwise specified. J Nerv Ment Dis 1994; 182:461–464.
29. Hammond DC, Garver RB, Mutter CB, Crasilneck HB, Frischholz E, Gravitz MA, Hibler NS, Olson J, Scheflin A, Speigel H, Wester W: Clinical Hypnosis and Memory: Guidelines for Clinicians and for Forensic Hypnosis. Chicago: American Society of Clinical Hypnosis Press, 1995.
30. Lynn SJ, Rhue JW (Eds.): Theories of Hypnosis: Current Models and Perspectives. New York: Guilford, 1991.
31. Brown D, Fromm E: Hypnotherapy and Hypnoanalysis. Hillsdale, NJ: Laurence Erlbaum, 1986.
32. Frischholz E, Spiegel D: Hypnosis is not therapy. Bull Br Soc Clin Exp Hyp 1983; 6:3–8.
33. Frankel FH: Hypnosis: Trance as a Coping Mechanism. New York: Plenum Medical Books, 1976.
34. McConkey KM: The effects of hypnotic procedures on remembering: the experimental findings and their implications for forensic hypnosis. In E Fromm, MR Nash (Eds.), Contemporary Hypnosis Research. New York: Guilford, 1992, pp. 405–426.
35. Laurence JR, Perry CW: Hypnotically created memory among highly hypnotizable subjects. Science 1983; 222:523–524.
36. Laurence JR, Perry CW: Hypnosis, Will, and Memory: A Psycho-legal History. New York: Guilford, 1988.
37. McConkey KM, Sheehan PW: Hypnosis, Memory, and Behavior in Criminal Investigation. New York: Guilford, 1995.
38. Orne MT: The use and misuse of hypnosis in court. Int J Clin Exp Hypn 1979; 27:311–341.
39. Scheflin AW, Shapiro JL: Trance on Trial. New York: Guilford, 1989.
40. Loftus E, Ketcham K: The Myth of Repressed Memory: False Memories and Allegations of Sexual Abuse. New York: St. Martins, 1994.
41. Ofshe RJ, Watters E: Making Monsters: False Memory, Psychotherapy, and Sexual Hysteria. New York: Scribners, 1994.
42. Frischholz EF, Lipman LS, Braun BG, Sachs RG: Psychopathology, hypnotizability, and dissociation. Am J Psychiatry 1992; 149:1521–1525.
43. Spiegel D, Hunt T, Dondershine HF: Dissociation and hypnotizability in posttraumatic stress disorder. Am J Psychiatry 1988; 145:301–305.
44. Stutman RK, Bliss EL: Posttraumatic stress disorder, hypnotizability, and imagery. Am J Psychiatry 1985; 142:741–743.
45. Kluft RP: Varieties of hypnotic interventions in the treatment of multiple personality. Am J Clin Hypn 1982; 24:230–240.
46. Kluft RP: Hypnosis with multiple personality disorder. Am J Prev Psychiatry Neurol 1992; 3:19–27.
47. Maldonado J, Spiegel D: The treatment of posttraumatic stress disorder. In SJ Lynn,

JW Rhue (Eds.), Dissociation: Clinical and Theoretical Perspectives. New York: Guilford, 1994, pp. 215–241.

48. Spiegel D: Dissociation and trauma. *In* A Tasman, SM Goldfinger (Eds.), American Psychiatric Press Review of Psychiatry, Vol. 10. Washington, DC: American Psychiatric Press, 1991, pp. 261–275.

49. Erdelyi MH: Repression, reconstruction, and defense: history and integration of the psychoanalytic and experimental frameworks. *In* JL Singer (Ed.), Repression and Dissociation. Chicago: University of Chicago Press, 1990, pp. 1–31.

50. Freud S: The ego and the id. *In* J Strachery (Ed. and Trans.), The Standard Edition of the Complete Psychological Works of Sigmund Freud, Vol. 19. London: Hogarth Press, 1961, pp. 3–66. (Original work published in 1923)

51. Hilgard JR: Divided Consciousness: Multiple Controls in Human Thought and Action. New York: Wiley, 1977.

52. Spiegel D: Dissociating damage. Am J Clin Hypn 1986; 29:123–131.

52a. Spiegel D: Hypnosis, dissociation, and trauma: hidden and over observers. *In* JL Singer (Ed.), Repression and Dissociation. Chicago: University of Chicago Press, 1990, pp. 121–142.

53. Rumelhart DE, McClelland JL (Eds.): Parallel Distributed Processing: Explorations in the Microstructure of Cognition. Vol. I, Foundations. Cambridge, MA: MIT Press, 1986.

54. Kluft RP: The psychodynamic psychotherapy of multiple personality disorder. *In* JP Barber, P Crits-Cristoph (Eds.), Dynamic Therapies for Psychiatric Disorders (Axis I). New York: Basic Books, 1995, pp. 332–385.

55. Freud S: A note on the unconscious in psycho-analysis. *In* J Strachey (Ed. and Trans.), The Standard Edition of the Complete Psychological Works of Sigmund Freud, Vol. 12. London: Hogarth Press, 1958, pp. 255–266. (Original work published in 1912)

56. Putnam FW: Dissociation as a response to extreme trauma. *In* RP Kluft (Ed.), Childhood Antecedents of Multiple Personality. Washington, DC: American Psychiatric Press, 1985, pp. 65–97.

57. Cardena E, Spiegel D: Dissociative reactions to the San Francisco Bay Area earthquake of 1989. Am J Psychiatry 1993; 150:474–478.

58. Classen C, Koopman C, Spiegel D: Trauma and dissociation. Bull Menninger Clin 1993; 2:179–194.

59. Koopman C, Classen C, Spiegel D: Predictors of posttraumatic stress symptoms among survivors of the Oakland/Berkeley firestorm. Am J Psychiatry 1994; 151:888–894.

60. Belli RF, Loftus EF: Recovered memories of childhood abuse: a source monitoring perspective. *In* SH Lynn, JW Rhue (Eds.), Dissociation: Clinical and Theoretical Perspectives. New York: Guilford, 1994, pp. 415–433.

61. Erdelyi MH: Dissociation, defense, and the unconscious. *In* D Spiegel (Ed.), Dissociation: Culture, Mind and Body. Washington, DC: American Psychiatric Press, 1994, pp. 3–20.

62. Erdelyi MH: The recovery of unconscious (inaccessible) memories: laboratory studies of hypermnesia. *In* G Bower (Ed.), The Psychology of Learning and Motivation: Advances in Research and Theory, Vol. 18. New York: Academic Press, 1984, pp. 95–127.

63. Payne DG: Hypermnesia and reminiscence in recall: a historical and empirical review. Psychol Bull 1987; 101:5–27.

64. Roediger HL, Thorpe LA: The role of recall time in producing hypermnesia. Mem Cogn 1978; 6:296–305.

65. Ballard PB: Oblivescence and reminiscence. Br J Psychol (Monogr Suppl) 1913; 1:1–82.

66. Cardena E: The domain of dissociation. *In* SJ Lynn, JW Rhue (Eds.), Dissociation: Clinical and Theoretical Perspectives. New York: Guilford, 1994, pp. 15–31.

67. Della Femina D, Yeager CA, Lewis DO: Child abuse: adolescent records vs. adult recall. Child Abuse Negl 1990; 14:227–231.
68. Herman JL, Schatzow E: Recovery and verification of memories of childhood sexual trauma. Psychoanal Psychol 1987; 4:1–14.
69. Briere J, Conte J: Self-reported amnesia for abuse in adults molested as children. J Traumatic Stress 1993; 6:221–231.
70. Loftus EF, Polonsky S, Fullilove MR: Memories of childhood sexual abuse: remembering and repressing. Psychol Women Q 1994; 18:67–84.
71. Loftus E: The reality of repressed memories. Am Psychol 1993; 48:518–537.
72. Cameron C: Women survivors confront their abusers: issues, decisions, and outcomes. J Child Sex Abuse 1994; 3(1):7–35.
73. Roesler TA, Wind TW: Telling the secret: adult women describe their disclosures of incest. J Interpers Violence 1994; 9:327–338.
74. Feldman-Summers S, Pope KS: The experience of ''forgetting'' childhood sexual abuse: a national survey of psychologists. J Consult Clin Psychol 1994; 62:636–639.
75. Burgess A, et al: Memory presentations of childhood sexual abuse. Paper presented at the 11th International Conference on Dissociation, Chicago, November, 1994.
76. Albach F, Moorman PP, Bermond B: Memory recovery of childhood sexual abuse. Dissociation (in press).
77. Frankel FH: Discovering new memories in psychotherapy—childhood revisited, fantasy, or both? N Eng J Med 1995; 333:591–594.
78. Holmes DS: The evidence for repression. In JL Singer (Ed.), Repression and Dissociation. Chicago: University of Chicago Press, 1990, pp. 85–102.
79. Singer JL (Ed.): Repression and Dissociation. Chicago: University of Chicago Press, 1990.
80. Ditto PH, Lopez DF: Motivated skepticism: use of differential decision criteria for preferred and non-preferred conclusions. J Pers Soc Psychol 1992; 63:568–584.
81. Holmes DL: Repression: theory versus evidence. Paper presented at the University of Kansas Medical Center's Conference on Childhood Sexual Abuse and Memories: Current Controversies, Kansas City, Kansas, April 1995.
82. Loftus E: The nature of memory: what we know. Paper presented at the University of Kansas Medical Center's Conference on Childhood Sexual Abuse and Memories: Current Controversies, Kansas City, Kansas, April 1995.
83. Loftus E: Eyewitness memory: implications for the dissociative disorders field. Paper presented at the meeting of the International Society for the Study of Dissociation, International Fall Conference, Orlando, FL, September 1995.
84. Pedzek K, Roe C: Memory for childhood events: how suggestible is it? Consciousness Cogn 1994; 3:374–387.
85. Kuhn TS: The Structure of Scientific Revolutions (2nd ed., enlarged). Chicago: University of Chicago Press, 1971.
86. Terr L: Childhood traumas: an outline and overview. Am J Psychiatry 1991; 148:10–20.
87. Kluft RP: Current controversies surrounding multiple personality disorder. In L Cohen, J Berzoff, M Elin (Eds.), Dissociative Identity Disorder. Northvale, NJ: Aronson, 1995, pp. 347–377.
88. Sargent W, Slater E: Amnestic syndromes in war. Proc R Soc Med 1941; 34:757–764.
89. Whitfield CL: Memory and Abuse: Remembering and Healing the Effects of Trauma. Deerfield Beach FL: Heath Communications, Inc., 1995.

II

CURRENT CONCEPTS OF MEMORY

3

Neuroanatomical Correlates of the Effects of Stress on Memory: Relevance to the Validity of Memories of Childhood Abuse

J. DOUGLAS BREMNER
STEVEN M. SOUTHWICK
DENNIS S. CHARNEY

The recent controversy surrounding the validity of memories of childhood abuse has centered on the question of whether memories of abuse can remain dormant for many years before they come to the surface in the form of delayed recall. Authors on one side of the controversy suggest that memories of abuse can be not available to conscious recall secondary to a mechanism described clinically as amnesia or "repression."[1,2] The other side of the controversy claims that psychotherapists practicing a form of psychotherapy known as *recovered memory therapy* have suggested episodes of abuse to their patients which never in fact occurred, through leading questions or excessive insisting.[3]

The fact that many individuals forget episodes of childhood abuse is well established. As many as 38% of individuals who experienced abuse severe enough to result in a visit to the hospital emergency room had no memory of the event 20 or more years later.[1,4] An important question is whether there are special mechanisms involved in the loss of memory for episodes of extreme childhood abuse in traumatized patients that are not normally operative.[5,6]

Findings from studies of the neurobiology of memory may provide insight into questions about delayed recall of childhood abuse. Traumatic stress has been shown in animal studies to result in long-term changes in brain regions involved in memory.[7,8]

Neuromodulators released during stress have both strengthening and diminishing effects on memory traces, depending on the dose and the particular type of neuromodulator. Dissociative amnesia, defined as gaps in memory that are not due to ordinary forgetting, is associated clinically with traumatic stress, amd empirical studies have shown an increase in this symptom in patients with posttraumatic stress disorder (PTSD).[9] Changes in brain regions involved in memory may underlie many of the symptoms of stress-related psychiatric disorders, including symptoms of amnesia. This chapter will review the controversy surrounding the validity of childhood memories of abuse from the standpoint of the neurobiology of memory. We feel that this approach may shed some light on the controversy surrounding the so-called false memory syndrome.

Are Normal Memories Subject to Modification?

There has been considerable interest in the potential vulnerability of memory traces to modification. In a typical example of a study addressing this question, subjects were shown a series of slides that told a story involving a stop sign. These slides were followed by the reading of a similar verbal narrative in which the reference to the stop sign was replaced by a reference to a yield sign. When subjects were tested on recall of material related to the slides, they were more likely to (incorrectly) report having seen a yield sign than subjects who did not receive the misleading information. The authors of this study concluded that misleading information led to an ''overwriting'' of the original memory trace.[10] Memory can also involve a shift in recall towards facts that fits one's expectations. For example, in a story in which the Six Million Dollar Man is said to be too weak to carry a can of paint, children tested 3 weeks later had a shift in their memory toward a recall that was more congruous with their pre-testing knowledge.[11]

Other authors have argued against the overwriting hypothesis. They point out that if subjects do not remember the original information, they may make a guess based on their recall of the misleading information. This would mean that their chances of getting the correct answer are less than that due to chance alone. In a study by McCloskey and Zaragoza,[12] subjects were assessed with a test in which they saw slides, which included one of a hammer, were then given misleading verbal information involving a screwdriver, and then a forced-choice test of what they had seen in the slides, the choice being between a hammer and an item to which they had previously not been exposed (a wrench). The authors argue that if there is a true overwriting phenomenon with misleading verbal material, then subjects exposed to misleading information should have a decrement in recall in comparison with subjects who have not been previously exposed to such information. They in fact found that there was no decrement in recall in this paradigm in subjects for whom the misleading item was not one of the possible choices in the forced-choice test of recall.[12] The effects of ''source amnesia,'' or the forgetting of the location where the original memory was encoded, was examined in another study by testing subjects for the source of their memories as well as for the recalled item. There was no difference in recall in this paradigm between subjects who had been exposed to misleading information versus controls[13] (although see Lindsay[14]). Suggestibility effects may be due to the forgetting of the source of the memory, rather than an overwriting phenomenon. Based on a review of these studies, there is not sufficient evidence to conclude that suggestive information does or does not result in the rewriting of memory.[14–16]

Effects of Stress on Memory in Normal Persons

Studies of normal memory may not be entirely applicable to those of memory for stressful events. John F. Kennedy's assassination raised the observation that most people had an enhanced awareness of where they were and what they were doing at the time they received news of his death. This led to a hypothesis formulated by Brown and Kulik[17] that certain events that are surprising and consequential (emotionally charged), which they described as "flashbulb memories," lead to an enhancement of memory for personal circumstances surrounding the event. These include such facts as what the person was wearing and what they were doing at the time they received the news. Studies of the explosion on January 28, 1986, of the space shuttle *Challenger* have shown a relationship between emotional upsetness and recall of personal circumstances upon hearing the news[18,19] (but see Neisser and Harsch[20]). Experimental paradigms have also been used to examine differences in memory of details during stressful compared to nonstressful situations. Studies of subjects who experienced traumatic slides involving injury or threat have found a more enhanced recall of central details of the slide and a reduced recall of peripheral details, in comparison with the recall of details of neutral slides.[21–23]

Studies of the effects of stress on memory in children have focused on the visit to the doctor, since it entails the touching of private areas, or procedures such as blood-drawing or injections, all of which are routine events in a doctor's office, but which are also similar to the types of events occurring in childhood abuse. These studies have shown that small children are remarkably resistant to suggestion.[24–30] Children undergoing physical exam have been shown to be very reliable in the reporting of genital contact, in both open-ended and direct questioning; they answered questions about the genital exam with better recall than for the nongenital physical exam.[25,27] Most of the children did not report genital contact unless they were directly asked.[27] These studes have implications for clinical treatment of childhood abuse, in that it can be expected that the lack of direct questioning during the history-taking about abuse experiences will probably result in many unreported cases of abuse. Stressful events such as innoculation have been associated with an enhancement of memory and a resistance to misleading suggestions. The stress of innoculation was also associated with a relative enhancement of memory for central details related to the procedure.[24] In summary, the findings are consistent with an enhancing effect of stress on memory, especially on recall of central details.

Brain Mechanisms Involved in Normal Memory Function

These studies have examined both the potential fallibility of memory and the effects of stress on memory in normal persons. Findings from these studies may not be applicable to situations in which there is severe childhood abuse. For many patients, childhood abuse may be associated with long-term alterations in brain systems involved in memory. We will now briefly review the mechanisms involved in normal memory function. This will serve as a background to a discussion about the effects of stress on memory.

Memory formation involves encoding, or the initial laying down of the memory trace, storage, or consolidation, and retrieval. Consolidation occurs over several weeks or more, during which time the memory trace is susceptible to modification.[31,32] Memory function can be divided into declarative, or *explicit* memory, and nondeclarative, or *implicit* or *procedural* memory.[33] Explicit memory includes free recall of facts and lists, and working memory, which is the ability to store information in a visual or verbal buffer while performing a particular operation utilizing that information. In contrast, implicit memory is demonstrated only through tasks or skills in which the knowledge is embedded. Forms of implicit memory include priming, conditioning, and tasks or skills.

Memory is mediated by several connected subcortical and cortical brain regions. The amygdala, hippocampus, and adjacent cortical areas, including perirhinal, entorhinal, and parahippocampal cortex; medial thalamus, fornix, and mammillary bodies have been shown to play an important role in memory. Other regions involved in memory are the prefrontal cortex, including what is known as the *dorsolateral prefrontal cortex* (middle frontal gyrus, principal sulcus region, or Area 46); orbital gyrus, and anteromedial prefrontal cortex (including the anterior cingulate cortex), as well as the parietal association cortex. In addition, memories are stored in the primary cortical sensory and motor areas that correspond to the particular sensory modality related to the memory. These brain regions interact with one another in the mediation of memory function.

The hippocampus plays an important role in explicit memory. Hippocampal lesions impair acquisition of spatial information as measured by a number of tasks, for instance, the ability of rats to learn to swim to a submerged water platform.[34,35] Lesion studies have been performed in monkeys in order to reproduce the anterograde explicit memory impairment seen in individuals with surgical resection of the medial temporal lobes.[33] Lesions occurring within the hippocampal formation (dentate gyrus, hippocampus proper, subicular complex, and entorhinal cortex), amygdala, and surrounding perirhinal and parahippocampal cortices have been termed the $H + A +$ *lesion,* where H refers to the hippocampus, A to the amygdala, and $+$ to the surrounding areas. Monkeys with $H + A +$ lesions have been shown to be severely impaired in delayed matching to sample memory tasks (a test of the working-memory type of explicit memory function), during which the animal has to remember where an object is located after a time delay, but is normal in acquiring and retaining motor skills.[36] Monkeys with the $H +$ lesion were also found to have impaired explicit memory, although not to the degree of the $H + A +$ monkeys. Furthermore, damage to the amygdala alone was not associated with declarative memory impairment,[37] whereas damage to the cortical areas adjacent to the amygdala, including the perirhinal cortex and parahippocampal gyrus (which has important efferent and afferent connections with the hippocampus), was associated with pronounced explicit memory impairment.[38,39] These studies suggest that the explicit memory impairment associated with the $H + A +$ lesion is due to damage to the hippocampal region (dentate, hippocampus proper, subicular complex, and entorhinal cortex) and to the adjacent perirhinal cortex and parahippocampal gyrus. In addition to mediating the working-memory type of explicit memory function involved in the delayed matching to sample task, the hippocampus, but not the amygdala, plays an important role in the memory of where an object is located in space.[40]

Findings in human subjects are consistent with those in monkeys, which demonstrate a role for the hippocampus and adjacent cortex in explicit recall. Case studies, such as the famous case of H.M., have shown a relationship between severe deficits in explicit memory measured with free verbal recall and bilateral resection of the medial temporal lobes (i.e., hippocampus and adjacent structures).[41] Patients with Korsakoff's amnesia, in which damage occurs specifically to the hippocampus and dorsal-medial nucleus of the thalamus because of a thiamine deficiency, exhibit a specific and severe deficit in explicit memory measured by free verbal recall. In addition, in patients with hypoxic encephalopathy following cardiac arrest, which is associated with glutamate toxicity to the brain, the most common cognitive impairment is a deficit in explicit memory function measured by free verbal recall. Following the interruption of oxygen to the brain that occurs with a cardiac arrest, the brain region that is most susceptible to damage is the CA1 region of the hippocampus. Positron emission tomography (PET) studies of cerebral blood flow with $[^{15}O]H_2O$ also indicate a role for the hippocampus in explicit memory with the finding of an increase in right hippocampal blood flow during a stem-completion explicit memory task.[42] In summary, several lines of evidence from preclinical and clinical studies have demonstrated a role for the hippocampus and adjacent structures in explicit recall.

The thalamus is a gateway for sensory information relayed to multiple brain areas, including the amygdala and primary sensory neocortical areas.[43,44] A portion of the thalamus, the dorsal-medial nucleus, also plays a role in explicit memory tasks of free verbal recall. In one case, the patient N.A. received a fencing injury to the mediodorsal thalamic nucleus. He showed normal intelligence and general cognitive abilities, could remember events from before the accident, and was able to converse normally. However, he was unable to learn the names of new people or learn new information. These findings show that the medial thalamus is involved in explicit memory.

The amygdala is an important mediator of emotional memory. Monkeys with amygdala lesions have been shown to be less fearful than normal (i.e., they have alterations in emotional memory) but are without impairment in explicit (cognitive) memory, whereas monkeys with lesions of the hippocampus or adjacent cortex had normal fear responses (i.e., abnormal emotional memory) but severe impairments in explicit (cognitive) memory.[45] The paradigm of conditioned fear has been used as an animal model for stress-induced abnormalities of emotional memory.[46,47] Noise bursts elicit the acoustic startle response, which is used in the measurement of the conditioned fear response. In the fear-potentiated startle paradigm, a normally neutral stimulus (or something which typically has no effect on the animal, such as a bright light), is paired with an aversive stimulus, such as electric shock. With repetitive pairing of the light and the shock, a learning process occurs (conditioning) in which the light alone eventually causes an increase in the startle response (referred to as *fear-potentiated startle*). The shock in this example is termed the *unconditioned stimulus,* because no training was required for it to have the effect of potentiating startle; the light is referred to as the *conditioned stimulus,* because the training trials pairing it with the shock were required for it to develop the capacity for potentiating the startle response.[46,47]

The neuroanatomy and neurophysiology of conditioned fear responses in animals have been well characterized (see Davis[46,47]). Lesions of the central nucleus of the amygdala have been shown to completely block fear-potentiated startle,[48,49] whereas electrical stimulation of the central nucleus increases acoustic startle.[50] The central nucleus of the amygdala projects to a variety of brain structures via the stria terminalis and the ventral amygdalofugal pathway. One pathway is from the central nucleus to the brainstem startle reflex circuit (nucleus reticularis pontis caudalis).[51] Lesions of this pathway at any point (caudal lateral hypothalamus-subthalamic area, substantia nigra, central tegmental field) block the development of fear-potentiated startle, whereas lesions of fibers which project outward from the central nucleus of the amygdala to sites other than the brainstem startle circuit have no effect.[52] The excitatory neurotransmitters play an important role in fear conditioning mediated by the amygdala, as demonstrated by the fact that antagonists of the N-methyl-D-aspartate (NMDA) receptor infused into the amygdala block the acquisition (but not the expression) of the fear-potentiated startle response.[53,54]

Considerable evidence suggests that the dorsolateral prefrontal cortex (principal sulcus, or middle frontal gyrus) is involved in the working memory type of explicit memory function.[55] In nonhuman primates, working memory is assessed by delayed-response tasks, in which monkeys perform tasks based on previously received information after a short time delay. These tasks typically involve learning a "set of rules," which is considered an important component of the memory function mediated by the dorsolateral prefrontal cortex. Lesions of the dorsolateral prefrontal cortex result in deficits in working memory tasks, but explicit memory for features of the stimuli remain unaffected.[55] PET [^{15}O]H$_2$O studies of cerebral blood flow in normal human subjects also demonstrate a role for the dorsolateral prefrontal cortex in both the encoding and retrieval of explicit memory traces[42,56,57,58] and attention.[59]

The anteromedial (or ventromedial) prefrontal cortex includes the anterior cingulate gyrus and is functionally and anatomically distinct from the dorsolateral prefrontal cortex. In the late nineteenth century the famous patient named Phineas Gage had a projectile metal spike pass through his frontal cortex, with damage specifically to the anterior cingulate, anteromedial prefrontal cortex, and parts of the orbitofrontal cortex. After the accident, the patient had normal memory recall and cognitive function, but his behavior deteriorated to irresponsibility, profanity, and a lack of social conventions, which indicated a deficit in the planning and execution of socially suitable behavior. This case suggests that the anteromedial frontal cortex (including the anterior cingulate) is responsible for socially appropriate behavior and the processing of emotionally related stimuli.[60] PET [^{15}O]H$_2$O studies show an activation of the anterior cingulate occurring along with visual and verbal association tasks[56] and the Stroop paradigm.[59]

The orbitofrontal cortex is another frontal cortical area important to the effects of stress on memory. The orbitofrontal cortex is the primary sensory cortical area for smell. It also plays a role in the fear response, extinction, and certain types of memory. Lesions of the orbitofrontal cortex result in deficits in explicit memory of visual features of objects, but not in explicit memory for delayed-response tasks (i.e., working memory), which functionally differentiates it from the dorsolateral prefrontal cortex.[55] Studies of rats, however, in which olfaction is the primary stimulus, have shown deficits in delayed-response tasks in association with lesions of the orbitofrontal cortex.[61] Lesions of the medial orbitofrontal cortex in rats result in a significant delay in extinction to conditioned stimuli in the tone–footshock pairing paradigm, which suggests that this region plays a role in extinction of conditioned stimuli.[62]

Parietal cortex has been demonstrated to play an important role in spatial memory and attention. Single-cell recordings from alert monkeys have shown an activation of the parietal cortex when monkeys are required to attend to a visual location.[63] In PET [^{15}O]H$_2$O studies of sustained vigilance and attention in healthy volunteers, subjects were asked to perform tasks of sustained visual attention (maintaining passive visual fixation on a mark on a screen while detecting pauses) and somatosensory attention (maintaining attention on their great toe while detecting pauses in a series of touches). Regardless of modality of sensory input, sustained attention was associated with increases in blood flow in the right prefrontal and superior parietal cortex.[64] Tasks of working memory have also shown activation of the right parietal cortex.[58]

In addition to the hippocampus and other subcortical structures, explicit memory storage also takes place in sensory brain areas in which an event is first experienced.[65]

Visual information is stored in the occipital cortex, tactile information in the sensory cortex, auditory information in the middle temporal gyrus, and olfactory information in the orbitofrontal cortex. PET [^{15}O]H$_2$O studies of word presentation have shown an activation of the striate (primary visual) and extrastriate cortex (visual association cortex) in association with visual word presentation, and activation of the middle temporal gyrus (primary auditory cortex), temporal-parietal cortex, and inferior cingulate cortex along with explicit memory tasks involving verbal word presentation.[56]

Explicit memory formation is not instantaneous. After the laying down of the original memory trace, a process that can take from weeks to months occurs, called *consolidation,* during which the stored memory is subject to modification or deletion. Studies of rats suggest that explicit memory formation can be affected for weeks after the laying down of the original memory trace. Electroconvulsive treatments (ECT) after training sessions impair memory for the training experience. As the interval between the ECT and the training session increases, the severity of memory impairment decreases.[66] Studies of humans who have received ECT suggest that the process of memory consolidation has a much longer time course. ECT results in an impairment of recall of television programs occurring 1 to 2 years before the administration of ECT, while memory of older programs is normal.[67] These findings suggest that modification of the original memory traces can occur for a considerable period of time after the original event.

Although the hippocampus and adjacent structures are important in encoding and retrieval, they do not play a major role in the long-term storage of explicit memory. Monkeys with intact hippocampus exhibited a pattern of remembering recently learned objects more than they did objects learned in the past. Monkeys with lesions of the hippocampus were impaired in the recall of recently learned objects, although their recall of objects learned in the distant past was normal.[68] The evidence is consistent with the fact that memories are stored in the primary neocortical sensory and motor areas and later evoked in those same cortical areas.[69] It has been hypothesized[68] that the role of the hippocampus is to bring together memory elements from diverse neocortical areas at the time of retrieval of explicit memory.

The neocortex may also play a role in some types of implicit memory function. Patients with anterograde amnesia (i.e., deficits in explicit memory, or the recall of things such as names and facts) do not necessarily lose all aspects of short-term memory function. These patients show evidence of intact implicit memory function. Procedural (or ''implicit'') memory is accessible only through performance, by engaging skills or operations in which the knowledge is embedded, as demonstrated by priming. An example of priming is providing the first few letters of the forgotten word and asking the subject to say the first word that comes to mind. Priming can improve memory performance in amnesic patients. Priming effects require only the intactness of the cortical sensory area in which the memory was originally stored.[65]

Effects of Stress on Brain Regions Involved in Memory

Efficient recall of memories associated with previous stressors is crucial for survival. For instance, if one encounters a dangerous animal, the rapid recall of the memory of a previous encounter with a dangerous animal of the same type may be life saving. Brain regions involved in the recall of memory simultaneously activate the body's stress response system, leading to increased release of stress-related neurotransmitters and neuropeptides. These in turn modulate the encoding of memory, which results in a type of feedback loop of the body's stress response system on memory storage.

Brain regions involved in memory also play a prominent role in the execution of the stress response. In the early part of this century the observation was made that, with the removal of the cerebral cortex, a hyperexcitability of anger developed, which was termed *sham rage*.[69,70] Animals in the sham-rage state were quick to attack, and behaved as if they were experiencing a profoundly threatening situation. Papez[71] proposed that the hypothalamus, thalamus, hippocampus, and cingulate are responsible for the behaviors of the decorticate cat. Kluver and Bucy[72,73] noted that removal of the temporal lobe (including hippocampus and amygdala) resulted in "psychic blindness," or the absence of anger and fear. These observations led to the development of the concept of the limbic brain, in which the brain regions listed above (and others, including the orbitofrontal cortex) mediate the stress response.[74] The circuits constructed by these authors are no longer valid, based on the current evidence, although the individual brain regions described above as being part of the limbic system play an important role in the effects of stress on memory function. There is considerable literature claiming that stress also results in alterations in memory function. Therefore, the brain regions that are responsible for memory function and the stress response are in turn affected by exposure to traumatic stress. We review below the effects of stress on brain regions involved in memory.

Stress has effects on the hippocampus, which leads to both changes in its cytoarchitecture as well as to deficits in explicit recall.[75] Twenty-one days of restraint stress has been shown to be associated with deficits in spatial memory as measured by the radial arm maze.[76] A release of glucocorticoids follows exposure to stress, and the hippocampus is a major target organ for glucocorticoids in the brain. In addition, the hippocampus appears to play an important role in the pituitary–adrenocortical response to stress.[77] Studies of monkeys who died spontaneously following exposure to severe stress from improper caging and overcrowding were found on autopsy to have multiple gastric ulcers, which is consistent with exposure to chronic stress, and hyperplastic adrenal cortices, which is consistent with sustained glucocorticoid release.[78] They also suffered damage to the CA2 and CA3 subfields of the hippocampus. Follow-up studies suggested that hippocampal damage was associated with direct exposure of glucocorticoids to the hippocampus.[79] Studies in a variety of animal species[80,81] have shown that direct glucocorticoid exposure results in a loss of pyramidal neurons[82,78] and dendritic branching[83,84] which are steroid- and tissue-specific.[85,86] Glucocorticoids appear to exert their effect by increasing the vulnerability of hippocampal neurons to endogenously released excitatory amino acids.[87–90] The same paradigm of stress exposure which increases glucocorticoids and causes loss of apical dendritic branching in the CA3 region of the hippocampus[84] is associated with deficits in spatial memory.[76] This suggests that the effects of glucocorticoids on the hippocampus have functional implications.

The hippocampus also plays an important role in emotional memory of the context of a fear-inducing situation. In conditioned fear response experiments where a tone (conditioned stimulus) is paired with an electric footshock (unconditioned stimulus), reexposure of the animal to the tone will result in conditioned fear responses (increase in "freezing" responses, which is characteristic of fear), even in the absence of the shock. In addition, reintroduction to the context of the shock, or the environment where the shock took place (the testing box), even in the absence of the shock or the tone, will result in conditioned fear responses. Lesions of the amygdala before fear conditioning block fear responses to both simple stimuli (tone) and to the context of the footshock. Lesions of the hippocampus, on the other hand, do not interfere with acquisition of conditioned emotional responses to the tone in the absence of the shock, although they do interfere with acquisition of conditioned emotional responses to the context.[91] Lesions of the hippocampus 1 day after fear conditioning (but not as much as 28 days after fear conditioning) also abolish context-related fear responses, but not the fear response related to the cue (tone), while lesions of the amygdala block fear responses to both the cue and the context.[92] These studies suggest that the hippocampus has a time-limited role in fear responses to complex phenomena with stimuli from multiple sensory modalities, but not to stimuli from simple sensory stimuli.

Stress also has effects on amygdala function. The amygdala integrates information necessary for the proper execution of the stress response, including (internal) emotion and information from the external environment.[93–95] Information from the environment that has emotional significance is transmitted through the dorsal thalamus to sensory cortical receiving areas, and from there to the amygdala.[96] Emotional responses to auditory stimuli are also mediated by direct projections from the medial geniculate in the thalamus to the amygdala, which suggests that the cerebral cortex is not necessary for emotional responses to stimuli.[97] Evidence suggests that the lateral nucleus of the amygdala is the site of convergence of stimuli from multiple sensory modalities, including somatosensory and auditory stimuli. This suggests that this region may be the site where information from unconditioned stimuli (footshock) and conditioned stimuli (tone) converge, and are translated into a final common pathway of the conditioned emotional response.[98] The amygdala then activates the peripheral sympathetic system, which plays a key role in the stress response, through the lateral nucleus of the hypothalamus and the central gray, leading to increased heart rate and blood pressure, as well as activating other aspects of the body's stress response system. Projections from the central nucleus of the amygdala to brainstem regions, including the parabrachial nucleus, dorsal motor vagal complex, and nucleus of the solitary tract, mediate the cardiovascular response to stress (increased heart rate and blood pressure).[99] Repeated exposure to stress can result in an exaggerated startle response, which indicates an increased sensitivity of amygdala function.

Very little is known about the effects of stress on dorsolateral prefrontal cortical function. Studies are currently underway using the Wisconsin Card Sort Test, which is felt to represent a measure of dorsolateral prefrontal cortical function, in PTSD patients and controls (R. Yehuda, personal communication, 1994). We have found a differential effect of yohimbine on dorsolateral prefrontal cortex metabolism in patients with PTSD in comparison with controls.

Studies have demonstrated that the anteromedial prefrontal cortex (including the anterior cingulate) plays an important role in the stress response. Lesions of the anteromedial prefrontal cortex (including the anterior cingulate) in the rat interfere with conditioned emotional responses to fear-eliciting stimuli. Specifically, these lesions result in a decrease in freezing behaviors and conditioned cardiovascular responses (increased heart rate) with fear-inducing stimuli. Lesions of the cingulate gyrus increase plasma levels of adrenocorticotropin (ACTH) and corticosterone in response to restraint stress. This suggests that this area is a target site for the negative feedback effects of glucocorticoids on stress-induced hypothalamic–pituitary–adrenal (HPA) activity. In other words, the cingulate has a braking effect on the HPA axis system response to stress.[100]

Little is known about the effects of stress on parietal cortex function. Since the parietal cortex is involved in attention, it is reasonable to predict that the increase in focused attention which occurs during stressful situations is associated with activation of the parietal cortex. As reviewed above, studies in normal human subjects have found differences in recall during stressful as compared with nonstressful situations, with an increase of focused attention on central details of stressful situations.

Stress-Induced Neuromodulation of Memory Traces

Neurotransmitters and neuropeptides released during stress have a modulatory effect on memory function. Several neurotransmitters and neuropeptides are released during stress which have an effect on learning and memory, including norepinephrine, epinephrine, adrenocorticotropic hormone (ACTH), glucocorticoids, corticotropin-releasing factor (CRF), opioid peptides, endogenous benzodiazepines, dopamine, vasopressin, and oxytocin.[101] Brain regions involved in memory, including the hippocampus and adjacent cortex, amygdala, and prefrontal cortex, are richly innervated by these neurotransmitters and neuropeptides.

Epinephrine has a modulatory effect on memory function. Studies of the effects of epinephrine (and other neuromodulators) have used the one-trial passive (inhibitory) avoidance test of memory. In this paradigm, the animal is placed in the starting chamber of an alley with two compartments and punished with footshock as it enters the second compartment. The amount of time that passes (or the latency) before the animal enters the second chamber when it is placed there on the second day is used as an index of retention of the training experience. Removal of the adrenal medulla, which is the site of most of the body's epinephrine, results in a blocking of passive avoidance behavior, which is restored by the administration of adequate amounts of epinephrine.[102] Post-training administration of epinephrine after a learning task influences retention, the rate of which resembles an inverted U-shaped curve: retention is enhanced at moderate doses and impaired at high doses.[103–105] Low-dose (0.2 μg) injections of norepinephrine into the amygdala facilitate memory function in an inhibitory avoidance task, while higher doses (0.5 μg) impair memory function.[106] Depletion of norepinephrine with DSP-4 has no effect on acquisition of place-learning, although it does have a significant effect on retention.[107] Stimulation of the locus coeruleus, site of most of the noradrenergic cell bodies in the brain, produces a significant improvement in performance of acquisition and extinction of a reinforced task, whereas lesions of the locus coeruleus suppress this effect.[108] Other studies have shown an impairment in acquisition of fear-conditioned learning[109] with noradrenergic depletion. The acetylcholine antagonist, scopolamine, impairs memory as measured by acquisition and retention of an inhibitory avoidance task, as well as by place-learning.[107] The combined blockade of the cholinergic and noradrenergic systems with scopolamine and propranolol, respectively, which only had effect when administered in combination, profoundly impaired inhibitory avoidance as well as spatial learning.[110] In summary, epinephrine and norepinephrine released during stress act to enhance the formation of memory traces.[37,111]

ACTH and glucocorticoids also affect learning and memory. Low doses of ACTH given immediately after a new learning task enhance retention, while a 10-fold higher dose has the opposite effect.[103] The effects of ACTH on learning and memory have also been tested through the measurement of its effect on the acquisition of conditioned fear responses. As reviewed above, animals are exposed to a conditioned stimulus (a tone) and an unconditioned stimulus (footshock). The animal must learn to exit from a box when the conditioned stimulus (the tone) comes on. ACTH enhances the acquisition of learning in this paradigm. ACTH also delays extinction of the avoidance response, i.e., it takes longer for the animal to realize after the association between the tone and the shock is ended that it does not have to exit the box when the tone comes on to avoid the shock.[112] The effects of ACTH on learning and memory are mediated through the hippocampus and amygdala.[113] Glucocorticoids, in contrast, enhance extinction in the conditioned fear paradigm.[112] The neuropeptide CRF, which stimulates release of ACTH from the pituitary and hence, glucocorticoids from the adrenal, has anxiogenic effects when administered into the cerebral ventricles.[114]

Other neurotransmitters and neuropeptides released during stress have effects on learning and memory. Both the dopamine and acetylcholine brain systems play a role in enhancing memory formation.[115] When administered after training in a learning task opiate receptor agonists impair retention, whereas opiate receptor antagonists, such as naloxone, enhance retention.[116] Opiate antagonists (naloxone) enhance retention of recently acquired information when injected into the amygdala.[117] Vasopressin injected 3 hours before or after a new learning paradigm increases resistance to extinction. The time course of vasopressin's effects suggests that it affects the consolidation phase of new learning. Vasopressin also facilitates passive avoidance behavior,[118] while oxytocin has the opposite effect. Gamma-aminobutyric acid (GABA) is the main inhibitory neurotransmitter in the brain and has receptor sites for benzodiazepines, which play a role in the stress response. GABA antagonists such as bicuculline, which block the action of GABA, impair memory retention following administration into the amygdala, as measured by the inhibitory avoidance task, whereas GABA agonists have the opposite effect.[119] The GABA antagonist picrotoxin enhances the extinction of conditioned fear.[105]

Recent studies have begun to address the question of neuromodulation of memory function with stress in human subjects. In one recent study, the β-adrenergic antagonist, propranolol, or placebo, was administered 1 hour before a neutral or an emotionally arousing (stress-related) story in healthy human subjects. Propranolol, but not placebo, interfered with the recall of the emotionally arousing story, but not the neutral story. This study suggests that activation of β-adrenergic receptors in the brain enhances the encoding of emotionally arousing memories.[120]

Findings related to neuromodulation of memory function are of importance for understanding the symptomatology of PTSD. The increased release of neurotransmitters and neuropeptides with modulatory actions on memory function during stress probably plays a role in deficits in encoding and retrieval, as well as in the enhancement of specific traumatic memories, which is part of the clinical presentation of PTSD. Chronic abnormalities in the function of these neurotransmitter and neuropeptide systems in PTSD may contribute to the abnormalities in memory seen in these patients. For instance, vasopressin has been shown to facilitate traumatic recall in patients with PTSD.[121] We have reviewed above how neuromodulators may be involved in the mechanisms of stress sensitization and the pathological retrieval of traumatic memories in patients with PTSD. We hope that an extension of preclinical findings on the effects of stress-related neuromodulators on memory function to clinical populations will enhance our understanding of memory alterations in PTSD.[6,8,122]

Stress-related Alterations in Brain Memory Systems in Patients with Stress-related Psychiatric Disorders

There is emerging evidence that stress has effects on explicit memory function in humans which involve deficits in both encoding and retrieval. Patients with a history of exposure to stressors such as childhood abuse exhibit alterations in memory, including nightmares, flashbacks, intrusive memories, and amnesia of the traumatic event(s). Studies of war veterans have documented incidents of alterations in memory function on the battlefield, such as the forgetting of one's name or identity and the forgetting of events that has just taken place during the previous battle.[123,124] In one study it was found that immediately after a major campaign, about 5% of the soldiers who had been combatants had no memory for the events that had just occurred.[125] Follow-up studies of WW II combat veterans have found that many veterans continue to suffer from "blackouts" or loss of memory many years after their period of service.[126] We have reported an increase in the dissociative symptom of amnesia (in addition to increased depersonalization, derealization, and identity disturbance) as measured with the SCID-D (Structured Clinical Interview for DSMIIIR–Dissociative Disorders) in Vietnam combat veterans with PTSD in comparison with Vietnam combat veterans without PTSD.[9] Episodes of amnesia in these patients took the form of gaps in memory which lasted from minutes to hours or days. Individual patients reported a range of experiences, from driving on the highway and suddenly noticing that three hours had passed, to walking down a street in Boston and then finding themselves in a motel room in Texas, with no idea of how they got there.

Physiological or emotional states may trigger recall of certain memories. For instance, one patient who was a Vietnam veteran with PTSD was involved in a house fire. He had to go back into the burning house in order to rescue other people who were trapped inside. He had had previous experiences pulling comrades from a burning helicopter while in Vietnam, an event for which he was previously amnestic. After the house fire incident he had a sustained flashback to the original event in Vietnam, and all he could say was "got to get them out, got to get them out!". This case illustrates how particular physiological or emotional states may facilitate recall of events for which there previously was amnesia, in a manner similar to state-dependent learning.[127] It also illustrates how traumatic recall often occurs in dissociated states that are reminiscent of the state in which the event originally was experienced, as we review below. In a similar fashion, victims of childhood sexual abuse may have no recall of their abuse until they are subsequently victimized as adults by rape. The emotional state which this involves is similar to the emotional state at the time of the original victimization; this emotional state may be associated with a triggering of recall of the original episode of childhood abuse. It may be that during states of arousal, release of neuromodulators such as norepinephrine leads to pathological recall of traumatic memories for which the patient may have been previously amnestic.

Evidence from other studies of traumatized patients is also consistent with that of abnormalities of explicit memory function involving encoding. Studies of concentration camp survivors from the Second World War have found high rates of impairment in explicit memory function.[128] In one group of 321 Danish survivors of WW II concentration camps who experienced high levels of psychiatric symptomatology and were seeking compensation for disability, 87% of the individuals complained of memory impairment suggestive of deficits in explicit recall 10 or more years after release from internment. Severe intellectual impairment was also found upon testing in 61% of the group.[129] Korean prisoners of war have been found to have an impairment of explicit memory tasks of free verbal recall as measured by the Logical Memory component of the Wechsler Memory Scale (WMS), whereas Korean veterans without a history of containment were not impaired.[130] We have measured explicit memory function with the WMS-Logical (for verbal memory) and WMS-Figural (for visual memory) components in Vietnam combat veterans with PTSD ($N = 26$) and controls matched for factors which could affect memory function ($N = 15$). PTSD patients had a significant decrease in free verbal recall (explicit memory) as measured by the WMS-Logical component, without deficits in IQ as measured by the Wechsler Adult Intelligence Scale-Revised.[131] PTSD patients also had deficits in explicit recall as measured by the Selective Reminding Test (SRT) for both verbal and visual components. We have subsequently found deficits in explicit memory tasks of free verbal recall as measured by the WMS-Logical component in adult survivors of childhood abuse seeking treatment for psychiatric disorders.[132] Studies have found deficits in explicit short-term memory as assessed by the Auditory Verbal Learning Test (AVLT) in Vietnam combat veterans with PTSD, whereas such deficits were not found in National Guard veterans without PTSD.[133] The California New Learning Test also revealed these deficits in Vietnam veterans with combat-related PTSD in comparison with controls.[134] Studies of female Vietnam combat nurses with PTSD are currently in progress (J. Wolfe personal communication, 1994). Deficits in academic performance have also been shown in Beirut adolescents with PTSD in comparison with Beirut adolescents without PTSD (P. Saigh, personal communication, 1994). These studies suggest deficits in encoding on explicit memory tasks. However, other studies of patients with PTSD have shown enhanced explicit recall of trauma-related words relative to neutral words in comparison with controls.[135] In summary, these findings show deficits in encoding on explicit memory tasks, deficits in retrieval, as well as enhanced encoding or retrieval of specific trauma-related material.

Studies using neuroimaging techniques have found that stress in humans may be associated with changes in brain structure, including the morphology of the hippocampus. As reviewed above, increased circulating glucocorticoids appear to be toxic to the hippocampus. An increase in glucocorticoids has been shown in soldiers undergoing the stress of bombardment.[136] Studies using computed tomography (CT) and magnetic resonance imaging (MRI) in human subjects suggest that a history of exposure to therapy, or depression may be associated with changes in brain structure.[137–140] Studies of concentration camp survivors from World War II seeking compensation for disability utilized pneumoencephalography and reported ''[cerebral] atrophy of varying degrees . . . in the majority [of the individuals].''[129] Other authors who have used pneumoencephalography to measure brain structure in concentration camp survivors reported ''diffuse encephalopathy'' in 81% of cases (reviewed in Thygesen et al.[129]).

We compared hippocampal volume measured with MRI in Vietnam combat veterans with PTSD (N = 26) and in healthy subjects (N = 22) who were matched for factors that could affect hippocampal volume, including age, sex, race, years of education, height, weight, handedness, and years of alcohol abuse. Patients with combat-related PTSD had an 8% decrease in right hippocampal volume in comparison with controls (p < 0.05) (Fig. 3-1), but no significant decrease in volume of comparison structures, including the temporal lobe and caudate. Deficits in free verbal recall (explicit memory) as measured by the Wechsler Memory Scale-Logical component, percent retention, were associated with decreased right hippocampal volume in the PTSD patients (r = 0.64; p < 0.05). There was not a significant difference between PTSD patients and controls in left hippocampal volume, or in volume of the comparison regions measured in this study, left or right caudate and temporal lobe volume (minus hippocampus).[141] We recently have analyzed data which shows a statistically significant 12% decrease in left hippocampal volume in 17 patients with a history of PTSD related to severe childhood physical and sexual abuse, as compared with 17 controls matched on a case-by-case basis with the patients (Bremner et al., unpublished data, 1996). In summary,

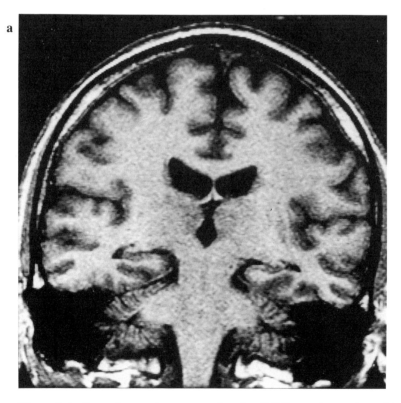

Figure 3–1. Coronal magnetic resonance imaging (MRI) scan in a patient with posttraumatic stress disorder (PTSD) (*a*) and a normal control (*b*). The hippocampus is visually smaller in the PTSD patient compared to the control.

this evidence is consistent with that of alterations in hippocampal morphology being associated with deficits in explicit memory function in patients with PTSD.

Other aspects of the alterations in memory function seen in PTSD may be mediated by the hippocampus. Electrical stimulation of the temporal lobe (including the hippocampus and adjacent cortical regions, parahippocampal gyrus, amygdala, and temporal lobe neocortex) in patients with epilepsy resulted in the subjective experience of a number of symptoms that are similar to those seen in PTSD. Eighteen out of 35 patients experienced symptoms of some kind. These included the subjective sensation of fear (7 patients), complex visual hallucinations (flashbacks) (5 patients), memory recall (5 patients), deja vu (4 patients), and emotional distress (3 patients).[142] In another study, electrical stimulation of the hippocampus and amygdala in epileptic patients was also associated with visual and auditory hallucinations, and dream-like and memory-like hallucinations, which are descriptively similar to flashbacks reported by patients with PTSD.[143] We have found an increase in dissociative symptomatology and disruption of delayed word recall in normal subjects following intravenous administration of keta-

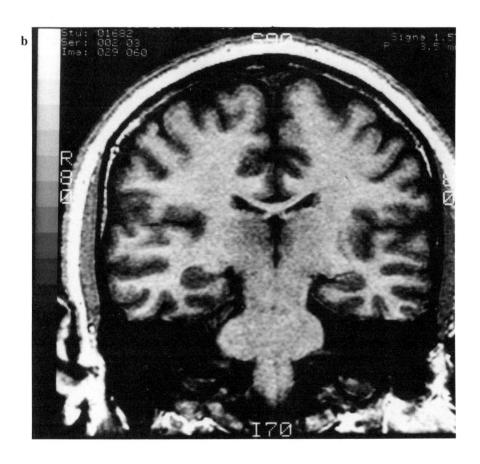

hydrochloride, a noncompetitive antagonist of the NMDA receptor.[144] The NMDA receptor, which is highly concentrated in the hippocampus, is involved in memory function at the molecular level (i.e., long-term potentiation [LTP]).

The neurophysiology of the thalamus is of interest from the standpoint of trauma-related symptomatology such as dissociation.[145] During slow-wave sleep, thalamic nuclei exhibit slow spindle oscillations that disrupt transmission of sensory information to cortical and limbic structures, while in wakefulness, the thalamus fires in a relay mode that facilitates transmission of sensory information to cortical regions. During rapid eye movement (REM) sleep (the sleep stage during which dreaming occurs), there is a phasic enhancement of thalamocortical cells,[146] which suggests that dreams (and other internally generated experiences) may arise as a result of thalamocortical projections that bypass the slow spindle oscillations of the thalamus blocking transmission of sensory information from the outside to the cortex.[147] Consistent with this process is the fact that patients with paramedian thalamic infarcts have a profound sense of detachment, reduced responsivity to external stimuli, and sleep-like posturing without the electrophysiological correlates of non-REM sleep. Dissociative states such as flashbacks in PTSD patients, which are also characterized by a feeling of unreality and detachment, may be due to alterations in thalamic function that result in a blocking of the transmission of sensory information from the outside. This is combined with the generation of internal images derived from recalled memories which have the unreal quality typical of dream or dissociative states.

Evidence from preclinical investigations indicates that the amygdala is involved in abnormalities of emotional memory manifested by, for instance, conditioned emotional responses, which are prominent in the clinical presentation of patients with PTSD. There is evidence that the amygdala mediates alterations in emotional memory as manifested by conditioned responses and other phenomena in humans (in addition to animals). For example, electrical stimulation of the amygdala in healthy human subjects has been shown to elicit feelings of anxiety.[148] Amygdala stimulation of human subjects is also accompanied by activation of the stress response system, as manifested by increases in peripheral catecholamines, a phenomenon that is also seen in animals during conditioned fear responses.[149] Exaggerated startle response (which has been demonstrated to be mediated by the amygdala in animals) is an important feature of the clinical presentation of patients with PTSD, and empirical investigations have shown alterations of startle to be associated with PTSD.[150] We have not found a difference in amygdala volume measured with MRI between patients with combat-related PTSD and healthy controls (Bremner et al., unpublished data, 1996).

Investigations have also addressed alterations in emotional memory as demonstrated by conditioned emotional responses in patients with PTSD. The conditioned emotional response can be studied in humans in the laboratory by using the psychophysiology paradigm. Lawrence Kolb[151] noted that patients with PTSD have a heightened physiological responsiveness to reminders of the original trauma that resemble conditioned responses. These conditioned responses to cues related to the original trauma (combat films and sounds, scripts of traumatic events) parallel those seen in the conditioned fear paradigm in animals. Studies have used measurements of heart rate and blood pressure as indexes of sympathetic function (the psychophysiology paradigm) to examine the relationship between traumatic reminders, subjective experience, and physiological reactivity.[152] Increases in heart rate and systolic blood pressure following exposure to combat sounds have been found in Vietnam veterans with combat-related PTSD but not in non-veteran healthy subjects, non-PTSD combat veterans,[153,154] and Vietnam veterans with other psychiatric disorders.[154] Increases in plasma epinephrine, pulse, blood pressure, and subjective distress following combat stimuli have been reported in PTSD patients but not in healthy controls.[155] PTSD patients have also been found to have a higher heart rate, skin conductance, and frontalis electromyogram than controls after hearing ''scripts'' of the subjects's combat experiences read to them.[156] An increase in heart rate responses and skin conductance following exposure to loud tones is also seen in patients with PTSD, but not in healthy controls, patients with other anxiety disorders, and patients without PTSD but with a history of past traumatic experiences.[157] This heightened responsiveness to reminders of the original trauma, or conditioned emotional stimuli, is probably mediated by the amygdala.

Abnormalities in the Stroop test, which are associated with activation of the cingulate cortex, have been associated with PTSD. Delays in color-naming PTSD-related words such as ''body-bag'' are involuntary, and such delays provide quantitative measures of the intrusive cognition which is an important part of PTSD. Vietnam combat veterans with PTSD have been found to take longer to color-name ''PTSD'' words than to color-name obsessive, positive, or neutral words; this delay was correlated with severity of PTSD symptomatology as measured by the Mississippi Scale.[158] Stroop interference has also been shown in patients with PTSD that is related to the trauma of rape.[159,160] These studies therefore make Stroop interference one of the more replicated findings in PTSD.

The anterior cingulate is also involved in abnormalities of emotional memory. Inducing fear by increasing the number of dangerous animals in a word list presented to human subjects results in an increase in blood flow in the anterior cingulate.[64] Studies of human patients with brain lesions have shown that damage to the anterior one-third of the frontal cortex often results in seizures during which the individual experiences intense feelings of fear or anguish. This suggests that the anteromedial prefrontal cortex plays a role in fear-related behavior. In addition, some patients have been observed to experience visual hallucinations during seizures,[161] which are reminiscent of the flashbacks seen in victims of trauma.

The orbitofrontal cortex may be involved in abnormalities of emotional memory that are seen in patients with a history of childhood abuse. Studies of human patients with brain lesions have shown that lesions of the orbitofrontal cortex also result in symptoms of intense fear during seizures. Some case reports have described a relationship between damage to the orbitofrontal cortex and visual hallucinations that appear to be similar to the flashbacks which are characteristic of PTSD.[162] Yohimbine is an alpha-2 noradrenergic antagonist which causes an increase in brain norepinephrine release and increased symptoms of PTSD.[163] Through assessment by PET [[18F]2-fluoro-2-deoxyglucose (FDG), we have found a differential response of cerebral metabolism in PTSD patients and controls after the administration of yohimbine.[164] The greatest magnitude of difference was seen in the orbitofrontal cortex. Differences were also seen in the prefrontal, temporal, and parietal cortex. The orbitofrontal cortex as well as other brain regions are involved in implicit memory function. Patients with PTSD have been shown to have a more enhanced implicit recall (i.e., recall following priming) of trauma-related words than of neutral words in comparison with controls.[135] These findings may have implications for the greater intrusiveness of trauma-related memories over normal memories in patients with PTSD.

Extinction

Extinction is also relevant to understanding the effects of stress on memory in patients with PTSD. The mechanism of extinction involves cortical inhibition of amygdala function. Victims of childhood abuse clinically exhibit a failure of extinction to trauma-related stimuli. For instance, an individual who was locked in a closet may continue to show anxiety reactions when they are in a close space, even when there is no real threat of danger. The neocortex mediates extinction of emotional memory. For instance, the auditory neocortex suppresses conditioned fear responses mediated by the amygdala to stimuli that are not specific to the original conditioned stimulus (i.e., it prevents stimulus generalization).[165] The auditory cortex is also involved in extinction through the suppression of amygdala responsiveness.[166]

Stress Sensitization

Stress sensitization refers to the phenomenon where repeated exposure to a stressor results in an amplification of responsiveness to subsequent stressors. For example, acute stress results in an increased release of norepinephrine in the hippocampus as well as in other brain regions. Animals with a history of exposure to prior stressors become sensitized to exposure to subsequent stressors, so that there is an accentuation of norepinephrine release in the hippocampus with a subsequent stressor.[167] As reviewed above, norepinephrine (in addition to other neurotransmitters and neuropeptides) modulates memory formation and retrieval. This raises the possibility that stress sensitization, acting through neuromodulators such as norepinephrine, may be associated with alteration in memory encoding and retrieval, which may have implications for understanding the mechanisms of traumatic recall in PTSD.

The mechanism of stress sensitization illustrates how the amygdala mediates the development of stress-induced abnormalities of emotional memory. In stress sensitization, repeated exposure to a stressor such as footshock results in the potentiation of the startle response with reexposure to a subsequent footshock. Enhanced release of neuromodulators in the amygdala that affect memory function, such as epinephrine or norepinephrine, may mediate the abnormalities of emotional memory that are seen following exposure to repeated stressors. Repeated exposure to stress will also potentiate responsiveness to cues associated with the original stressors, as well as the number of cues that can act as conditioned stimuli. This produces the phenomenon of stimulus generalization, in which a wide range of stimuli in the environment can result in conditioned responsiveness. As is seen both in animals in the laboratory model of conditioned fear as well as in patients with PTSD, avoidant behavior develops in an attempt to stay away from these stimuli in the environment, leading to conditioned responses.

Stress sensitization has clinical applications for PTSD. We have found that exposure to the stressor of childhood physical abuse increases the risk for the development of combat-related PTSD.[168] Israeli veterans with a history of previous combat-related acute stress reactions have also been found to be at increased risk for reactivation of combat-related stress reactions in comparison with combat veterans without a history of stress reaction in response to combat.[169] In addition, other clinical examples exist of how a history of exposure to prior stress increases the risk for stress-related symptomatology upon reexposure to stressors.[170]

A Working Model for the Neurobiology of Memory Alterations in Survivors of Childhood Abuse

A special mechanism of memory which explains delayed recall of episodes of childhood abuse may be found in amnesia. Dissociative amnesia is not typically a normal phenomenon of memory and has been found to be increased in patients with PTSD.[9] Amnestic symptoms in these patients ranged from gaps of memory lasting from minutes to hours to days. Some patients reported driving down the highway from Boston to New Haven, and suddenly realizing that they had covered 2 hours of the trip and had no recall of what had happened during that time. One patient said that he was walking down a street in Boston, and the next thing he knew he was in a motel room in Texas. Another patient disappeared from an inpatient psychiatric unit, and found himself in the woods somewhere in Illinois, in the middle of the night, wearing combat fatigues. A patient of one of the authors with a history of childhood sexual abuse reported that she was on the telephone at her day hospital program, and the next thing she knew she was at home in bed. These clinical case examples provide a feeling for the wide range of phenomena that characterize dissociative amnesia in patients with a history of exposure to extreme psychological trauma. A number of other recent studies have documented the existence of dissociative amnesia in patients with PTSD.[171–176]

Based on what is known about the effects of stress on brain systems involved in memory, there is evidence that mechanisms other than ''normal forgetting'' are probably operative in the delayed recall of childhood abuse. As noted above, the hippocampus and adjacent cortices have been hypothesized to bind together information from multiple sensory cortices into a single memory at the time of retrieval. For instance, an episode of sexual abuse is marked by the smell of the perpetrator, the sounds involved in the abuse, the visual appearance of the perpetrator and the scene where the abuse takes place, and the tactile sensations. All of these individual features are stored in the primary sensory cortical areas to which they correspond; for instance, smell is stored in the olfactory cortex. When a similar situation recurs, the hippocampus and adjacent cortex activate cortical areas and bring together the diverse sensory elements to recreate the memory. Abnormalities of hippocampal function in PTSD may affect this normal function of the hippocampus in bringing together memory elements from diverse neocortical sensory areas. This may account for the abnormal intrusion of some traumatic memories into consciousness, the disintegration of dissociated traumatic memories, and the total lack of recall (amnesia) for other events.

Neuropeptides and neurotransmitters released during stress can modulate memory function (Fig. 3-2). These neuromodulators act at the level of the hippocampus, amygdala, and other brain regions involved in memory. Disorders such as PTSD may be associated with long-term alterations in the function of these neuromodulators, which would in turn be associated with alterations in memory in these patients that would not occur in normal persons. Exposure to subsequent stressors could also be associated with altered release of neuromodulators, resulting in altered memory recall in PTSD patients.

Mechanisms involving state-dependent recall may also be applicable to amnesia for abuse.[127] *State-dependent recall* refers to the phenomenon whereby an affective state similar to that at the time of encoding leads to a facilitation of memory retrieval. For instance, memories encoded during a state of sadness will have a facilitated retrieval during similar states of sadness. Similar situations can occur for other emotional states. To extend this concept to victims of abuse, it can be seen that particular emotions will predominate at the time of the original abuse, such as extreme fear or sadness. These emotional states occur infrequently during a routine adult life that is free of stressors. The recurrence of the extreme fear or sadness that occurred during the original abuse during psychotherapy or with exposure to a subsequent stressor may lead to a delayed recall of the original abuse experiences. A clinical example of this would be the victim of sexual abuse who has no recall of her experiences of sexual abuse until she is raped as an adult, which leads to a recall of the original trauma.

Concluding Remarks

We have examined the question of the validity of memories of childhood abuse as it relates to the current controversy surrounding the false memory syndrome from both theoretical and biological perspectives. Studies in cognitive psychology have provided evidence for an enhancement of central details related to stressful events and for the

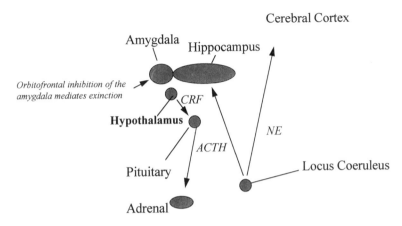

Figure 3–2. Diagrammatic representation of the effects of traumatic stress on brain regions and systems involved in memory. Input to the amygdala from orbitofrontal cortex and temporal cortex is involved in extinction of conditioned fear, which is mediated by the amygdala. Release of corticotropin releasing-factor (CRF) from the hypothalamus causes release of ACTH from the pituitary, which in turn results in release of cortisol from the adrenal. CRF and cortisol play an important role in the stress response, modulate memory function, and are altered in PTSD. The hippocampus is involved in short-term memory and fear responses for context. High levels of cortisol associated with stress may damage the hippocampus and lead to altered memory function in PTSD. Locus coeruleus, site of norepinephrine (NE) cell bodies, is also involved in stress. Alterations in NE function are associated with PTSD, and may underlie sensitization and alterations in memory in PTSD patients.

exclusion of peripheral details in normal human subjects. Much has been made in the popular press about the potential effects of suggestion on memory. However, a review of this literature does not support the conclusion that suggestions can lead to a rewriting of original memory traces.

Patients with PTSD have been shown to have an increase in self-reported dissociative amnesia, which is defined as gaps in memory not due to normal forgetting. Other aspects of memory function are deficient in PTSD patients, including verbal recall. Both preclinical and clinical studies support the idea that traumatic stress is associated with alterations in brain regions involved in memory, resulting in functional memory deficits. Other concepts such as state-dependent memory, stress sensitization, and modulation of memory traces during and after encoding by neurotransmitters and neuropeptides released at high levels during stress, provide potential explanations for delayed recall of memories of childhood abuse. These mechanisms are probably only applicable to patients with disorders such as PTSD secondary to abuse, and not to the entire range of individuals who are exposed to childhood abuse, including those who do not develop abuse-related psychiatric disorders.

Studies to date have provided only an incomplete picture of how biological mechanisms may explain phenomena such as delayed recall of childhood abuse and dissociative amnesia. We do not mean to imply that definitive biological mechanisms have been elucidated which could explain these phenomena. Rather, this chapter is a critical review of the current status of the topic, and through it we have sought to raise awareness about how the neurobiology of the effects of stress on memory may be applicable to these questions. Future studies should shed additional light on the neurobiology of memory in individuals with a history of exposure to childhood abuse.

References

1. Williams LM: Recall of childhood trauma: a prospective study of women's memories of child sexual abuse. J Consult Clin Psychol 1994; 62:1167–1176.
2. Williams LM: What does it mean to forget child sexual abuse? A reply to Loftus, Garry, and Feldman (1994). J Consult Clin Psychol 1994; 62:1182–1186.
3. Loftus EF, Polonsky S, Fullilove MT: Memories of childhood sexual abuse: remembering and repressing. Psychol Women Q 1994; 18:67–84.
4. Loftus EF, Garry M, Feldman J: Forgetting sexual trauma: what does it mean when 38% forget? J Consult Clin Psychol 1994; 62:1177–1181.
5. Bremner JD, Krystal JH, Southwick SM, Charney DS: Functional neuroanatomical correlates of the effects of stress on memory. J Traumatic Stress 1995; 8:527–554.
6. Pitman RK: Posttraumatic stress disorder, hormones and memory [editorial]. Biol Psychiatry 1989; 26:221–223.
7. Charney DS, Deutch AY, Krystal JH, Southwick SM, Davis M: Psychobiologic mechanisms of posttraumatic stress disorder. Arch Gen Psychiatry 1993; 50:294–299.
8. Bremner JD, Davis M, Southwick SM, Krystal JH, Charney DS: The neurobiology of posttraumatic stress disorder. *In* JM Oldham, MG Riba, A Tasman (Eds.), Reviews of Psychiatry, Vol. 12. Washington, DC: American Psychiatric Press, 1993, pp. 182–204.
9. Bremner JD, Steinberg M, Southwick SM, Johnson DR, Charney DS: Use of the Structured Clinical Interview for DSMIV-Dissociative Disorders for systematic assessment of dissociative symptoms in posttraumatic stress disorder. Am J Psychiatry 1993; 150:1011–1014.
10. Loftus EF, Miller DG, Burns HJ: Semantic integration of verbal information into a visual memory. J Exp Psychol Hum Learn Mem 1978; 4:19–31.
11. Ceci SJ, Caves RD, Howe MJA: Children's long-term memory for information that is incongruous with their prior knowledge. Br J Psychol 1981; 72:443–450.
12. McCloskey M, Zaragoza M: Misleading postevent information and memory for events: arguments and evidence against memory impairment hypotheses. J Exp Psychol Gen 1985; 114:1–16.
13. Lindsay DS, Johnson MK: The eyewitness suggestibility effect and memory for source. Mem Cogn 1989; 17:349–358.
14. Lindsay DS: Misleading suggestions can impair eyewitnesses' ability to remember event details. J Exp Psychol Learn Mem Cogn 1990; 16:1077–1083.
15. Loftus EF, Schooler J, Wagenaar W: The fate of memory: comment on McCloskey and Zaragoza. J Exp Psychol Gen 1985; 114:375–380.
16. McCloskey M, Zaragoza M: Postevent information and memory: reply to Loftus, Schooler and Wagenaar. J Exp Psychol Gen 1985; 114:381–387.
17. Brown R, Kulik J: Flashbulb memories. Cognition 1977; 5:73–99.

18. Bohannon JN: Flashbulb memories for the space shuttle disaster: a tale of two theories. Cognition 1988; 29:179–196.

19. Bohannon JN III, Symons VL: Flashbulb memories: confidence, consistency and quantity. *In* E Winograd, U Neisser (Eds.), Affect and Accuracy in Recall: Studies in "Flashbulb Memories." Cambridge: Cambridge University Press, 1992, pp. 65–94.

20. Neisser U, Harsch N: Phantom flashbulbs: false recollections of hearing the news about Challenger. *In* E Winograd, U Neisser (Eds.), Affect and Accuracy in Recall: Studies in "Flashbulb Memories." Cambridge: Cambridge University Press, 1992, pp. 9–31.

21. Loftus EF, Loftus GR, Messo J: Some facts about "Weapon Focus." Law Hum Behav 1987; 11:55–62.

22. Christianson S, Loftus EF: Memory for traumatic events. Appl Cogn Psychol 1987; 1:225–239.

23. Christianson SA, Loftus EF: Remembering emotional events: the fate of detailed information. Emotion Cogn 1991; 5:81–108.

24. Goodman GS, Hirschman JE, Hepps JE, Rudy L: Children's memory for stressful events. Merrill-Palmer Q 1991; 37:109–158.

25. Goodman GS, Aman C: Children's use of anatomically detailed dolls to recount an event. Child Dev 1990; 61:1859–1871.

26. Rudy L, Goodman GS: Effects of participation on children's reports: implications for children's testimony. Dev Psychol 1991; 27:527–538.

27. Saywitz KJ, Goodman GS, Nicholas E, Moan SF: Children's memories of a physical examination involving genital touch: implications for reports of child sexual abuse. J Consult Clin Psychol 1991; 59:682–691.

28. Ornstein PA, Gordon BN, Larus D: Children's memory for a personally experienced event: implications for testimony. Appl Cogn Psychol 1992; 6:49–60.

29. Ceci SJ, Ross DF, Toglia MP: Suggestibility of children's memory: psycholegal implications. J Exp Psychol Gen 1987; 116:38–49.

30. Ceci SJ, Bruck M: Suggestibility of the child witness: a historical review and synthesis. Psychol Bull 1993; 113:403–439.

31. McGaugh JL: Involvement of hormonal and neuromodulatory systems in the regulation of memory storage: endogenous modulation of memory storage. Annu Rev Neurosci 1989; 12:255–287.

32. Squire LR, Moore TY: Dorsal thalamic lesion in a noted case of human memory dysfunction. Ann Neurol 1979; 6:503.

33. Squire LR, Zola-Morgan S: The medial temporal lobe memory system. Science 1991; 253:1380–1386.

34. Morris RGM, Garrud P, Rawlins JNP, O'Keefe J: Place navigation impaired in rats with hippocampal lesions. Nature 1982; 297:681–683.

35. Sutherland RJ, Kolb B, Whishaw IQ: Spatial mapping: definitive disruption by hippocampal or medial frontal cortex damage in the rat. Neurosci Lett 1982; 31:271–276.

36. Mishkin M: Memory in monkeys severely impaired by combined but not separate removal of amygdala and hippocampus. Nature 1978; 173:297–298.

37. Zola-Morgan S, Squire LR, Amaral DG: Lesions of the amygdala that spare adjacent cortical regions do not impair memory or exacerbate the impairment following lesions of the hippocampal formation. J Neurosci 1989; 9:1922–1936.

38. Zola-Morgan S, Squire LR, Amaral DG, Suzuki WA: Lesions of perirhinal and parahippocampal cortex that spare the amygdala and hippocampal formation produce severe memory impairment. J Neurosci 1989; 9:4355–4370.

39. Murray EA, Mishkin M: Visual recognition in monkeys following rhinal cortical abla-

tions combined with either amygdalectomy or hippocampectomy. J Neurosci 1986; 6: 1991–2003.

40. Parkinson JK, Murray EA, Mishkin M: A selective mnemonic role for the hippocampus in monkeys: memory for the location of objects. J Neurosci 1988; 8:4159–4167.
41. Scoville WB, Milner B: Loss of recent memory after bilateral hippocampal lesions. J Neurol Psychiatry 1957; 20:11–21.
42. Squire LR, Ojemann JG, Miezin FM, Petersen SE, Vidden TO, Raichle ME: Activation of the hippocampus in normal humans: a functional anatomical study of memory. Proc Natl Acad Sci USA 1992; 89:1837–1841.
43. Turner BH, Mishkin M, Knapp M: Organization of amygdaloid projections from modality-specific association areas in the monkey. J Comp Neurol 1980; 191:515–543.
44. Turner BH, Herkenham M: Thalamoamygdaloid projections in the rat: a test of the amygdala's role in sensory processing. J Comp Neurol 1991; 313:295–325.
45. Zola-Morgan SM, Squire LR, Alvarez-Royo P, Clower RP: Independence of memory functions and emotional behavior: separate contributions of the hippocampal formation and the amygdala. Hippocampus 1991; 1:207.
46. Davis M: Pharmacological and anatomical analysis of fear conditioning using the fear-potentiated startle paradigm. Behav Neurosci 1992; 100:814–824.
47. Davis M: The role of the amygdala in fear and anxiety. Annu Rev Neurosci 1992; 15:353–375.
48. Hitchcock JM, Davis M: Lesions of the amygdala, but not of the cerebellum or red nucleus, block conditioned fear as measured with the potentiated startle paradigm. Behav Neurosci 1986; 100:11–22.
49. Hitchcock JM, Sananes CB, Davis M: Sensitization of the startle reflex by footshock: blockade by lesions of the central nucleus of the amygdala or its efferent pathway to the brainstem. Behav Neurosci 1989; 103:509–518.
50. Rosen JB, Davis M: Enhancement of acoustic startle by electrical stimulation of the amygdala. Behav Neurosci 1988; 102:195–202.
51. Rosen JB, Hitchcock JM, Sananes CB, Miserendino MJ, Davis M: A direct projection from the central nucleus of the amygdala to the acoustic startle pathway: anterograde and retrograde tracing studies. Behav Neurosci 1991; 105:817–825.
52. Hitchcock JM, Davis M: Efferent pathway of the amygdala involved in conditioned fear as measured with the fear-potentiated startle paradigm. Behav Neurosci 1991; 105:826–842.
53. Campeau S, Miserendino MJD, Davis M: Intra-amygdala infusion of the N-methyl-D-aspartate receptor antagonist AP5 blocks the acquisition but not expression of fear-potentiated startle to an auditory conditioned stimulus. Behav Neurosci 1992; 106:569–574.
54. Miserendino MJD, Sananes CB, Melia KR, Davis M: Blocking of acquisition but not expression of conditioned fear-potentiated startle by NMDA antagonists in the amygdala. Nature 1990; 345:716–718.
55. Goldman-Rakic PS: Topography of cognition: parallel distributed networks in primate association cortex. Annu Rev Neurosci 1988; 11:137–156.
56. Petersen SE, Fox PT, Posner MI, Mintun M. Raichle ME: Positron emission tomographic studies of the cortical anatomy of single-word processing. Nature 1988; 331:585–589.
57. Tulving E, Kapur S, Craik FIM, Moscovitch M, Houle S: Hemispheric encoding/retrieval asymmetry in episodic memory: positron emission tomography findings. Proc Natl Acad Sci USA 1994; 91:2016–2020.
58. Jonides J, Smith EE, Koeppe RA, Awh E, Minoshima S, Mintun MA: Spatial working memory in humans as revealed by PET: Nature 1993; 363:623–625.
59. Pardo JV, Pardo PJ, Janer KW, Raichle ME: The anterior cingulate cortex mediates process-

ing selection in the Stroop attentional conflict paradigm. Proc Natl Acad Sci USA 1990; 87:256–259.

60. Damasio H, Grabowski T, Frank R, Galaburda AM, Damasio AR: The return of Phineas Gage: clues about the brain from the skull of a famous patient. Science 1994; 264:1102–1105.

61. Otto T, Eichenbaum H: Complementary roles of the orbital prefrontal cortex and the perirhinal-entorhinal cortices in an odor-guided delayed-nonmatching-to-sample task. Behav Neurosci 1992; 106:762–775.

62. Morgan MA, LeDoux JE: Medial orbital lesions increase resistance to extinction but do not affect acquisition of fear conditioning. Proc Soc Neurosci 1994; 2:1006.

63. Posner MI, Petersen SE, Fox PT, Raichle ME: Localization of cognitive operations in the human brain. Science 1988; 240:1627–1631.

64. Pardo JV, Fox PT, Raichle ME: Localization of a human system for sustained attention by positron emission tomography. Nature 1991; 349:61–64.

65. Squire LR: Mechanisms of memory. Science 1986; 232:1612–1619.

66. McGaugh JL, Herz MJ: Memory Consolidation. San Francisco: Albion, 1972.

67. Squire LR, Slater PC, Chace PM: Retrograde amnesia: Temporal gradient in very long term memory following electroconvulsive therapy. Science 1975; 187:77–79.

68. Zola-Morgan SM, Squire LR: The primate hippocampal formation: evidence for a time-limited role in memory storage. Science 1990; 250:288–290.

69. Cannon WB: Again the James-Lange and the thalamic theories of emotion. Psychol Rev 1931; 38:281–295.

70. Cannon WB, Britton SW: Pseudoaffective medulliadrenal secretion. Am J Physiol 1925; 7:283–294.

71. Papez JW: A proposed mechanism of emotion. AMA Arch Neurol Psychiatry 1937; 38:725–743.

72. Kluver H, Bucy PC: "Psychic blindness" and other symptoms following bilateral temporal lobectomy in rhesus monkeys. Am J Physiol 1937; 119:352–353.

73. Kluver H, Bucy PC: Preliminary analysis of functions of the temporal lobes in monkeys. Arch Neurol Psychiatry 1939; 42:979–1000.

74. MacLean PD: Psychosomatic disease and the visceral brain. Recent developments bearing on the Papez theory of emotion. Psychosom Med 1949; 11:338–353.

75. McEwen BS, Angulo J, Cameron H, Chao HM, Daniels D, Gannon MN, Gould E, Mendelson S, Sakai R, Spencer R, Woolley C: Paradoxical effects of adrenal steroids on the brain: protection versus degeneration. Biol Psychiatry 1992; 31:177–199.

76. Luine V, Villages M, Martinex C, McEwen BS: Repeated stress causes reversible impairments of spatial memory performance. Brain Res 1994; 639:167–170.

77. Sapolsky RM, McEwen BS: Why dexamethasone resistance? Two possible neuroendocrine mechanisms. In AF Schatzberg, CB Nemeroff (Eds.), The Hypothalamic-Pituitary-Adrenal Axis: Physiology, Pathophysiology, and Psychiatric Implications. New York: Raven Press, 1988, pp. 159–169.

78. Uno H, Tarara R, Else JG, Suleman MA, Sapolsky RM: Hippocampal damage associated with prolonged and fatal stress in primates. J Neurosci 1989; 9:1705–1711.

79. Sapolsky RM, Uno H, Rebert CS, Finch CE: Hippocampal damage associated with prolonged glucocorticoid exposure in primates. J Neurosci 1990; 10:2897–2902.

80. Sapolsky RM, Packan DR, Vale WW: Glucocorticoid toxicity in the hippocampus: in vitro demonstration. Brain Res 1988; 453:367–371.

81. Kerr DS, Campbell LW, Hao SY, Landfield PW: Corticosteroid modulation of hippocampal potentials: increased effect with aging. Science 1989; 245:1505–1509.

82. Sapolsky R, Krey L, McEwen B: Prolonged glucocorticoid exposure reduces hippocampal neuron number: implications for aging. J Neurosci 1985; 5:1221–1226.
83. Wooley CS, Gould E, McEwen BS: Exposure to excess glucocorticoids alters dendritic morphology of adult hippocampal pyramidal neurons. Brain Res 1990; 531:225–231.
84. Watanabe Y, Gould E, McEwen BS: Stress induces atrophy of apical dendrites of hippocampal CA3 pyramidal neurons. Brain Res 1992; 588:341–345.
85. Sapolsky RM: A mechanism for glucocorticoid toxicity in the hippocampus: increased neuronal vulnerability to metabolic insults. J Neurosci 1985; 5:1228–1232.
86. Packan DR, Sapolsky RM: Glucocorticoid endangerment of the hippocampus: tissue, steroid and receptor specificity. Neuroendocrinology 1990; 51:613–618.
87. Sapolsky R, Pulsinelli W: Glucocorticoids potentiate ischemic injury to neurons: therapeutic implications. Science 1985; 229:1397–1400.
88. Sapolsky R: Glucocorticoid toxicity in the hippocampus: synergy with an excitotoxin. Neuroendocrinology 1986; 43:440–446.
89. Armanini MP, Hutchins C, Stein BA, Sapolsky RM: Glucocorticoid endangerment of hippocampal neurons is NMDA-receptor dependent. Brain Res 1990; 532:7–1.
90. Virgin CE, Taryn PTH, Packan DR, Tombaugh GC, Yang SH, Horner HC, Sapolsky RM: Glucocorticoids inhibit glucose transport and glutamate uptake in hippocampal astrocytes: implications for glucocorticoid neurotoxicity. J Neurochem 1991; 57:1422–1428.
91. Phillips RG, LeDoux JE: Differential contribution of amygdala and hippocampus to cued and contextual fear conditioning. Behav Neurosci 1992; 106:274–285.
92. Kim JJ, Fanselow MS: Modality-specific retrograde amnesia of fear. Science 1992; 256:675–677.
93. Parent MB, Tomaz C, McGaugh JL: Increased training in an aversively motivated task attenuates the memory-impairing effects of posttraining N-methyl-D-aspartate-induced amygdala lesions. Behav Neurosci 1992; 106:789–797.
94. Nahm FKD, Tranel D, Damasio H, Damasio AR: Cross-modal associations and the human amygdala. Neuropsychologia 1993; 8:727–744.
95. Cahill L, McGaugh JL: Amygdaloid complex lesions differentially affect retention of tasks using appetitive and aversive reinformcement. Behav Neurosci 1990; 104:532–543.
96. Turner BH, Herkenham M: Thalamoamygdaloid projections in the rat: a test of the amygdala's role in sensory processing. J Comp Neurol 1991; 313:295–325.
97. Iwata J, LeDoux JE, Meeley MP, Arneric S, Reis DJ: Intrinsic neurons in the amygdaloid field projected to by the medial geniculate body mediate emotional responses conditioned to acoustic stimuli. Brain Res 1986; 383:195–214.
98. Romanski LM, LeDoux JE: Bilateral destruction of neocortical and perirhinal projection targets of the acoustic thalamus does not disrupt auditory fear conditioning. Neurosci Lett 1992; 142:228–232.
99. Frysztak RJ, Neafsey EJ: The effect of medial frontal cortex lesions on cardiovascular conditioned emotional responses in the rat. Brain Res 1994; 643:181–193.
100. Diorio D, Viau V, Meaney MJ: The role of the medial prefrontal cortex (cingulate gyrus) in the regulation of hypothalamic-pituitary-adrenal responses to stress. J Neurosci 1993; 13:3839–3847.
101. De Wied D, Croiset G: Stress modulation of learning and memory processes. Methods Achiev Exp Pathol 1991; 15:167–199.
102. Borrell J, De Kloet ER, Versteeg DHG, Bohus B: Inhibitory avoidance deficit following short-term adrenalectomy in the rat: the role of adrenal catecholamines. Behav Neurol Biol 1983; 39:241.

103. Gold PE, van Buskirk R: Facilitation of time-dependent memory processes with posttrial epinephrine injections. Behav Biol 1975; 13:145–153.

104. Liang KC, Juler RG, McGaugh JL: Modulating effects of posttraining epinephrine on memory: involvement of the amygdala noradrenergic system. Brain Res 1986; 368:125–133.

105. McGaugh JL, Castellano C, Brioni J: Picrotoxin enhances latent extinction of conditioned fear. Behav Neurosci 1990; 104:264–267.

106. Liang KC, McGaugh JL, Yao HY: Involvement of amygdala pathways in the influence of post-training intra-amygdala norepinephrine and peripheral epinephrine on memory storage. Brain Res 1990; 508:225–233.

107. Decker MW, McGaugh JL: Effects of concurrent manipulations of cholinergic and noradrenergic function on learning and retention in mice. Brain Res 1989; 477:29–37.

108. Velly J, Kempf E, Cardo B, Velley L: Long-term modulation of learning following locus coeruleus stimulation: behavioral and neurochemical data. Physiol Psychol 1985; 13:163–171.

109. Selden NRW, Robbins TW, Everitt BJ: Enhanced behavioral conditioning to context and impaired behavioral and neuroendocrine responses to conditioned stimuli following ceruleocortical noradrenergic lesions: support for an attentional hypothesis of central noradrenergic function. J Neurosci 1990; 10:531–539.

110. Decker MW, Gill TM, McGaugh JL: Concurrent muscarinic and β-adrenergic blockade in rats impairs place-learning in a water maze and retention of inhibitory avoidance. Brain Res 1990; 513:81–85.

111. McGaugh JL: Significance and remembrance: the role of neuromodulatory systems. Psychol Sci 1990; 1:15–25.

112. De Wied D, Jolles J: Neuropeptides derived from pro-opiocortin: behavioral, physiological and neurochemical effects. Physiol Rev 1982; 62:976.

113. Van Wimersma Greidanus TJB, Croiset G, Bakker B, Bouman H: Amygdaloid lesions block the effect of neuropeptides (vasopressin, ACTH (4-10)) on avoidance behavior. Brain Res Bull 1979; 3:227.

114. Britton DR, Koob G, Vale W: Intraventricular corticotropin-releasing factor enhances behavioral effects of novelty. Life Sci 1982; 31:363–367.

115. Gasbarri A, Introini-Collison IB, Packard MG, Pacitti C, McGaugh JL:Interaction of cholinergic-dopaminergic systems in the regulation of memory storage in aversively motivated learning tasks. 1993; 627:72–78.

116. Castellano C: Effects of morphine and heroin on discrimination learning and consolidation in mice. Psychopharmacology 1975; 42:235–242.

117. Introini-Collison IB, Nagahara AH, McGaugh JL: Memory-enhancement with intra-amygdala posttraining naloxone is blocked by concurrent administration of propanolol. Brain Res 1989; 476:94–101.

118. Gaffori O, De Wied D: Time-related memory effects of vasopressin analogues in rats. Pharmacol Biochem Behav 1986; 25:1125.

119. Brioni JD, Nagahara AH, McGaugh JL: Involvement of the amygdala GABAergic system in the modulation of memory storage. Brain Res 1989; 487:105–112.

120. Cahill L, Prins B, Weber M, McGaugh JL (1994): β-adrenergic activation and memory for emotional events. Nature 1994; 371:702–703.

121. Andreasen NC: Posttraumatic stress disorder: psychology, biology, and the Manichean warfare between false dichotomies. Am J Psychiatry 1995; 152:963–965.

122. Pitman RK, Orr SP, Lasko NB: Effects of intranasal vasopressin and oxytocin on physio-

logic responding during personal combat imagery in Vietnam veterans with posttraumatic stress disorder. Psychol Res 1993; 48:107–117.

123. Henderson JL, Moore M: The psychoneurosis of war. N Engl J Med 1944; 230:274–278.

124. Grinker RR, Spiegel JP: War Neuroses in North Africa. New York: Josiah Macy Jr. Foundation, 1943.

125. Torrie A: Psychosomatic casualties in the Middle East. Lancet 1944; 29:139–143.

126. Archibald HC, Tuddenham RD: Persistent stress reaction after combat. Arch Gen Psychiatry 1965; 12:475–481.

127. Bower GH: Mood and memory. Am Psychol 1981; 36:129–148.

128. Helweg-Larsen P, Hoffmeyer H, Kieler J, Thaysen EH, Thaysen JH, Thygesen P, Wulff MH: Famine disease in German concentration camps: complications and sequels. Acta Med Scand 1952; 274:235–460.

129. Thygesen P, Hermann K, Willanger R: Concentration camp survivors in Denmark: persecution, disease, disability, compensation. Dan Med Bull 1970; 17:65–108.

130. Sutker PB, Winstead DK, Galina ZH, Allain AN: Cognitive deficits and psychopathology among former prisoners of war and combat veterans of the Korean conflict. Am J Psychiatry 1991; 148:67–72.

131. Bremner JD, Scott TM, Delaney RC, Southwick SM, Mason JW, Johnson DR, Innis RB, McCarthy G, Charney DS: Deficits in short-term memory in post-traumatic stress disorder. Am J Psychiatry 1993; 150:1015–1019.

132. Bremner JD, Randall PR, Capelli S, Scott T, McCarthy G, Charney DS: Deficits in short-term memory in adult survivors of childhood abuse. Psychiatry Res 1996 (in press).

133. Uddo M, Vasterling JT, Brailey K, Sutker PB: Memory and attention in posttraumatic stress disorder. J Psychopathol Behav Assess 1993; 15:43–52.

134. Yehuda R, Keefer RSE, Harvey PD, Levengood RA, Gerber DK, Geni J, Siever LJ: Learning and memory in combat veterans with posttraumatic stress disorder. Am J Psychiatry 1995; 152:137–139.

135. Zeitlin SB, McNally RJ: Implicit and explicit memory bias for threat in posttraumatic stress disorder. Behav Res Ther 1991; 29:451–457.

136. Howard JM, Olney JM, Frawley JP, Peterson RE, Smith LH, Davis JH, Guerra S, Dibrell WH: Studies of adrenal function in combat and wounded soldiers. Ann Surg 1955; 141:314–320.

137. Bentson J, Reza M, Winter J, Wilson G: Steroids and apparent cerebral atrophy on computed tomography scans. J Comput Assist Tomogr 1978; 2:16–23.

138. Okuno T, Ito M, Konishi Y, Yoshioka M, Nakano Y: Cerebral atrophy following ACTH therapy. J Comput Assist Tomogr 1980; 4:20–23.

139. Kellner CH, Rubinow DR, Gold PW, Post RM: Relationship of cortisol hypersecretion to brain CT scan alterations in depressed patients. Psychol Res 1983; 8:191–197.

140. Starkman MN, Gebarksi SS, Berent S, Schteingart DE: Hippocampal formation volume, memory dysfunction, and cortisol levels in patients with Cushing's syndrome. Biol Psychiatry 1992; 32:756–765.

141. Bremner JD, Randall P, Scott TM, Bronen RA, Seibyl JP, Southwick SM, Delaney RC, McCarthy G, Charney DS, Innis RB: MRI-based measurement of hippocampal volume in combat-related posttraumatic stress disorder. Am J Psychiatry 1995; 152:973–981.

142. Gloor P, Olivier A, Quesney LF, Andermann R, Horowitz S: The role of the limbic system in experiential phenomena of temporal lobe epilepsy. Ann Neurol 1982; 12:129–144.

143. Halgren E, Walter RD, Cherlow DG, Crandall PH: Mental phenomena evoked by electrical

stimulation of the human hippocampal formation and amygdala. Brain 1978; 101:83–117.

144. Krystal JH, Karper LP, Seibyl JP, Freeman GK, Delaney R, Bremner JD, Heninger GR, Bowers MB Jr, Charney DS: Subanesthetic effects of the noncompetitive NMDA antagonist, ketamine, in humans. Arch Gen Psychiatry 1944; 51:199–214.

145. Krystal JH, Bennett A, Bremner JD, Southwick SM, Charney DS: Toward a cognitive neuroscience of dissociation and altered memory functions in posttraumatic stress disorder. *In* MJ Friedman, DS Charney, AY Deutch (Eds.), Neurobiological and Clinical Consequences of Stress: From Normal Adaptation to PTSD. New York: Raven Press, pp. 239–269.

146. Steriade M, Datta S, Pare D, Oakson G, Curro Dossi R: Neuronal activities in brain-stem cholinergic nuclei related to tonic activation in thalamocortical systems. J Neurosci 1990; 19:2541–2559.

147. Llina RR, Pare D: Of dreaming and wakefulness. Neuroscience 1991; 44:521–535.

148. Chapman WP, Schroeder HR, Guyer G, Brazier MAB, Fager C, Poppen JL, Solomon HC, Yakolev PI: Physiological evidence concerning the importance of the amygdaloid nuclear region in the integration of circulating functions and emotion in man. Science 1954; 129:949–950.

149. Gunne LM, Reis DJ: Changes in brain catecholamines associated with electrical stimulation of amygdaloid nucleus. Life Sci 1963; 11:804–809.

150. Butler RW, Braff DL, Rausch JL, Jenkins MA, Sprock J, Geyer MA: Physiological evidence of exaggerated startle response in a subgroup of Vietnam veterans with combat-related PTSD. Am J Psychiatry 1990; 147:1308–1312.

151. Kolb LC: The post-traumatic stress disorder of combat: a subgroup with a conditioned emotional response. Mil Med 1984; 149(3):237–243.

152. Prins A, Kaloupek DG, Keane TM: Psychophysiological evidence for autonomic arousal and startle in traumatized adult populations. *In* MJ Friedman, DS Charney, AY Deutch (Eds.), Neurobiological and Clinical Consequences of Stress: From Normal Adaptation to PTSD. New York: Raven Press, 1995, pp. 291–314.

153. Blanchard EB, Kolb LC, Gerardi RJ, Ryan P, Pallmeyer TP: Cardiac response to relevant stimuli as an adjunctive tool for diagnosing post-traumatic stress disorder in Vietnam veterans. Behav Ther 1986; 17:592–606.

154. Malloy PF, Fairbank JA, Keane TM: Validation of a multimethod assessment of post-traumatic stress disorders in Vietnam veterans. J Consult Clin Psychol 1983; 51:488–494.

155. McFall ME, Murburg MM, Ko GN, Veith RC: Autonomic responses to stress in Vietnam combat veterans with posttraumatic stress disorder. Biol Psychiatry 1990; 27:1165–1175.

156. Pitman RK, Orr SP, Forgue DF, de Jong JB, Claiborn JM: Psychophysiologic assessment of posttraumatic stress disorder imagery in Vietnam combat veterans. Arch Gen Psychiatry 1987; 44:970–975.

157. Shalev AY, Orr SP, Peri T, Schreiber S, Pitman RK: Physiologic responses to loud tones in Israeli patients with posttraumatic stress disorder. Arch Gen Psychiatry 1992; 49:870–874.

158. McNally RJ, English GE, Lipke HJ: Assessment of intrusive cognition in PTSD: use of the modified Stroop paradigm. J Traumatic Stress 1993; 6:33–41.

159. Foa EB, Feske U, Murdock TB, Kozak MJ, McCarthy PR: Processing of threat-related information in rape victims. J Abnorm Psychol 1991; 100:156–162.

160. Cassiday KL, McNally RJ, Zeitlin SB: Cognitive processing of trauma cues in rape victims with posttraumatic stress disorder. Cogn Ther Res 1992; 16:283–295.

161. Goldensohn E: Structural lesions of the frontal lobe: manifestations, classification, and prognosis. *In* P Chauvel, AV Delgado-Escueta, E Halgren, J Bancaud (Eds.), Advances in Neurology. Vol. 57. New York: Raven Press, 1992, pp. 435–447.

162. Fornazzari L, Farcnik K, Smith I, Heasman GA, Ichise M: Violent visual hallucinations in frontal lobe dysfunction: clinical manifestations of deep orbitofrontal foci. J Neuropsychiatry Clin Neurosci 1992; 4:42–44.

163. Southwick SM, Krystal JH, Morgan CA, Johnson D, Nagy LM, Nicolaou A, Heninger GR, Charney DS: Abnormal noradrenergic function in posttraumatic stress disorder. Arch Gen Psychiatry 1993; 50:266–274.

164. Bremner JD, Innis RR, Ng CK, Staib L, Duncan J, Zubal G, Krystal JH, Rich D, Southwick SM, Capelli S, Dey H, Soufer R, Charney DS: PET measurement of cerebral metabolism following a noradrenergic challenge in patients with posttraumatic stress disorder and in healthy subjects. Arch Gen Psychiatry 1997 (in press).

165. Jarrell TW, Gentile CG, Romanski LM, McCabe PM, Schneiderman N: Involvement of cortical and thalamic auditory regions in retention of differential bradycardiac conditioning to acoustic conditioned stimuli in rabbits. Brain Res 1987; 412:285–294.

166. LeDoux JL: Emotional memory: in search of systems and synapses. Ann NY Acad Sci 1993, pp. 149–157.

167. Abercrombie ED, Keller RW Jr, Zigmond MJ: Characterization of hippocampal norepinephrine release as measured by microdialysis perfusion: pharmacological and behavioral studies. Neuroscience 1988; 27:897–904.

168. Bremner JD, Southwick SM, Johnson DR, Yehuda R, Charney DS: Childhood physical abuse in combat-related posttraumatic stress disorder. Am J Psychiatry 1993; 150:235–239.

169. Solomon Z, Garb R, Bleich A, Grupper D: Reactivation of combat-related posttraumatic stress disorder. Am J Psychiatry 1987; 144:51–55.

170. Bremner JD, Southwick SM, Charney DS: Etiologic factors in the development of posttraumatic stress disorder. *In* CM Mazure, (Ed.), Stress and Psychiatric Disorders. Washington, DC: American Psychiatric Press, 1994, pp. 149–186.

171. Bremner JD, Southwick SM, Brett E, Fontana A, Rosenheck R, Charney DS: Dissociation and posttraumatic stress disorder in Vietnam combat veterans. Am J Psychiatry 1992; 149:328–332.

172. Carlson EB, Rosser-Hogan R: Trauma experiences, posttraumatic stress, dissociation, and depression in Cambodian refugees. Am J Psychiatry 1991; 148:1548–1552.

173. Koopman C, Classen C, Spiegel D: Predictors of posttraumatic stress symptoms among survivors of the Oakland/Berkeley, Calif., firestorm. Am J Psychiatry 1994; 151:888–894.

174. Loewenstein RJ, Putnam F: A comparison study of dissociative symptoms in patients with partial-complex seizures, MPD, and PTSD. Dissociation 1988; 1:17–23.

175. Marmar CR, Weiss DS, Schlenger WE, Fairbank JA, Jordan BK, Kulka RA, Houg RL: Peritraumatic dissociation and posttraumatic stress in male Vietnam theater veterans. Am J Psychiatry 1994; 151:902–908.

176. Spiegel D, Hunt T, Dondershine HE: Dissociation and hypnotizability in posttraumatic stress disorder. Am J Psychiatry 1988; 145:301–305.

4

Inaccuracy and Inaccessibility in Memory Retrieval: Contributions from Cognitive Psychology and Neuropsychology

WILMA KOUTSTAAL
DANIEL L. SCHACTER

People depend on memory in countless facets of their everyday lives. Fortunately, human memory systems are capable of encoding and retrieving large amounts of reasonably accurate information about past events. But memory is far from perfect. We do not retain all that we experience; forgetting is a ubiquitous feature of memory. And not everything that we do remember is entirely accurate; memories often contain a degree of distortion. Our memories thus can fail because information is either lost or temporarily inaccessible, or because what is remembered does not correspond well to what actually happened.[1,2]

Both kinds of memory failure are highly relevant to recent debates about traumatic memory. On the one hand, people who have suffered sexual abuse or other traumatic experiences may be unable to remember those traumas at a later time. The forgotten traumas may be lost forever or may be temporarily inaccessible. How might such forgetting occur? How could people fail to remember highly significant experiences, and how might they recover such experiences after years or even decades have intervened? On the other hand, people may sometimes ''remember'' abusive experiences that never actually occurred. What accounts for the lack of correspondence between such distorted recollections and past reality? How might people come to believe that they had been subjected to painful, even horrific, abuse by trusted family members and

Preparation of this chapter was supported by National Institute on Aging Grant AG08441.

others in positions of authority and respect, if that abuse never actually occurred? Although these questions have generated considerable controversy,[3-7] there are good reasons to suppose that both the forgetting of actual abuse and illusory recollections of nonexistent abuse are real phenomena, each of which requires careful analysis and systematic study.[8]

In an effort to come to terms with these questions, clinicians, researchers, and others involved in this debate have turned to a number of different areas of research that might provide helpful concepts and relevant evidence. This chapter focuses on these two sets of questions with regard to the retrieval of normal or nontraumatic events. In examining results from empirical research in cognitive psychology and neuropsychology we ask: What factors—in the usual course of events—make it especially difficult to retrieve or to remember an event or stimulus? And what types of factors, again in the normal course of things, affect the correspondence between memory and reality, rendering it more or less likely that what we remember will be remembered accurately? Are there particular circumstances under which even memory of relatively neutral and simple stimuli or experiences is especially vulnerable to inaccuracy or distortion, or to inaccessibility and retrieval failure? To answer these questions, we will draw on studies that have used traditional laboratory methodologies, which typically involve encoding lists of words or pictures, and on more naturalistic investigations of autobiographical memories for everyday experiences.

The chapter is divided into two main sections. In the first section, we identify several broad, often interrelated, factors that may impede or prevent memory retrieval. Detrimental effects due to incongruent retrieval environments, interference arising from prior and subsequent learning, and the costs of simply not retrieving—or of intentionally forgetting—adequately encoded and processed information, are among the factors we review here. In the second section, we point to several broad factors that may contribute to memory distortion, including memory intrusions and false recognition. For example, a failure to recognize the source of one's experiences may result in various kinds of misattributions, including the ''mis-taking'' of imagined or self-generated occurrences for actually perceived events. Likewise, pragmatic or logical inferences concerning objects or events generated—on the basis of one's own general knowledge—at the time of initially encountering and comprehending a stimulus or event may later lead one to falsely recognize or recall those objects or events.

Throughout the two main sections, as well as in a briefer concluding section, we argue that both memory accessibility and memory accuracy are *multiply determined*. Whether individuals are able to gain conscious access to information that is at least potentially available in memory,[9] and whether the information that they access is retrieved ''correctly,'' or in a manner that corresponds to the original event or experience and with an awareness of its true source or origins, depends on a multitude of factors and conditions. Some of the more important of those conditions are outlined below.

Mechanisms or Sources of Inaccessibility

Absence of Sufficiently Informative Cues to Guide or Permit Retrieval

Conscious or deliberate retrieval of past experiences is actively guided by information that is currently in consciousness and by an individual's understanding of what it is she is seeking to remember. Several researchers (e.g., Ackerman,[10] Morton et al.,[11] and Norman and Bobrow[12]) have proposed that retrieval involves two phases: an initial stage in which one generates what is called a "description" or a representation of some of the critical features of the sought-for information, and a second phase involving access to the sought-for information. The likelihood of successful access to a given memory depends on two factors: the degree to which the description that is generated *matches critical features* that are present in the target memory, and the degree to which the description *uniquely specifies* that memory from among other similar memories.

The degree of "match" between a description and the features that are present in the memory trace might be conceptualized in various ways, and could be seen as varying along several dimensions. One important factor in determining the degree of match, however, is simply the amount of "overlap" between the features in the description and the features in memory.[13,14] If many attributes are common to both the initial encoding and the description (or more generally, the initial encoding and the entire retrieval context), there is a high degree of overlap; if relatively few attributes or features are common to both the original encoding context and the description (or retrieval context), then there is a low degree of overlap. From this perspective, it might be expected that, all else being equal, a retrieval situation that provides very little information to guide retrieval would be less likely to result in successful access than a retrieval situation that provides more information. Findings from both list-learning studies and from investigations of autobiographical memory provide support for this very rough (and thus far strictly quantitative) notion of "match."

The three types of tests most commonly used in list-learning studies to test intentional retrieval—free recall, cued recall, and recognition—under many conditions align themselves along a continuum such that retrieval is lowest with free recall, somewhat higher in cued recall, and highest in recognition. Whereas in free recall an individual is provided only with a broad specification of the temporal–spatial context surrounding the to-be-remembered item or event, both cued recall and recognition tests provide, in addition, some item-specific information—most commonly, parts of the particular targets that were presented during a study episode (cued recall) or the entire target item (recognition). This item-specific information may help to guide or focus retrieval, in some cases prompting retrieval of memories that would not have been retrieved spontaneously or independently. Note that although this item-specific information might itself have been part of the original event, such as a word or picture from a larger set of items that was presented earlier, it need not be. For example, if subjects had studied a set of pictures drawn from several semantic categories, such as types of furniture, fruits, and tools, the recall cues might consist of the names of the categories of items that were studied even if these had never been presented when subjects first encountered the pictures.

A more naturalistic investigation of autobiographical memory by Wagenaar[15] also provides support for the notion that with regard to retrieval cues (and again, all else being equal), more extensive cuing is better than less. Wagenaar initially recorded one or two life events per day for a period of several years, for each incident recording who was involved, what happened, where it happened, and when. He later attempted to recall the items, cuing himself with only one of these types of cues or a combination of two or three of the cues (e.g., who and what but not where or when, or what, where, and when but not who). Combining across retention intervals ranging from as brief as 6 months to as long as 6 years, he found that he remembered more with an increasing number of cues: retrieval in the presence of triple cues exceeded that for double cues, which in turn exceeded that for single cues.

One reason why the provision of more cuing information may allow retrieval where less information was insufficient is that more extensive information is also to some degree positively correlated with how *distinctive* the cues are. Roughly speaking, distinctiveness refers to the number of to-be-remembered items that can be subsumed under a given retrieval cue: a cue that is low in distinctiveness does not strongly or uniquely specify a to-be-remembered item but instead is congruent with either many to-be-remembered items or with many items that the individual knows from contexts other than the relevant context. Distinctiveness is therefore sometimes conceptualized in terms of how many items are mapped to a particular retrieval cue, with fewer mappings corresponding to greater distinctiveness. If too many items can be mapped to a given retrieval cue, the cue is said to be "overloaded,"[16,17] meaning that its functional cuing power or effectiveness is not very great. Whereas an overloaded cue is likely to provide only a weak and diffuse guide to retrieval, a highly distinctive cue is likely to provide stronger and more focused retrieval guidance.

One way to increase cue distinctiveness is to tailor cues to conform to each subject's own (sometimes idiosyncratic) learning history with regard to the to-be-remembered material. An experiment employing this approach in an incidental learning task—that is, a situation in which subjects are not told that their memory will be tested but in which they encounter the material "incidentally," usually under the guise of some other required activity—provides a dramatic illustration of how distinctive cues can influence accessibility.[18] Subjects were visually presented with 600 words (nouns), with one of two kinds of instructions. Half of the subjects were asked to generate one property for each word that, according to their own experience, comprised an appropriate description of the target item. The remaining subjects were asked to generate three such properties for each word. After presentation of the words (which took approximately 4.5 hours!) subjects were unexpectedly given the properties that they had generated and asked to use these (self-generated, idiosyncratic) descriptions as retrieval cues to help recall the words in response to which the properties had originally been generated. Subjects who were asked to generate three properties for each word and were given these three properties as retrieval cues demonstrated a remarkably high level of retention: they recalled an average of 90% of the 600 words. Subjects who were asked to generate only one property per word recalled considerably fewer words, but even these single, self-provided retrieval cues yielded a surprisingly high retention rate, with an average of 62% of the words recalled.

Mismatch of Encoding and Retrieval Contexts

Mismatch of Intrinsic Semantic Context

The examples considered thus far have involved primarily quantitative considerations of the sufficiency or amount of cue information that is available to permit or guide retrieval. But there is a further question that is equally important: holding the amount of cue information constant, what effect does the *relation* between the information that was encoded and the information present in the retrieval context have upon the likelihood of recall or recognition? Another experiment[18] that again employed the characterizations that subjects themselves provided in response to the studied stimuli, but where the subject was later given either her own characterizations or the properties that were generated by another subject as retrieval cues, begins to address this question. The properties that individuals had themselves generated were clearly more effective than those generated by someone else. For example, subjects given the three properties that they themselves had generated recalled 91% of the items during immediate testing whereas subjects given three properties that had been generated by someone else recalled only about 55% of the items.

This decrement in the amount that subjects recalled when they were given the properties generated by another subject as retrieval cues rather than the properties that they themselves had generated illustrates the costs of a mismatch between the *intrinsic semantic context* of an item at study and its context during attempted retrieval.[14] *Intrinsic semantic context* refers to aspects that are important to the meaning of the stimulus itself, that is, to how the stimulus is interpreted or conceptualized.[19] Although each of the subjects was presumably following instructions when he generated properties for the nouns that were presented, the attributes or characteristics that any one subject, based on his experience, believed to comprise appropriate descriptions of the target items would not entirely match or fit the attributes or characteristics that seemed to be apt to another subject. Mismatches between the properties that a given subject had observed and generated for himself and the properties that another subject had generated would tend to more or less severely mislead subjects in their attempt to recall the nouns.

The importance of intrinsic semantic context has also been demonstrated under conditions where the experimenter provides the semantic context during initial acquisition and then manipulates that context during retrieval. For example, subjects who are first presented with nouns accompanied by a particular adjective (e.g., ''soda cracker'') are less likely to recognize those nouns if they are accompanied by a different adjective that changes its meaning (e.g., "graham cracker") or if the nouns are simply presented alone, without their previously accompanying adjectives, than if precisely the same adjectival context as was initially present is again present during recognition testing.[20] Largely similar results have been observed with words that are associatively related (e.g., "love–hate"),[21] and with photographs of faces. Subjects who first encountered photographs of male–female "couples" (the photographs were, in fact, randomly paired individuals of roughly comparable ages) with instructions to rate each pair for perceived marital compatibility were later significantly more likely to recognize the photographs of these individuals if they were accompanied by the same partner as was present during their first encounter with the item, than if the photographs were presented with no partner or with a different partner than at study.[22]

Mismatch of Intrinsic Physical Context

Sensory and perceptual aspects of a stimulus that are necessarily processed simply by virtue of attending to the stimulus, but that do not influence the meaning or interpretation of the stimulus, can be construed as a form of intrinsic *physical* context. For example, in order to read a type-written word, we will process information concerning the type of font in which the word is printed even though, ordinarily, the particular font that is employed will not affect how we interpret the word. Considering this type of intrinsic physical context, it has often (though not always) been found that subjects attempting to consciously or explicitly remember an event do not benefit from a reinstatement of the exact physical features of the stimulus that were present during initial encoding (or stated conversely, there is little or no decrement in performance as a function of mismatch on this type of intrinsic physical context). For example, subjects' level of cued recall has been found to be essentially identical regardless of whether the cues are presented in the same voice or in a different voice than at study,[23] and recognition memory was unaffected by changing the stimulus modality (visual or auditory) from study to test[24] (see Hayman and Rickards[24] for review). This contrasts with the situation when memory is tested implicitly, with indirect methods in which conscious recollection of the prior study episode is not required. Here changes in the intrinsic physical features of the stimulus often result in decreased facilitation from prior exposure,[23,25,26] although even in this case not all types of changes are detrimental (see Schacter[27] for discussion).

Mismatch of Extrinsic Physical Context

Physical reinstatement.
Extrinsic physical context might be seen as comprised of the sensory and perceptual characteristics of the encoding environment that are relatively more peripheral or extrinsic to the target information itself,[19] such as features concerning the particular room

in which a list of words was learned, the time at which it was learned, or what the experimenter was wearing. Although these kinds of sensory and perceptual details do not, strictly speaking, need to be processed in order to perceive the target stimuli, and may be processed largely independently of the targets, to the degree that these features *are* processed and stored, they may contribute to a greater or lesser degree of overlap between features in the encoding and retrieval environments. Thus physically reinstating some of these features during retrieval might be expected to enhance memory accessibility over that observed when reinstatement does not occur.

The advantage shown in memory performance when encoding and retrieval contexts are the same compared to when they are different has been termed the *context-dependency effect*. Context effects on free recall performance can be of considerable magnitude (see Smith[28] for review). For example, in a classic study by Godden and Baddeley,[29] the subjects, who were scuba divers, learned lists of words either on land or while under water. Testing also took place either on land or underwater, with subjects either tested in the same environment as during initial learning or in the opposite environment. Subjects who experienced a mismatch between the learning and testing environment recalled approximately 40% fewer words than subjects for whom the learning and testing environments were the same. A replication of this study using a yes/no recognition test in which the studied words were embedded among an equal number of nonstudied distractor items did not find such a context-dependency effect[19] (but also see Canas and Nelson[30]).

The degree to which free recall may be facilitated by the reinstatement of physical context may be moderated by other factors, however. For example, in a study of list learning, Smith[31] found that whereas free recall showed the usual contextual reinstatement effect when initial learning occurred in only one room, no context-dependency effect was observed when learning occurred in three different rooms and subjects were tested in either one of those three rooms, or in a totally different room. One-room same-context subjects recalled 42% more words than one-room different-context subjects, but the recall performance of multiple-room same-context subjects and multiple-room different-context subjects did not differ. These findings seem to indicate that contextual change during learning may help to ''immunize''[31] material from the detrimental effects of contextual change at test, making the target information less contextually bound.

Mental reinstatement.

Might the benefits obtained through the physical reinstatement of context also be obtained if that reinstatement occurs *mnemonically,* through a deliberate attempt to remember the context, rather than perceptually (through physical reinstatement of the context)? At least two alternatives seem possible here.[32] On the one hand, it is possible that the physical reinstatement of a context cues the individual's mental representation of the context, thereby making contextual associations more available; without the physical reinstatement, there may be less ''support'' for the retrieval of the encoding context, and thus contextual associations will be less accessible. This suggests that mental reinstatement would be less effective than physical reinstatement. On the other hand, it is possible that individuals who are in a physically different retrieval environment from that in which they were at study are equally capable of accessing the study context (and contextual associations) as those who are present in the same environment, but that individuals in a different context are simply less likely to adopt this as a strategy. This suggests that the mnemonic disadvantage arising from a different retrieval context could be overcome by instructing subjects to mentally reinstate the context.

List-learning studies have provided evidence consistent with each of these possibilities.[32,33] The latter (equally capable but less likely) alternative has been supported when subjects learned materials in only one encoding context and then were tested in that same context or in a different context. Subjects tested in a different room from that in which they had encountered the study materials a day earlier, showed essentially equivalent levels of free recall as shown by subjects who were tested in the same room as at encoding when either of two forms of mental reinstatement were encouraged: simply thinking back to the acquisition room by trying to recall objects, sounds, feelings, and so on from the original context, or thinking back in this manner plus viewing slides of the original room. In contrast, when subjects were tested in the different room without mental reinstatement instructions, or with instructions to think of another room that was completely unrelated to that in which the list was originally learned, the usual decrement in recall due to the changed context was observed. However, physical reinstatement proved superior to mental reinstatement when multiple contexts (several different rooms) were present during acquisition, possibly because under these conditions the contexts themselves were more difficult to remember.

The technique of mental reinstatement has also been the object of considerable research in investigations of eyewitness memory. For example, Malpass and Devine[34] used an extensive guided interview to help witnesses reinstate the events and general context of a staged vandalism that they had witnessed 5 months earlier. The interview encouraged subjects to recall their feelings and immediate reactions as well as their memory of the room, the vandal, and the events that had occurred. Witnesses given the guided memory instructions were more likely to correctly identify the vandal from a photographic lineup (60% correct identifications) than were witnesses given only simple choice instructions without mental reinstatement (40% correct identifications).

Encouraging witnesses to try to reevoke both the environmental context and the personal context that was present during a crime is also an important component in the cognitive interviewing schedule developed by Geiselman, Fisher, and colleagues to enhance eyewitness memory.[35–38] Compared with standard interviewing procedures, the cognitive interview has been found to increase the number of correct items that witnesses retrieve concerning simulated violent crimes without increasing the number of incorrect items.[35,36] Instructing eyewitnesses to mentally reinstate the environmental and personal context present during the crime is one of four general retrieval strategies (or retrieval mnemonics) included in the cognitive interview. Instructions in this strategy alone led to significantly higher levels of recall than when no instructions were given. However, encouraging both mental reinstatement and complete reporting (another of the general retrieval strategies in which subjects are instructed to report all of the details they can remember, even if they are incomplete or seem unimportant) led to significantly more correct responses than either alone.[36]

Nonetheless, as with list-learning studies, caution is necessary in making broad generalizations as to the effectiveness of mental reinstatement of context. For example, one study used a variant of the cognitive interviewing schedule that included, in addition to the usual components, a requirement that subjects review written descriptions of the event (a robbery) that they had provided immediately after watching the videotaped event as well as a series of photographs of the scene of the crime. Contextual reinstatement enhanced identification accuracy only when the robber had been disguised, but had little effect when the robber was not disguised.[39] Similarly, Geiselman and colleagues[35] found that the cognitive interview format was superior to a standard interview procedure only for two of the crime scenarios that they used (a bank robbery and a liquor store holdup) but not for two other scenarios (a family dispute and a search through a warehouse). Inasmuch as the robbery and holdup scenarios tended to portray several events occurring simultaneously and at a rapid pace, whereas the dispute and search scenarios portrayed more sequentially occurring events at a relatively slower pace, it appears that context reinstatement might be relatively more beneficial when information was poorly encoded initially (e.g., due to the presence of a disguise in the former study, or the rapid and concurrent events in the latter study) than when information is more adequately encoded initially (e.g., no disguise, or less rapidly occurring events).[28,40,41]

Mismatch of Internal Subjective and Physiological Environment

In addition to semantic and physical attributes, the ensemble of attributes that comprises a memory may include features relating to an individual's internal subjective state, for example, affective and evaluative responses, and aspects concerning the individual's internal physiological environment. These attributes are important to state-dependent memory, where recall is enhanced by inducing a subjective or physiological state at retrieval that matches the state that was present at encoding (for reviews see Blaney[42] and Eich[43,44]). As with other forms of mismatch, the consequences of mismatch on internal subjective factors tend to be more strongly manifested in free recall than in cued recall or recognition. Also, the degree to which state-dependent effects are observed may depend on the nature of the to-be-retrieved event, particularly whether it is internally or externally generated.[45,46] Internally generated events, or events produced by the subject's own thinking, reasoning, and imagining, may be more closely associated with, and affected by, the subject's mood and general internal state than are external events, with the consequence that incongruencies of mood and the like between encoding the retrieval contexts would have a greater adverse effect on internally generated events than external events.

To the extent that this latter point is true, it may reflect a more general pattern, noted by Baddeley,[47,48] that context dependency tends to be greater when a stimulus and contextual information are encoded *interactively* rather than *independently*. In interactive encoding the context actually changes the way in which the stimulus is perceived (as when one's thoughts or imaginings are likely to be perceived differently depending on one's mood). In contrast, contextual information that is processed independently or noninteractively is encoded and stored with the stimulus but does not alter the way that the stimulus is perceived. Baddeley[19,47,48] has suggested that this distinction may help to reconcile conflicting findings concerning whether context effects are obtained in recognition: context effects in recognition occur when subjects interrelate a stimulus and its context in a meaningful way (e.g., as when subjects in the experiment by Winograd and Rivers-Bulkeley[22] were encouraged to assume that the photographs of individuals presented side by side were of married couples, or with the noun–adjective pairs in the ''soda cracker'' study), but are less likely to occur when a stimulus and its context have little semantic bearing upon one another (e.g., whether a list of words is presented under water or on land, as in the experiment of Godden and Baddeley[19]). Because interactive encoding of contextual information alters what is learned, its reinstatement during retrieval is beneficial in guiding the subject back to the interpretation of the stimulus that occurred initially, and this may help recognition. In contrast, reinstatement of contextual information that was encoded independently will not alter the interpretation of the stimulus. Nonetheless, even the reinstatement of independently encoded context may facilitate recall by changing the area in memory that is likely to be searched, thereby increasing the likelihood of accessing a trace.[48]

Mismatch of Subjective Organization and Retrieval Plans

Under free recall conditions, individuals do not engage in random retrieval of the to-be-remembered items; rather, items are often retrieved in meaningful sequences, showing associative clustering,[49] category clustering (e.g., recalling animal names separately[50]), temporal grouping,[51,52] or more subjective forms of organization that derive from the individual's attempts to actively process and retrieve information.[53] Thus one could imagine situations in which the purported retrieval cues provided in cued recall might disrupt the forms of organization and associative thinking that would otherwise naturally occur under free recall conditions. Further, if the detrimental effects of this mismatch between the retrieval cues and the individual's subjective organization or retrieval plan were not entirely offset or compensated for by the benefits derived from the additional information provided in the retrieval cues, a person might even retrieve less information with the cues than without them.

An experiment using the misleading question paradigm[54] that is often used to investigate eyewitness memory provides an example of the harmful effects of this type of mismatch on memory accessibility—and also on memory accuracy. Many studies that have shown detrimental effects of misleading post-event information on observers' memory have presented the test items used to probe memory in a *random* order. Bekerian and Bowers[55] hypothesized that randomly ordering the items during testing might make various cues concerning the overall theme of the incident, its setting and context, and its place in a larger episodic structure less salient or explicit than would otherwise be the case, thereby misleading subjects into a less-than-optimal retrieval strategy. Consistent with this hypothesis were their findings that a markedly greater proportion of subjects given inconsistent post-event information responded incorrectly to a critical item when the test items were presented in a random order (40%) than when the test items were presented sequentially (13%). Indeed, the latter proportion was very similar to that shown by subjects who were given consistent post-event information. Encouraging subjects to try to recall events in a systematic temporal order (either from earlier events to later events or vice versa) is also one of the retrieval mnemonics used in the cognitive interviewing schedule, and it may contribute to the enhanced eyewitness accounts obtained with that technique[37] (cf. Mismatch of Extrinsic Physical Context above).

The possibility that the cues present in the retrieval environment might fit uncomfortably with an individual's spontaneous or learned manner of organizing to-be-remembered information, and so impair access to that information, has also been postulated as a potential culprit in a counterintuitive finding known as the *part-set cuing effect*. This counterintuitive finding is that providing some of the items from a larger set of to-be-remembered items, allegedly as hints or cues to facilitate retrieval of the remaining members of the set, sometimes has the opposite effect, such that significantly fewer of the to-be-remembered items are produced when the cues are present than when they are absent. Inhibitory effects due to part-set cuing have been observed both in list-learning studies, in which subjects attempt to recall words from a recently studied list either with or without some of the words from that list as alleged cues,[56-59] and in studies of long-term semantic memory, in which individuals attempt to recall well-learned information, such as the names of the states or counties of their native country, with or without some of the items from the to-be-remembered set as cues.[60,61]

One possible account of these inhibitory effects on retrieval is that presenting the part-set cues either immediately prior to recall or during recall itself leads individuals to adopt a retrieval framework that is incongruent with the subjective framework that they employed during initial exposure. To the extent that the provided cues capture an individual's attention and encourage her to adopt an organizational framework that is different from or incongruent with the organizational schemes she adopted during study, retrieval may be impeded.

Support for an organizational account of part-set cuing inhibition[62,63] has been found both in list-learning studies and in studies of semantic memory. For example, in one study[64] subjects studied a list of common words and then were presented with half of those items as part-set cues, either in a random order relative to the order in which they had been studied or in an order that was congruent with the study list order (every second item presented sequentially). Significant inhibition was observed only with the randomly ordered cues. Similarly, a comparison of subjects' recall of items from long-term memory (the names of U.S. states) under conditions of part-set cuing with a measure of the preexperimental retrieval probabilities of those items showed that part-set cuing altered the priority with which items tended be recalled. If the part-set cues were comprised of the names of states that were highly likely to be recalled under free recall conditions (as determined preexperimentally for the population that was being studied), then these high-probability items were even more likely to occur in the first half of subjects' protocols than would otherwise have been the case. However, if the part-set cues were comprised of states that had an initially low-recall probability in the preexperimental sample, then the output dominance of the high-recall probability items was decreased—now these items were less likely than usual to occur in the first half of subjects' protocols than would otherwise have been the case[61] (cf. Brown and Hall[65]).

Presence of Competing (Inordinately Dominant) Retrieval Cues

Might providing some items from a larger set of to-be-remembered items make those items in some sense too strong, so that they block or impede access to the other items? For example, might the part-set cues bias the meaning or associative context that is present at retrieval (cf. Anderson and Bjork[66] and Mismatch of Intrinsic Semantic Context above), making it more difficult to retrieve noncued items that lie outside of that semantic context? Or might the provided and nonprovided items directly compete with one another in some way, so that increasing the likelihood of retrieving some items from the list actually decreases the likelihood of retrieving other items?

Several studies also provide support for a dominance or competition-at-retrieval account of part-set cuing.[57–59] According to one such account,[58] the initial likelihood of retrieving a particular item depends on two factors. One factor concerns the relationship of various retrieval cues (semantic, associative, or other subgroupings of items) to a higher-order spatiotemporal or contextual representation of the entire list of to-be-remembered items; the second factor concerns the relationship of specific list items to these retrieval cues. The probability that a given item (X) will be accessed depends both on how strongly X is associated with its own retrieval cue and on how strongly that retrieval cue is associated with the higher-order contextual representation of the whole list. More specifically, the likelihood of accessing X, given that one has accessed its retrieval cue, is equal to the strength of the association of X to the cue, divided by the sum of strengths of association of all items to that cue. This so-called ratio rule also governs the relationship between the retrieval cues and the general list cue. The account makes two further assumptions. First, it is assumed that retrieving an item strengthens the association between that item and the retrieval cue. Second, it is assumed that retrieval occurs with replacement, such that recall attempts may sometimes yield already retrieved items. This combination of hypotheses leads to the expectation that retrieval of a word should increase its own probability of retrieval and at the same time reduce the probability that other words associated with the same retrieval cue will be recalled. Consistent with this expectation, findings have shown that whereas the provision of a single cue or the name of a category often facilitates retrieval of items within that category, providing additional instances within a given category often has an *inhibitory* effect on the retrieval of the remaining items in the category, with this inhibitory effect tending to be stronger, the greater the proportion of provided instances.[57-59] Also, even when facilitation occurs for the cued categories, inhibition of the noncued categories may be observed.[67]

More generally, the presence of retrieval blocks in semantic memory, such as the tip-of-the-tongue phenomenon, has often been found to be associated with competitive interlopers.[68] Words that are similar to the sought-for item but which, for various reasons, may be more dominant than the target, tend to interfere with retrieval of the desired item. For example, based on diary reports of instances of retrieval blocks in everyday life, Reason and Lucas[69] found that between 50% and 70% of the instances reported involved what they (after Cinderella's less fair but more dominant older sisters) termed *an ugly sister*—a word or name other than the target that was known to be wrong but that kept recurring in a tenacious and intrusive fashion. The diarists judged that these intrusive items had been encountered more recently, and more frequently, than either the targets or other words that did *not* block retrieval; ugly sisters were also judged to be more highly associated with the target than were nonblocking words. Whereas these instances of blocked recall were most often overcome through some *external* factor (e.g., accidentally hearing or seeing the target, or asking another person), instances that did not involve an ugly sister were more often overcome by *internal* strategies (e.g., forming an image or recalling contextual information). Overall, about 50% of the tip-of-the-tongue states were alleviated through a search procedure, about 25% involved external prompting of some form, and about 25% involved spontaneous retrieval of the sought-for information.

Termination of Active Retrieval Attempts

Attempts to actively search memory do not usually continue indefinitely. Researchers have postulated that active memory search is sometimes curtailed, even though sought-for items have not yet been retrieved because, after some unspecified number of consecutive trials have yielded no new information, a termination or stopping rule is activated.[58,61] Yet, given that the accessibility of memories varies—sometimes in an upward direction—it might be that if active retrieval efforts were continued, access to additional items would be attained.

One way to examine the effects of termination of active retrieval attempts is to give subjects repeated tests for the same information, without reexposing them to the originally studied information. Researchers using this repeated test approach can track two kinds of events: the number of items that are not recalled on one trial but which are recalled on subsequent trials (item *gains*) and the number of items that are recalled on early trials but that are not recalled on later trials (item *losses*). They can also examine the relation between these two types of events at an *overall* level, asking if, overall, item gains exceed item losses. Instances where individual items that were not present on an earlier trial are retrieved on a later trial have been designated by the term *reminiscence*; cases in which there are item gains of this form and the overall level of such gains exceeds the overall level of item losses, resulting in a *net increase* in the level of recall over trials, have been designated as *hypermnesia*.[70]

List-learning studies involving repeated testing without reexposure to the original information have convincingly demonstrated that both reminiscence and hypermnesia often occur (see Erdelyi,[71] Payne,[72] and Payne and Wenger[73] for reviews). Although initially it appeared that hypermnesia could be observed only with pictorial materials,[70] subsequent researchers have also reported hypermnesia with verbal materials, including both lists of words[74,75] and prose passages.[76] This net gain in the number of items recalled across successive tests is often accompanied by an increase in the rate or speed with which the information is recalled, with items that were recalled on one test tending to be retrieved more quickly on subsequent tests. This finding shows the benefits of retrieval strengthening for these items (cf. section on disuse below), but it also has implications for the nonretrieved items because more rapid access to already retrieved items allows additional time to attempt retrieval of hitherto unrecalled items.[75,77,78]

Recent work has shown that an important factor in determining whether hypermnesia will be observed is the length of the retention interval between tests. Generally speaking, when the intervals between successive tests are brief (on the order of minutes), a net improvement, or hypermnesia is found, but when the intervals are long (on the order of 1 week), a net loss (overall forgetting) is seen.[76] Recent work in which subjects' self-efficacy expectancies about their memory abilities were manipulated through the use of false feedback has also pointed to the possible role of motivational factors in producing hypermnesia. Whereas subjects who had been given false feedback indicating exceptionally good memory performance showed a rate of forgetting (item losses) across recall attempts that was very similar to that of subjects who were given no feedback, they *gained* more items than did individuals given no feedback and therefore showed greater hypermnesia.[79]

Within the domain of autobiographical memory research, there is anecdotal evidence which suggests that attempts at retrieval may be terminated at a point that could underestimate the amount of information in memory that might eventually have become accessible had the duration of the search been extended. For example, both Wagenaar[15] and Williams and Santos-Williams[80] pointed to the often strenuous and tiring nature of attempts to search autobiographical memory, with the former researcher observing that he himself found the process of attempting long-term retrieval ''somewhat torturous'' and the latter investigators making an essentially similar remark on behalf of their subjects[80] (also see Whitten and Leonard[81]).

The work of Williams and colleagues[80,82] also illustrates both the potentially positive consequences (increased recovery of valid memories) and the likely hazards (increased intrusion of invalid memories) of an especially extended and intensive effort to remember information from one's past. The subjects—four female adults who had been out of high school for from 4 to 19 years—were asked to think aloud as they attempted to recall the first and last names of their classmates from high school. Subjects' retrieval attempts were tape recorded and continued for several hours over many weeks in sessions of approximately 1 hour. Over the course of the experiment, the number of correct names that were retrieved continued to increase; however the occurrence of incorrect names (fabrications) also increased with continued attempts at recollection. (Correct names were verified by reference to subjects' high school yearbooks for their senior year and during debriefing at the conclusion of the experiment.) The variability in both the level of accurate recall and of fabrications is noteworthy. Hit rates ranged from as low as 12% (Subject 3) to as high as 35% (Subject 1), and the ratio of hits to intrusions from as low as 1.5 to 1 (Subject Three, 4 years out of high school with a graduating class of 750 members who, across ten sessions, recalled 93 correct names and gave 69 fabrications) to the extreme where intrusions actually exceeded correct recalls (Subject Four, 19 years out of high school, with a graduating class of 318 members who, across six sessions, recalled 83 correct names and gave 90 fabrications). Clearly, the outcome of continued efforts to remember was neither uniform across subjects nor uniformly positive within subjects.

Interference

Several of the factors that have been discussed in the preceding sections might also be conceptualized as demonstrations of interference phenomena, that is, as illustrations of how engaging in activities or tasks of various kinds, including other memory activities, may adversely affect a target memory, rendering it less accessible and/or less accurate than it might otherwise have been. For example, the inhibitory effects observed in the part-set cuing paradigm could be viewed as a manifestation of *retroactive interference*—that is, as a case where later learning retroactively interferes with earlier learning. However, unlike many, more typical, manifestations of retroactive interference where the interfering information consists of new information that is highly similar to the originally learned material, in this case, the retroactive interference derives from the presentation of material that is actually part of the originally learned material.[61] The misleading question paradigm used to investigate eyewitness testimony likewise comprises an example of retroactive interference.

Instances of *proactive interference*, that is, situations where earlier learning interferes proactively with the learning and/or retrieval of information acquired at a later point in time, are also possible. If, for example, subjects are asked to study several sets of words, with each set first followed by a brief period of distractor activity and then by a recall test of the words for the immediately preceding trial, their recall performance across trials typically rapidly declines: they recall fewer items on the second trial than on the first trial, fewer still on the third trial, and so on.[83,84] If, however, the semantic content of the to-be-remembered words is suddenly shifted (e.g., from one taxonomic category to another, or from words with primarily positive evaluative connotations to words that are primarily negative), recall performance on the shift trial is restored to almost the same level as on the first trial. Changes in the physical features of the to-be-remembered items (such as word length or the colors of the slides on which the words are presented) tend to have a much less pronounced effect.[85]

Both the initial decrement in recall performance (reflecting a buildup of proactive interference or inhibition) and the sudden improvement in performance (reflecting a release from proactive interference or inhibition) have been conceived as due to the similarity of the to-be-remembered items. This may in turn be conceptualized as yet another demonstration of the important role played by cue distinctiveness or cue overload effects in determining the likelihood and ease with which items can be recalled (cf. Absence of Sufficiently Informative Cues to Guide or Permit Retrieval, above): the to-be-remembered items following a shift in meaning might be viewed as mapped to retrieval cues that are less weighted down by previous (and now irrelevant) items than was true for the items prior to the shift.

Consistent with such an account is the observation that release from proactive inhibition does not necessarily depend on subjects' being aware at the time of initially encountering or encoding the material that a shift has occurred, but such awareness at the time of retrieval does seem to be necessary.[86,87] Although most often demonstrated using simple verbal materials such as digits[88] or words,[89] the buildup and release from proactive inhibition has also been observed with more complex stimulus materials, such as television news items (involving, for example, a shift from news items dealing with home politics to items concerning foreign politics, or from politics to sports), and both under immediate recall and delayed recall conditions.[90,91] There is also evidence that the detrimental effects on retrieval accessibility due to proactive interference can be reduced through designating earlier learned materials as ''to-be-forgotten''[92–95] (also see the discussion of directed or instructed forgetting below).

Disuse: Limited Retrieval Capacity and the Costs of Lack of Retrieval Strengthening

The critical importance of the act of retrieving information in determining the future accessibility of that information has been demonstrated repeatedly and across a wide variety of materials and methods, ranging from studies of semantic memory[96] to autobiographical memory[97,98] to list-learning studies of hypermnesia and part-set cuing (see discussion of retrieval cues and attempts above). Recalling an item at one time increases the likelihood that it will be recalled at a later time, with the benefits derived from repeated retrievals being greatest if they take the form of an expanding rehearsal procedure: initial retrievals occurring relatively more closely together in time and subsequent retrievals occurring at increasingly longer intervals.[96]

However, recalling some information but not other information that is associated with the same cue or cues also places the nonretrieved information at greater risk of being forgotten. At least three different (not necessarily independent) accounts of how this increased risk might come about have already been considered. Recalling some items associated with a given retrieval cue but not others (particularly if recall is prompted by externally provided cues) may (*a*) disrupt retrieval organization, thereby rendering nonrecalled items less accessible; (*b*) lead to the retrieval-strengthened items becoming inordinately dominant, thereby blocking the retrieval of associated items; or (*c*) make successive retrieval attempts less likely to yield new, as-yet-unretrieved items, and so result in a termination of active search.

Recent work by Michael Anderson and colleagues,[99,100] in which a retrieval practice paradigm was used, has suggested that yet still another factor, involving the inhibition or suppression of related information, might also be operative. They found that retrieval practice on some items from a particular category of studied items (e.g., fruit) improved recall of those items on a subsequent test, but often at the expense or cost of the unpracticed items. More importantly, this cost to the unpracticed items was observed even when the test was structured so as to provide highly specific retrieval cues for the unpracticed items (e.g., if "orange" was an unpracticed item, subjects might be given "fruit or___" as a cue). Further, under these conditions, the cost to the unpracticed items was greatest when the unpracticed items were strongly associated to the category cue; if the unpracticed items were only weakly associated to the category cue, little inhibition (or even slight facilitation) was observed. These findings suggest that, at least under some circumstances, the impairment of nonretrieved items following retrieval strengthening of other items arises from a process of suppression in which competitors for access to retrieval are inhibited, with stronger competitors (those more likely to gain access to retrieval resources) being more strongly suppressed than their weaker (and less potentially interfering) counterparts.

Directed (Instructed) Forgetting

The notion that individuals might intentionally or voluntarily try to forget certain materials, particularly those of an unpleasant sort, is perhaps one of the most familiar potential sources of memory inaccessibility. Although most likely conceived of as falling within the research domains of personality and psychopathology, intentional or voluntary forgetting has, in fact, also been subject to considerable investigation in cognitive psychology and social psychology (for reviews see Bjork,[101,102] Johnson, [103] and Kihlstrom and Barnhardt[104]). Cognitive psychologists have been interested in the outcome of designating some (usually neutral) information as *to-be-forgotten* and other information as *to-be-remembered,* for a variety of reasons. These range from efforts to determine the degree to which individuals can successfully segregate different kinds of information in memory, by selectively rehearsing, elaborating, and retrieving only the to-be-remembered items, to efforts to determine whether designating some information as irrelevant may result in the actual suppression or inhibition of that information.

A factor that has emerged as particularly important in determining whether individuals can effectively forget stimuli which (at least allegedly) are no longer relevant concerns the manner in which the individual is told that some stimuli can be forgotten. If individuals are presented with both to-be-remembered items and to-be-forgotten items in an intermixed fashion, with the instruction to either remember or to forget given soon after they have encountered each item, their subsequent ability to remember the to-be-forgotten items is impaired, often quite dramatically. Several considerations suggest that, under these conditions, individuals encode the to-be-forgotten items less well than the to-be-remembered items, less often rehearsing and semantically elaborating upon these items than on items that are designated to-be-remembered. The magnitude of the difference in memory performance for the to-be-remembered and to-be-forgotten items, its clear emergence on both recall tests and during recognition testing, as well as subjects' post-experimental accounts of how they approached the task, all point to preferential encoding and elaboration of the to-be-remembered items as a likely and substantial contributing factor[105–107] (see Johnson[103] for review).

In an alternative approach to directed forgetting, individuals first study an entire set or block of items and only then—quite unexpectedly—are told that those items are practice items and so can be forgotten. This approach, too, yields evidence of reduced accessibility of the to-be-forgotten items. However, evidence for impaired access to the to-be-forgotten material under this directed forgetting procedure generally emerges only on recall tests and not in recognition, and the difference between to-be-remembered and to-be-forgotten items is often of a smaller magnitude than under the first procedure. Although the directed forgetting effects observed under this alternative approach are in some respects less dramatic, they are also more theoretically challenging. Whereas encoding factors might, in a few instances, contribute to an advantage of to-be-remembered items over to-be-forgotten items even under this procedure, here most of the evidence points to factors that are operative at retrieval rather than encoding. One reason to believe that the locus of the forgetting effect under this procedure is primarily at retrieval involves the nature of the task itself. Individuals are unaware that some items will be designated as to-be-forgotten until some time after they have encountered the stimuli, at which time they have already exerted strong efforts to remember those same items. A second reason to posit a retrieval-based account is that impaired performance on the forget-cued items is found only under retrieval conditions that involve little or no re-exposure to the to-be-forgotten items,[105–109] such as free recall, but not under retrieval conditions where portions of the to-be-forgotten information are also re-encountered, such as during recognition testing.

Although the precise retrieval mechanisms that lead to impaired access to the to-be-forgotten items under this second procedure are still unclear, it appears that this decreased accessibility may be of a quite diffuse or general form, not only reducing an individual's ability to access the to-be-forgotten information itself, but also more general spatial–temporal contextual information associated with the to-be-forgotten stimuli. Geiselman, Bjork, and Fishman[110] found that subjects were especially inaccurate at remembering when the to-be-forgotten items that they produced during free recall had occurred (in the first or second block of study items). In a recent experiment in our laboratory, we found a largely parallel effect during recognition testing.[107] One possibility is that no longer relevant or otherwise to-be-forgotten information may be rendered less accessible through inhibition that focuses on hierarchically structured "control" or "access" nodes, including representations of spatial–temporal information. This inhibitory process might be similar to the process of "response-set suppression" proposed by earlier interference theorists[111,112] and to the process of retrieval inhibition recently advanced by Wheeler[113] to account for the phenomenon of spontaneous recovery, or memory improvement over time without repeated testing. Alternatively, it may be that decreased access to contextual information is simply a by-product of a global deactivation of the set of behavioral goals and intentions that were initially activated at the outset of the list but were then rendered obsolete by the forget-instruction.[114–116] These and other possibilities require additional empirical and theoretical work.

Neural Bases of Forgetting: Medial Temporal Lobe and Amnesia

Although the detailed neural substrates of organic amnesia continue to be the subject of intensive investigation in which a variety of neuroimaging and neurophysiological techniques is used, the profoundly detrimental behavioral effects of lesions to the medial temporal lobe and associated structures have been known for many years (for historical and contemporary reviews see Schacter,[27,117] Squire,[118] and Squire and Zola-Morgan[119]). Patients with damage to the hippocampus and other medial temporal lobe/diencephalic structures have been found to experience a radical impairment in the ability to intentionally and voluntarily recollect experiences, both in their everyday lives and in a wide variety of experimental tasks, that involve a diverse array of stimulus materials and procedures.

Nonetheless, organic amnesia patients also provide some of the most compelling demonstrations of the highly conditional nature of the inaccessibility of memories in that these profound memory deficits emerge only when test instructions require explicit memory for prior experiences. If instead, memory is tested in a way that allows patients to reveal the effects of past experiences implicitly or indirectly, without requiring intentional or deliberate reference to those past experiences, their performance is often unimpaired. Thus despite revealing marked deficits on such tasks as free recall, cued recall, and recognition, which require explicit and conscious recollection of prior events or stimuli, amnesic patients show normal or nearly normal levels of repetition priming—that is, facilitation on tasks such as perceptual identification or stem completion arising from prior exposure to words, objects, or other stimuli (for recent reviews and discussions see Schacter[27,120] and Roediger and McDermott[121]). These patients also show normal or near-normal levels of retention of past experience on various other types of tasks that do not require accessing declarative knowledge of one's past, such as classical conditioning, solving cognitive puzzles or tasks, and procedural and motor skill learning.

Mechanisms or Sources of Inaccuracy or Distortion

Failures of Source Monitoring

Information enters the cognitive system from a variety of sources. At perhaps the coarsest and most basic level, we can distinguish between information that is generated internally, by ourselves (e.g., our thoughts, imaginings, behavior, and dreams), and information that originates externally, entering our cognitive system from the outside world rather than by our own doing. Yet even at this very coarse and fundamental level, differentiating between sources of information is not always an easy task, though it is often a very important one. More fine-grained discriminations concerning the origins of our memories, as when we must discriminate between two or more possible external sources of a remembered event (e.g., was it Joe or Sue who said that?) or between two or more possible internal sources of a remembered event (e.g., did I only wish that I had said *Y,* or did I in fact really say it?), are, of course, also possible and frequently necessary.

A crucial assumption underlying research and theorizing about the role of source monitoring in memory is that the source of a memory is not simply ''given'' with the memory as an abstract tag or label. This assumption holds regardless of whether source monitoring involves reality monitoring, wherein one determines whether an event was internally or externally generated,[122,123] or involves a more fine-grained type of discrimination between two or more external sources, or two or more internal sources. Specifying the conditions or circumstances under which a memory was acquired involves evaluative and attributional processes, or *inferences,* that operate on the retrieved information.[124,125] These processes, which may operate either relatively automatically or under more deliberative or strategic guidance and are influenced by both internal and situational cues, rely upon the fact that memories derived from different sources often have different qualitative characteristics. Whereas memories for perceived events generally contain many perceptual details (e.g., sound, color), contextual information (details concerning time and place), and semantic information, memories originating in one's thinking or imagination tend to have relatively less information of these forms and more information about an individual's internal cognitive environment at the time of the event, such as why or when one happened to notice certain things. Information about such cognitive operations thus often plays an important role in helping individuals to discriminate one possible internal source of a memory (e.g., words or actions they were asked to imagine speaking or performing) from another internal source (e.g., words or actions which they actually spoke or performed).[124,126,127]

However—and this is a critical point—these differences in the types of attributes that are salient for memories derived from different kinds of sources describe only what is usually or most often the case; they are general tendencies rather than invariably true, and particular circumstances may occur that minimize or blur such differences. For example, a high degree of semantic similarity between items from different sources might be expected to make source discriminations more difficult—a fact that contributes to a variety of instances of memory distortion. These range from confusions due to misleading eyewitness questioning,[128] to high rates of false recognition in paradigms that require "old" versus "new" source discriminations and in which the nonpresented lure or distractor items are close semantic associates of actually presented items (see discussion on associative factors below), to cases where the nonpresented items comprise highly plausible inferences that might be drawn from meaningfully processing the stimulus situation (see discussions of verbatim vs. gist representations, and schemas below; for review see Schacter[8]).

More generally, if events do not emerge from memory bearing a tag designating their origins but rather receive a source determination on the basis of attributional and decision processes, then various factors that might interfere with those processes (for example, limited attentional resources) might be expected to increase the likelihood of errors: events and their (alleged) sources might become incorrectly conjoined. Particularly given that our memory for events themselves is but a compilation of features or attributes of various sorts[129–131,85] that may be more or only less tightly bound or associated with one another,[132–134] a diverse array of source-monitoring failures is possible. Thus, for example, experimental evidence has shown that, under certain conditions, individuals may carry out any of the following processes that could lead to inaccurate or distorted source attributions. Individuals may:

1. *Perceive (and claim) as original, information that objectively derives from memory* When this occurs unintentionally, assuming the form of inadvertent or involuntary plagiarism, such that information that was in fact generated by another person (or even oneself at some earlier time) is subjectively perceived as original, it is called *cryptomnesia*. Several intriguing historical examples of cryptomnesia exist, involving such individuals as Friedrich Nietzsche and Helen

Keller (for reviews see Bowers and Hilgard,[135] and Taylor[136]). Cryptomnesia has also been demonstrated experimentally.[137,138]

2. *Mistake recently learned information for information that was acquired much earlier* A striking example of this form of source misattribution has been observed in individuals who are under a suggestion for posthypnotic amnesia.[139–141] Subjects who have apparently only just learned relatively obscure or recondite items of general knowledge (e.g., the color of a heated amethyst) during the hypnosis session itself may claim, while under the suggestion of posthypnotic amnesia, to have acquired this knowledge much earlier, from various sources in their past (e.g., a geology class). Such source amnesia has also been observed in nonhypnotized normal subjects when newly learned information was tested after a retention interval of many weeks,[142] and in organic amnesia patients and the elderly using fictional materials that could never previously have been learned (see, respectively, Schacter et al.,[143] and McIntyre and Craik[144]). Another clear illustration of this form of source misattribution is the so-called false fame effect.[145] In the false fame effect, individuals who have been exposed, under the guise of a different task, to nonfamous names in one phase of an experiment later incorrectly judge these names as being famous. That is, they incorrectly perceive these names as having accrued *pre-experimental* familiarity (or fame) in a context and for reasons that have nothing to do with the experimental setting in which they were, in fact, first encountered.

3. *Incorrectly attribute information from one external source to another external source* Perhaps a less dramatic, but nonetheless frequent and potentially quite harmful, form of source-monitoring error involves the incorrect attribution of information that was acquired from one external source (e.g., Journal X) to another external source (e.g., Journal Y). This type of error is close to what Schacter, Harbluk, and McLachlan[143] referred to as *source forgetting,* wherein individuals correctly recollect that information was presented within a given spatiotemporal context (such as an experiment) but misattribute the information at a more specific level, judging, for example, that an item was presented by one person in the experimental situation when it was presented by another person. Correctly identifying the general spatiotemporal context in which a person was encountered, but then incorrectly identifying that person's precise role within that context, can be a very costly error in instances of eyewitness testimony. In such cases, innocent bystanders at a crime may be misidentified as the perpetrator of the crime, or exposure to a given individual in a very different context but at approximately the same time as the crime can lead to the misidentification of the latter as the culprit.[146] More generally, such misattributions may arise whenever memory for various forms of contextual information is examined, such as determining the list in which an item occurred or which of two items occurred more recently, or when information from a particular spatiotemporal or life context is required (e.g., the name of one's first grade teacher) that might readily be con-

fused with information from another context (e.g., one's second grade teacher). Whitten and Leonard[81] found that university students who mistakenly recalled one of their teachers from their pre-university years most often pointed to transpositions of this form—involving a mismatch of a teacher and grade—as the cause of their error. Students also pointed to other types of situational confusions as giving rise to their errors, such as one student who explained that he had wanted a particular teacher to be his 12th-grade teacher but that teacher had been reassigned to teach a different grade, or students who reported their sibling's or friend's teachers rather than their own. Attempts to intentionally forget information, particularly when a whole series of items or a large block of items is targetted as to-be-forgotten, appear to make this form of source error especially likely[110,107] (cf. discussion of directed forgetting above).

4. *Mistake the fictional for the real*   Both anecdotal and experimental evidence suggests that information embedded within a fictional context may sometimes illegitimately influence subjects' opinions and beliefs outside of that context, so that the fictional is mistaken for the real, or opinions are altered in a direction consistent with false facts embedded in the fictional information (for reivew see Johnson et al.[124]). For example, subjects who were introduced to false information within the context of a story (e.g., "most forms of mental illness are contagious") subsequently were slower to decide whether, in everyday life, these statements were true or false than if the stories had contained correct information.[147] These findings suggest that at least under some conditions, individuals may have difficulty isolating or compartmentalizing the fictional from the real.

5. *Mistakenly attribute the effects of past experience to processes or factors other than memory*   Under certain conditions, past experiences may exert an effect on an individual's judgments or decisions, usually by facilitating or enhancing them in some manner, and yet not only does the actual source of these effects go unremarked (as often happens in various forms of implicit memory), but some outside or extraneous factor is mistakenly thought to be their cause or source instead. That is, some other factor or process is credited for effects that are really due to memory. For example, in one study subjects were asked to listen to sentences presented against a background of white noise and to rate the loudness of the background noise. Subjects judged the noise level to be lower when the sentence was one that they had heard previously in the experiment than when the sentence was a new sentence had not been presented earlier, even though the actual level of the background noise was the same.[148] An essentially similar result was obtained when subjects were asked to rate the duration for which individual words were presented. Words that had been presented earlier were judged to have a longer duration than words that had not previously been presented.[149] Although these two particular instances of misattribution might seem relatively harmless or innocuous, the occurrence of a similar outcome when the task involved judging whether statements were true or false,[150] such that previously presented items

were judged as more likely to be true than nonpresented items, suggests that, at least under certain conditions, this kind of source misattribution might assume more pernicious guises.

6. *Misattribute the effects of other (nonmemory-related) cognitive processes to memory*   If individuals can make source-monitoring errors such that they deny memory its due, crediting a nonmemorial extraneous source for what really belongs to memory, they can also make the converse error: making false alarms or intrusions due to a nonmemorial factor and claiming for memory what does not belong to memory. An example of this converse pattern is found in what has been called the *revelation effect,* first reported by Peynircioglu and Watkins.[151] If an item on a recognition test is presented in a way that initially distorts or impedes its perception but then is fully revealed before a recognition decision has to be made, subjects show a positive response bias: for both old (studied) words and for new (nonstudied) words they are more likely to call the item old if it was revealed than if it was presented in normal format. This tendency to more often correctly recognize revealed than nonrevealed old items *and* to more often falsely recognize revealed than nonrevealed *new* items has been observed across several types of revelation procedures (e.g., when test words are presented letter by letter or in initially rotated form, or the word as a whole is presented in transposed form).[152–155] Interestingly, however, this tendency does not generalize to tasks that do not involve episodic memory (e.g., judging categorized items for their degree of prototypicality or their frequency of general usage).

Associative Factors: Relatively Specific or Restricted Effects of Preexisting Semantic Associations

When we hear or see a given word, various other words that are semantically associated with that word may be elicited, sometimes consciously and overtly (as when we are asked to produce the first word that comes to mind in response to the target word), but more often covertly, or implicitly. These associates might be words that are at the same level of usage as the target word—so-called parallel associates—including, for example, antonyms, synonyms, or functional associates such as cup–saucer, table–chair, or key–lock, wherein the associative relationship derives from functional contiguity. Alternatively, these associates might be words from a higher-order semantic level than the target word, including, for example, category responses such as ''animal'' when the target word is ''horse'' and possibly also less obvious forms of class membership, such as ''four-footed animals.''[131] An important aspect involved in the recall or retrieval of such associative attributes is that, like any memories, they do not come labeled as to their source. Deciding that a given word was actually presented or was only thought about in response to some other word is a discrimination that depends on other attributes that are present in memory (cf. Underwood[130]). When these other attributes are insufficient to allow a discrimination, errors will result.

One type of error that may occur is false recognition. Subjects might be expected to incorrectly identify distractor items that are similar to the target items because they are unable to discern the directionality of the associative relationship: does this word now seem highly familiar in relation to the study context because the word occurred during the study list, or because I thought of this word in response to another word that (unlike this word) really was a target word? Underwood[156] documented this kind of error by using a continuous recognition paradigm in which new and old words were intermixed and the subject's task was to indicate whether each item had occurred earlier in the list. An unusually high number of false alarms was observed when the lure or distractor items were related to previously studied items, including, for example, antonyms and superordinates. Underwood[156] suggested that these false recognition errors are attributable to ''implicit associative responses'' (compare with Bousfield et al.[157]) that people made when they first studied a target word. Consistent with such an associative response account, Vogt and Kimble[158] found that subjects were especially likely to falsely recognize related lure items that the subjects themselves had (2 months earlier) ranked as highly associated to the presented items. Recent work[159] using a standard yes/no recognition test to explore associatively related errors also produced findings consistent with the notion that such false alarms might arise from associative responses that occurred only covertly or implicitly. In this study,[159] heightened susceptibility to false recognition did not depend on the individual's having consciously attended the target word when it was first presented. Following a dichotic listening task, subjects falsely recognized lure or distractor items that were semantically related to previously presented items significantly more often than they falsely recognized unrelated new items, regardless of whether those items had been presented but to-be-remembered items on an attended channel or as simultaneously presented but to-be-ignored items on an unattended channel.

Some of the lure words used by Underwood involved ''converging associates,'' that is, pairs or larger sets of words that, on the basis of word association norms, are known to elicit a particular associate. For example, ''sugar,'' ''bitter,'' and ''candy'' all tend to elicit the response ''sweet,'' which was one of the experimental words. Such convergent associations appear to play a critical role in the genesis of another type of error that may arise as a result of preexisting semantic associations: intrusions in free recall. When subjects are asked to study several words, each of which is known to frequently elicit a given word as an associate, these associations, which are themselves never actually presented, are often incorrectly given (intruded) as studied items during free recall.[160–162] For example, Deese[160] found that subjects recalled these never-presented critical items with an average frequency of approximately 24%—a rate nearly eight times greater than that observed for other (unrelated) intrusions. Using a modified version of Deese's paradigm, Roediger and McDermott[162] recently observed such intrusions for as many as 55% of the sets of converging associates that subjects studied.

Deese found that the likelihood with which these never-presented critical new items occurred as intrusions in free recall was quite variable, depending on the particular items that were used. Some items elicited very high rates of intrusions, for example, "sleep" (44%) and "needle" (42%), whereas other items produced relatively few intrusions, for instance, "whistle" (4%) and "butterfly" (0%). The rate at which items occurred as intrusions in free recall was found to be very strongly and positively correlated with how often the critical words (on average) were given as the first associate that came to mind to the study list words.

When subjects are tested on recognition as well as in free recall under variants of the Deese[160] paradigm, they often claim to recognize the (nonpresented) experimental lure items with a high level of confidence. They also claim to specifically recollect or "remember" some particular aspect of the original stimulus situation that was present during the (purported) occurrence of the distractor items, rather than attributing their recognition decisions to a general feeling of familiarity or of "knowing."[161,162] This pattern of a high frequency of remembering false alarms contrasts with what has usually been found in other work with the remember/know recognition procedure, where false alarms are typically more often accompanied by know-responses than by remember-responses.[152,163–165] Upon more specifically querying subjects about the types of information that they claimed to remember, Norman and Schacter[161] found that what subjects were remembering largely consisted of semantically associated information which—though it may have been elicited in response to the presented items—in fact, provided no grounds for inferring the physical presentation of the experimental lure items.

Verbatim versus Gist

Numerous experiments have shown that subjects not only often retain the semantic gist of materials but also mistakenly recognize and recall gist-like substitutions of the original event, reporting the latter as having been directly experienced.[166,167] Although most often reported for verbal materials, the often-cited observations of surprisingly high recognition–memory for pictures[168,169] may also, in part, reflect gist-like rather than verbatim-like retention or precise memory for details. Subjects who had studied pictures of scenes and were then asked to decide whether these pictures had been presented previously were more likely to falsely recognize an item if some relatively less important detail had been changed (false alarms of 40%) than if a more central detail in the picture had been altered (false alarms of only 6%), even though this manipulation did not involve different degrees of physical change in the picture.[170, cf.171] The false alarms and intrusions observed in Underwood's[156] continuous recognition paradigm and in the Deese paradigm could also be viewed as exemplifying errors arising from gist-like processing. A subject who provides the word "sweet" as an (alleged) study item given that she had, in actuality, studied some dozen or more words that were associatively related to "sweet" is certainly responding in a manner consistent with the gist of the study episode, even though it is incorrect when the retrieval requirements demand a literal or verbatim standard.

In the Deese paradigm, both Roediger and McDermott[162] and Norman and Schacter[161] found that intrusions of the critical lure words (the words that were not actually presented but for which several associatively related items had been presented) tended to occur during the later portions of the allotted recall time rather than earlier. Several observations have pointed to the moderating role of the length of the retention interval between initial exposure to information and the requirement for retrieval in determining whether errors due to gist-like processing emerge, with such errors being more likely with longer retention intervals.[172–175] Recent work by Reyna, Brainerd, and Kiernan[176,177, cf.178,179] is also consistent with this suggestion. They propose that during initial encoding and comprehension, both the surface forms of the inputs (verbatim traces) and the meanings and senses corresponding to those forms (gist traces) are used. Although both forms of traces are also stored, verbatim traces are lost more quickly and more readily than gist traces (both as a function of time and as a function of interference). Hence performance on retention tests is often more strongly dependent on gist traces than on verbatim traces.

Condensation or Generalization across Episodes: Generic Memories versus Specific Memories

Although, strictly speaking, no two events are exactly the same, some events quite closely resemble other events that we have already experienced. These events may share many common features or attributes. If there is a high proportion of such shared or common attributes between two or more events, and particularly if there are relatively few attributes that are especially distinctive of any one event, then differentiating between those events in memory may be very difficult, or perhaps impossible. In this situation, individuals may retrieve memories containing information that is "true" or "correct" for the general class or kind of events that they are recollecting but that is not necessarily true for (or applicable to) a specific memory.[180,181] On the basis of his analysis of the evidence in the Watergate case, Neisser[182] concluded that John Dean's testimony in the Watergate trial was largely of this sort: accurate at a gist-like level but not at a more specific, micro-level. Through an analysis of her own memory for autobiographical events over a period of several years, Linton[183] observed a largely similar process. Details of particular or unique events either tended to disappear with time or to become amalgamated with other, similar events.

The potential contribution of such generic memories to memory distortion, particularly false recognition, has also been demonstrated by Barclay and colleagues.[184,185] In examining subjects' long-term recognition memory for autobiographical events which they had initially judged to be memorable or noteworthy and had recorded in diary-type records, these investigators found that subjects falsely recognized nearly *one-half* of the foil or distractor items when those items were drawn from the subjects' own records but their reported evaluation of the events had been changed or descriptive details of the described events were altered. False alarms to records written by another person were considerably less frequent. These researchers suggested that this difference in the rate of false alarms derived from the greater degree of consistency that the subjects' own altered records had with the general theme or gist of their lives than was true for records that were written by other subjects. A subsequent study [185] ruled out the possibility that false alarms were attributable to the greater syntactical similarity (rather than semantic content) of the altered foils. Subjects very frequently made false alarms to items that were semantically similar to originally recorded events, even if those events were written in a style different from their own (80%) but much less often gave false recognition responses for items that were written is a *style* similar to their own but that differed in meaning (10%).

Schemas: Effects of Relatively More Complex Preexisting Patterns of Associations

Schemas may be thought of as general knowledge structures,[186,187] or as patterns of activation among learned associations,[188,189] that are based on past experience. Of varying degrees of complexity or abstractness (we may have a schema for what comprises a ''room'' or an ''animal'' as well as for what constitutes a ''novel'' or ''justice''), schemas may influence not only memory but also perception, comprehension, and action much more generally. Often facilitative in their effects (operating so as to guide attention, encoding, and retrieval), schemas may also result in memory errors. For example, schemas may encourage individuals to draw inferences of either a pragmatic or logical sort, which then are mistakenly identified as actual occurrences. The statement, ''John was pounding a nail'' may lead to the pragmatic inference that John used a hammer, which then later results in the incorrect recognition of the item ''hammer.''[190] Using one's past experience to fill in unspecified or ambiguous details by assuming or generating *default values* that represent what is most often or usually the case can clearly facilitate both comprehension and communication. Yet it may also engender source-monitoring problems: Did I really hear or see X or did I only infer it? Thus, for example, nearly one-third of subjects who briefly waited in what appeared to be a graduate student's office incorrectly reported that the room contained books when it did not (a highly plausible but nonetheless incorrect inference) and 10% of the subjects recalled a (nonexistent) filing cabinet. On a recognition test, nearly one-quarter of the items that subjects most often judged as having been present in the room were, in fact, not present; all but one of these objects had been independently ranked as highly likely to appear in a room similar to the experimental room.[191]

Schema-related errors may also entail gross distortions of more complex situations, such as a narrative of a romantic relationship. Individuals' attempts to accommodate presented information with their prior knowledge and expectations concerning a relationship led them to negate events that actually occurred (an engaged couple's bitter argument about whether they should have children became "They didn't disagree" or "They didn't discuss it"), and to describe occurrences that never took place ("They underwent counseling," "They discussed it and decided upon adoption as a compromise").[175] Schemas concerning the self and self-characteristics may also induce various forms of memory distortions, particularly selectivity in free recall, with schema-consistent information recalled more frequently than schema-inconsistent information.[192–195]

Taken together, the findings from each of the last three sections concerning verbatim versus gist processing, condensation or generalization across episodes, and the effects of schemas on memory, clearly suggest that, with the passage of time and with ongoing experience, the essential features of everyday experience may be abstracted, thereby producing more or less generic, and more or less reconstructed, autobiographical recollections.[196,197] Nonetheless, several additional considerations also suggest that we cannot construe memory as entirely reconstructive but only partially so.[198] These considerations include the high level of accuracy with which subjects in the experiments by Barclay and colleagues[184,185] recognized unchanged records of events from their lives; the more general fact that we can and often do recollect particularized events[199] that include apparently irrelevant details;[200] and the degree to which we generally successfully monitor reality, remembering what actually occurred rather than merely what (given the general themes, thrusts, and patterns of our lives) could or might have occurred.[184] Thus, although memory is susceptible to error due to gist-like, abstractive, and schematic processing, it is not always or invariably vulnerable to errors from these sources.

Disturbances in the Subjective Quality of Memory Awareness

Although a feeling or sense of familiarity appears to be an essential component of remembering, the diversity of possible source misattributions described previously clearly indicates that whatever the nature of the phenomenological or subjective state that we denote as "familiarity," it is also subject to misconstrual or misplacement. An individual may have an "illusion of remembrance,"[201] attributing mental content or experiences to familiarity when, objectively speaking, there are no grounds for that judgment—all the while remaining oblivious of the error.

What might happen if an individual became aware of the discrepancy between their subjective experiences and the "objective" state of affairs? Awareness of that discrepancy may, in part, underlie the disconcerting response that people may have to the feeling of déjà vu—the sentiment that something that one is currently experiencing or observing has been experienced or observed before, even though one also knows, from the nature of the case, that this is impossible. Various and often ingenious explanations of this phenomenon have been proposed (for recent reviews see Berrios[202] and Sno[203]). The sheer range and multiplicity of these interpretations and assimilations of the experience to other normal and pathological states underscores the difficulties involved in isolating the subjective correlates of memory from other ongoing cognitive processes (e.g., perception, imagination, attention) and from contributions due to various disorders or pathology (e.g., temporal lobe epilepsy, psychogenic fugues, schizophrenia, organic amnesia). Thus Sno, Linszen, and DeJonghe[204] have proposed the concept of a *continuum* of experiences of inappropriate familiarity. Situated at one end of the continuum are less severe instances of disturbances in familiarity experiences, such as minor forms of déjà vu (involving transient experiences in which the individual is simultaneously aware that it is impossible that their current experience could be identical to that undergone previously and where reality testing is only negligibly affected). Situated at the other end of the continuum are markedly pathological forms of inappropriate familiarity involving delusions of familiarity (the so-called reduplicative paramnesias, where reality testing is persistently or repeatedly impaired, and where an individual believes that a time, place, or person has been duplicated; also see section on pathological distortion).

Attentional Resources, Memory Monitoring, and Meta-memory Assumptions

Considerable evidence from both laboratory and autobiographical studies points to the presence of, and the need for, mnemonic monitoring or vigilance in "normal" memory functioning. For example, in their study of long-term autobiographical memory retrieval, Williams and Hollan[82] observed that subjects used several different techniques, in a quite complex and integrated manner, in an effort to verify the accuracy of names that they retrieved as possibly belonging to their high school classmates. Sometimes subjects treated a particular piece of information as only a possibility until it was confirmed by an independent recovery of the same information (coincident recovery). Sometimes they used an indirect confirmation technique in which they attempted to use the recovered information to recover additional information, and then treated the recovery of this further information as confirmation of the original information. On still other occasions, they used a technique of consistency checking, attempting to confirm if the newly recovered information was congruent with information that was already known (cf., the double checks and self-corrections reported by Whitten and Leonard[81]). Similarly, Johnson and colleagues found that subjects often referred to supporting memories to justify their belief that particular autobiographical events actually occurred in their past rather than having been only dreamt or imagined. For example, subjects noted other related events that they remembered as having occurred prior to the target event (e.g., purchasing clothing for an occasion) or consequences or sequelae of the event (e.g., conversations with others about the event) as supporting the veridical nature of their memories.[205]

Yet the decisions reached via these types of reasoning and attempted memory monitoring processes are not always accurate, as attested by the large number and diverse variety of errors that may nonetheless occur: the frequency with which various kinds of source attribution errors arise, the large number of fabricated names that were produced by subjects in the Williams et al.[80,82] experiment, and so on. Indeed, such decision processes and attempted monitoring may themselves prove to be misleading, as when individuals might misattribute their own dreams to another person on the basis of general beliefs about the "type of thing" that they normally dream,[206] or when an attempt to make remembered details more coherent or consistent with each other may itself induce distortions and further divergences from the original event.[76,175,207]

Considered from a broader perspective, memory distortions in the form of false recognitions and intrusions could be viewed as instances of cognitive failure, and therefore susceptible to the same sorts of factors that induce cognitive failures in other domains such as perception, skilled action, or problem solving. Reason[208] has noted that different individuals show relatively stable and consistent patterns of susceptibility to cognitive failures across these domains. Individuals who report frequent action slips also tend to report many memory lapses, recognition errors, and so on, and the reported frequency of these errors does not change radically across intervals of as long as 16 months. Further, across all these domains, errors are most commonly due to strong habit intrusions, which suggests that what goes awry in memory failure may often be a failure to suppress tendencies that should be suppressed.[208] It may be partially for these reasons that suggestibility effects in memory—the likelihood of incorporating and incorrectly reporting post-event information into accounts of an event—can be reduced by forewarning individuals regarding the possibility of misinformation[209,210] or by requiring individuals to make more stringent source judgments (specifying whether information was actually observed or was only suggested) rather than simple yes/no recognition decisions.[211, cf.212] Spiro's[175] finding that subjects made fewer schema-consistent intrusions and distortions under explicit instructions to remember than under more naturalistic or interactive incidental encoding instructions might have a similar explanation: intentional encoding instructions could help to dampen or keep inferential processes in check, and might also encourage subjects to isolate the experimental materials from prior knowledge and expectations. Increased vigilance derived from forewarnings might also enhance the encoding of the source of information. Nonetheless, it is also possible that under certain conditions, individuals do not recognize the need for vigilance or have insufficient motivation to exercise vigilance and thus still are susceptible to misinformation effects.[213, cf.214] Similarly, conditions such as high attentional load[215–218] or particular personality traits[212,219, cf. 220] may render subjects less able to employ strategic monitoring processes that could prevent source misattribubutions, or more cautious decisions deriving from such monitoring might be over-ridden by instructional or situational pressures that lead subjects to make a guess, regardless of their confidence.[221,222, cf.180] Finally, the warning that stringent source and decision monitoring is necessary may simply arrive too late. The misleading information may be so inextricably assimilated to the subject's memory of actual events that, even with explicit and emphatic directions as to what misinformation should be excluded, they still recall events and details that were only suggested as having, in fact, occurred.[223]

Pathological Distortion

Some of the most forceful and convincing demonstrations of the necessity for memory monitoring derive from cases where memory function is pathologically disrupted. Perhaps foremost among such cases are instances of confabulation: cases where individuals, due to a variety of neurological and psychiatric factors, provide incorrect and sometimes blatantly bizarre accounts of their past (or present) experiences. Because the confabulating individual typically clearly believes his own account, despite its demonstrable falsity, Moscovitch[218] has characterized confabulation as "honest lying." Generally involving frontal lobe damage and possibly basal forebrain damage as well,[224] many cases of confabulation appear to involve disturbances in source monitoring.[218,225] The confabulating individual may confuse the temporal-spatial origins or other attributes of different events that actually occurred or, particularly in the case of more bizarre confabulations, mistakenly incorporate aspects of fantasies, dreams, or incidental aspects of their present environment into what they believe are accounts of "actual events." Other instances of confabulation, again particularly those involving more blatantly bizarre and improbable construals, likely involve, in addition to disruptions in source monitoring, disturbances of other higher-order cognitive processes that normally monitor and evaluate the plausibility and coherence of mental contents.[225–227] For example, patients with the rare form of confabulatory-like phenomenon known as *reduplicative paramnesia* (also called *Capgras syndrome*), who believe that one or more members of their family or intimate acquaintances have been replaced by exceedingly similar-seeming duplicates of their real family members, appear to be fully aware of the sheer implausibility of this state of affairs, but nonetheless tenaciously persist in this belief.[228] Similarly, some frontal lesion patients will persistently maintain highly implausible and internally inconsistent accounts of their personal and family lives, despite strong and abundant evidence to the contrary.[48,218]

Other instances of memory distortion due to neurological dysfunction, particularly frontal lobe dysfunction, may involve unusually high levels of intrusions during free recall [229–231] and/or high rates of false alarms during recognition testing.[229,231] B.G., a patient who suffered a right frontal lobe infarction, and who has been studied extensively in our laboratory, provides a remarkable example of such false recognition.[227,232] Although B.G. performs poorly on tests that are sensitive to frontal lobe pathology, such as the Wisconsin Card Sorting Task, he is not globally amnesic (e.g., his hit rate during recognition testing is often within the range of his age matched control subjects), nor does he spontaneously confabulate. Yet, across a wide variety of stimuli and test conditions, B.G. shows a pathologically high level of false recognition. He claims, often far more frequently than his age-matched controls, to recognize and remember stimuli that were not presented. Although the precise nature of the factors leading to this deficit remain unclear, the overall pattern of his performance suggests that B.G. often accepts certain broad or general features or characteristics of a stimulus as evidence that he has encountered the item previously when those features are insufficient to permit that judgment.

Finally, frontal lobe deterioration associated with normal aging[233] may be associated with an increased likelihood of memory distortion. Under some conditions, elderly subjects are more susceptible to source-monitoring errors.[234–236] They may also be more likely than college-aged subjects to indicate that falsely recognized items are accompanied by a specific recollection of an item's earlier occurrence (a ''remember'' response) rather than a simple feeling of familiarity (a ''know'' response).[236]

Conclusion

In this chapter we have considered, and illustrated, a wide range of factors that may render memory retrieval either especially difficult or especially susceptible to distortion and error. With this approach we have sought to emphasize the multiply determined and highly conditionalized nature of memory accessibility and memory accuracy. Given particular combinations of factors we may observe exceptionally good memory performance (a high level of accessibility and a high degree of accuracy); given other combinations of factors we may observe apparently paradoxical effects (instances where patterns that are generally true fail to obtain or the opposite pattern to what might be expected is observed); given still yet other combinations we may observe what is, after all, still most often the case: good-to-moderately good and to some degree fluctuating accessibility and mostly accurate performance. For instance, presenting an individual with very distinctive cues concerning a to-be-remembered stimulus may result in surprisingly high levels of recall, but providing some of the items from a larger set of to-be-remembered items may actually impede recall of the remaining items. Similarly, extending one's retrieval efforts beyond a normal termination point may result in the recovery of additional (otherwise available but unaccessed) information; yet, depending on the circumstances and the degree of monitoring exercised during this extended retrieval, the number of items retrieved may be offset by many intrusions.

A possible drawback of this approach, however, is that it may be difficult to conceptually relate or condense all of the factors that have been delineated. Accordingly we would like to conclude by offering three broader and more integrative principles that might be viewed as spanning (or undergirding) the more specific sources of inaccessibility and inaccuracy that we have outlined.

First, memory for events, even events of a very simple and neutral form, is dependent on a diverse array of factors and influences, only some of which directly involve the memory representation or trace itself. Memory retrieval is a highly interactive occurrence, dependent not only on various characteristics of the memory representation (e.g., the number and nature of the attributes or features concerning the target event that are available in memory) but also on characteristics of the retrieval environment in which memory is being "queried" (e.g., the specificity or richness of the cues that are available to help guide or prompt memory). Memory retrieval also depends on the nature of an individual's intentions with respect to the available retrieval cues (e.g., whether or not the individual is engaged in a voluntary effort to remember, and the duration and degree of effort expended in the attempt to intentionally remember), and the nature of an individual's awareness concerning the relation between the available retrieval cues and the target event (e.g., whether or not the individual is aware that the retrieval cues are relevant to the target event).[237,238]

Second, memory for an event (again, even of a very simple and neutral form, such as might be involved in recalling a word that was presented in a list) does not involve simply finding that event as an independently existing corpus in memory;[130] rather, the representation of an event consists of an ensemble or collection of features or attributes, including sensory–perceptual attributes, temporal–spatial information, semantic associations, and so on, which, at the time of retrieval, may be more or only less tightly associated or bound with one another.[132–134] Accessing a particular target memory and differentiating it from other (possible highly similar) memories depends on the particular attributes or configuration of attributes that are present in the target memory, and it is possible that some attributes may become dissociated from a given event or incorrectly conjoined with another (possibly quite similar) event.

Third, memory for events (once again including those of a very simple and neutral sort) is not necessarily accompanied by a subjective or phenomenological experience of remembering, nor is memory for an event invariably correctly associated with information concerning the temporal–spatial and other contextual circumstances of its occurrence. The correct assignment of a given event or experience to a particular time, place, and set of circumstances in one's past depends on evaluative and attributional processes which may, under some conditions, go awry, resulting in various forms of mistaken identifications as to the source of one's experiences.

References

1. Koriat A, Goldsmith M: Memory metaphors and the real-life/laboratory controversy: the correspondence versus the storehouse conceptions of memory. Behav Brain Sci 1996; 19:167–228.

2. Thomson DM: Context and false recognition. *In* GM Davies, DM Thomson (Eds.), Memory in Context: Context in Memory. Chichester: Wiley, 1988, pp. 285–304.
3. Lindsay DS, Read JD: Psychotherapy and memories for childhood sexual abuse: a cognitive perspective. Appl Cogn Psychol 1994; 8:281–338.
4. Loftus EF: The reality of repressed memories. Am Psychol 1993; 48:518–537.
5. Loftus EF, Ketcham K: The Myth of Repressed Memory: False Memories and Allegations of Sexual Abuse. New York: St. Martin's Press, 1994.
6. Ofshe R, Watters E: Making Monsters: False Memories, Psychotherapy, and Sexual Hysteria. New York: Scribner's, 1994.
7. Pendergrast M: Victims of Memory: Incest Accusations and Shattered Lives. Hinesburg, VT: Upper Access, 1995.
8. Schacter DL: Memory distortion: history and current status. *In* DL Schacter, JT Coyle, GD Fischbach, MM Mesulam, LE Sullivan (Eds.), Memory Distortion. Cambridge, MA: Harvard University Press, 1995, pp. 1–46.
9. Tulving E, Pearlstone Z: Availability versus accessibility of information in memory for words. J Verbal Learn Verbal Behav 1966; 5:381–391.
10. Ackerman BP: Descriptions: a model of nonstrategic memory development. *In* HW Reese (Ed.), Advances in Child Development and Behavior, Vol 20. New York: Academic Press, 1987, pp. 143–183.
11. Morton J, Hammersley RH, Bekerian DA: Headed records: a model for memory and its failures. Cognition 1985; 20:1–23.
12. Norman DA, Bobrow DG: Descriptions: an intermediate stage in memory retrieval. Cogn Psychol 1979; 11:107–123.
13. Flexser A, Tulving E: Retrieval independence in recognition and recall. Psychol Rev 1978; 85:153–171.
14. Reddy BG, Bellezza FS: Encoding specificity in free recall. J Exp Psychol Learn Mem Cogn 1983; 9:167–174.
15. Wagenaar WA: My memory: a study of autobiographical memory over six years. Cogn Psychol 1986; 18:225–252.
16. Watkins OC, Watkins MJ: Buildup of proactive inhibition as a cue-overload effect. J Exp Psychol Hum Learn Mem 1975; 104:442–452.
17. Watkins MJ: Engrams as cuegrams and forgetting as cue overload: a cueing approach to the structure of memory. *In* CR Puff (Ed.), Memory Organization and Structure. New York: Academic Press, 1979, pp. 347–372.
18. Mäntylä T: Optimizing cue effectiveness: recall of 500 and 600 incidentally learned words. J Exp Psychol Learn Mem Cogn 1986; 12:66–71.
19. Godden D, Baddeley AD: When does context influence recognition memory? Br J Psychol 1980; 71:99–104.
20. Light LL, Carter-Sobell L: Effects of changed semantic context on recognition memory. J Verbal Learn Verbal Behav 1970; 9:1–11.
21. Tulving E, Thomson DM: Retrieval processes in recognition memory: effects of associative context. J Exp Psychol 1971; 87:116–124.
22. Winograd E, Rivers-Bulkeley NT: Effects of changing context on remembering faces. J Exp Psychol Hum Learn Mem 1977; 3:397–405.
23. Schacter DL, Church BA: Auditory priming: implicit and explicit memory for words and voices. J Exp Psychol Learn Mem Cogn 1992; 18:915–930.
24. Hayman CAG, Rickards CA: A dissociation in the effects of study modality on tests of implicit and explicit memory. Mem Cogn 1995; 23:95–112.
25. Gabrieli JDE, Fleischman DA, Keane MM, Reminger SL, Morrell F: Double dissociation

between memory systems underlying explicit and implicit memory in the human brain. Psychol Sci 1995; 6:76–82.

26. Roediger HL III, Blaxton TA: Retrieval modes produce dissociations in memory for surface information. *In* DS Gorfein, RR Hoffman (Eds.), Memory and Cognitive Processes: The Ebbinghaus Centennial Conference. Hillsdale, NJ: Erlbaum, 1987, pp. 349–379.

27. Schacter DL: Priming and multiple memory systems: perceptual mechanisms of implicit memory. *In* DL Schacter, E Tulving (Eds.), Memory Systems 1994. Cambridge, MA: MIT Press, 1994, pp. 233–268.

28. Smith SM: Environmental context-dependent memory. *In* GM Davies, DM Thomson (Eds.), Memory in Context: Context in Memory. Chichester: Wiley, 1988, pp. 13–34.

29. Godden D, Baddeley AD: Context-dependent memory in two natural environments: on land and underwater. Br J Psychol 1975; 66:325–331.

30. Canas JJ, Nelson DL: Recognition and environmental context: the effect of testing by phone. Bull Psychonomic Soc 1986; 24:407–409.

31. Smith SM: Enhancement of recall using multiple environmental contexts during learning. Mem Cogn 1982; 10:405–412.

32. Smith SM: Remembering in and out of context. J Exp Psychol Hum Learn Mem 1979; 5:460–471.

33. Smith SM: A comparison of two techniques for reducing context-dependent forgetting. Mem Cogn 1984; 12:477–482.

34. Malpass RS, Devine PG: Guided memory in eyewitness identification. J Appl Psychol 1981; 66:343–350.

35. Geiselman RE, Fisher RP, MacKinnon DP, Holland HL: Eyewitness memory enhancement in the police interview: cognitive retrieval mnemonics versus hypnosis. J Appl Cogn Psychol 1985; 70:401–412.

36. Geiselman RE, Fisher RP, MacKinnon DP, Holland HL: Enhancement of eyewitness memory with the cognitive interview. Am J Psychol 1986; 99:385–401.

37. Fisher RP, Geiselman RE: Enhancing eyewitness memory with the cognitive interview. *In* MM Gruneberg, PE Morris, RN Sykes (Eds.), Practical Aspects of Memory: Current Research and Issues, Vol. 1. Memory in Everyday Life. Chichester; Wiley, 1988, pp. 34–39.

38. Geiselman RE: Improving eyewitness memory through mental reinstatement of context. *In* GM Davies, DM Thomson (Eds.), Memory in Context: Context in Memory. Chichester: Wiley, 1988, pp. 245–266.

39. Cutler BL, Penrod SD, Martens TK: Improving the reliability of eyewitness identification: putting context into context. J Appl Psychol 1987; 72:629–637.

40. Cutler BL, Penrod SD: Context reinstatement and eyewitness identification. *In* GM Davies, DM Thomson (Eds.), Memory in Context: Context in Memory. Chichester: Wiley, 1988, pp. 231–244.

41. Deffenbacher KA: A maturing of research on the behaviour of eyewitnesses. Appl Cogn Psychol 1991; 5:377–402.

42. Blaney PH: Affect and memory: a review. Psychol Bull 1986; 99:229–246.

43. Eich JE: The cue-dependent nature of state-dependent retrieval. Mem Cogn 1980; 8:157–173.

44. Eich JE: Searching for mood dependent memory. Psychol Sci 1995; 6:67–75.

45. Eich JE, Metcalfe J: Mood-dependent memory for internal versus external events. J Exp Psychol Learn Mem Cogn 1989; 15:443–455.

46. Eich JE, Macaulay D, Ryan L: Mood dependent memory for events of the personal past. J Exp Psychol Gen 1994; 123:201–215.

47. Baddeley A: Domains of recollection. Psychol Rev 1982; 89:708–729.
48. Baddeley A: Human Memory: Theory and Practice. Needham Heights, MA: Allyn and Bacon, 1990.
49. Jenkins JJ, Russell WA: Associative clustering during recall. J Abnorm Soc Psychol 1952; 47:818–821.
50. Bousfield WA: The occurrence of clustering in the recall of randomly arranged associates. J Gen Psychol 1953; 49:229–240.
51. Mandler G, Dean PJ: Seriation: development of serial order in free recall. J Exp Psychol 1969; 81:207–215.
52. Riegel KF: The recall of historical events. Behav Sci 1973; 18:354–363.
53. Tulving E, Patkau JE: Concurrent effects of contextual constraint and word frequency on immediate recall and learning of verbal material. Can J Psychol 1962; 16:83–95.
54. Loftus EF, Miller D, Burns H: Semantic integration of verbal information into a visual memory. J Exp Psychol Hum Learn Mem 1978; 4:19–31.
55. Bekerian DA, Bowers JM: Eyewitness testimony: were we misled? J Exp Psychol Hum Learn Mem 1983; 9:139–145.
56. Mueller CW, Watkins MJ: Inhibition from part-set cuing: a cue-overload interpretation. J Verbal Learn Verbal Behav 1977; 16:699–709.
57. Roediger HL III: Inhibition in recall from cueing with recall targets. J Verbal Learn Verbal Behav 1973; 12:644–657.
58. Rundus D: Negative effects of using list items as recall cues. J Verbal Learn Verbal Behav 1973; 12:43–50.
59. Watkins MJ: Inhibition in recall with extralist "cues." J Verbal Learn Verbal Behav 1975; 14:294–303.
60. Brown J: Reciprocal facilitation and impairment in free recall. Psychonomic Sci 1968; 10:41–42.
61. Karchmer MA, Winograd E: Effects of studying a subset of familiar items on recall of the remaining items: the John Brown effect. Psychonomic Sci 1971; 25:224–225.
62. Basden DR: Cued and uncued free recall of unrelated words following interpolated learning. J Exp Psychol 1973; 98:429–431.
63. Basden DR, Basden BH, Galloway BC: Inhibition with part-list cuing: some tests of the item strength hypothesis. J Exp Psychol Hum Learn Mem 1977; 3:100–108.
64. Sloman SA, Bower GH, Rohrer D: Congruency effects in part-list cuing inhibition. J Exp Psychol Learn Mem Cogn 1991; 17:974–982.
65. Brown AS, Hall LA: Part-list cueing inhibition in semantic memory structures. Am J Psychol 1979; 92:351–362.
66. Anderson MC, Bjork RA: Mechanisms of inhibition in long-term memory: a new taxonomy. *In* D Dagenbach, TH Carr (Eds.), Inhibitory Processes in Attention, Memory, and Language. San Diego: Academic Press, 1994, pp. 265–325.
67. Parker RE, Warren L: Partial category cueing: the accessibility of categories. J Exp Psychol 1974; 102:1123–1125.
68. Brown R, McNeill D: The 'tip of the tongue' phenomenon. J Verbal Learn Verbal Behav 1966; 5:325–337.
69. Reason JT, Lucas D: Using cognitive diaries to investigate naturally occurring memory blocks. *In* JE Harris, PE Morris (Eds.), Everyday Memory, Actions and Absent-Mindedness. London: Academic Press, 1984, pp. 53–70.
70. Erdelyi MH, Becker J: Hypermnesia for pictures: incremental memory for pictures but not words in multiple recall trials. Cogn Psychol 1974; 6:159–171.

71. Erdelyi MH: The recovery of unconscious (inaccessible) memories: laboratory studies of hypermnesia. Psychol Learn Motivation 1984; 18:95–127.

72. Payne DG: Hypermnesia and reminiscence in recall: a historical and empirical review. Psychol Bull 1987; 101:5–27.

73. Payne DG, Wenger MJ: Improving memory through practice. *In* DJ Herrmann, H Weingartner, A Searleman, C McEvoy (Eds.), Memory Improvement: Implications for Memory Theory. New York: Springer-Verlag, 1992, pp. 187–209.

74. Payne DG, Roediger HL III: Hypermnesia occurs in recall but not in recognition. Am J Psychol 1987; 100:145–165.

75. Roediger HL III, Thorpe LA: The role of recall time in producing hypermnesia. Mem Cogn 1978; 6:296–305.

76. Wheeler MA, Roediger HL III: Disparate effects of repeated testing: reconciling Ballard's (1913) and Bartlett's (1932) results. Psychol Sci 1992; 3:240–245.

77. Payne DG: Hypermnesia for pictures and words: testing the recall level hypothesis. J Exp Psychol Learn Mem Cogn 1986; 12:16–29.

78. Roediger HL III, Payne DG, Gillespie GL, Lean DS: Hypermnesia as determined by level of recall. J Verbal Learn Verbal Behav 1982; 21:635–655.

79. Klein SB, Loftus J, Fricker SS: The effects of self-beliefs on repeated efforts to remember. Soc Cogn 1994; 12:249–261.

80. Williams MD, Santos-Williams SM: Method for exploring retrieval processes using verbal protocols. *In* RS Nickerson (Ed.), Attention and Performance, Vol. 8. Hillsdale, NJ; Erlbaum, 1980, p. 673, footnote.

81. Whitten WB II, Leonard JM: Directed search through autobiographical memory. Mem Cogn 1981; 9:566–579.

82. Williams MD, Hollan JD: The process of retrieval from very long-term memory. Cogn Sci 1981; 5:87–119.

83. Brown J: Some tests of the decay theory of immediate memory. Q J Exp Psychol 1958; 10:12–21.

84. Peterson LR, Peterson MJ: Short-term retention of individual verbal items. J Exp Psychol 1959; 54:157–173.

85. Wickens DD: Encoding categories of words: an empirical approach to meaning. Psychol Rev 1970; 77:1–15.

86. Gardiner JM, Craik FIM, Birtwistle J: Retrieval cues and release from proactive inhibition. J Verbal Learn Verbal Behav 1972; 11:778–783.

87. O'Neil ME, Sutcliffe JA, Tulving E: Retrieval cues and release from proactive inhibition. Am J Psychol 1976; 89:535–543.

88. Reutener DB: Class shift, symbolic shift, and background shift in short-term memory. J Exp Psychol 1972; 93:90–94.

89. Wickens DO, Clark SE: Osgood dimensions as an encoding class in short-term memory. J Exp Psychol 1968; 78:580–584.

90. Gunter B, Berry C, Clifford BR: Proactive interference effects with television news items: further evidence. J Exp Psychol Hum Learn Mem 1981; 7:480–487.

91. Gunter B, Clifford BR, Berry C: Release from proactive interference with television news items: evidence for encoding dimensions within televised news. J Exp Psychol Hum Learn Mem 1980; 6:216–223.

92. Barnhardt TM: Directed Forgetting Effects in Implicit and Explicit Memory. Ph.D. dissertation, University of Arizona, 1993.

93. Bray NW, Hersh RE, Turner LA: Selective remembering during adolescence. Dev Psychol 1985; 21:290–294.

94. Bray NW, Justice EM, Zahm DN: Two developmental transitions in selective remembering strategies. J Exp Child Psychol 1983; 36:43–55.
95. Goernert PN: The antecedents of retrieval inhibition. J Gen Psychol 1992; 119:237–245.
96. Landauer TK, Bjork RA: Optimal rehearsal patterns and name learning. *In* MM Gruneberg, PE Morris, RN Sykes (Eds.), Practical Aspects of Memory. London: Academic Press, 1978, pp. 625–632.
97. Linton M: Memory for real-world events. *In* DA Norman, DE Rumelhart (Eds.), Explorations in Cognition. San Francisco: Freeman, 1975, pp. 376–404.
98. Linton M: Real world memory after six years: an in vivo study of very long term memory. *In* MM Gruneberg, PE Morris, RN Sykes (Eds.), Practical Aspects of Memory. Orlando, FL: Academic Press, 1978, pp. 3–24.
99. Anderson MC, Bjork RA, Bjork EL: Remembering can cause forgetting: retrieval dynamics in long-term memory. J Exp Psychol Learn Mem Cogn 1994; 20:1063–1087.
100. Anderson MC, Spellman BA: On the status of inhibitory mechanisms in cognition: memory retrieval as a model case. Psychol Rev 1995; 102:68–100.
101. Bjork RA: The updating of human memory. Psychol Learn Motivation 1978; 12:235–259.
102. Bjork RA: Retrieval inhibition as an adaptive mechanism in human memory. *In* HL Roediger III, FIM Craik (Eds.), Varieties of Memory and Consciousness: Essays in Honour of Endel Tulving. Hillsdale, NJ: Erlbaum, 1989, pp. 309–330.
103. Johnson HM: Processes of intentional forgetting. Psychol Bull 1994; 116:274–292.
104. Kihlstrom JF, Barnhardt TM: The self-regulation of memory: for better and for worse, with and without hypnosis. *In* DM Wegner, JW Pennebaker (Eds.), Handbook of Mental Control. Englewood Cliffs, NJ: Prentice Hall, 1993, pp. 88–125.
105. Basden BH, Basden DR, Gargano GJ: Directed forgetting in implicit and explicit memory tests: a comparison of methods. J Exp Psychol Learn Mem Cogn 1993; 19:603–616.
106. Basden BH, Basden DR, Coe WC, Decker S, Crutcher K: Retrieval inhibition in directed forgetting and posthypnotic amnesia. Int J Clin Exp Hypn 1994; 42:184–203.
107. Koutstaal W: Beyond Content: The Fate—or Function?—of Contextual Information in Directed Forgetting. Ph.D. Dissertation, Harvard University, 1996.
108. Bjork RA, Bjork EL: Dissociations in the impact of to-be-forgotten information. Paper presented at the annual meeting of the American Psychological Association, San Francisco, 1991.
109. Goernert PN, Larson ME: The initiation and release of retrieval inhibition. J Gen Psychol 1994; 121:61–66.
110. Geiselman RE, Bjork RA, Fishman DL: Disrupted retrieval in directed forgetting: a link with posthypnotic amnesia. J Exp Psychol Gen 1983; 112:58–72.
111. Postman L, Stark K, Fraser J: Temporal changes in interference. J Verbal Learn Verbal Behav 1968; 7:672–694.
112. Postman L: Interference theory revisited. *In* J Brown (Ed.), Recall and Recognition. New York: Wiley, 1976, pp. 157–181.
113. Wheeler MA: Improvement in recall over time without repeated testing: spontaneous recovery revisited. J Exp Psychol Learn Mem Cogn 1995; 21:173–184.
114. Beckmann J: Ruminative thought and the deactivation of an intention. Motivation and Emotion 1994; 18:317–334.
115. Cohen JD, O'Reilly RC: A preliminary theory of the interactions between prefrontal cortex and hippocampus that contribute to planning and prospective memory. *In* MA Brandimonte, GO Einstein, MA McDaniel (Eds.), Prospective Memory: Theory and Applications. Hillsdale, NJ: Lawrence Erlbaum, 1996, pp. 267–295.
116. Kuhl J: A theory of action and state orientations. *In* J Kuhl, J Beckmann (Eds.), Volition

and Personality: Action- and State-Oriented Modes of Control. Seattle, Göttingen: Hogrefe, 1994, pp. 9–46.

117. Schacter DL: Implicit memory: history and current status. J Exp Psychol Learn Mem Cogn 1987; 13:501–518.

118. Squire LR: Declarative and nondeclarative memory: multiple brain systems supporting learning and memory. *In* DL Schacter, E Tulving (Eds.), Memory Systems 1994. Cambridge, MA: MIT Press, 1994, pp. 203–231.

119. Squire LR, Zola-Morgan S: The medial temporal lobe memory system. Science 1991; 253:1380–1386.

120. Schacter DL, Chiu CYP, Ochsner KN: Implicit memory: a selective review. Annu Rev Neurosci 1993; 16:159–182.

121. Roediger HL III, McDermott KB: Implicit memory in normal human subjects. *In* H Spinnler, F Boller (Eds.), Handbook of Neuropsychology, Vol. 8. Amsterdam: Elsevier, 1993, pp. 63–131.

122. Johnson MK: Reality monitoring: an experimental phenomenological approach. J Exp Psychol Gen 1988; 117:390–394.

123. Johnson MK, Raye CL: Reality monitoring. Psychol Rev 1981; 88:67–85.

124. Johnson MK, Hashtroudi S, Lindsay DS: Source monitoring. Psychol Bull 1993; 114:3–28.

125. Kelley CM, Jacoby LR: The construction of subjective experience: memory attributions. Mind Lang 1990; 5:49–68.

126. Hashtroudi S, Johnson MK, Chrosniak LD: Aging and source monitoring. Psychol Aging 1989; 4:106–112.

127. Johnson MK, Raye CL, Foley HJ, Foley MA: Cognitive operations and decision bias in reality monitoring. Am J Psychol 1981; 94:37–64.

128. Weingardt KR, Loftus EF, Lindsay DS: Misinformation revisited: new evidence on the suggestibility of memory. Mem Cogn 1995; 23:72–82.

129. Bower G: A multicomponent theory of the memory trace. *In* KW Spence, JT Spence (Eds.), Psychology of Learning and Motivation, Vol 1. New York: Academic Press, 1967, pp. 229–325.

130. Underwood BJ: Attributes of memory. Psychol Rev 1969; 76:559–573.

131. Underwood BJ: Attributes of memory. Glenview, IL: Scott, Foresman, 1983.

132. Damasio AR: Time-locked multiregional retroactivation: a systems-level proposal for the neural substrates of recall and recognition. Cognition 1989; 33:25–62.

133. Johnson MK, Chalfonte BL: Binding complex memories: the role of reactivation and the hippocampus. *In* DL Schacter, E Tulving (Eds.), Memory Systems 1994. Cambridge, MA: MIT Press, 1994, pp. 311–350.

134. Kesner RP, Jackson-Smith P: Neurobiology of an attribute model of memory: role of prefrontal cortex. *In* I Gormezano, EA Wasserman (Eds.), Learning and Memory: The Behavioral and Biological Substrates. Hillsdale, NJ: Erlbaum, 1992, pp. 251–273.

135. Bowers KS, Hilgard ER: Some complexities in understanding memory. *In* HM Pettinati (Ed.), Hypnosis and Memory. New York: Guilford, 1988, pp. 3–18.

136. Taylor FK: Cryptomnesia and plagiarism. Br J Psychiatry 1965; 111:1111–1118.

137. Brown AS, Halliday HE: Cryptomnesia and source memory difficulties. Am J Psychol 1991; 104:475–490.

138. Brown AS, Murphy DR: Cryptomnesia: delineating inadvertent plagiarism. J Exp Psychol Learn Mem Cogn 1989; 15:432–442.

139. Cooper LM: Spontaneous and suggested posthypnotic source amnesia. Int J Clin Exp Hypn 1966; 14:180–193.

140. Evans FJ: Contextual forgetting: posthypnotic source amnesia. J Abnorm Psychol 1979; 88:556–563.

141. Evans FJ, Thorn WAF: Two types of posthypnotic amnesia: recall anmesia and source amnesia. Int J Clin Exp Hypn 1966; 14:162–179.

142. Shimamura AP, Squire LR: The relationship between fact and source memory: findings from amnesic patients and normal subjects. Psychobiology 1991; 19:1–10.

143. Schacter DL, Harbluk JL, McLachlan DR: Retrieval without recollection: an experimental analysis of source amnesia. J Verbal Learn Verbal Behav 1984; 23:593–611.

144. McIntyre JS, Craik FIM: Age differences in memory for item and source information. Can J Psychol 1987; 41:175–192.

145. Jacoby LL, Kelley C, Brown J, Jasechko J: Becoming famous overnight: limits on the ability to avoid unconscious influences of the past. J Pers Soc Psychol 1989; 56:326–338.

146. Read JD, Tollestrup P, Hammersley RH, McFadzen E, Christensen A: The unconscious transference effect: are innocent bystanders misidentified? Appl Cogn Psychol 1990; 4:3–31.

147. Gerrig RJ, Prentice DA: The representation of fictional information. Psychol Sci 1991; 2:336–340.

148. Jacoby LL, Allan LG, Collins JC, Larwill LK: Memory influences subjective experience: noise judgments. J Exp Psychol Learn Mem Cogn 1988; 14:240–247.

149. Witherspoon D, Allan LG: The effect of a prior presentation on temporal judgments in a perceptual identification task. Mem Cogn 1985; 13:101–111.

150. Begg I, Armour V: Repetition and the ring of truth: biasing comments. Can J Behav Sci 1991; 23:195–213.

151. Peynircioglu ZF, Watkins MJ: Effect of unfolding stimulus presentation on recognition memory. *In* MM Gruneberg, PE Morris, R Sykes (Eds.), Practical Aspects of Memory: Current Research and Issues, Vol. 2. Chichester: Wiley, 1988, pp. 518–523.

152. LeCompte DC: Recollective experience in the revelation effect: separating the contributions of recollection and familiarity. Mem Cogn 1995; 23:324–334.

153. Luo CR: Enhanced feeling of recognition: effects of identifying and manipulating test items on recognition memory. J Exp Psychol Learn Mem Cogn 1993; 19:405–413.

154. Peynircioglu ZF, Teckan AI: Revelation effect: effort or priming does not create the sense of familiarity. J Exp Psychol Learn Mem Cogn 1993; 19:382–388.

155. Watkins MJ, Peynircioglu ZF: The revelation effect: when disguising test items induces recognition. J Exp Psychol Learn Mem Cogn 1990; 16:1012–1020.

156. Underwood, BJ: False recognition produced by implicit verbal responses. J Exp Psychol 1965; 70:122–129.

157. Bousfield WA, Whitmarsh GA, Danick JJ: Partial response identities in verbal generalization. Psychol Rep 1958; 4:703–713.

158. Vogt J, Kimble GA: False recognition as a function of associative proximity. J Exp Psychol 1973; 99:143–145.

159. Bentin S, Kutas M, Hillyard SA: Semantic processing and memory for attended and unattended words in dichotic listening: behavioral and electrophysiological evidence. J Exp Psychol Hum Percept Perform 1995; 21:54–67.

160. Deese J: On the prediction of occurrence of particular verbal intrusions in immediate recall. J Exp Psychol 1959; 58:17–22.

161. Norman KA, Schacter DL: False recognition in younger and older adults: exploring the characteristics of illusory memories. Mem Cogn (in press).

162. Roediger HL III, McDermott KB: Creating false memories: remembering words not presented in lists. J Exp Psychol Learn Mem Cogn 1995; 21:803–814.

163. Gardiner JM: Functional aspects of recollective experience. Mem Cogn 1988; 16:309–313.
164. Gardiner JM, Java RI: Recollective experience in word and nonword recognition memory. Mem Cogn 1990; 18:23–30.
165. Wippich W: Implicit and explicit memory without awareness. Psychol Res 1992; 54:212–224.
166. Bransford JD, Franks JJ: The abstraction of linguistic ideas. Cogn Psychol 1971; 2:331–350.
167. Sulin RA, Dooling DJ: Intrusion of a thematic idea in retention of prose. J Exp Psychol 1974; 103:255–262.
168. Shepard RN: Recognition memory for words, sentences, and pictures. J Verbal Learn Verbal Behav 1967; 6:156–163.
169. Standing L: Learning 10,000 pictures. Q J Exp Psychol 1973; 25:207–222.
170. Mandler JM, Ritchey GH: Long-term memory for pictures. J Exp Psychol Hum Learn Mem 1977; 3:386–396.
171. Friedman A: Framing pictures: the role of knowledge in automatized encoding and memory for gist. J Exp Psychol Gen 1979; 108:316–355.
172. Dooling DJ, Christiaansen RE: Episodic and semantic aspects of memory for prose. J Exp Psychol Hum Learn Mem 1977; 3:428–436.
173. Reder LM: Plausibility judgment versus fact retrieval: alternative strategies for sentence verification. Psychol Rev 1982; 89:250–280.
174. Spiro RJ: Remembering information from text: the ''state of the schema'' approach. *In* RC Anderson, RJ Spiro, WE Montague (Eds.), Schooling and the Acquisition of Knowledge. Hillsdale, NJ: Erlbaum, 1977, pp. 137–165.
175. Spiro RJ: Accommodative reconstruction in prose recall. J Verbal Learn Verbal Behav 1980; 19:84–95.
176. Brainerd CJ, Reyna VF: Learning rate, learning opportunities, and the development of forgetting. Dev Psychol 1995; 31:251–262.
177. Reyna VF, Kiernan B: Development of gist versus verbatim memory in sentence recognition: effects of lexical familiarity, semantic content, encoding instructions, and retention interval. Dev Psychol 1994; 30:178–191.
178. Hintzman DL, Curran T: Retrieval dynamics of recognition and frequency judgments: evidence for separate processes of familiarity and recall. J Mem Lang 1994; 33:1–18.
179. Hintzman DL, Curran T, Oppy B: Effects of similarity and repetition on memory: registration without learning? J Exp Psychol Learn Mem Cogn 1992; 18:667–680.
180. Koriat A, Goldsmith M: Memory in naturalistic and laboratory contexts: distinguishing the accuracy-oriented and quantity-oriented approaches to memory assessment. J Exp Psychol Gen 1994; 123:297–315.
181. Wagenaar WA, Groeneweg J: The memory of concentration camp survivors. Appl Cogn Psychol 1990; 4:77–87.
182. Neisser U: John Dean's memory: a case study. *In* U Neisser (Ed.), Memory Observed. San Francisco: Freeman, 1982, pp. 139–159.
183. Linton M: Ways of searching and the contents of memory. *In* DC Rubin (Ed.), Autobiographical Memory. Cambridge: Cambridge University Press, 1986, pp. 50–67.
184. Barclay CR, Wellman HM: Accuracies and inaccuracies in autobiographical memories. J Mem Lang 1986; 25:93–103.
185. Barclay CR, DeCooke PA: Ordinary everyday memories: some of the things of which selves are made. *In* U Neisser, E Winograd (Eds.), Real Events Remembered: Ecological Approaches to the Study of Memory. New York: Cambridge University Press, 1987, pp. 91–125.

186. Bless H, Fiedler K: Affective states and the influence of activated general knowledge. Pers Soc Psychol Bull 1995; 21:766–778.
187. Hastie R: Schematic principles in human memory. *In* ET Higgins, P Herman, MP Zanna (Eds.), Social Cognition: The Ontario Symposium, Vol. 1. Hillsdale, NJ: Erlbaum, 1981, pp. 39–88.
188. Rumelhart DE, Smolensky P, McClelland JL, Hinton GE: Schemata and sequential thought processes in PDP models. *In* JL McClelland, DE Rumelhart (Eds.), Parallel Distributed Processing: Explorations in the Microstructure of Cognition, Vol. 2. Cambridge, MA: MIT Press, 1986, pp. 7–57.
189. McClelland JL: Constructive memory and memory distortions: a parallel-distributed processing approach. *In* DL Schacter, JT Coyle, GD Fishbach, MM Mesulam, LE Sullivan (Eds.), Memory Distortion. Cambridge, MA: Harvard University Press, 1995, pp. 69–90.
190. Johnson MK, Bransford JD, Solomon S: Memory for tacit implications of sentences. J Exp Psychol 1973; 98:203–205.
191. Brewer WF, Treyens JC: Role of schemata in memory for places. Cogn Psychol 1981; 13:207–230.
192. Barclay CR, Subramaniam G: Autobiographical memory and self-schemata. Appl Cogn Psychol 1987; 1:169–182.
193. Kuiper NA, Rogers TB: Encoding of personal information: self-other differences. J Pers Soc Psychol 1979; 37:499–514.
194. Markus H: Self-schemata and processing information about the self. J Pers Soc Psychol 1977; 35:63–78.
195. Swann WB, Read SJ: Acquiring self-knowledge: the search for feedback that fits. J Pers Soc Psychol 1981; 41:1119–1128.
196. Barclay CR: Schematization of autobiographical memory. *In* DC Rubin (Ed.), Autobiographical Memory. New York: Cambridge University Press, 1986, pp. 82–89.
197. Barclay CR: Remembering ourselves. *In* GM Davies, RH Logie (Eds.), Memory in Everyday Life. Amsterdam: Elsevier, 1993, pp. 285–309.
198. Brewer WF: Memory for randomly sampled autobiographical events. *In* U Neisser, E Winograd (Eds.), Remembering Reconsidered: Ecological and Traditional Approaches to the Study of Memory. New York: Cambridge University Press, 1988, pp. 21–90.
199. Larsen SF: Commentary: memory of schemata, details and selves. *In* GM Davies, RH Logie (Eds.), Memory in Everyday Life. Amsterdam: Elsevier, 1993, pp. 310–315.
200. Brewer WF: What is autobiographical memory? *In* DC Rubin (Ed.), Autobiographical Memory. Cambridge: Cambridge University Press, 1986, pp. 25–49.
201. Whittlesea BWA: Illusions of familiarity. J Exp Psychol Learn Mem Cogn 1993; 19:1235–1253.
202. Berrios GE: Déjà vu in France during the 19th century: a conceptual history. Compr Psychiatry 1995; 36:123–129.
203. Sno HN, Linszen DH: The déjà vu experience: remembrance of things past? Am J Psychiatry 1990; 147:1587–1595.
204. Sno, HN, Linszen DH, DeJonghe F: Déjà vu experiences and reduplicative paramnesia. Br J Psychiatry 1992; 161:565–568.
205. Johnson MK, Foley MA, Suengas, AG, Raye CL: Phenomenal characteristics of memories for perceived and imagined autobiographical events. J Exp Psychol Gen 1988; 117:371–376.
206. Johnson MK, Kahan TL, Raye CL: Dreams and reality monitoring. J Exp Psychol Gen 1984; 113:329–344.

207. Owens J, Bower GH, Black JB: The "soap opera" effect in story recall. Mem Cogn 1979; 7:185–191.
208. Reason JT: Absent-mindedness and cognitive control. *In* JE Harris, PE Morris (Eds.), Everyday Memory, Actions and Absent-Mindedness. London: Academic Press, 1984, pp. 113–132.
209. Greene E, Flynn MS, Loftus EF: Inducing resistance to misleading information. J Verbal Learn Verbal Behav 1982; 21:207–219.
210. Warren A, Hulse-Trotter K, Tubbs E: Inducing resistance to suggestibility in children. Law Hum Behav 1991; 15:273–285.
211. Lindsay DS, Johnson MK: The eyewitness suggestibility effect and memory for source. Mem Cogn 1989; 17:349–358.
212. Gauld A, Stephenson GM: Some experiments related to Bartlett's theory of remembering. Br J Psychol 1967; 58:39–49.
213. O'Sullivan JT, Howe ML: Metamemory and memory construction. Consciousness Cogn 1995; 4:104–110.
214. Wilson TD, Brekke N: Mental contamination and mental correction: unwanted influences on judgments and evaluations. Psychol Bull 1994; 116:117–142.
215. Jacoby LL: A process dissociation framework: separating automatic from intentional uses of memory. J Mem Lang 1991; 30:513–541.
216. Jacoby LL, Woloshyn V, Kelley CM: Becoming famous without being recognized: unconscious influences of memory produced by dividing attention. J Exp Psychol Gen 1989; 118:115–125.
217. Moscovitch M: Memory and working-with-memory: a component process model based on modules and central systems. J Cogn Neurosci 1992; 4:257–267.
218. Moscovitch M: Cognitive resources and dual-task interference effects at retrieval in normal people: the role of the frontal lobes and medial temporal cortex. Neuropsychology 1994; 8:524–534.
219. Reardon R, Doyle SM: The self-concept and reality judgments: memory, memory monitoring, and internal-external correspondence. Soc Cogn 1995; 13:1–24.
220. Schacter DL, Kagan J, Leichtman MD: True and false memories in children and adults: a cognitive neuroscience perspective. Psychol Public Policy Law 1995; 1:411–428.
221. Neisser U: Time present and time past. *In* M Gruneberg, P Morris, R Sykes (Eds.), Practical Aspects of Memory: Current Research and Issues, Vol. 2. Chichester: Wiley, 1988, pp. 545–560.
222. Warnick DH, Sanders GS: Why do eyewitnesses make so many mistakes? J Appl Soc Psychol 1980; 10:362–366.
223. Lindsay, DS: Misleading suggestions can impair eyewitnesses' ability to remember event details. J Exp Psychol Learn Mem Cogn 1990; 16:1077–1083.
224. DeLuca J: Predicting neurobehavioral patterns following anterior communicating artery aneurysm. Cortex 1993; 29:639–647.
225. Johnson MK: Reality monitoring: evidence from confabulation in organic brain disease patients. *In* GP Prigatano, DL Schacter (Eds.), Awareness of Deficit After Brain Injury: Clinical and Theoretical Issues. New York: Oxford University Press, 1991, pp. 176–197.
226. Dalla Barba G: Confabulation: knowledge and recollective experience. Cogn Neuropsychol 1993; 10:1–20.
227. Schacter DL, Curran T: The cognitive neuroscience of false memories. Psychiatric Ann 1995; 25:726–730.
228. Alexander MP, Stuss DT, Benson DF: Capgras syndrome: a reduplicative phenomenon. Neurology 1979; 29:334–339.

229. Delbecq-Derouesné J, Beauvois MF, Shallice T: Preserved recall versus impaired recognition. Brain 1990; 113:1045–1074.
230. Parkin AJ, Leng NRC, Stanhope N, Smith AP: Memory impairment following ruptured aneurysm of the anterior communicating artery. Brain Cogn 1988; 7:231–243.
231. Parkin AJ, Bindschaedler C, Harsent L, Metzler C: Pathological false alarm rates following damage to the frontal lobes. 1996, submitted for publication.
232. Schacter DL, Curran T, Galluccio LD, Milberg WP, Bates JF: False recognition and the right frontal lobe: a case study. Neuropsychologia 1996; 34:793–808.
233. Squire LR: Memory and Brain. New York: Oxford University Press, 1987.
234. Schacter DL, Kaszniak AW, Kihlstrom JF, Valdiserri M: The relation between source memory and aging. Psychol Aging 1991; 6:559–568.
235. Schacter DL, Osowiecki D, Kaszniak AW, Kihlstrom JF, Valdiserri M: Source memory: extending the boundaries of age-related deficits. Psychol Aging 1994; 9:81–89.
236. Schacter DL, Koutstaal W, Johnson MK, Gross MS, Angell KE: False recollection induced via photographs: a comparison of older and younger adults. Psychol Aging (in press).
237. Schacter DL: Searching for Memory: The Brain, The Mind, and The Past. New York: Basic Books, 1996.
238. Tulving E: Elements of Episodic Memory. Oxford: Oxford University Press, 1983.

5

Psychoanalysis, Memory, and Trauma

ROBERT M. GALATZER-LEVY

> "I did this," says my Memory. "I cannot have done this," says
> my Pride and remains inexorable. In the end—Memory yields."
>
> Nietzsche, *Beyond Good and Evil*

During the hot Vienna summer of 1882 physician Josef Breuer observed his young patient, Anna O.: "She would take up the glass of water she longed for, but as soon as it touched her lips she would push it away. . . . This had lasted for some six weeks, when one day during hypnosis she grumbled about her English lady-companion whom she did not care for, and went on to describe, with every sign of disgust, how she had once gone into that lady's room and how her little dog—horrid creature!—had drunk out of a glass there. The patient had said nothing, as she had wanted to be polite. After giving further energetic expression to the anger she had held back, she asked for something to drink, drank a large quantity of water without any difficulty and woke from her hypnosis with the glass at her lips; and thereupon the disturbance vanished, never to return"[1] (pp. 34–35). Breuer and Freud observed that when hysterical patients remembered, with affect, the circumstances in which a symptom arose, that symptom disappeared. Thus began the study of the relationship between bad events, memory, and symptoms.

Psychoanalysts try to understand human actions in terms of personal meanings, intents, and wishes. These meanings, intents, and wishes may or may not be available to awareness. Until recently, psychoanalytic discussion often used the language that described mental function in terms of physical concepts like energy and force. But the major contributions of psychoanalysis have been to clinical theory. The greatest success of psychoanalysis is making psychological events comprehensible as intentional and meaningful (if unconscious) acts.[2]

The major sources of psychoanalytic information are clinical encounters, which often last for years. As a result, psychoanalysis provides an extraordinarily rich picture of people in the therapeutic process. However, generalizing these findings to other contexts may be problematic. In particular, psychoanalysts have explored how patients construct and use autobiographical memory in forming symptoms, understanding their worlds, interacting with others and the process of cure. Psychoanalysis addresses a limited, but important, aspect of memory.

Contemporary discussions about the relationship between bad events, memory, and psychological suffering commonly borrow psychoanalytic terms and concept. Often the terms and ideas are misused or used idiosyncratically. Psychoanalytic investigations are said to provide data for positions they do not actually support. Long discarded ideas, and even ideas they never espoused, are attributed to analysts. Analysts, simultaneously, and equally inaccurately, are blamed for creating a system that supports false memories and for suppressing the reality of child abuse. We need to clarify the underlying psychoanalytic ideas, the bases on which they are asserted, and their relationship to related ideas about memory and trauma. This chapter describes a group of psychoanalytic concepts important to thinking about memory and to the impact of untoward experience on memory. Psychoanalysis is a large discipline. Controversy about fundamental issues continues. This chapter draws on a range of widely current contemporary psychoanalytic ideas. But the reader should note that some of these ideas would draw dissent even in analytic circles.

Psychoanalysis and Memory

Memory is central to psychoanalysis but Freud did not publish a systematic theory of memory. LaPlanche and Pontalis[3] have culled a theory of memory from his writings. Freud regarded memory traces as discrete pieces of information (declarative statements, images, etc.). His main interest was how people connected, stratified, and interrelated memories. He viewed memory as a complex archive in which the individual memories are arranged in several ways: chronological order, links in chains of association, and degree of accessibility to consciousness. Freud believed people automatically record perceptions as memories. How available a memory is to awareness depends on the person's current active interests and the extent to which the memory is actively barred from consciousness. Memories are ordinarily descriptively unconscious. Some memories are available to awareness as needed. These are called *preconscious*. Other memories are actively barred from awareness. They are said to be *dynamically unconscious*. Freud asserted that the common absence of more than sporadic memories from before school age, a phenomenon he called *infantile amnesia*, resulted from active repression of early anxiety-arousing experience.

Freud's early study of hysteria led him to believe that repressed memories can produce psychopathology. At first he believed that these memories reflected actual experiences. Early in the development of psychoanalysis he came to regard many such memories as largely the residues of childhood fantasy. The first generation of psychoanalysts viewed specific repressed memories and ideas as central to understanding psychopathology. Attempts to lift repression or at least to satisfactorily *reconstruct*, i.e., to accurately describe early psychological events based on current function, were central to psychoanalytic treatment.[4,5] With increasing clinical experience, analysts found that psychopathology usually does not arise from isolated distressing experiences. The way a person processes experiences, long-lasting experiences of relations to others, and the overall quality of the supporting environment emerged as more important.[6–8] Psychoanalysts became less interested in the recovery of particular past experiences and fantasies. They recognized that cathartic recollection of past events was far less important than other analytic activities, including the exploration of how the patient protects himself from psychological distress, the modification of harsh unconscious moral standards, and other forms of experience with the analyst. Contemporary analysts are much less interested in detailed reconstruction of past events than earlier analysts were.[6,9]

Freud's early observations of neurotic people's symptoms and associations seemed consistent with histories of childhood abuse. Initially he concluded that all neurosis resulted from abuse. However, both his clinical experience and self-analysis led him to doubt this conclusion. It implied that very many people were victims of extensive and often bizarre abuse in a way that Freud found inconsistent with his observations of adult behavior. Writers like Jeffrey Masson interpret Freud's rejection of this hypothesis as one example among many of bad faith by psychoanalysts, who, to maintain their own positions of power, emphasize other than manifest sources for evidence of child abuse.[10] If nothing else is clear from the study of memory and trauma, it is that people in good faith can disagree about the relationship between external events and what is remembered. It is beyond the scope of this chapter to address the bad-faith idea in depth. Neither the evidence put forward for Freud's bad faith nor the idea that his changed position was inconsistent with the data available to him support close scrutiny.[11]

At the same time that Freud noted the inconsistency of the "seduction hypothesis" with his knowledge of ordinary people's actions, he found an alternative explanation for his data. Instead of interpreting the evidence of memory as indicating past external events, he asserted that it memorialized childhood fantasies and wishes which, being unacceptable to the more mature child, the child repressed. Typically, these wishes and fantasies involved bodily function and relations within the family. On the basis of clinical experience, self analysis, examination of literary and anthropological materials, and informal child observation, Freud described several common forms of early fantasy and wish that shape later psychological function. The most important and thoroughly described of these ideas is the boy's Oedipus complex. In the classical formulation, the boy wishes to take his father's place (as the boy understands that place) in relationship to the mother. He is frightened to do so because he both wishes to maintain a loving relationship with his father and fears his father's violent retribution. All of this goes on in the context of the concrete, bodily centered fantasy life of a 3- to 5-year-old. The boy notes his own sexual arousal in response to erotic fantasies. He combines this with his idea of the role of the penis in intimacy and his sense of pride in having a penis. He may conclude that his father will destroy or damage his penis in

revenge for sexual interest in the mother. The child's elaborated, fantastical constructions are remembered but not differentiated from material reality and they form another
source for "memories" of horrendous happenings. Subsequent repression of these
memories makes them unavailable to modification, so they persist in the unconscious
outside awareness but they still affect psychological function (see below.) In a *tour de
force* of interpretation that has so reshaped Western thought that in the late twentieth
century many of his findings are clichés, Freud concluded that we can understand
many psychological activities, including psychopathology, social structures, morality,
dreams, jokes, and artistic creation, as the adult's attempt to deal with ever-present
repressed wishes and memories from early childhood.

Contemporary analysts emphasize a wider range of experience as important to psychological development than Freud did. However, they continue to believe that the
presently remembered past, whether generated primarily internally or in response to
external events, shapes current psychological functioning. When people bar ideas from
interaction with new experience and thought, the original ideas may continue to affect
current function without the learning from experience that ordinarily would lead those
ideas to come in line better with new experience. Thus analysts continue to believe in
the impact of memory. Note that we are speaking strictly of memories. The relationship
of those memories to actual events continues to be a tricky issue in psychoanalytic
thinking.

Psychoanalysis regards memory as plastic. Because the significance of memory lies
in its meaning, we expect that memory changes with the capacity to appreciate new
meanings. Freud used the term *Nachträglichkeit* (unfortunately, customarily translated
as *deferred action*) to refer to the way people revise experiences, impressions, and
memories to fit in with fresh experiences or with the attainment of a new developmental
level. For example, Freud[12] described how his patient, the Wolf Man, dreamed at age 4
of the still wolves with large tails. Freud interpreted this dream as originating from his
patient's observation of parental sexual activity when the patient was 18 months old.
When the patient reached an oedipal level of development, he reshaped the memory in a
manner consistent with the child's current understanding of the world and his current
interests, emphasizing the frightening movement of the observed intercourse through
the stillness of the wolves and his view of the father's penis as their tails. Whether we
find Freud's particular example credible, the experience of reinterpreting elements of a
memory and changing the memory, at least in its significance, is a common happening.
Sometimes the memory's manifest content may be retained but its significance alone
changes—e.g., the memory of a pain in the arm becomes the memory of the first
symptoms of heart disease. But surprisingly often the memory's contents are transformed to correspond to the subject's new understanding. For example, a wholly absent
element of the scene is added because it bolsters the significance of the memory. A
patient in analysis had long recalled his emotional pain during a specific incident when a
sibling mercilessly teased him. However, it was only when the analysis turned to the
question of his parent's failure to protect the patient from his sibling that he "recalled"
that his father had been in the same room, ensconced behind a newspaper.

Arnold Modell[13] suggests that we can understand both psychological distress and the curative impact of emotional, re-engaged past experience in terms of effective and failed *Nachträglichkeit*. A memory may become problematic in two ways. Reinterpreted in light of a new world view, previously unobnoxious recollections may become severely distressing. For example, a woman transformed the innocuous memory of her father's road trips with a sister into a recollection of recurrent planned abuse of the sister after she confronted her own clear experiences of being abused by her father. At the other end of the spectrum, memories that are not brought into contact with current information may retain a terrifying quality that would not persist if the memory were reworked by using current knowledge. For example, consider "primal scenes," the child's observation of the parents' sexual activity. From the point of view of the young child, who is unclear about sexual anatomy and interpreting observations through her own experience, the vigorous motions, sounds, facial expressions, and postures of sexual intercourse suggest some sort of assault in which one party or another is injured. These memories commonly remain problematic. Because they are so frightening, they are repressed. As a result, they are separated from newer understandings of sexuality. At the same time, they unconsciously shape the subject's view of sexuality. One view of the therapeutic value of the exploration of memory is that it allows a reworking of memories, bringing them into relationship with the mass of experience. Note that in both these instances the subject transforms memory through psychological activity. Memories are plastic. They are not simply recordings of past events. This plasticity is in the service of making memory useful in current psychological life.

Trauma

Consistent with the psychoanalytic focus on people's internal worlds, psychoanalysts define trauma not in terms of external events but through the effects of events on the subject. Psychoanalysts use the term to refer to events whose intensity is such that the person is overwhelmed to the point of not functioning in any ordinary psychological mode. As Anna Freud[14] states, *traumatic* refers to "shattering, devastating, causing internal disruption by putting ego functioning and ego mediation out of action" (p. 238). At the time of trauma, the traumatized person cannot give himself a minimal sense of safety or organization because of the intensity of the experience. He feels overwhelming anxiety, helplessness, or at least the threat of those states. Subsequent events reminiscent of the trauma are likely to precipitate again its psychological dangers. In studying psychoanalytic ideas about trauma, readers should keep in mind that analysts usually mean something more specific than a very unpleasant experience. Some analysts have followed common parlance in using it to refer to any significant untoward event. But Cooper[15] observes, by maintaining a narrower definition, psychoanalysts can speak clearly about a specific set of phenomena.

The psychoanalytic definition of trauma involves not only the event but also the subject's response to that event. No event, no matter how obviously unpleasant or bad, is intrinsically traumatic. Nor is the external observer's assessment of an event as apparently minor a guarantee that it is not traumatic. Because people vary in the tools they have to deal with untoward happenings, events in and of themselves are not traumatizing. They can only be judged traumatizing in relation to a person's internal capacities to deal with the event, the personal history that gives the event meaning, the availability of social support to deal with the event, and the areas of current anxiety that overlap with the event. For some children who cannot regulate the intensity of stimuli, ordinary noises and scenes may be traumatic. People can often manage great loss or pain without trauma when other people provide adequate emotional support. For a child in the midst of a developmental phase in which bodily mutilation holds great terrors, a surgical procedure may prove traumatic. However, the same procedure would not overwhelm the same child earlier or later in development. For the young child who cannot maintain an adequate picture of a caretaker for more than a few hours, day-long separation from the caretaker may prove traumatic. Yet a separation of the same duration for a child who can maintain such an image longer will not be traumatic.

As psychoanalytic theory focused on a wider range of contributions to psychological distress, analysts viewed trauma as a less important pathogenic factor than it had been. Terms like *stress trauma, cumulative trauma,* and *overstimulation* were introduced to describe how chronic environmental failures to meet children's psychological needs impaired development.[16,17] Besides terminological confusion, these views led to punctate trauma being viewed in a different, richer light. Analysts increasingly focused on the way in which the experience of other people provides solace, organization, and support in the face of difficulty.[18,19] Analysts saw that trauma often resulted from the context of chronic environmental failures and disturbed development in which the specific event occurred. Erik Erikson,[20] for example, reexamined Freud's understanding of the case of "Dora." Freud had observed that Dora's traumatization by the sexual advances of a family friend resulted from the meaning of this approach in terms of childhood erotic fantasies. Erikson extended this analysis. He observed that Dora's parents and supposed friends chronically but subtly exploited her to arrange their sexual satisfactions. To that end, they interfered with her ordinary adolescent attempts to clarify the actualities of her world. Similarly, the commonest childhood traumas occur through chronic environmental failures. The untoward event is but a dramatic concrete situation that arises from ultimately more important chronic failures. The following illustrates this situation.

Case Study

A woman sought analysis because of chronic depression, obesity and inability to be sexually involved except through phone sex. She developed a transference in which she mistrusted her analyst's motives. One day she reported an almost hallucinatory experience that the lipstick she applied before the session tasted like semen. She agreed with the analyst that it was puzzling that she should be so certain of this as she had no conscious recollection of having ever tasted semen. At the same time she felt the analyst was denigrating her experience by his observation. The next night the patient dreamed that she was trying to tell her mother and aunt about something that was very distressing but they responded only with jokes and laughter. Ultimately, the patient and analyst concluded that she had been sexually abused by her uncle. But far more important than the specific sexual experiences was a chronic, easily remembered environment in the household. The family avoided any statement or action that might distress the uncle, on whom the family relied financially. The patient recalled chronic hypocrisy in which these women's interests dominated the patient's childhood. They regularly sacrificed and demeaned her concerns to keep her brittle uncle content.

These differing foci in understanding trauma suggest different therapeutic approaches to traumatic events. Focus on the broad context of trauma uses the history of trauma as a road into pervasive themes of environmental and developmental deficits. Focus on the traumatic event itself leads to attention to reworking the particular happenings. Just as contemporary psychoanalysis pays attention to pervasive themes in personality, most psychoanalysts today, while respecting the impact of particular traumatic events, attend more closely to the broad contexts in which these events occur and from which they draw their meaning.

Psychoanalysts view trauma and pathogenic effects of trauma in several ways. Consistent with his view that early development shaped later psychological function, Freud held that neurosis-inducing trauma occurred before age 6. The child represses these early traumata, which gain their power from their close relationship to the child's sexual and aggressive drives. These traumata lead to *fixation,* an unconscious tendency to recreate the traumatic event and, simultaneously, to avoid knowing about it. Although it is tempting to posit that this "repetition compulsion" arises from attempts to rework and thus master the traumatic experience, Freud avoided this rather optimistic conclusion and stuck closer to his clinical experience that there seemed to be some primary tendency to repeat the trauma. Both tendencies have great psychological force and are largely independent of other features of the personality.

Later analysts asked how, besides creating fixations, trauma was pathogenic. In isolation, the fact of having been unable to manage intense stimulation at a given moment would not necessarily be harmful. It is the memory and meaning of such experience that leads to the many disturbances associated with trauma. We may classify these into three types: changes in the subject's view of himself and others that result from trauma, changes that result from unsuccessful attempts to manage these meanings, and situations in which the memory of trauma itself is not problematic but stands in place of memory of a wider range of formative experiences.

The direct effects of trauma and its memory are several-fold. The experience of being exposed to overwhelming bad experiences may directly result in a tendency to physiological arousal that occurs in response to lesser stimuli. This tendency leaves the subject with the problem of managing startle responses and other physiological arousal in response to ordinary environmental happenings. The traumatic event may create a constant awareness of the possibility of bad happenings. Though such a view may, in some sense, be more realistic than the more optimistic view that many people enjoy, it carries with it a chronic sense of fear and distress. Trauma may shatter the ordinary sense of being able to manage difficulties of living, the feeling of effectiveness in the world, and confidence that one can manage experience. Trauma that results directly from mistreatment by caretakers or their substitutes (or even is perceived as the result of bad faith) deprives the subject of the sense that others may be relied upon to act in his interest. The sense of trust is badly damaged. Finally, when another has treated the traumatized person as inhuman, the subject may come to view himself as less than human. If I matter so little to another that they can hurt me in this way, that shows that I am valueless or not human.

Attempts to protect against the memory of trauma through various mechanisms of defense result in secondary symptomatology. The person may constrict experience to avoid retraumatization and stimulation of painful memories. For example, the sexually abused person may avoid intimate relationships that stimulate memories of abuse. She may attempt to deal with the sense of helplessness by unconsciously reenacting the traumatic situation in an attempt at mastery. Or she may reenact it so that, rather than suffering as passive victim, she actively controls the situations by causing rather than suffering maltreatment herself.

Very often analysts can relate discrete traumatic events to psychopathology not through a direct causative connection but because the factors that allowed the trauma to occur have other pathogenic effects. Recognizing this is important because the dramatic character of specific bad events may obscure the larger context in which they occur. As investigators progressively clarify people's developmental needs for others across the life course,[19,21] it becomes clear that the absence of needed interactions may be more damaging than specific noxious experiences. Furthermore, specific bad events are more likely to occur when needed interactions are absent or disturbed. For example, a middle-aged woman entered analysis because of chronic low self esteem and discomfort in relations with men, ''who always turn out to be bastards.'' With much sense, she attributed her negative feelings to the many times her drunken father had beaten her for almost no reason (making a noise at dinner or simply being nearby when he became enraged). Yet the analysis revealed another set of experiences that contributed even more powerfully to her view of herself and the world. The patient's mother suffered from a chronic severe depression and rarely expressed any interest in the child. In fact, the patient viewed herself most centrally not as the object of angry aggression but as a person of no interest or value. Unable to find an adequate engaged, enthusiastic response to herself from her mother, her sense of being of value was severely impaired. In this context, the beatings assumed a new meaning. Neither the patient nor her mother saw themselves as valuable enough nor sufficiently effective to protect the youngster from repeated violence. It was this sense of incompetence and valuelessness related to the bleak relationship with the mother that shaped the patient's pathology, not just the experience of being beaten.

The most dramatic sequelae of trauma, posttraumatic stress disorders, are characterized by a major reshaping of the personality. They alter the experience of oneself and the world. Large parts of psychological life are given over to issues associated with the trauma. Dreams center on the trauma. Other aspects of living are constricted. Irritability and rage become predominant affects. Those who suffer from posttraumatic stress disorder are generally unable to limit the access of memories of traumatic events to awareness. They suffer not from repressed memories but from an inability to use ordinary mechanisms of defense to control the impact of traumatic events on their current psychological lives.

Mechanisms of Defense

Freud found that we regulate awareness to reduce psychological distress. One solution to the problem that ideas, wishes, and memories can cause anxiety, depression, guilt, and shame is to fully or partly bar them from awareness or, in some other way, to alter their relationship to other ideas and affects. This regulation is likely to be imperfect because people often have strong reasons to remain aware of the distressing material. For example, a person may want to be unaware of a morally unacceptable sexual wish and simultaneously want the pleasure of imagining its satisfaction. Furthermore, the person may lack adequate tools to control awareness, so that despite efforts to limit awareness, distressing material continues to come to mind. Psychoanalysts call the means by which awareness is regulated *mechanisms of defense*.[22]

We may broadly divide the mechanisms of defense into two categories. *Repressive defenses* aim to keep objectionable ideas from awareness altogether. *Splitting defenses* keep ideas available to consciousness but alter their meaning by changing their connections to other conscious ideas. Examples of repressive defenses include the motivated forgetting of painful experiences (repression) and the belief that some other person, but not oneself, has hostile motives (projection). Examples of splitting defenses include disavowing the emotion associated with an event or knowing and also denying the significance of one's behavior. Other splitting defenses include maintaining two, unintegrated views of the same person and maintaining information dissociated from the context or emotions that would give it meaning. *Dissociation* is sometimes differentiated from other forms of splitting by its aim. While splitting is often used to maintain a pristine image of a person or a situation, dissociation is an effort to protect the individual from memories of trauma, which may stimulate overwhelming affects and fantasies.[23]

Analysts recognize two types of repression. Those experiences that never found representation in words but nonetheless are retained as active determinants of current function are said to be subject to *primary repression*. They are often retained as either procedural memories or difficult-to-articulate feeling states. Because they were never part of the declarative memory, analysts have called them "unrememorable and unforgettable."[24] *Secondary repression* (which analysts commonly call simply *repression*) refers to the forcing from awareness of ideas or memories that have representation in words. Past experience may be memorialized in several ways other than conscious memory. Though both may be remnants of the past, their evaluation and the impact of awareness of them is expectably different. When a person has repressed an idea or memory, simply bringing it to and maintaining it in awareness should set in motion the ordinary processes that integrate it with the rest of psychological life. However, in other instances, while awareness of historical factors contributing to past psychological function may provide useful insight into the current situation, awareness need not be curative. For example, consider a person who has secondarily repressed memories of sexual assault and as a result, fears sexuality without understanding why. The derepression of these memories would result in their integration with other aspects of experience and the realization, for example, that sexual activity is not necessarily associated with victimization. In contrast, although the person who feels unable to calm herself as a result of similar experiences, may find knowing part of the history of that sense helpful, we would not expect that knowledge in itself to relieve the need for the development of methods to soothe herself. The difference arises because in the former situation, repression has essentially led to an uncorrected cognitive error that equates sexuality with danger. In the latter situation, the individual lacks a means to soothe herself and must develop this capacity.

Action is an especially important defense. Rather than remembering an event or fantasy in words or images, people sometimes compulsively reenact it, unaware that the action has any particular meaning. Commonly, parents treat their children almost identically to the way their caretakers treated them, without any awareness that they are doing so.[25] Traumas are commonly memorialized as action schema even when verbal and pictorial memories are absent. The actions often include the formerly passive victim enacting the role of an active perpetrator and thus may contribute to the transmission of abuse across generations. As a defense, action allows the partial expression of the underlying experience without the need to avow its meaning. Defenses are commonly used in combination and are mutually reinforcing.

In terms of defense, the most characteristic feature of trauma is the relative failure of defensive operations both at the time of the trauma and subsequently. Much of the phenomenology of posttraumatic stress disorders can be described as the failure of defensive operations. For example, we may regard flashbacks as resulting from the breakdown of repressive defenses and the flooding of awareness with vivid reexperiencing of past events that occurs in the face of stimuli that invite the recollection of painful happenings.

Psychoanalytic terms are notoriously confusing because analysts who wish to emphasize various aspects of psychological situations use terms in varying ways. Additionally, as might be expected in a century-old discipline, the meaning of terms has changed over time.[26] In studying a psychoanalytic text, the reader should take pains to learn how the author is using these terms. Unfortunately this is not only a matter of academic interest. When, for example, the term *repression* is used without reference to its particular psychoanalytic meaning, conclusions that are valid for the term as used in one context may be misapplied in another. This is nowhere more evident than in debates about the recovery of repressed memory. As Cohler[27] observes, ''recovered'' memories are not the result of the emergence into consciousness of what was previously unconscious, because unconscious mental content can only be available to consciousness through its derivatives. Analytic work generally recovers the significance of always available memories, whose meanings and associated affects have been denied or disavowed. It is the connection between symptom and memory that is reestablished, not the memory itself. Thus the phenomenon analysts refer to as *lifting repression* is very different from recovered memory. Unfortunately, lack of clarity about the use of the word repression has led to discussions of these very different phenomena as though they were one and the same.

In this chapter we describe common psychoanalytic usage. As used by psychoanalysts, *repression* refers to the active operation by which people try to bar thoughts, images, and memories from awareness because awareness would produce anxiety, guilt, depression, or shame. *Denial* involves operating on a basis as if what the subject knew to be true was not. People commonly do things that damage their health, even though they are aware and believe that the action is harmful, but they put aside this knowledge as a determinant of actual behavior. *Dissociation* achieves similar ends by keeping ideas whose juxtaposition would cause distress separated from one another. For example, a person who cheats on an examination but wants to be honest, can maintain the image of himself as honest by avoiding bringing together the memory of cheating with the idea that cheating is dishonest. The ideas remain available to awareness, but by keeping them separate, the person spares himself the emotional distress that would result from recognizing that his action was an instance of dishonest behavior. Generally, dissociated material is kept at arm's length from the main body of experience and thought. In *disavowal,* distress is diminished by separating a particular idea from its associated affect. The subject may even be aware that most people would respond to a similar memory or idea with strong emotions but reports none or little of this feeling.

Mechanisms of defense are often not fully successful. As a result material barred from awareness reemerges in disguised and distorted form. These expressions include jokes, slips of the tongue, dreams, and symptoms. For example, a patient dreamed of a beautiful but dangerously hot fire on a hearth. His associations led to a fireplace in the bedroom of his family's summer home and to how his own bedroom was only separated from that bedroom by a curtain. The patient and analyst concluded that the fire was a disguised representation of the patient's experience of hearing his parent's sexual activities. A particularly important form of emergence of barred ideas occurs in *trans-*

ference. Transference occurs when the experience of another is shaped by attributing a role to them from the ideas that are outside awareness. Originally, the term referred to the emergence of repressed early childhood fantasies in which the patient cast the analyst in the role of some important figure of childhood. Analysts now recognize transference as a ubiquitous phenomenon. In it the relationships that are enacted need not reflect only early childhood experience or fantasy. They may reflect, among other things, current psychological needs, transformations of roles, and experiences of the other not as a person in the ordinary sense but as an environmental state or aspect of a person. We recognize transferences as arising in every aspect of life, not only psychoanalytic therapy. What is different about therapeutic transference is the commitment to clarifying, understanding, and using it therapeutically. The idea of transference has sometimes been used to attempt to explain away reports of mistreatment, especially by psychotherapists. While misperceptions of others' actions are always possible, patients are no more likely to misperceive the concrete actions of their therapists than they are of anyone else with whom they have an intense relationship. An example of transference should help to clarify the concept. (The clinical examples included in this paper are designed to illustrate its ideas. The data that lead to their conclusions are not presented and the rapid movement from manifest content to underlying meaning does not reflect the way contemporary psychoanalysts draw conclusions.)

Case Study

A young woman whose parents divorced when she was four was unconsciously enraged at her parents and critical of herself for not keeping the family together. She feared the damage her rage might cause and tried hard to "be good" by keeping angry wishes from awareness. She did this by passively accepting everything. The rage reemerged as unforgiving self-criticism. She expected others to be as critical of her. So she was often convinced that her performance enraged supervisors at work and that they were ever ready to fire her. The early experience of helpless rage at the destruction of her family thus found expression in the belief that those in authority were angrily attacking her.

Because of the wide range of defensive operations, the manifestations of unconscious memories are confused and confusing. As with other ideas, defenses against memory arise because of the current meanings of those memories. It is not the past that the analyst tries to understand but the *presently remembered past*. Analyst and patient are always dealing with material within a currently active matrix of meaning. We organize whatever we remember through its meaning. Memories are never isolated. They emerge as part of the dialogue between analyst and patient. They are shaped by current needs, which include defense against distress, the state of the transference, and therapeutic goals. Contemporary analysts are more likely to ask what role a reported memory (whether true or false) plays in the current interaction of analyst and patient than to try to puzzle out the impact of the reported events on the person's development. Many contemporary analysts regard the narrative value of a memory, the extent to which it contributes to a more cogent and useful life story, as more significant than the extent to which the memory reflects material history.[28] The multiple determinants of what is remembered and when it is remembered imply that psychoanalysis and related therapies are neither designed to recapture the material past nor are they particularly well suited to this end.

How do mechanisms of defense interact with memory? When any psychological material is defended against, that material is processed differently than it would otherwise be. Freud noted that the processing of information differs, depending on the extent to which the ideas are available to awareness. In *primary process thinking,* which is characteristic of dynamically unconscious activity, many aspects of rationality are absent. Propositions and their negations are essentially equivalent, just as the underlying iconography in signs representing "smoking" and "no smoking" are the same. Things and their representation are closely linked in primary process mentation. Words are not treated as arbitrary signs but are immediately connected to the thing itself. For example, objects whose names rhyme or are homonymous may be treated as similar (a hare may represent hair). Finally, and most important for this discussion, the distinction between what has been thought and what has been externally observed is largely obliterated. Fantasies and actual events are treated alike. Thus, learning the extent to which memories uncovered from repression represent actual occurrences is difficult or impossible. Repressed material is processed differently from material available to consciousness. Consider the example of transference given above. The ordinary information that would differentiate supervisor from parent if the idea were in awareness is not used to correct the tempting equation of parent and supervisor based on their similiarities.

Ideas and memories that are dissociated or split off from the main mass of thinking are also largely uninfluenced by new experience and so remain unaltered by experiences that might otherwise transform their meaning. This tends to be more confusing to the person who uses splitting defenses and to those who interact with such people. How can a person explicitly have acknowledged a situation and at the same time continue to act as though the situation did not exist? Without answering the question adequately, psychoanalysts acknowledge and describe these phenomena and recurrently find that they function to protect the person from painful feelings. It may be in part because it seems so odd that a person can at the same time know something and not integrate what is known with other conscious ideas that memory recovery advocates commonly refer to ideas of this type as repressed, even though these ideas do not fit the psychoanalytic usage of this term.

The equation of dissociated or split-off ideas with repressed ones confuses discussions of recovered memories. There is considerable evidence[29] that materially accurate repressed memories cannot be recovered from the unconscious. People with demonstrated histories of significant trauma generally demonstrate the opposite of repression, i.e., memories of the traumatic event invade their awareness inappropriately. Memories of trauma do commonly exist in a dissociated state, making them functionally unavailable for reworking and for integration with the rest of psychological life. From what we know of defense mechanisms in other contexts, it can be expected that a person might maintain a memory available to consciousness but act inconsistently with the memory. If people truly repress memories and then have them return to awareness in the same manner as ordinary recollections, this is an extremely rare event. Proust's madeleine did not unlock the door to totally unavailable memories but instead ushered him into a coherent attention to the meanings of seemingly unrelated recollections of sense impressions.

Defenses restrict the interaction of the material that is defended against with other ideas and experiences. As a result, they limit processes by which people integrate a particular experience with the mass of personal experiences. Psychological insults ordinarily initiate at least two processes—learning from the experience and repairing the psychological damage that has resulted from the event. If the person defensively removes a memory of a material reality from interaction with other aspects of psychological life, both processes are likely to be truncated. If it is too painful to recall injury in a dangerous situation, then learning to avoid that situation from the bad experience becomes impossible. In addition, if a person attempting to avoid painful memories of past events avoids recognizing the similarities between situations that involve common dangerous elements, that opportunity to learn from these new experiences is lost. Ultimately, the person not only fails to learn from the original bad experience but also from similar ones, and so she fails to learn from these experiences too. Internal and external solace and understanding ordinarily result from the juxtaposition of the dangerous idea with other ones. Putting together the fact of recent mistreatment with memories of being treated with respect or reminders that the current situation differs from the older, very disturbing one, lessens the impact of the bad event. However, if through an unconscious effort to protect myself from the danger of fully knowing about the event, such interactions are avoided, the potential solace and reconsideration become impossible.

The finding that traumatized people tend to be repeatedly involved in episodes similar to the traumatic event can be understood in many ways. This phenomenon and its devasting impact ultimately so impressed Freud that he posited a primary repetition compulsion. He closely related this compulsion to an inherent tendency to self-destruction, a death instinct. While few analysts concur with Freud in this regard, the power of this tendency to repeat bad happenings is enormous. Often analysts can understand the repetition as an effort to master actively what patients passively experienced. Now the patient can create the experience in the hope of having it occur differently. Or she may switch roles in the experience so that the once helpless victim now is the masterful perpetrator. We may also understand repetition as a compromise: we remember an event without calling it fully into memory, thereby partly achieving the ends of recalling the event without fully experiencing the psychological distress that would result from recall. Repetition may also occur because the defense against the original untoward experience and related experience results in lacunae in the person's knowledge of potentially dangerous situations, so that the apparent repetition arises from bad judgment.

Analysts' attitudes toward memories are primarily determined by pragmatic therapeutic considerations. If the presently experienced past causes unneeded distress because the patient has not integrated it with the person's overall experience, one goal of treatment is to achieve greater integration. The analyst principally focuses on the psychic (or narrative) reality of the patient. The question of what actually occurred is important in this context, only because it elucidates and supports the reworking of psychic reality. Two related issues are often confused. One is the reconstruction or recollection of past events concerning material reality. The other is that distress suffered from untoward happenings is often exacerbated when people who should provide comfort and protection deny the material reality. For many people, the worst aspect of bad events is that important others deny the material reality. A therapist who believes that a memory of abuse does not reflect a material reality may repeat the original experience in which important others denied the material reality. This is why some analysts recommend validating the patient's view of the situation. They underline the value of ways victims of abuse can find support for belief in the actuality of the occurrences.[30] This therapeutic recommendation has at least two disadvantages. It obscures the patient's needs by assuming one understands them in advance and it muddies the question of the actuality of the events that the patient discusses.

Determining the material reality of memories is not a major task of psychoanalysis. So it is not surprising that analysts do not agree on the relationship of memories and reconstructions to the material past. Nor have they developed methods adequate to differentiate material from psychic reality. In practice, most analysts take a common-sense approach to these issues. When a patient directly reports memories of trauma or abuse, the analyst assumes that the memories are veridical unless evidence contradicts that assumption. Such evidence may emerge during the careful exploration of the memories. Practically, analyst and patient may come to the conclusion that actual abuse occurred because overwhelming circumstantial evidence points to such abuse. A common analytic outcome is the capacity to live with uncertainty, even about aspects of one's own life. Unlike many "recovered memory" therapists, analysts do not believe that symptoms or other later-life phenomena are invariably related to early happenings. Analysts do not attempt to convince patients that certain events must have occurred. They do offer interpretations, the analyst's best understanding of the current situation. However, the analyst judges the validity of her interpretation not only by the evidence favoring it in advance. She also judges it by the patient's response, i.e., whether the interpretation leads to further understanding and deepening of the analytic work. These criteria are valuable in terms of analysis as therapy and differentiate analysis from therapies in which the therapist informs the patient of the truth of the situation. However, these criteria for the validity of psychoanalytic interpretation within the treatment context are again, not necessarily related to questions of material reality. Although analysts are sometimes accused of inadvertently gaining patients' compliance through suggestion,[31] such criticism ignores the central feature of psychoanalytic practice. In analysis, analyst and patient carefully explore their interactions to understand such influences. The transference-based distortion of information passed between any two people is universal. Psychoanalysis involves no more transference than any equivalently intense interpersonal relationship. Where it differs from other relationships is in its dedication to understanding and resolving such transference. Thus, the analytic situation is a particularly good one for teasing out the impact of suggestion and compliance on the analysand's reports and conclusions.

Some analysts believe that specific features of the patient's symptoms and memories strongly suggest that they refer to material reality. Person and Klar[32] argue that "repressed memories and conscious fantasies often can be distinguished insofar as they may be 'stored' or encoded differently; consequently the sequelae of trauma and fantasy can often, though not always be disentangled" (p. 1058). They accept the assertion that dissociation is a response to traumatic life events. They claim that when characteristic features of dissociation are present, the analyst may infer a history of actual trauma. These features include intrusive recollections (in nightmare or flashback); recollections in state-dependent situations; depersonalized states (including fugues) in which anxiety is unassociated with the patient's current situation; compulsive reenactments (including reenactments with role reversals); elaborated fantasy around the trauma; and transferences in which dissociation is evident as manifest by sudden breaks in the transferential flow. Even these authors are careful to observe that such findings are not definitive indicators of external trauma. Their argument rests heavily on the problematic assertion that the presence of symptoms observed as common sequelae of external trauma strongly suggests that trauma has occurred. This view, which various recovered memory advocates commonly take in extreme form, involves a simple logical error of the same type that Freud initially made in asserting a universal traumatic etiology to hysteria, namely, that if A is a known cause of B, then whenever B occurs, it must be the result of A.

Although critics have faulted analysts both for denying the significance of actual abuse and for promulgating ideas that support the veracity of false allegations, neither position is consistent with psychoanalytic ideas about memory. Freud discovered that fantasies could be experienced as profoundly dangerous and could shape development. This served to correct his earlier belief that the scenarios of abuse constructed from patients' current actions and memories necessarily resulted from actual maltreatment. Analysts have also found that it is the meaning of maltreatment to the individual, not the event in itself, that causes much of the lasting impact of bad happenings. Neither idea denies that actual abuse occurs nor the profundity of its impact. They only show that plausible reconstructions of past events can easily confuse material and psychological reality. The primary function of analysis is clarifying the impact of the presently remembered past. Analysts recognize that the effects of primary process mentation are such that clear assertions that particular events occurred are not often possible. Sometimes the convergence of analytic and extra-analytic data, or internal features of the analytic data themselves, strongly suggest conclusions about actual events. But generally, psychoanalysis is not an adequate method for reconstruction of past actualities. It is not even claimed to be a general method for understanding past psychological states.

This view departs from Freud. Freud, trained in nineteenth century embryology and neurology, tried to construct an embryology of mental life from examination of adult psychological functions. He analogized his work to archaeological and neurological investigation, assuming that the partial ablation of the higher functions revealed earlier functioning. The limits of his method are obscured because, from the beginning, Freud supplemented it with child observation and common sense. Clinical data only support the conclusion that current phenomena can be reasonably *interpreted* as arising from a posited history and that the emotional construction of this history in the company of the analyst in many instances reduces psychological distress. The direct observation of infants and children and the correlations of these observations with memories and other memorializations of past experience in adults points to an expectably complex interaction between early material events and their residues in adult life.

Summarizing the data that show how suggestion can profoundly influence memory, Brenneis[33] emphasizes the analyst's dilemma. The analyst is caught between the patient's need for a psychological witness to personal suffering and the analyst's knowledge of the unreliability of reconstructions of material events. He observes that either emphasizing skepticism about recovered or reconstructed memories or readily accepting the material reality of events leads to clinical problems. He notes that, '[a]t some points, we may find ourselves forced to choose between bearing false witness or failing to bear true witness without knowing with any certainty which we are doing'' (p. 1050). Although Brenneis is speaking in a psychoanalytic clinical context, his use of legal language suggests a solution to the dilemma. Lawyers, and scientists too, carefully distinguish the degree to which propositions are regarded as true. For certain purposes, a ''preponderance of evidence'' may be adequate, while other situations demand proof ''beyond a reasonable doubt.'' Similarly, a researcher may say that an observed difference was significant with a certain probability, e.g., that the likelihood that the different observation resulted from chance is less than 1%. The levels of proof required in various situations depend on the consequences of the decision, recognition of the many factors likely to shape the decision, and the expectable level of certainty within a discipline. So, too, the clinician should appropriately ask not only what problems there are in reaching a conclusion but also to what use the conclusion is put. If the consequence of the clinician's belief in the material reality of the abuse is limited to increased appreciation of the patient's suffering and the patient's increased sense of having an ally to deal with that suffering, the situation is very different from one in which the patient or clinician uses that belief as the basis for legal and other actions. An ideal analytic situation includes careful exploration of the meaning for the patient of the analyst's belief or skepticism. However, in less intensive therapies or at times in analysis when other issues are more pressing, such exploration may not be practical. In the vast majority of clinical situations, analyst and patient understand from the beginning the ends to which their exploration is likely to be used, i.e., the understanding of the patient's presently remembered past and the freedom that comes with that understanding. When, as a result of analytic work, the patient wishes to take action on what has been "uncovered," it becomes the analyst's job to explore the full meaning of that wish. It is particularly important that the analyst recognize the great limitations of the analytic method for producing evidence of the kind appropriate to nonanalytic contexts.

Analysts have learned from hard experience that the personal needs of the analyst can shape the understanding of the patient and analytic material. The analyst is not immune to the same unconscious forces that affect patients. She is only partly protected from them by professional understanding of the situation and a personal analysis aimed at increasing awareness of potential interference with analytic functioning. The question of the significance of the therapist's attitude toward the possibility of actual mistreatment should be the object of careful attention. It may be that the question of whether events actually occurred arises because therapists share the subtle cultural bias that suffering that is not related to material occurrences is in some way less real and less deserving of empathic response, so that the material reality of events becomes a marker of the degree to which the patient is deserving of empathy.[34]

Conclusion

Psychoanalysis provides a unique method and conceptual framework for understanding the personal meanings of memory and trauma. On the basis of the wish to avoid psychological distress, it describes how individuals shape their experiences, including memories. Designed as a therapeutic tool, which uses the exploration of personal history as a means for constructing richer and more satisfactory personal narratives, psychoanalysis is only secondarily a tool for exploring the impact of specific events on development. It does not even provide a reliable method for reconstructing early psychological states. Therapists who base their work on psychoanalytic concepts should not claim that those concepts support ideas like the potential recovery of repressed memories of actual traumatic events.

References

1. Breuer J, Freud S: Studies in Hysteria. *In* J. Strachey (Ed. and Trans.), The Standard Edition of the Complete Psychological Works of Sigmund Freud, Vol. 2. London: Hogarth Press, 1955, pp. 1–311. (Original work published 1895).
2. Klein G: Psychoanalytic Theory: An Exploration of Essentials. New York: International Universities Press, 1976.

3. LaPlanche J, Pontalis JB. The Language of Psychoanalysis. D. Nicholson-Smith (Trans.) New York: Norton, 1973, pp. 247–249.

4. Greenacre P: A historical sketch of the use and disuse of reconstruction. Psychoanal Study Child 1980; 35:35–40.

5. Glover E: The Technique of Psychoanalysis. New York: International Universities Press, 1955.

6. Reed G: On the value of explicit reconstruction. Psychoanal Q 1993; 62:52–73.

7. Khan M: Ego distortion, cumulative trauma, the role of reconstruction. Int J Psychoanal 1964; 45:272–279.

8. Bollas C: The Shadow of the Object. New York: Columbia University Press, 1987.

9. Blum HP: The value of reconstruction in adult psychoanalysis. Int J Psychoanal 1980; 61(1):39–52.

10. Masson J: The Assault on Truth: Freud's Suppression of the Seduction Hypothesis. New York: Farrar, Straus, and Giroux, 1984.

11. Lothane Z: Love, seduction, and trauma. Psychoanal Rev 1987; 74:83–105.

12. Freud S: Notes upon a case of obsessional neurosis. *In* J. Strachey (Trans. & Ed.), The Standard Edition of the Complete Psychological Works of Sigmund Freud, Vol. 10. London: Hogarth Press, 1957, pp. 158–250. (Original work published 1909).

13. Modell A: Other Times, Other Realities: Toward a Theory of Psychoanalytic Treatment. Cambridge, MA: Harvard University Press, 1990.

14. Freud A: Comment on psychic trauma. *In* The Writings of Anna Freud. New York: International University Press, 1967, vol. 5, pp. 221–241.

15. Cooper A: Toward a limited definition of psychic trauma. *In* Rothstein, A. (Ed.) Reconstruction of Trauma: Its Significance in Clinical Work. Madison, CT: International Universities Press, 1986, pp. 41–58.

16. Khan M: The principle of cumulative trauma. *In* The Privacy of the Self. London: Hogarth Press, 1963, pp. 42–59.

17. Winnicott D: The Maturational Process and the Facilitating Environment. New York: International Universities Press, 1965.

18. Kohut H: The Analysis of the Self. New York: International Universities Press, 1971.

19. Galatzer-Levy R, Cohler B: The Essential Other: A Developmental Psychology of the Self. New York: Basic Books, 1993.

20. Erikson E: Reality and actuality: an address. J Am Psychoanal Assoc 1962; 10:451–474.

21. Stern D: The Interpersonal World of the Infant. New York: Basic Books, 1985.

22. Freud A: The Ego and the Mechanisms of Defense (Rev ed.). New York: International University Press, 1966.

23. Davies J, Frawley M: Dissociative processes and tranference-countertransference paradigms, in the psychoanalytically oriented treatment of adult survivors of childhood sexual abuse. Psychoanal Dialogs 1991; 2:5–36.

24. Frank A: The unrememberable and the unforgettable. Passive primal repression. Psychoanal Study Child 1969; 24:48–77.

25. Fraiberg S, Adelson E, Shapiro V: Ghosts in the nursery. J Am Acad Child Psychiatry 1975; 14:387–421.

26. Klumpner G: The Language of Psychoanalysis: A Thesaurus of Psychoanalytic Terms. Madison, CT: International University Press, 1994.

27. Cohler B: Memory recovery and the uses of the past: a commentary on Lindsay and Reed from a psychoanalytic perspective. Appl Cogn Psychol 1994; 8:365–378.

28. Schafer R: Retelling a Life: Narration and Dialogue in Psychoanalysis. New York: Basic Books, 1992.

29. Lindsay S, Read D: Psychotherapy and memories of childhood sexual abuse: a cognitive perspective. [Special issue: Recovery of Memories of Childhood Sexual Abuse] Appl Cogn Psychol 1994; 8:281–338.

30. Herman J: Trauma and Recovery. New York: Basic Books, 1991.

31. Grünbaum A: Validation in the Clinical Theory of Psychoanalysis: A Study in the Philosophy of Psychoanalysis. Madison, CT: International Universities Press, 1994.

32. Person E, Klar H: Establishing trauma: the difficulty distinguishing between memories and fantasies. J Am Psychoanal Assoc 1994; 42:1055–1081.

33. Brenneis C: Belief and suggestion in the recovery of memories of childhood sexual abuse. J Am Psychoanal Assoc 1994; 42:1027–1053.

34. Galatzer-Levy R: Children, bad happenings and meanings. J Am Psychonanal Assoc 1994; 42:997–1000.

6

The Nature and Development of Children's Event Memory

MICHELLE D. LEICHTMAN
STEPHEN J. CECI
MARJORIE B. MORSE

In a routine report on the Boston evening news, an investigative reporter spoke with a family whose house had been burned to the ground just hours before. Still clearly shaken, the mother described her horror at awakening to smoke emanating from the ground floor of her home, her fright in realizing her children were asleep in the next room, her actions in removing them from the home, and her present feelings of relief at their safety and dismay at the material loss. When the microphone was trained on the family's 5-year-old son, his first response was a stunned pause. He was then able to answer the reporter's inquiries with the information that he felt "happy, because my baby sister's o.k." and "sad, because I don't know where my toys are." A younger baby, apparently around 6 months, cried in the arms of her father, who had not been home at the time that the fire was discovered.

From a developmental perspective, this brief news clip captures the essence of a fascinating problem. Simply put, how does the process of remembering personally relevant, emotionally laden experiences change across development? This question, and a host of others that swirl around it, is currently of great interest to researchers.[1-4] In part, such interest stems from theoretical advancements over the past two decades that have underscored the importance of contextual variables in shaping performance on cognitive tasks. No longer satisfied with models of memory derived solely from laboratory observations, researchers have created a significant body of empirical work directed at understanding real-world memories.[5,6] A critical aspect of the context in which any event memory occurs is its original emotional significance, as well as the emotional impact of the retrieval experience.

Interest in the development of personally relevant event memories also stems from children's increasingly common participation in the American legal system. In cases ranging from civil suits to felony trials, children are testifying as witnesses in record numbers, and their eyewitness memory capabilities are under scrutiny in the popular as well as scientific arenas.[7,8] A rise in reported cases of sexual abuse, in which a child may be both the victim and the sole witness, has been of particular import.[8–11]

Returning to our description of the family on the evening news, we can discern several lines of scientific inquiry reflected by their experience of the traumatic fire. First, there are clearly baseline differences in the abilities of the various family members to remember what has just occurred, and further, to report on it. While the mother can provide a coherent, chronologically ordered, relatively full description of the event, the 5-year-old's response is quite comprehensible, yet in this instance, relatively impoverished. Evidently, the infant is unable to participate in the questioning, and her emotional behavior cannot be clearly read as related to the recent experience. How will she later recall this event, if at all?

Second, the experience and the context of the event may be quite different for the various members of this family, and as a result the memories that they hold of it will eventually differ. Obviously, the physical perspectives of the participants connect only loosely in this case; for example, because of their heights, the eye-level view of the participants differs, the point at which they became aware of the event differs, and so does their physical mobility during the event. The father, who only learned about some of the critical details of the fire episode when he joined the family after they had left the house, may later have memories of these details that are shaped by the explanations of his wife.

As an equally important part of context, we might consider that the psychological state and cognitive status that the individuals bring to the event vary considerably. For example, the individual's mood, degree of sleepiness, and ability to understand what is happening will certainly be important elements of memory. Likewise, the social and motivational components of the event will influence how it is remembered. Here, for instance, the mother's motivation to rush her children out of the house, versus the 5-year-old's more limited understanding of the implications of not doing so, could direct their attention and cause divergence in their memories. If we consider that subsequent changes in such contextual factors at the time of remembering may also affect how the event is recalled, the picture is further complicated. For example, when the now 5-year-old child is a teenager remembering this event, his new memorial report is likely to reflect not only his past experience, but also his intervening cognitive advancements and new motivations.

While some social and cognitive factors (such as the aforementioned motivations) tend to change considerably across situations, it is also important to note that stable individual differences may help guide memory. For example, if the mother in this case were a highly visual thinker, her memories of the fire episode in years to come might center around vivid visual detail.

Our goal in this chapter is to provide an overview of literature pertinent to the question of how memory functions in children, with an eye toward memory for salient, emotional events. To this end, we first provide a brief synopsis of how normal memory is approached by developmental researchers, delineating the various functional components of the memory system that develop. As part of this discussion, we consider the issue of memory in the earliest years of life, and describe work that illustrates the striking abilities demonstrated by very young children in storing and retrieving information about the past. We then discuss research, conducted primarily with preschoolers, that has explored social and cognitive factors influencing the nature and accuracy of children's memorial reports. We conclude with a commentary on the limitations of current developmental knowledge, including a particular caution about individual differences.

The Developmental Approach to Early Memory

As other chapters in this volume imply (see Chapters 4 and 7, this volume), the study of memory has a venerable place in the history of psychology. From a contemporary perspective, it is interesting to note that the earliest theorists approached memory from contextual and functional perspectives, focusing on the higher purposes served by memory in an organism's functioning. The subject of the earliest psychological experiments was often the entire organism, viewed as a seamless whole emerging from the interaction of biological, social, and cognitive processes.[12-14] Memory itself held a privileged position, conceived of as a central ingredient in all higher forms of intelligence and cognition.

This perspective became obscured as research advances prompted more contemporary memory theorists to subspecialize into developmental, social, cognitive, and biological factions.[15] Across these various areas, dialogue about memory eventually became substantially fragmented, with different levels of discourse characterizing the work in each discipline. However, over the past 15 years, renewed appreciation for the impact of context on cognition has contributed to the narrowing of these interdisciplinary gaps.[16,17] It has become clear, for example, that models of memory that cannot account for the recollection of affective information are insufficient.[18,19] Likewise, applied concerns, such as those addressing the ability of children to report on personally relevant incidents in forensic settings, have brought memory again into focus as an interactive part of the broader developmental process. Thus, studies directed at integrating models of diverse aspects of human psychological functioning are no longer uncommon.[20,21]

Consistent with the impression held by parents and others who interact regularly with children, researchers have generally found that across childhood, the use of memory becomes more effective. However, this point requires immediate qualification. The typical tasks in which such developmental improvements are confirmed involve free or prompted recall, as opposed to recognition measures.[22,23] They often involve the use of deliberate, conscious processes, requiring children to memorize or otherwise purposefully use their memories.[24–26] In addition, the most evident developmental trends are seen in explicit memory tasks, which alert the subjects at retrieval that they are remembering.[27] Implicit memory tasks, such as word-priming tasks which demonstrate that subjects are remembering without awareness, show far less developmental variance.[28,29] It is important to note that the particular parameters of any given task may often be set to obscure developmental trends; for example, if items to be remembered have been overlearned by children of all ages, or if delay intervals are extremely short, 2-year-olds and 5-year-olds may emerge with similar performance on a given task.

What mechanism accounts for this general trend toward more effective memory across childhood? The contemporary history of research on memory development has been influenced by the notion that the unfolding of memory is the result of changes in a number of distinct areas. Children's basic capacities, knowledge base, strategic behaviors, and metacognition have been widely studied as part of the attempt to account for progressively better memory across childhood.[19,30–32] Each of these factors, and their interactions, contributes to the way in which we understand the normal progression of memory.

Basic capacities can be identified as memory processes that are frequently used and speedily executed. These are fundamental components of more complex memorial processes, aptly described as the "hardware" of the memory system.[33] Some of the basic processes that have been the source of much developmental literature include the ability to recognize, or sense that stimuli experienced in the past are familiar, the ability to associate stimuli with behavioral responses, and the capacity for symbolism invoked in recall tasks. Related issues concern the speed with which children are able to process information, and the functional memory capacity that they possess at various points across development.[19,33–35] Finally, an influential recent literature has focused on differences in the strength and probable decay trajectory of memory traces across childhood.[36,37] Such differences have been shown to account for a large variety of outcomes on memory tasks, as well as having a broad influence on other aspects of cognitive development.[38,39] While the focus of this discussion is not on the large body of literature specifically debating the relative importance of each of these basic processes, their critical contribution to the ultimate fate of any event memory is important to recognize.

Perhaps less obviously than basic processes, children's knowledge contributes quite directly to their ability to remember. Here, we refer to both children's knowledge of the world, in general, and to their knowledge about the local stimuli being remembered, in particular. This kind of knowledge, which is alternately referred to in the literature as *declarative, semantic,* or *factual,* has been repeatedly shown to influence memory performance. For instance, some experiments have manipulated the normally occurring positive correlation between age and knowledge, ensuring that younger children know more about a particular set of stimuli than do older individuals. Under such circumstances, memory differences between the age-groups either wash out, or actually tilt in favor of the younger children.

In a classic study, Chi[40] demonstrated this by identifying a group of 10-year-olds who were more knowledgeable about chess than was a group of university graduate student subjects. When asked to memorize the placement of pieces on a chess board, the younger subjects outrecalled the graduate students, despite the superior memory span of the latter group when tested with digits. Moreover, the 10-year-olds encoded the information in larger chunks, which allowed them to store more information in short-term memory at one time. Nevertheless, the younger children's superiority was limited: only actual configurations from real chess matches could be recalled at high levels. Thus, when Chi scrambled the pieces on a chess board into meaningless positions, 10-year-old chess experts did not perform as well as the graduate students. Apparently, the younger children's superiority was due to their ability to code entire game configurations (e.g., "this board looks like the opponent tried a knight's tour strategy"), and scrambling the pieces resulted in novel constellations of chess pieces that did not conform to anything in their knowledge.

Since Chi demonstrated the importance of relevant knowledge on memory performance, numerous others have followed in the same vein,[41–44] for example, showing that eighth graders who possess a great deal of knowledge about soccer outperform other eighth graders on various types of soccer-related memory tests (gist, rote recall), as well as on tests of other forms of cognition that focus on soccer (such as comprehension of soccer stories), regardless of the strength of their overall general aptitude. This is true even though higher aptitude eighth graders outperform the group with soccer knowledge on non-soccer stories and other more general cognitive indices (e.g., IQ). In short, it appears that much of the variance among individuals on a host of cognitive tasks can be localized at the level of knowledge differences.[42] When lower IQ individuals are given ample background knowledge on recall, comprehension, and problem-solving tasks, they often end up performing as well as higher IQ individuals.[45]

Thus, the size of a person's knowledge base in the area being studied is a potent factor in accounting for developmental differences in memory. Because older individuals virtually always have a larger reservoir of knowledge about experimental stimuli than do their younger counterparts, they are provided a large advantage on many tasks. Their ample knowledge allows them to process items more deeply and more easily than children, whose knowledge is impoverished by comparison.

Apart from knowledge, the growth of strategies explains some developmental differences in memory, especially between ages 6 and 10. Memory strategies are planful, goal-oriented behaviors that may assist at all points during the memory process. Stated simply, older children and adults know much more about how to maximize the efficiency of their own memory systems than do young children. For example, older individuals know what strategies are appropriate for a given occasion, and when it is optimal to deploy them. When the structure of mnemonic tasks minimizes the use of strategies, developmental differences in performance are likely to be reduced in the same manner as they are when task-relevant knowledge is equalized for adults and children.[46] Likewise, when younger children are taught adult strategies, their memory performance improves, although rarely to adult levels. For instance, teaching 5-year-olds to use spatial coding strategies or mental rehearsal strategies aids their recall and recognition memory,[47,48] though adults usually continue to outperform them. Ordinarily, children who have been taught to use strategies do not use them spontaneously. They need to be induced to do so, even though these strategies convey an advantage when they are used. Young children therefore appear to lack knowledge not only about how to deploy the strategies but about their usefulness.

Another variable that has been universally accepted as an important source of developmental differences in memory is *metacognitive awareness,* which refers to children's ability to introspect about and understand their own cognitive processes. *Metamemory,* an important part of metacognition, involves knowledge about how one's own memory functions and what factors may enhance its efficiency. As children develop, they gain greater access to the contents of their own memories, realizing, for instance, when it is appropriate to apply new strategies to refresh their memory traces and when they have rehearsed enough. It is not sufficient merely to know how to execute a memory strategy.[49] Metacognitively mature thinking also requires recognizing the attributes of a situation that permit various strategies to be used profitably. Indeed, studies have shown that this type of recognition typically develops later than the simple ability to employ a strategy. For example, Schneider[25] found that while second graders could use categorization strategies for the facilitation of recall to some extent, they were unaware of the importance of such strategies for this purpose. Fourth graders, on the other hand, used categorization strategies deliberately to help themselves remember. In considering the issue of metamemory, we must not be oversimplistic in characterizing the relationship between the possession of knowledge and the ability to utilize it. Some research has pointed to the conclusion that the amount of knowledge one has about strategies is unrelated to the tendency to use relevant knowledge on actual tasks.[50]

In addition to advances in their understanding of mnemonic processes, children also develop other metacognitive skills during middle childhood that may partially account for developmental differences in memory. An example of such a metacognitive skill is *source monitoring,* which refers to the ability to correctly remember the sources of one's knowledge and beliefs. For instance, a child may remember a specific fact about the eating habits of dinosaurs, but may not remember whether she heard it from a parent, from a teacher, or from a television program. Children's skills at source monitoring increase as they develop and, as a result, their memory for and understanding of the sources of information and knowledge that they have learned becomes more robust and reliable. Moreover, when children learn to correctly match learned pieces of information with their sources, the memory of these sources will serve both as additional retrieval cues, which will assist them in the recall of this knowledge, and as factors through which related pieces of information may be associated and interconnected in memory.

Studies on source-monitoring ability have uncovered clear developmental differences, demonstrating that very young children, in particular, have a high degree of source confusion.[51-53] For example, Gopnik and Graf[54] conducted a study in which children learned the contents of six drawers by seeing, hearing about, or inferring the contents of each drawer. Children were then asked to recall the source of their knowledge about the items in each drawer. The results showed clear developmental trends toward improvement, with 73% of 5-year-olds, 54% of 4-year-olds, and 30% of 3-year-olds making no errors in source monitoring.

Similar developmental trends in source monitoring were found in a study by Foley and Johnson.[55] In this work, children aged 6 and 9 and college-aged students were asked to either do, imagine doing, or watch someone else do simple bodily movements such as touching their nose and pointing their finger. In this study, the younger children had more trouble remembering the source of each simple action than did older children and college-aged subjects. In addition, Foley and Johnson[55] found that certain types of events and actions were more likely to result in source confusion than were others. The differences in source-monitoring ability between 6-year-olds, 9-year-olds, and adults were greatest when subjects were asked to distinguish between actions that they had imagined doing from actions that they had actually performed. Thus, when subjects both performed and imagined a set of actions, they had a harder time remembering this distinction than when they performed and watched others perform the actions. This suggests that young children may be particularly likely to confuse events and actions they imagined with those that actually occurred.

Developmental differences in metacognitive abilities such as mnemonic strategy use and source monitoring determine age differences in the amount of information that is retained and retrieved, as well as the richness with which pieces of information are associated in memory. Metacognition is the executive control mechanism for the entire memorial system, driving decisions as diverse as those resulting in mid-task switches in strategies and updated inferences about the origins of information. Certainly, until children acquire metamemorial insight to an adequate degree, they do not know when to use the strategies that they possess. This is the main reason that teaching strategies to preschoolers has been less than satisfactory, and that virtually all current educational technologies incorporate metamnemonic insight as a component.[56,57] In addition, until children develop an understanding of the importance of remembering the sources of their knowledge, their ability to retrieve such knowledge from memory will be limited.

In short, knowledge about the world, knowledge of strategies, and knowledge of the way our own memories work are all factors that contribute to both developmental and individual differences in remembering. Differences in the efficiency of these factors distinguish high functioning from low performance on memory, learning, and cognitive batteries.

Long-term Memory in the First Years of Life

The various components of the developing memory system that we have just discussed can be clearly tracked once children have reached school age, and often before. By that point in development, children have been socialized to respond to adult demands, they can participate in language-based tasks, they can answer direct questions, and in many other ways, they can provide clues about the organization and substantive contents of their event memories. Among the most elusive issues currently under consideration by developmentalists is the proper way to characterize long-term memory before this point.

From a theoretical perspective, the development of such memory during infancy and early childhood is particularly alluring, because it touches on the adult experience of infantile amnesia. That is, memories of events in the very earliest years of life typically cannot be retrieved by human beings as they reach later childhood and adulthood.[58,59] American adults, for instance, on average date their first-event memory around the time that they were 3.5 years of age.[58] In contrast, events occurring after this point in life are more readily accessed over the long term. Although this phenomenon has received considerable attention from theorists, its causes remain a matter of debate.[60,61] Pertinent to our present discussion, one factor that has traditionally contributed to the difficulty in understanding infantile amnesia is a limited comprehension of how long-term memory develops across the years of infancy and preschool.

From an applied perspective, the issue of early memory appears as interesting as from a theoretical view. Clearly, therapeutic models often revolve around retrieving or understanding early life relationships and events.[62–65] In courtroom situations, children and adults are also often called to testify about events that occurred during the first 4 years of their lives.[2,7,8] Judges and juries are increasingly required to decide on the validity of testimony from older children remembering their first 2 years, or from preschoolers recalling events after a year's delay. In recent years, many such cases have entered into the dialogue over childhood memory in the legal arena.[2,11,66–69]

Ongoing empirical work by developmentalists that is directed at memory during the first years of life profits from both these theoretical and applied lines of inquiry. Traditionally, little attention was devoted by the research community to this topic because of a prevailing view that the infant was an organism with little capacity to make sense of its environment.[13,70] It was generally believed that information about events could not be meaningfully encoded for long-term storage during the first years of life and would thus stand no chance of retrieval from the memory system upon later prompting. For this reason, the largest body of work on memory development during the first years of life concerns only short-term processes,[71,72] with retention intervals commonly limited to under several minutes.[73]

Happily, over the past 15 years, several clever new methodologies have been developed to study infants and toddlers. These methods have produced a body of provocative evidence that forces reconsideration of the potential of memory during the first 3 years.[74,75] In short, current evidence suggests that memories can be laid down earlier in life and remain accessible to retrieval for longer periods than was previously thought possible.[76–78]

But what is the precise nature of these very early long-term memories? Occasional anecdotal evidence has appeared in laboratories indicating the ability to retrieve, in verbal form and after a significant delay, specific information acquired during experiences at just 16–17 months of age.[79] However, most of the evidence reflects a more elusive kind of memory that may be laid down during the experiences of this period of life and before.

We know that from the time children are able to use language to narrate stories about past events, such stories are similar in structure and representation to those of adults, although their content may differ considerably.[80–82] By the age of 4 years, studies indicate that children can encode memory traces for aspects of events that may be responsive to prompting after 2 years or longer.[83,84] Although anecdotal, a few reports have also documented the spontaneous verbal recall of specific past events by children in the 2- to 3-year-old range, from 6 months to 2 years after they occurred.[85] The central problem, of course, is to determine the extent of memory for those events encountered before language has been mastered. The different methodological constraints posed by studying memory in prelinguistic children, in contrast with those who are verbally proficient, have contributed to the fact that memory in these two groups has rarely been studied empirically in comparable ways.

Nonetheless, a number of investigators have directed their efforts at unearthing evidence of long-term memory in infancy, independent of the paradigms that are useful with older subjects. The first evidence of such memory comes from experiments on long-term recognition, many of them employing habituation paradigms. This kind of experimental paradigm generally uses infants' looking behavior as an indicator of their differential attention to novel and familiar stimuli. The habituation methodology is predicated on the notion that infants eventually grow "bored" of stimuli that they recognize as old and will respond with renewed attention when presented with equivalent stimuli that are either novel or have been forgotten. Studies based on habituation have revealed delayed recognition from several days to several weeks for various photographs and abstract designs in 5- to 7-month olds.[86–88]

Even more impressive evidence of recognition over long delays has been demonstrated using a mobile conjugate reinforcement paradigm. In this paradigm, retention is indexed by the anticipatory production of a conditioned foot-kicking response when the context of the original contingency learning is reinstated. Using the conjugate reinforcement technique, long-term memory of conditioned responding for up to 8 days has been demonstrated in 3-month-olds, and 6-month-olds have evidenced memory for up to 21 days.[74,89]

Studies of this nature are fascinating in the glimpse they provide of otherwise obscured aspects of infant cognition. However, some theorists have questioned what they reveal about how early long-term processes map onto "true" long-term memory. Here, we refer to the kind of memory that we all recognize, both empirically and introspectively, as existing in adulthood and supporting our sense of the past and our accompanying ability to recount it.[70] To qualify as true memory, long-term memory must involve an actual mental representation of the past, moving beyond the simple ability to provide a conditioned or habitual response at the reinstatement of a past context.[90–92] While there is some disagreement about what qualifies as convincing evidence of this kind of representation, demonstrations of reproductive memory certainly come closer to providing such evidence than do many other demonstrations of infant memory.[91] Unlike recognition tasks, these require the acting out (or reproducing) of aspects of an event on the part of the subject, which is presumed to rely on some manner of mental representation.[92,93]

Evidence for reproductive memory processes during the first years of life comes from several research paradigms. As an example of early reproductive processes, infants as young as 5 months have demonstrated the ability to use event sequences or routines for prediction after delays of several days to weeks.[94,95] Findings from other work indicate that when provided with materials cueing them to reproduce 3-step action sequences, children who were 21 months at exposure could do so accurately after a 6-week delay,[96] and, in a follow-up, those as young as 18 months could do so 8 months later. Fourteen-month-olds, who were included in the same experimental condition as the 18-month-olds, failed to demonstrate memory of this sort.[77] However, ofter experiments have shown increased evidence of surprise in infants across the period from 9 to 18 months when expectations established by a past event are violated.[97]

Studies of deferred imitation appear to offer more rigorous demonstrations of reproductive memory. This type of task generally requires that young subjects produce an unusual behavior that was either observed or carried out in the past. Such work has shown memory in 9-month-olds for the actions of a researcher after 24 hours, and memory in 14-month-olds for more sophisticated modeled actions after 1 week.[75,78] In a recent study with 192 14- and 16-month-olds, Meltzoff[98] has demonstrated significant deferred imitation of experimenter-modeled actions after both 2- and 4-month intervals. Even when infants were only allowed to watch an experimenter perform target activities (i.e., they were not allowed to engage in these activities themselves during the encoding sessions), these infants engaged in the activities reliably more at testing as a function of having been exposed to them much earlier. Thus, an impact of the early experience was seen on behavior even though this experience did not involve habitual or conditioned learning, and even though it did not allow reinforcement of the pairing between the visual stimulus (i.e., the novel object) and the target response. Using a deferred imitation paradigm after an even longer delay interval, McDonough and Mandler[99] provided suggestive evidence that 2-year-olds could remember and behaviorally demonstrate a particular novel action that they either observed or performed when they were only 11 months of age.

The nature of delayed imitation tasks makes it plausible to consider that mental representation, which may carry with it the same phenomenology as in adulthood, controls this process. Further evidence for reproductive memory in the early years has been provided by Perris, Myers, and Clifton.[76] Subjects who had participated in an auditory localization experiment at 6.5 months, which required them to reach for a sounding object in a dark or lit room, were brought back to the original laboratory context and reintroduced to the procedure at either 1.5 or 2.5 years of age. Those in the older group showed behavioral memory of the early experience by reaching out and grasping the object more than controls, and by acting less startled and more persistent in the testing situation than controls. Similar results were not obtained for the younger subjects, although the experimental design leaves open the possibility that this was primarily due to very high levels of reaching by control subjects in this age-group.

Also testing after a very long delay interval, Myers and Speaker[100] looked at the memory of 32-month-olds for an experience last encountered at 14 months. Subjects were initially in a study by Perris,[101] in which 10-month-olds learned to operate a toy on four occasions, and were tested 4 months later. That study indicated familiarity and fast relearning of the original toy operation by the experimental subjects, when contrasted with controls. In Myers and Speaker's[100] follow-up, children who had been involved in only one training session were contrasted with those who had been involved in five sessions and were also contrasted with matched controls. The results indicate that any prior experience resulted in greater interest in the target toy, more touching of the toy, and more successful responses to verbal prompts to operate it. Notably, however, only children with multiple past experiences were able to operate the toy without demonstration, revealing memory for a sequence of actions they had learned 18 months earlier.

In a further study of reproductive memory processes, Leichtman[79] presented 147 subjects between 4 months and 3 and a half years of age with 50 minutes of puppet interaction, distributed over 5 consecutive days. The behaviors of the subjects when represented with the puppet after many months were evaluated against the behaviors of 64 control subjects. The results of this study indicated that a substantial proportion of subjects, beginning with those as young as 6 months at exposure, could demonstrate behavioral effects of their prior experience with the puppet. This was particularly interesting because they were tested after extremely long delay intervals of 3 or 6 months. Almost certainly, many of the memory-referent behaviors produced by children below 1.5 years were of an unconscious nature, and were not linguistically accessible. Starting from around 6 months of age (at the time of exposure), these included indications of memory at testing such as looking inside the puppets' mittens, significantly more speedy removal of the mittens relative to controls, and persistence in searching again and again for the treat. In this study, the youngest subjects to produce spontaneous references in language to the past experience after 3 and 6 months were 17- and 18-months-old, respectively, at the time of exposure. This fairly early spontaneous verbal reference was quite unusual, however; only 12% of children between 1.5 and 2 years of age at exposure made this kind of spontaneous mention after 3 months, and even fewer did so after the longer delay. These numbers increased with age of exposure, to approximately 45% of children in the 2- to 3-year-old group at exposure, and a similar percentage who were 3–4 years old when they first encountered the puppet.

Taken together, the corpus of empirical evidence now emerging with regard to memorial processes in children between several months and 3 years of age makes the compelling point that these subjects' memories are indeed sensitive to events occuring around them. Moreover, in some cases, subjects are capable of demonstrating the influence of prior events after considerable delays, when exposed to an adequate retrieval context. Considering the history of research on early long-term memory, the findings reported recently concerning this issue are striking.

The Nature and Accuracy of Children's Memories

Considerable work on adult memory over the past two decades has raised questions about people's ability to reliably remember and report on events, and about their ability to discern whether particular memories that they hold are inaccurate.[102–107] Much of this work has focused on the effects of misleading post-event information, with many studies employing some version of the paradigm originally developed by Loftus and her colleagues.

In studies of the misinformation effect, subjects are first exposed to an event, usually involving the viewing and/or hearing of information from slides, pictures, films, or a live episode. After some delay interval, subjects are exposed to new erroneous or misleading information pertaining to that event, but the conflict between this misleading information and the original information is not pointed out to them. After further delay, there is a retrieval or testing phase in which the subject's memory for the original event is assessed by either recall or recognition tasks. Taken together, findings across a wide variety of studies have indicated that adults perform more poorly on memory tasks when they have been exposed to such misleading information than when they go directly from the original event to the testing phase (i.e., with no misleading information). Findings of this sort are consistent with the notion that post-event information may have an impact on the original information in such a way as to either compete with or even alter underlying traces and the subsequent recollection of the event. That is, there may be cases in which post-event information simply impedes the process of remembering the initial event (i.e., retrieval competition), as well as cases in which it damages the original memory trace (i.e., trace alteration).[108] In short, adults' memories appear to be subject to considerable distortion in contexts contrived by either experimenters or nature to interfere with optimal performance.

Following these findings of memory distortion in adulthood, a burgeoning literature on children's suggestibility has appeared. Two central developmental questions posed in the research literature consider broadly whether children's reports are susceptible to distortion from elements outside the scope of the reported-on event, and how the degree of their suggestibility compares with that of older subjects. The answers to these questions are of particular import, as they enrich our understanding of the potential mechanisms involved in the process of suggestibility at all ages.

In a review of research on children's suggestibility, 83% of studies comparing preschool-aged children's suggestibility with older children's suggestibility reported larger effects for the former.[2] To understand this effect, it is useful to consider experimental data provided by Ceci, Ross, and Toglia.[109] In research using children from ages 3 through 12 years, subjects were read a picture story about several events that happened to a protagonist. The day after this initial phase, subjects were interviewed about the story by an experimenter, who subtly included misinformation about the story details during interviews with experimental subjects, but provided no such misinformation to controls. Two days after this biasing, children were given two-item forced choice recognition tests pertaining to the story elements. In each pair of pictures presented during testing, one item reflected what had actually been in the original story, while the other reflected the misleading detail that had been suggested a day later. The results indicated that the mean recognition of the correct original item was quite high for control subjects in all age groups (mean proportion correct ranged from .84 for 3- and 4-year-olds to .95 for the oldest group). In contrast, 3- and 4-year-olds who were subjected to the misleading information achieved a mean of .37 correct, 5- and 6-year-olds a mean of .58, 7- to 9-year-olds a mean of .67, and the oldest subjects a mean of .84. Thus, the youngest group was disproportionately affected by the intervening suggestion, a fact that is reflected in the significant age X condition interaction that was achieved.

Like this study of the effects of misinformation on story recall, many subsequent experiments have looked at factors that might have an impact on accuracy. Often, the experimental paradigms in these studies have not taken into account a variety of factors that appear in real-world circumstances in which children's memory is an issue, in particular, those factors present in legal cases.[110–112] In one study, we attempted to partially redress this problem by incorporating at least two factors that are problematic in the legal arena.[113]

First, we included negative stereotypes, such as those that are sometimes inculcated in the real world regarding potential perpetrators, in the pre-event phase of our study. Stereotypes are naive theories about personal characteristics, which function to organize and structure experience by directing individuals to look for expectancies in their environment and advising them on how to interpret such expectancies. Thus stereotypes are a form of schematic knowledge that helps organize memory by adding thematically congruent information that was not perceived, or sometimes by distorting what is perceived.[114,115] Prior to witnessing an event, a child may be provided with a particular stereotype about the person involved (e.g., he is very clumsy, doesn't shave, or takes things), and this may direct the child's attention to expectancy-congruent behaviors (e.g., in court cases, the defendant might be an estranged parent who has been previously criticized by the custodial parent in the child's presence, and the child may even have come to accept these criticisms as stable aspects of the absent parent's character). Hence, such behaviors may be remembered and reported dispropor-tionately.

Second, we included long delay intervals in our study, which were filled with regular questioning. Multiple repetitive interviews are an important element of many cases in which children testify, and these generally take place over the course of extensive retention intervals. Recent estimates indicate that by the time they get to court, children have been subjected to between 4 and 11 forensic interviews, on average, and in most cases they have experienced numerous other bouts of questioning from nonforensic interviews (e.g., family members, therapists, social workers, and other interested parties).[8,116] Nonetheless, most studies to date have focused on the suggestibility of children after a single suggestive interview.

The study we conducted involved the visit of a man we called Sam Stone to the classrooms of our subjects, a sample of 176 preschoolers 3 to 6 years of age. There were four conditions in the study, reflecting two manipulations posited to have an effect on the children's reports of the events that occurred during Sam Stone's visit. The manipulations were the laying down of a stereotype, and the subjection to repeated suggestive questions about Sam's visit. The stereotype about Sam Stone was provided prior to the children ever meeting him. This stereotype indicated that Sam Stone was a clumsy and bumbling friend of the experimenters, and over the course of numerous discussions children heard about "real" examples of his recent clumsiness. In the post-event manipulation, children were asked questions that included misleading informa-tion about Sam Stone's visit four times over the course of the 8 weeks following his visit. Importantly, during these misinforming interviews, two items received particular attention. Children were asked whether Sam had ripped a book, and whether he had dirtied a teddy bear. Children in all conditions were interviewed by an independent interviewer 10 weeks after the event, at which time they were asked an open-ended question about Sam Stone's visit ("Can you tell me what happened that day he came to your school?") and several probe questions ("I heard something about a teddy bear/book. Do you know anything about that?").

Thus, children were assigned to one of the following conditions: (1) control, in which no interviews contained suggestive questions; (2) stereotype, in which subjects were given pre-visit expectations about Sam Stone; (3) suggestion, in which interviews contained erroneous suggestions about misdeeds committed by Sam Stone; and (4) stereotype plus suggestion, in which subjects were given both pre- and post-visit manipulations. The results of the study indicated that during open-ended interviews after 10 weeks, control subjects provided accurate reports. That is, in the absence of stereotypes and leading questions, subjects in both the 3- to 4-year-old age-group and the 5-to 6-year-old age-group were accurate.

The results with respect to the other conditions were in line with past research regarding children's suggestibility. In each case, the younger group of children showed significantly more susceptibility to the suggestions provided than did the older children. In the stereotype condition, free narratives were devoid of errors, but when probed,

37% of the younger children's responses and 18% of those by older children indicated that Sam Stone was involved in destruction to one of the items. In the suggestion condition, 21% of the younger children and 14% of the older children made commission errors in free recall, and in reponse to probes, the error rates climbed to 53% for the youngest subjects and 38% for the oldest. Finally, when exposed to both suggestions and stereotypes, 46% of the younger and 30% of the older children wrongly asserted Sam's misdeeds in their free narratives, while this figure rose to 72% and 38% during probing. In each case, a subset of subjects was also asked as a final question whether they actually saw Sam do the misdeeds they asserted with their own eyes. In response, in the most potent (suggestion-plus-stereotype) condition, 44% of these children in the younger group said that they actually saw him do these things, while 11% in the older group said the same.

In short, it seems reasonable to conclude from these data that in the absence of external influences bearing upon them, even very young children can provide useful and accurate reports about some past events. However, researchers and other adults in the lives of children can evidently take an enormous toll on their report accuracy by indoctrinating them with expectations and/or pursuing them repeatedly with heavy-handed, leading interviews.

The underlying mechanisms that are responsible for the age-related differences in memory distortion effects that appeared in this and other studies are not yet completely clear. However, there are several cognitive and social-developmental possibilities under discussion among researchers. On the social side, it is important to note that children are sensitive to many of the essentially nonmnemonic factors that are thought to sometimes influence the reports of adults. For example, bribes, threats, fear of embarrassment, protection of loved ones, and desire to gain material rewards all have been shown to influence preschoolers' report accuracy.[117–120] A precise comparison between the level of distortion that children display in their reports in the presence of these external pressures and the level of distortion of adults under similar conditions has not been made in the literature. However, broadly speaking, such motivations appear to affect both children and adults, and a differential sensitivity to general demand characteristics suggests that young children may be comparatively more prone to memory distortion in the face of these motivations under some circumstances. For example, preschoolers have been shown to be more suggestible than older children, particularly when erroneous suggestions are made by adult authority figures,[109] which may be a result of their greater tendency to consider their own memories less reliable than an adult's and/or their desire to please adult interviewers by telling them what the child imagines they want to hear.

In the cognitive realm, one suggestion has been that developmental differences in the strength of memory traces make young children's memories especially vulnerable to featural disintegration or resistant to relearning at retrieval.[37,121,122] As conceptualized by some theorists, the incorporation of post-event information occurs as a function of the strength of the memory trace, with weak traces being especially vulnerable to featural dilution or blending (i.e., "destructive updating"), or total dissolution or erasure.[123] Trace theory indicates that age differences in suggestibility may occur because younger children encode weaker (and less "gist-like") traces, which are more vulnerable to featural disintegration or overwriting than those of older subjects. While a number of studies lend support to this position,[124,125] some theorists have also challenged the notion that suggestibility is related to trace strength.[122,126]

Another possible cause of developmental differences in suggestibility is the source misattribution factor introduced earlier as a component of metacognition. The line of reasoning here rests on the possibility that repeated suggestive questions may induce children to create images of events that have been suggested to them. At the time of later questioning, these children may have difficulty remembering the sources of their stored images. They may be unable to mentally identify whether the sources of the images are from the direct perception of the event of interest, or whether they are just products of internally generated images. Because we know that younger subjects have a harder time than older ones in distinguishing between the sources of their experiences in the real world, it could be that very young children's suggestibility is a result of their source confusions.

In a set of experiments designed to look at the contribution of source monitoring to suggestibility effects, we focused on 3- to 4-year-old preschoolers.[127,128] In the original study, once each week for 10 weeks, children received interviews in which they were asked to draw from a deck of large cards. Half of these cards had written descriptions of real events that had occurred in that particular child's life (obtained from their parents), and half of the cards had descriptions of events that never happened. During each session, the children drew each card separately until all of the cards had been drawn. After each drawing, the researcher read the event described to the child and asked the child to "think real hard, and tell me, did that ever happen to you?" After the child had answered this question with a "yes" or "no," he or she would move on to the next card. In the 11th week, a new interviewer interviewed the child, and asked a similar question for each card. In this final interview, however, the interviewer asked the child to elaborate. If the child said that an event had happened in her life, she was asked to tell the researcher all about it. Further, the children were asked detailed follow-up questions after these open-ended questions.

The results of this study show that by the final interview, more than a third of the children reported remembering an event that had never occurred, and in most cases these were events that they had denied remembering earlier. Moreover, the children's reports were striking: they were often internally consistent, full of vivid detail, and accompanied by a confident attitude. One indication of just how realistic the children's reports were is seen in the inability of experts to discriminate between true and false events. We asked hundreds of professionals in psychology, psychiatry, law enforcement, and social work to watch videotapes of three of the children's reports and rate each one on their credibility. Raters were asked to judge the validity of a number of specific claims made by the children, some of which were true and some of which were not (see Leichtman and Ceci[113]). Experts' performance levels did not reliably differ from chance on this task. This suggests that children who have been subjected to repeated, suggestive questioning over long periods of time may appear highly credible to experts. Their reports may be convincing because they are often coherent and highly detailed, accompanied by seemingly appropriate affect.

In an extension of this card-drawing paradigm, we also looked at how the emotional nature of an event might influence the child's susceptibility to incorporating it. Here the manipulation was a bit more heavy-handed; we actually encouraged children across the weekly sessions to visualize the events that they acquiesced to. The suggested events were either positive (getting a present), neutral (waiting for a bus), in which the child participated or watched, or negative (falling off a tricycle and cutting one leg). The results of this experiment show that while children were quite accurate from start to finish in reporting on the events that had actually occurred in their lives, the mean assent rate (or rate of commission errors) went up across interviews. In this study, the trend of increasing assents over time appeared similar for the 3- to 4-year-old and 5- to 6-year-old groups, although the total number of assents in the early interviews was on average slightly higher for younger subjects. Notably, all types of events were subject to this effect, although not equally so. The negative events were less easily incorporated, although commission errors pertinent to these were also committed, and false assents to negative events increased with time.

Although extensive treatment of emotional processes in relation to memory is out of our scope and appears elsewhere in this volume, in the present context it seems appropriate to mention just a few studies in this connection. The fact that children in the card-drawing paradigms[128] showed differential tendencies to incorporate positive and negative events into their reports raises the interesting question of how such emotional contexts affect the general accuracy of event memory across development.

Limited research has evaluated the effects of positive mood manipulations on the memorial processes of very young children. Research does suggest that such manipulations can affect strategy behaviors, such as sorting, as well as creative processes requiring memory, in much the same way that they do in adulthood.[129] In one study directly focused on mood and memory, Bartlett and Santrock[130] demonstrated that when children were provided with positive affect conditions throughout a memory task, their performance exceeded that obtained under moderately negative affective conditions. In this work, 5-year-olds listened to a story and subsequently underwent a variety of recall and recognition tests for words that had appeared in it. Children's emotional state was manipulated by the manner in which researchers interacted with them during initial encoding and at the time of retrieval, as well as by the emotional tone of stimulus materials presented (a positive story about a boy who played with his friends and was given cake versus a negative story about an injury incident to the same boy). The results showed that when children were provided with positive encoding and retrieval conditions, they recalled 4.3 words, on average. In contrast, when faced with negative encoding and retrieval conditions, they recalled an average of only 2.3 out of 6 critical words. Thus, when affective conditions were consistent from encoding to retrieval, positive affect was associated with superior free recall performance. No significant impact of the affect manipulation was obtained on recognition memory tests that followed, which suggests that negative affect had its deleterious influence in this case by rendering the memory less accessible to recollection, and not by destroying it.

The mechanism behind this demonstrated relationship between positive mood and memory is still under discussion. Because it is generally thought that the efficacy of a retrieval cue is contingent upon the extent to which it overlaps with information that was originally encoded,[131] some researchers have suggested that positive affect may often serve as a broad category within which information is organized in memory. From this perspective, positive affect facilitates the ability to see relationships between objects or ideas because it allows access to a particularly broad range of related concepts. It is also possible, however, that many of the findings pertinent to positive affect (as illustrated by the pattern of results in Bartlett and Santrock's work) can be accounted for by a more parsimonious explanation. When subjects are in a positive, relaxed frame of mind, they may be more willing than otherwise to take chances and to expend effort in ways that benefit their performance on various tasks, including those that index memory. This suggestion corresponds with a substantial adult literature that has accumulated, demonstrating that negative affect (in particular, sadness) may sap energy. The low energy level of depressive subjects helps explain their poor performance on memory tasks that require high levels of effortful processing, relative to their performance on those that require less processing.[132,133]

Although they often exert opposite effects on the mediating variables of energy and effort, negative and positive affect rarely show symmetrical opposite direct effects on memory processes. In the developmental research domain that has focused on negative affect in memory, a major issue of concern has been the relationship between stress and accuracy. Most pertinent to our developmental focus, Peters[120] conducted several studies of children's experiences of stress-inducing events and found that higher levels of anxiety led to less accurate recall. In one study, children's anxiety levels during their first or second visit to the dentist were rated by the dentist, the dental assistant, and a parent. After their trips to the dentist, the children were visited in their homes by a male research assistant who presented them with a lineup or photographs and asked them to pick out the dentist and the assistant. Later, children were also asked to identify the research assistant. Results showed that the most anxious children made the highest number of false identifications in the lineups, and that more false identifications were made during the recognition test for the dentist and assistant (high-stress event) than for the research assistant (low-stress event). Accuracy was found more often when the actual "perpetrator" was present in the lineup than if he or she was absent. Other studies that use a variety of stressful events, such as being rubbed on the head by a stranger, going to get immunizations at a clinic, and hearing a loud fire alarm, have revealed the same negative effect of stress on children's memory performance.[120] These studies also suggest that the stress level of the child during the actual lineup identification procedure has a negative impact on recognition. This finding demonstrates the importance of minimizing children's anxiety during lineup procedures to promote maximum memory performance. (For a review of studies on the impact of extreme stress on memory, see Ceci and Bruck.[2])

Although the above studies provide evidence that negative emotion impairs episodic memory, other developmental research has found either no relationship between stress and memory[134] or has found a facilitating effect of trauma on memory.[8,135,136] For instance, one study examined children's recollections of a playful interaction with an adult which shared some of the same features associated with child sexual abuse, such as touching, tickling, and taking photographs.[136] When later questioned both neutrally and suggestively about these events, a majority of the children gave accurate reports of the details of the interaction and resisted the incorporation into memory of misleading suggestions that they were kissed or touched inappropriately by the adult. Other studies have examined children's responses to suggestive questions about their experiences in doctor's offices, and similar patterns of results have been observed.[135]

Reconciliation of these findings regarding the role of emotion in the accuracy of event memory may turn on the specific parameters inherent in each type of study. In particular, negative emotion has been characterized in a variety of ways across studies, making the results difficult to group together for comparison. For example, markers of negative affect that have been considered include general mood states, mental stress levels, and emotional reactions to specific stimuli. Experiences such as receiving painful blood work, listening to a loud radio, and having one's head rubbed in an annoying manner may be as phenomenologically different as they are alike. The coerciveness and other demand characteristics of the interview environment also need to be considered as they interact with emotion. Real-world settings may provide children with an incentive to distort the truth originally in order to please the questioner, and once acquiescence to an inaccurate recollection has occurred, it may snowball. Some studies of children's memorial distortion that include negative affect manipulations do not provide an incentive for original distortion, and thus it is difficult to draw inferences about potential distortion under these circumstances.

In sum, there is a growing body of evidence that indicates a particular susceptibility among young children to the kinds of distorting effects of misinformation that have also been seen in older subjects. The age between 3 and 4 years seems to represent an especially vulnerable period, with 5- and 6-year-olds showing considerably more resistance to suggestion, although not as much as adults. While the mechanisms behind the developmental trends in suggestibility are continuing to be explored, research is making clear that the effects of misinformation and other potential jeopardizers of memorial accuracy do operate across a variety of situations. While some of these situations are most useful to consider primarily because they are theoretically informative, others incorporate elements encountered by clinicians and participants in the legal system who observe children's memorial reports. Important factors present in the real world that are now being paid experimental attention include repeated interviews, long delay intervals, stereotypes, and the emotional valence of the environments surrounding children at encoding and at retrieval.

Individual Differences

Historically, developmental researchers have taken a normative approach to the study of memory development. Their basic goal has been to understand how the functioning of memory processes, and the accuracy with which children recall information and events, changes as children grow older. In considering such data, researchers have traditionally ignored the variance in individual performance across time. For example, if we considered the same sample of children across several years, we might ask whether the individual 4-year-olds who perform best on a particular task are likely to emerge as the 6-year-olds who do so. Interesting results have emerged from the relatively rare work that has addressed this question. A longitudinal study conducted with German children, for example, followed their performance from ages 4 to 12 on tasks focused on memory-relevant processes such as recall, sorting, and clustering. An impressive array of results suggest that, indeed, the rank ordering of children within the sample in terms of performance tends to be quite unstable over the long term. In addition, this work shows that some individual children may demonstrate apparent regressions in performance on particular tasks across development, in defiance of normative group trends.[137,138] Thus, the maturational function reflecting any individual child's performance over time is not as well predicted by the function for the group that she belongs to as one might imagine.

Results such as these illustrate the potential insights gained from observing individual differences in addition to normative descriptions of the memory development process. In particular, it is of both theoretical and practical interest to understand stable individual differences in memory functioning and accuracy. From a theoretical perspective, clarifying the sources of individual differences strengthens researchers' vision of the various factors that may influence the quality and accuracy of recollection. Additionally, such knowledge could assist practitioners in both clinical and forensic settings in estimating the probable accuracy of particular children's event memories as well as in understanding the conditions that facilitate accurate recall.

Pertinent to children's accuracy, for example, one of the most provocative questions explored by developmentalists concerns individual differences in suggestibility. This issue reflects the complexity of the interactions among the biological, cognitive, and social factors that influence how well events are recalled. As we have already noted, it is well established that there is a normative developmental trend in suggestibility that favors the accuracy of older children and adults.

However, in many of the studies conducted on this topic, there have been some younger children who are more resistant to suggestion than some older children. This is to say that in addition to normative age effects, there are substantial individual differences. For example, Ceci and his colleagues[128] found that, when they asked children to repeatedly imagine experiencing events that never happened to them, individual differences in the tendency to acquiesce to the occurrence of these false events emerged and were stable across the 12-week questioning period. This suggests that individual children may differ in the extent to which the accuracy of their memories is likely to be affected by post-event suggestion.

What is responsible for these individual differences? Among the various candidates that we and others have proposed are differences within individuals with respect to theory of mind variables, IQ, social knowledge and ability, temperamental factors, visual imagery ability, and frontal lobe development.[7,139] Most recently, we have collected preliminary data pertinent to the role that two of these mechanisms—source monitoring and visualization—might play in determining individual differences in suggestibility.

The suggestibility task that we used in this study was somewhat similar to the card-drawing procedures described earlier.[128] Specifically, we used a very recent set of suggestibility data collected with a small sample of 23 subjects by Bruck and Ceci (experimental work currently in progress). The subjects in their study were questioned about four events over the course of the experiment. In this paradigm, children were questioned about the first two events once per week over a 5-week period, and then about the second set of two events over a separate 5-week period. The four events of interest were a false negative event (in which a man stole food from the daycare), a false positive event (in which children had helped a lady find a monkey in the park), a true negative event (about a real discipline or punishment the child had received) and a true positive event (in which the children had helped a visitor to their school). Four suggestive interviews were administered by one interviewer and a final interview was administered by a different person. The primary variable of interest at each point was whether children asserted, when asked, that the events described had happened to them.

To separately assess source-monitoring ability, we administered variations of both the drawer task developed by Gopnik and Graf,[54] and the do/imagine procedure designed by Foley and Johnson[55] to the same children who were in Bruck and Ceci's sample. As expected, results with this sample showed a significant correlation between children's performance on the divergent drawer and do/imagine source-monitoring tasks. More importantly, subjects' ability to monitor the source of their knowledge on both of these tasks was highly correlated with their ability to resist the suggestion of false events on the card-drawing task. Acquiescence in this case was operationalized by the number of sessions of visualizing false events that it took until each child asserted that these events had occurred. This predicted negative correlation between source-monitoring ability and acquiescence was seen for both positive and negative events.

Studies on both adults and children indicate that there are trait-like differences in the levels of absorption and vividness of people's imaginations.[140–143] We hypothesized that such differences in children's typical levels of imagery might contribute to their suggestibility, perhaps in interaction with their source-monitoring ability. Thus, if certain children were to imagine highly detailed and vivid representations of suggested events at the time that misleading information was introduced to them, at a later time they might be particularly vulnerable to confusing this information with information from real-world events. To evaluate this possibility, we adapted Betts's[140] imagery scale so that it would be appropriate for children in order to assess potential differences in the vividness of children's imagery. We asked children to generate several images in their heads (i.e., make pictures in their heads) of animals and other common objects. Children were trained in rating the clarity of images before doing the image task. After generating each image (if they could do so), children were asked if the image was very clear, a little clear, or not clear at all. Finally, children were asked perceptual detail questions about the images and we assessed whether they responded immediately, after a delay, or not at all. With the small sample of children for whom we have full data, the imagery scale appears to be valid (e.g., delay times for answers correlate with clarity ratings). However, overall imagery ratings appear to have low correlations with acquiescence to false events, and to overall event acquiescence on the suggestibility task. Imagery in this task appears neither to correlate with source monitoring abilities nor to interact with them in predicting suggestibility. Thus, it may be that the level of visualization does not contribute to source confusion during source monitoring in the manner we had envisioned. Instead, it may be that low and high imagers who are susceptible to suggestibility all simply tend to have equally clear images of suggested and experienced event memories when they reach the final interviews. We are continuing to empirically disentangle these possibilities.

Although we have just begun working on the question of how source monitoring and visual imagery contribute to memorial inaccuracies, our findings are consistent with the view that one component of suggestibility is the child's ability to introspect on the question of whether her visions of past events come from an actual memory of the world.

Conclusions

As we have delineated in this chapter, evidence that helps developmental researchers characterize the nature of children's memory comes from a number of divergent literatures. This is an exciting time in history to study memory development, for a number of reasons. The convergence of theoretical advancements that prompt us to integrate social–emotional perspectives on children's development with those from more traditionally cognitive domains gives us a fuller picture of memory in its natural context than we have ever had before. New methods targeted at capturing the characteristics of infant memory have given us a richer view of the capacities that the youngest subjects possess, to remember and to show us that they do. A large, critical mass of work that has accumulated over many years has flushed out much that is to be known about the various components of childhood memory, including the basic cognitive substrates that build event memories, and the strategies and monitoring that subserve them. Particularly as we approach the applied issues that surround the accuracy of children's reports, this body of knowledge provides a solid underpinning for our work.

Relative to the issue of accuracy, studies have now begun to offer us a vision of the phenomenon of report distortion and are provoking us to consider the factors that contribute to the likelihood that this may occur. We expect that as work continues in this burgeoning area, researchers will obtain more information about the specific ways that contextual factors have an impact on the process across situations. We also look forward to future studies that flesh out our understanding of the circumstances under which particular types of individuals tend to display accuracy problems in memory, and the characteristics of those individuals who tend to resist incorporating misleading, suggestive cues into their event memories.

A word remains to be said about the limits of applying the array of results we have reported in this chapter to particular cases of real-world memory. Research methods provide powerful tools that allow us to isolate the independent contributions of various factors to the process of remembering. For this reason, the work that has been conducted over the long history of studies of memory development can offer valuable information to clinicians and to the courts about how such factors are likely to affect the way in which memory occurs. However, as we have discussed elsewhere in detail,[144] methodological challenges still abound for those who wish to understand the way in which memories of personally relevant and highly emotional events change across the life course. In particular, it is on the whole quite difficult to capture empirically the confluence of factors that are present in many real-world settings. This is particularly true of those complex encoding and retrieval environments that are so often the cause of children's need to testify in court. In any real-world case, the particular host of emotional, social, and psychological variables that bears on an individual child's memory will be idiosyncratic. These factors will not correspond perfectly with those in any single experiment; often, researchers can only examine the various parameters that potentially impinge on event memory individually, or in some combination that represents less than perfect ecological validity. Nonetheless, research and theory provide an excellent guide for thinking about what may be occurring in real-world cases. The simple fact is, normative data cannot serve as a basis for a definitive "diagnosis" of the nature or accuracy of the event memories of a particular child. Especially illustrative of this is the case of individual differences in suggestibility. Our enthusiasm for the new line of research exploring these differences stems in part from the fact that they should tell us something about which children are likely to be susceptible to suggestion across various tasks. However, even if we are able to isolate with great accuracy the cognitive and social factors that are affecting this process, it is unlikely that social science alone will ever be able to determine with perfect precision whether an individual child in a particular situation is subject to these factors. In clinical and forensic settings, such diagnosis is often tempting and sometimes required, in cases in which it is unclear whether a child's report of the past is accurate. No matter how solid our understanding of individual differences, a thorough evaluation of contextual factors in conjunction with knowledge derived from social scientific studies is still likely to lead to the best understanding about what a child has experienced.

Much as we might desire to do so, it is impossible for us to predict exactly how the memories of the mother, child, and baby who experienced the housefire reported on the Boston news will remember it in years to come. The meaning of the event will undoubtedly change for each of them as their lives progress, and this will have an impact on the images and the emotions that they remember.

References

1. Doris JL (ed): The Suggestibility of Children's Recollections. Washington, D.C.: American Psychological Association, 1991.
2. Ceci SJ, Bruck M: The suggestibility of the child witness: a historical review and synthesis. Psychol Bull 1993; 113:403–439.
3. Goodman GS, Bottoms BL: Child Victims, Child Witnesses. New York: Guilford Press, 1993.
4. Stein NL, Leventhal B, Trabasso T (Eds.): Psychological and Biological Approaches to Emotion. Hillsdale, NJ: Lawrence Erlbaum, 1990.
5. Neisser U: Memory Observed: Remembering in Natural Contexts. New York: W.H. Freeman, 1982.
6. Rogoff B, Mistry J: The social and functional context of children's remembering. In R Fivush, JA Hudson (Eds.), Knowing and Remembering in Young Children. Cambridge: Cambridge University Press, 1982, pp. 197–222.
7. Ceci SJ, Bruck M: Jeopardy in the Courtroom. Washington, D.C.: American Psychological Association, 1995.
8. McGough L: Child Witness: Fragile Voices in the American Legal System. New Haven: Yale University Press, 1994.
9. Daro D, Mitchel L: Current Trends in Child Abuse Reporting and Fatalities: The Results of the 1989 Annual 50 States Survey. Washington, D.C.: National Commission for the Prevention of Child Abuse, 1990.
10. Eberle P, Eberle S: The Abuse of Innocence: The McMartin Preschool Trial. Buffalo, NY: Prometheus Books, 1993.
11. Manschel L: Nap Time. New York: Kensington, 1990.
12. Ebbinghaus H: Über das Gedächtnis. Leipzig: Duncker and Humblot, 1885.
13. James W: Principles in Psychology. New York: Dover, 1950.
14. Rosenfield I: The Invention of Memory: A New View of the Brain. New York: Basic Books, 1988.
15. Casey ES: Remembering: A Phenomenological Study. Bloomington: Indiana University Press, 1987.
16. Bronfenbrenner U: The Ecology of Human Development. Cambridge, MA: Harvard University Press, 1979.
17. Wozniak RH, Fischer KW (eds): Development in Context: Acting and Thinking in Specific Environments. Hillsdale, NJ: Erlbaum, 1993.

18. Leichtman MD, Ceci SJ, Ornstein PA: The influence of affect on memory: mechanism and development. *In* SA Christianson (Ed.), The Handbook of Emotion and Memory. Hillsdale, NJ: Erlbaum, 1992, pp. 181–199.
19. Weinert F, Schneider W (eds): Memory Performance and Competencies: Issues in Growth and Development. Mahwah, NJ: Lawrence Erlbaum, 1995.
20. Wyer RS, Srull TK: Memory and Cognition in its Social Context. Hillsdale, NJ: Erlbaum, 1989.
21. Rothbard JC, Shaver P: Continuity of attachment across the lifespan. *In* MB Sperling, WH Berman (Eds.), Attachment in Adults. New York: Guilford Press, 1994, pp. 31–71.
22. Nelson K, Gruendel J: Generalized event representations: basic building blocks of cognitive development. *In* M Lamb, A Brown (Eds.), Advances in Developmental Psychology, Vol. 1. Hillsdale, NJ: Erlbaum, 1981.
23. Fivush R, Hamond NR: Autobiographical memory across the preschool years: toward reconceptualizing infantile amnesia. *In* R Fivush, JA Hudson (Eds.), Knowing and Remembering in Young Children. New York: Cambridge University Press, 1990, pp. 223–248.
24. Bjorklund DF, Zeman BR: Children's organization and metamemory awareness in their recall of familiar information. Child Dev 1982; 53:799–810.
25. Schneider W: The role of conceptual knowledge and metamemory in the development of organizational processes in memory. J Exp Child Psychol 1986; 42:218–236.
26. Schneider W, Sodian B: Metamemory-memory behavior relationships in young children: evidence for a memory-for-location task. J Exp Child Psychol 1988; 45:209–233.
27. Schacter D: Understanding implicit memory. Am Psychol 1992; 47:559–569.
28. Ausley JA, Guttentag RE: Direct and indirect assessments of memory: implications for the study of memory development. *In* ML Howe, R Pasnak (Eds.), Emerging Themes in Cognitive Development, Vol. 1. Foundations. New York: Springer-Verlag, 1993, pp. 234–264.
29. Naito M: Repetition priming in children and adults: age-related dissociation between implicit and explicit memory. J Exp Child Psychol 1990; 50:462–484.
30. Brainerd CJ: Working memory and the developmental analysis of probability judgement. Psychol Rev 1981; 88:463–502.
31. Brown AL: The development of memory: knowing, knowing about knowing, and knowing how to know. *In* HW Reese (Ed.), Advances in Child Development and Behavior. New York: Academic Press, 1975, pp. 104–152.
32. Flavell JH: Developmental studies of mediated memory. *In* HW Reese, LP Lipsitt (Eds.), Advances in Child Development and Behavior. New York: Academic Press, 1970, pp. 181–211.
33. Siegler RS: Children's Thinking. Englewood Cliffs, NJ: Prentice Hall, 1991.
34. Salthouse TA: Processing capacity and its role in the relations between age and memory. *In* FE Weinert, W Schneider (Eds.), Memory Performance and Competencies: Issues in Growth and Development. Mahwah, NJ: Erlbaum, 1995, pp. 111–125.
35. Halford GS: The Development of Thought. Hillsdale, NJ: Lawrence Erlbaum, 1982.
36. Brainerd CJ, Reyna VF, Howe ML, Kevershan J: The last shall be first: how memory strength affects children's recall. Psychol Sci 1990; 1:247–252.
37. Brainerd CJ, Reyna VF, Howe ML, Kingma J: The development of forgetting and reminiscence. Monogr Soc Res Child Dev 1990; 55:3–4.
38. Brainerd CJ, Kingma J: Do children have to remember to reason? A fuzzy-trace theory of transitivity development. Dev Rev 1984; 4:311–377.
39. Brainerd CJ, Reyna VF: Acquisition and forgetting processes in normal and learning disabled children: a disintegration/reintegration theory. *In* JE Obrzut, GW Hynd (Eds.),

Neuropsychological Foundations of Learning Disabilities. New York: Academic Press, 1991, pp. 147–177.

40. Chi MTH: Knowledge structures and memory development. *In* RS Siegler (Ed.), Children's Thinking: What Develops? Hillsdale, NJ: Erlbaum, 1978, pp. 73–96.
41. Ceci SJ, Howe MJA: Semantic knowledge as a determinant of developmental differences in recall. J Exp Child Psychol 1978; 26:230–245.
42. Chi MTH, Ceci SJ: Content knowledge: its role, representation, and restructuring in memory development. *In* HW Reese (Ed.), Advances in Child Development and Behavior, Vol. 20. New York: Academic Press, 1987, pp. 91–142.
43. Lindberg M: Is knowledge base development a necessary and sufficient condition for memory development? J Exp Child Psychol 1980; 30:401–410.
44. Schneider W, Korkel J, Weinert F: Expert knowledge and general abilities and text processing. *In* W Schneider, F Weinert (Eds.), Interactions Among Aptitudes, Strategies, and Knowledge in Cognitive Performance. New York: Springer-Verlag, 1989, pp. 235–251.
45. Ceci SJ: On Intelligence . . . More or Less. Englewood Cliffs, NJ: Prentice Hall, 1990.
46. Kail R, Strauss M: The development of human memory: an historic overview. *In* R Kail, NE Spear (Eds.), Comparative Perspectives on the Development of Memory. Hillsdale, NJ: Erlbaum, 1984, pp. 3–22.
47. Ornstein P (ed): Memory Development in Children. Hillsdale, NJ: Erlbaum, 1978.
48. Kail R: The Development of Memory in Children (3rd Ed). New York: W.H. Freeman, 1990.
49. Schneider W, Pressley M: Memory Development Between 2 and 20. New York: Springer-Verlag, 1989.
50. Cavanaugh JC, Borkowski JG: Searching for metamemory-memory connections: a developmental study. Dev Psychol 1980; 16:441–453.
51. Gopnik A, Astington J: Children's understanding of representational change and its relation to the understanding of false belief and the appearance-reality distinction. Child Dev 1988; 59:26–37.
52. O'Neill DK, Gopnik A: Young children's ability to identify the sources of their beliefs. Dev Psychol 1991; 27:390–397.
53. Foley MA, Passalacqua C, Ratner HH: Appropriating the actions of another: implications for children's memory and learning. Cogn Dev 1993; 8:373–401.
54. Gopnik A, Graf P: Knowing how you know: young childrens' ability to identify and remember the sources of their beliefs. Child Dev 1988; 59:1366–1371.
55. Foley MA, Johnson MK: Confusions between memories for performed and imagined actions. Child Dev 1985; 56:1145–1155.
56. Glaser R: The emergence of theory within instructional research. Am Psychol 1990; 45:29–39.
57. Pressley M, Van Meter P: Memory strategies: natural development and use following instruction. *In* R Pasnak, ML Howe (Eds.), Emergent Themes in Cognitive Development, Vol. 2. Competencies. New York: Springer-Verlag, 1993, pp. 128–165.
58. Pillemer DB, While SH: Childhood events recalled by children and adults. *In* HW Reese (Ed.), Advances in Child Development and Behavior. Orlando: Academic Press, 1989, pp. 297–340.
59. Rubin DC: On the retention function for autobiographical memory. J Verbal Learn Verbal Behav 1982; 21:21–38.
60. Freud S: A General Introduction to Psychoanalysis. New York: Simon and Schuster, 1953. (Original work published 1920).

61. Howe ML, Courage ML: On resolving the enigma of infantile amnesia. Psychol Bull 1993; 113:403–439.

62. Fowler C: A pragmatic approach to early childhood memories: shifting focus from truth to clinical utility. Psychotherapy 1994; 31:676–686.

63. Powell DH: What we can learn from negative outcome in therapy: the case of Roger. [Special issue: What Can We Learn from Failures in Psychotherapy.] J Psychotherapy Integration 1995; 5:133–144.

64. Sarnoff CA: The use of fantasy, dreams, and play. *In* MH Etezady (Ed.), Treatment of Neurosis in the Young: A Pychoanalytic Perspective. Northvale, NJ: Jason Aronson, 1993, pp. 107–167.

65. Simonds SL: Bridging the Silence: Nonverbal Modalities in the Treatment of Adult Survivors of Childhood Sexual Abuse. New York: W. W. Norton, 1994.

66. Baxter J: The suggestibility of child witnesses: review. J Appl Cogn Psychol 1990; 3:1–15.

67. Loftus EF: The reality of repressed memories. Am Psychol 1993; 48:518–537.

68. Terri L: Too Scared to Cry: Psychic Trauma in Childhood. New York: Harper & Row, 1990.

69. Poole DA, White LT: Two years later: effects of question repetition and retention interval on the eyewitness testimony of children and adults. Dev Psychol 1993; 29:844–853.

70. Mandler JM: How to build a baby: II. Conceptual primatives. Psychol Rev 1992; 99:587–604.

71. Bornstein MH, Sigman MD: Continuity in mental development from infancy. Child Dev 1986; 57:251–274.

72. McCall RB: The development of intellectual functioning in infancy and prediction of later IQ. *In* JD Osofsky (Ed.), Handbook of Infant Development. New York: Wiley, 1979, pp. 707–741.

73. Werner JS, Perlmutter M: Development of visual memory in infants. *In* HW Reese, LP Lipsitt (Eds.), Advances in Child Development and Behavior, Vol. 14. New York: Academic Press, 1979, pp. 1–55.

74. Rovee-Collier C, Hayne H: Reactivation of infant memory: implications for cognitive development. *In* HW Reese (Ed.), Advances in Child Development and Behavior, Vol. 20. New York: Academic Press, 1987, pp. 185–238.

75. Meltzoff AN: Infant imitation and memory: nine-month-olds in immediate and deferred imitation tests. Child Dev 1988; 59:217–225.

76. Perris EE, Myers NA, Clifton RK: Long-term memory for a single infancy experience. Child Dev 1990; 61:1796–1807.

77. Bauer PJ, Hertsgaard L, Dow GAA: After 8 months have passed: memory for specific events by 1- to 2-year-olds. Poster presented at the Biennial International Conference on Infant Studies, Miami Beach, FL, May, 1992.

78. Meltzoff AN: Infant imitation after a 1-week delay: long-term memory for novel acts and multiple stimuli. Dev Psychol 1988; 24:470–476.

79. Leichtman MD: The developmental trajectory of early event memory: visual, auditory and olfactory components. Poster presented at The Biennial Meeting of the Society for Research in Child Development, New Orleans, LA, March, 1993.

80. Hudson JA: The emergence of autobiographic memory in mother-child conversation. *In* R Fivush, JA Hudson (Eds.), Knowing and Remembering in Young Children. New York: Cambridge University Press, 1990.

81. Nelson K: Event Knowledge: Structure and Function in Development. Hillsdale, NJ: Erlbaum, 1986.

82. Nelson CA (ed): Memory and Affect in Development, The Minnesota Symposia on Child Psychology, Vol. 26. Hillsdale, NJ: Erlbaum, 1993.

83. Fivush R: The functions of event memory: some comments on Nelson and Barcelou. *In* U Neisser, E Winograd (Eds.), Remembering Reconsidered: Ecological and Traditional Approaches to the Study of Memory. New York: Cambridge University Press, 1988, pp. 277–282.

84. Pillemer DB, Picariello ML, Pruett JC: Very long-term memories of a salient preschool event. Appl Cogn Psychol 1994; 8:95–106.

85. Fivush R, Gray JT, Fromhoff FA: Two-year-olds talk about the past. Cogn Dev 1987; 2:393–409.

86. Fagan JF: Infants' recognition memory for a series of visual stimuli. J Exp Child Psychol 1971; 14:453–476.

87. Topinka CV, Steinberg B: Visual recognition memory in 3 1/2 and 7 1/2 month old infants. Paper presented at the International Conference on Infant Studies, Providence, RI, 1978.

88. Strauss MS, Cohen LB: Infant immediate and delayed memory for perceptual dimensions. Paper presented at the International Conference on Infant Studies, New Haven, CT, May, 1980.

89. Rovee-Collier C, Patterson J, Hayne H: Specificity in the reactivation of infant memory. Dev Psychobiol 1985; 18:559–574.

90. Crowder G, Schab FR: Imagery for odors. *In* FR Schab, RG Crowder (Eds.), Memory for Odors. 1995, pp. 93–107.

91. Mandler JM: Recall of events by preverbal children. *In* A Diamond (Ed.), The Developmnt and Neural Bases of Higher Cognitive Functions. Ann NY Acad Sci 1990; 608:485–516.

92. Mandler JM: How to build a baby: on the development of an accessible representational system. Cogn Dev 1988; 3:113–136.

93. Mandler JM: The precocious infant revisited. SRCD Newsletter 1992; spring: 1–10.

94. Ceci SJ, Hembrooke H: The contextual nature of earliest memories. *In* JM Puckett, HW Reese (Eds.), Mechanisms of Everyday Cognition. 1993, pp. 117–136.

95. Smith PH: Five-month-old infant recall and utilization of temporal organization. J Exp Child Psychol 1984; 38:400–414.

96. Bauer PJ, Shore CM: Making a memorable event: effects of familiarity and organization on young children's recall of action sequences. Cogn Dev 1987; 2:327–338.

97. LeCompte CK, Gratch G: Violation of a rule as a method of diagnosing infants' level of object concept. Child Dev 1972; 43:385–396.

98. Meltzoff AN: What infant memory tells us about infantile amnesia: long-term recall and deferred imitation. [Special issue: Early Memory] J Exp Child Psychol 1995; 59:497–515.

99. McDonough L, Mandler JM: Very long term recall in two-year olds. Poster presented at the Biennial Meeting of the International Society of Infant Studies, Montreal, April 1990.

100. Myers N, Speaker E: Joy in a toy: infant experience reflected after 18 months. Poster presented at the Biennial Meeting of the Society for Research in Child Development, New Orleans, LA, March, 1993.

101. Perris EE: Memory for events during the first year of life. Doctoral Dissertation, University of Massachusetts, Amherst, MA.

102. Lindsay DS, Johnson MK: The eyewitness suggestibility effect and memory for source. Mem Cogn 1989; 17:349–357.

103. Loftus EF: Leading questions and the eyewitness report. Cogn Psychol 1975; 7:560–572.

104. Loftus EF: Eyewitness Testimony. Cambridge, MA: Harvard University Press, 1979.

105. Loftus EF, Miller DG, Burns HJ: Semantic integration of verbal information in visual memory. J Exp Psychol Hum Learn Mem 1978; 4:19–31.

106. Loftus EF, Schooler J, Wagenaar W: The fate of memory: comment on McCloskey and Zaragosa. J Exp Psychol Gen 1985; 114:375–380.

107. McCloskey M, Zaragoza M: Misleading postevent information and memory for events: arguments and evidence against memory impairment hypotheses. J Exp Psychol Gen 1985; 114:1–16.

108. Loftus EF, Hoffman HG: Misinformation in memory: the creation of new memories. J Exp Psychol Gen 1989; 118:100–104.

109. Ceci SJ, Ross DF, Toglia MP: Suggestibility of children's memory: psycholegal implications. J Exp Psychol Gen 1987; 116:38–49.

110. Cohen RL, Harnick MA: The susceptibility of child witnesses to suggestion. Law Hum Behav 1980; 4:201–210.

111. Howe ML, Courage ML, Bryant-Brown L: Reinstating preschoolers' memories. Dev Psychol 1993; 29(5):854–869.

112. Duncan EM, Whitey P, Kunen S: Integration of visual and verbal information in children's memories. Child Dev 1982; 53:1215–1223.

113. Leichtman MD, Ceci SJ: The effects of stereotypes and suggestions on preschoolers' reports. Dev Psychol 1995; 31:568–578.

114. Martin CL, Halverson CF: The efffects of sex-typing schemas on young children's memory. Child Dev 1983; 54:563–574.

115. Strangor C, McMillan D: Memory for expectancy-congruent and expectancy-incongruent information: a review of the social and social developmental literatures. Psychol Bull 1992; 111:42–61.

116. Gray E: Unequal Justice: The Prosecution of Child Sexual Abuse. New York: MacMillan, 1993.

117. Bussey K: Children's lying and truthfulness: implications for children's testimony. *In* SJ Ceci, M Leichtman, M Putnick (Eds.), Cognitive and Social Factors in Preschoolers' Deception. Hillsdale, NJ: Erlbaum, 1992, pp. 89–110.

118. Ceci SJ, Leichtman M, Putnick M (eds): Cognitive and Social Factors in Early Deception. Hillsdale, NJ: Erlbaum, 1992.

119. Lewis M, Stranger C, Sullivan M: Deception in three-year-olds. Dev Psychol 1989; 25:439–443.

120. Peters DP: The influence of stress and arousal on the child witness. *In* JL Doris (Ed.), The Suggestibility of Children's Recollections. Washington, D.C.: American Psychological Association, 1991, pp. 60–76.

121. Brainerd CJ, Reyna V: Memory loci of suggestibility development: comment on Ceci, Ross, and Toglia. J Exp Psychol Gen 1988; 118:197–200.

122. Howe ML: Misleading children's story recall: forgetting and reminiscence of the facts. Dev Psychol 1991; 27:746–762.

123. Ceci SJ, Toglia M, Ross D: On remembering . . . more or less. J Exp Psychol Gen 1988; 118:250–262.

124. Warren AR, Hulse-Trotter K, Tubbs E: Inducing resistance to suggestibility in children. Law Hum Behav 1991; 15:273–285.

125. King M, Yuille J: Suggestibility of the child witness. *In* SJ Ceci, D Ross, M Toglia (Eds.), Children's Eyewitness Memory. New York: Springer-Verlag, 1987, pp. 24–35.

126. Zaragoza M, Dahlgren D, Muench J: The role of memory impairment in children's suggestibility. *In* ML Howe, CJ Brainerd, VF Reyna (Eds.), Development of Long Term Retention. New York: Springer-Verlag, 1992, pp. 184–216.

127. Ceci SJ, Crotteau ML, Smith E, Loftus EF: Repeatedly thinking about a non-event: source misattributions among preschoolers. [Special issue: The Recovered Memory / False Memory Debate] Consciousness Cogn: Int J 1994; 3:388–407.

128. Ceci SJ, Loftus EF, Leichtman MD, Bruck, M: The possible role of source misattributions

in the creation of false beliefs among preschoolers. [Special issue: Hypnosis and Delayed Recall] Int J Clin Exp Hypn 1994; 2:304–320.

129. Isen AM: The influence of positive and negative affect on cognitive organization: some implications for the development. *In* N Stein, B Leventhal, T Trabasso (Eds.), Psychological and Biological Approaches to Emotion. Hillsdale, NJ: Erlbaum, 1990, pp. 75–94.

130. Bartlett JC, Santrock JW: Affect-dependent episodic memory in young children. Child Dev 1979; 50:513–518.

131. Tulving E, Thomson DM: Encoding specificity and retrieval processes in episodic memory. Psychol Rev 1973; 80:352–373.

132. Ellis HC, Thomas R, McFarland A, Lane W: Emotional mood states and retrieval in episodic memory. J Exp Psychol Learn Mem Cogn 1985; 11:363–370.

133. Hertel P: Improving memory and mood through automatic and controlled procedures of the mind. *In* DJ Herrmann, H Weingartner, A Searleman, C McEvoy (Eds.), Memory Improvement: Implications for Memory Theory. New York: Springer-Verlag, 1992, pp. 43–60.

134. Vandermaas MO: Does anxiety affect children's reports of memory for a stressful event? Appl Cogn Psychol 1993; 7:109–127.

135. Goodman GS, Hirschman JE, Hepps D, Rudy L: Children's memory for stressful events. Merrill Palmer Q 1991; 37:109–158.

136. Goodman GS, Rudy L, Bottoms B, Aman C: Children's concerns and memory: issues of ecological validity in the study of children's eyewitness testimony. *In* R Fivush, J Hudson (Eds.), Knowing and Remembering in Young Children. New York: Cambridge University Press, 1990, pp. 249–284.

137. Schneider W, Weinert FE: Universal trends and individual differences in memory development. *In* A de Ribaupierre (Ed.), Transition Mechanisms in Child Development: The Longitudinal Perspective. Cambridge: Cambridge University Press, 1989, pp. 68–106.

138. Schneider W, Sodian B: A longitudinal study of young children's memory behavior and performance in a sort-recall task. J Exp Child Psychol 1991; 51:14–29.

139. Schacter DL, Kagan J, Leichtman MD: True and false memories in children and adults: a cognitive neuroscience perspective. Psychol Public Policy Law 1995; 1:411–428.

140. Betts CH: The distribution and functions of mental imagery. New York: Teachers College Contribution to Education, 1909.

141. Sheehan PW: A shortened form of Bett's questionnaire upon mental imagery. J Clin Psychol 1967; 23:386–389.

142. Hilgard ER: Suggestibility and suggestions as related to hypnosis. *In* JF Schumaker (Ed.), Human Suggestibility: Advances in Theory, Research and Application. New York: Routledge, 1991, pp. 37–58.

143. Tellegen A, Atkinson G: Openness to absorbing and self-altering experiences ("absorption"), a trait related to hypnotic susceptibility. J Abnorm Psychol 1974; 83:268–277.

144. Ceci SJ, Leichtman MD, Bruck M: The suggestibility of children's eyewitness reports: methodological issues. *In* FE Weinert, W Schneider (Eds.), Memory Performance and Competencies: Issues in Growth and Development. Mahwah, NJ: Erlbaum, 1995, pp. 323–347.

7

An Integrative Developmental Model for Trauma and Memory

"How does one rid oneself of something buried far within: memory and the skin of memory? It clings to me yet. Memory's skin has hardened, it allows nothing to filter out of what remains, and I have no control over it. I don't feel it anymore"[1] (p.1).

Charlotte Delbo wrote those words about memory in *La Mémoire et les Jours* (*Memory and Days*), an autobiographical account of her experiences in a Nazi-run concentration camp. Delbo uses the image of a snake skin to create a compelling metaphor for the process of encapsulation. "How did I manage to extricate myself from [the memory of Auschwitz] when I returned?" she writes. "What did I do so as to be alive today? People often ask me that question, to which I continue to look for an answer, and still find none"[1] (p. 2).

Delbo's question constitutes the central focus of this chapter. Although on some deep human level her question is unanswerable, and will remain always so, clinicians are faced time and again with this question as they work with traumatized patients. This chapter thus presents an integrated developmental model for trauma and memory, with a focus on describing the neuropsychological mechanisms by which traumatic experiences are encapsulated across the following seven developmental domains: sensorimotor, linguistic, affective, cognitive, moral, psychosocial, and what I term the self-memory system. My developmental model recognizes that memory occurs within dynamic and parallel systems of information exchange which continuously move and change over time.[2–5] In developmental terms this means the way in which trauma is individually absorbed, memorialized, and expressed depends on the complex interplay of the biological and neuropsychological systems described in this section of the book, and on the actual state of the person as a whole. During the encapsulation process, external factors relating to the nature of the traumatic event interact with numerous internal, or developmentally dependent, factors.[6-10] These factors include the trauma victim's level of linguistic and motor ability,[8-10] physiological integrity,[11] stage of moral and psychological development,[6-10,12] and impulse control. Thus, aspects of the trauma victim's developmental history—including the extent, duration and timing of abuse—help determine how and to what degree traumatic memories are encapsulated in the seven domains listed above. Because encapsulated material always contains the developmental features and affects from the time when the trauma took place, I view these seven developmental domains as diagnostic tools for guiding the analytic psycho-therapist during treatment. Using an integrated developmental model, a therapist is able to recognize the traumatized patient's developmental strenghts; these strengths can be used to anchor weaker areas of development as treatment continues.

My developmental model of trauma integrates my clinical work in the trauma field with current theories about parallel distributed systems for information processing, or PDP.[2-5] A concept I have termed the *self-memory system* is the cornerstone of my developmental model because it is the subverbal, metaphysical plane on which the individual *experiences* trauma and attempts to make meaning of it through fantasy, dreams, symbolic representations, character adjustments, developmental disruptions, and somatic and psychic symptoms.

I propose that this self-memory system has its own parallel information structures for receiving affective impressions and for holding images, symbols, and representations. The self-memory system develops from the moment of birth, and under normal devel-opmental conditions is able to communicate fluidly and dynamically with the cognitive memory system and with the external world. It is subverbal, responding to the affective rather than the cognitive component of words and language. Consider the deep emo-tions that can be aroused by listening to opera, even when the words are sung in a language not spoken by the listener; these deep emotions are a representation of self-memory being "touched" by the tone, harmony and beauty of the language and music. While my theory of self-memory builds on previous work on the self as described by such researches as Epstein,[13-15] Kohut,[16] Noam,[17] and Wolf,[18] my model stresses the importance of the individual's meaning-making efforts, the individual's sense of mo-rality and drive toward spirituality, and the relationship of the self and its memories to language, literature, art, and history.

My model proposes that when it is faced with overwhelming trauma or abuse, the self-memory system separates wholly or partially from the cognitive memory system, truncating normal development by blocking the flow of information between develop-mental domains. The intense focus on the internal self that can occur when the two systems are split produces common dissociative symptoms such as amnesia, dream-like states, and psychosomatic complaints.[19] The depth and nature of the trauma, as well as the developmental integrity of the individual at the time of the trauma, determine to what degree this cognitive-self splitting will take place.

Although I discuss the self-memory system in scientific and psychodynamic terms, it is perhaps best evoked by the Ojibwa word for mirror, *wabimujichagwan,* which translates to "looking at your soul."[20] Deeply aesthetic, the self-memory system responds to the symbolism and beauty of high art, literature, theater, and dance. Self-memory differs from implicit memory in an important way: while both kinds of memory are nonverbal, the self-memory system is primarily concerned with meaning-making. Like the immunological system, the self-memory system is deeply embedded on a physiological level. Implicit memory, on the other hand, is an "image" of an event or a piece of previously learned knowledge. Self-memory, then, is the sum of the individual's representations of the individual's inner and outer world; it is a meaning-making system that is as deeply rooted physiologically and neurobiologically as the human immunological system.

I believe that the integrity of an individual's self-memory is best measured by the Rorschach Inkblot Test and other projective measures and neuropsychological instruments (see, for example, Levin[21]). The subverbal language of the self can be heard as the individual responds to the shapes, textures, colors, and spatial configurations of the Rorschach. Self-memory reveals itself during Rorschach testing in the form of emotion, memories, and fantasies, providing rich information about what has been memorialized in self-memory in terms of safety, trust, morality, guilt, attachment, and separation, and objects and their representational processes.[21] The Rorschach is exquisitely sensitive to the patient's developmental levels, artistic and aesthetic expressions, and his or her perceptions of self-memories.

The self-memory system is internal and personal, and as such, is exquisitely sensitive to the pain of trauma, neglect, and abuse. Similar to a person's native language, the self-memory system is laid down during the formative years from birth through young adulthood. During normal development, the self-memory system and the cognitive system work hand in hand to make meaning of experiences. I believe that under conditions of trauma, the cognitive and self-memory systems may separate in whole or in part. It is possible for cognition to proceed even when the two systems are detached from each other; this is the reason some dissociated patients can function at a high intellectual level in their academic or professional careers yet feel as if they are moving "in a fog" or feel as if they are "not really there." Karen C., a dissociated patient, garnered many athletic and academic awards in high school and college, yet reported in therapy that she went through life feeling as if "somebody else had accomplished all those things."

Time and again, Holocaust survivors describe this self-cognitive splitting in their fictional and nonfictional writing (see Delbo,[1] Appelfeld,[22] Langer,[23–25] and Wiesel[26]). Charlotte Delbo, the Parisian writer who was imprisoned in a Nazi-run concentration camp, describes how the prolonged horror of her experience forced a deep split between her self-memory and cognitive memory systems. In the following passage, Delbo admits that in order to write about Auschwitz she had to separate the affective horror of her memories from her core self, using only her intellect to describe her memories to her readers. This splitting between Delbo's cognitive and self-memory systems serves to keep a "snake skin" wrapped tightly around her encapsulated memories, allowing her to share these memories on an intellectual level, without a trace of emotion or upset. "[I] can talk to you about Auschwitz without exhibiting or registering any anxiety or emotion. Because when I talk to you about Auschwitz, it is not from deep memory that my words issue. They come from external memory, if I may put it that way, from intellectual memory, the memory connected with thinking processes."[1] (p. 3).

Delbo tells her readers that her experiences in Auschwitz are so deeply etched in her memory that she cannot forget one moment of them. When asked if she is living with Auschwitz, she replies: "No, I live next to it. Auschwitz is there, unalterable, precise, but enveloped in the skin of memory, an impermeable skin that isolates it from my present self"[1] (p. 2).

Delbo acknowledges that while the snake skin that encapsulates her memories of the Holocaust is tough, it "gives way" at times. This giving way, for Delbo, occurs most often when she is dreaming, a time when the self-memory system is engaged at its deepest and most symbolic level. In her vulnerable dream state, the encapsulated Auschwitz memories invade Delbo's self-memory system, causing a flood of affective horror so deep that she feels as though she is dying. Her heart beats wildly and she cries out in the dark. "[I]n those own dreams I see myself, yes, my own self such as I know I was: hardly able to stand on my feet, my throat tight, my heart beating wildly, frozen to the marrow, filthy, skin and bones; the suffering I feel is so unbearable, so identical to the pain endured there, that I feel it physically, I feel it throughout my whole body, which becomes a mass of suffering; and I feel death fasten on me, I feel that I am dying"[1] (p. 3).

Delbo's dissociation occurred when she was an adult. The following case study, in contrast, is an example of dissociation during early childhood and adolescence. Karen C., a 40-year-old patient, drank alcohol heavily from the time she was 8 years of age until her early thirties. Her family history includes a confirmed case of sexual abuse against her sister. Although Karen is unsure whether she herself was sexually abused as a child, she was deeply affected by the atmosphere of abuse which permeated her home. She entered therapy with me 2 years ago, exhibiting a trance-like demeanor and reporting that she went through her life "as if in a fog." She felt separated from other people in the day-to-day tasks of her career as a trial lawyer. Karen's affect and mood were dysphoric and she exhibited symptoms for anhedonia, fatigue, and confusion.

My theory is that there are significant gaps in both Karen's cognitive and self-memory systems because of the chronic childhood intoxication. Her self-memory system took on an identity of toxicity, drunkenness, and emotional flatness. Her descriptions of her adult life, such as "being in a fog," reflect this early self-memory of being drunk. Her self-memory simultaneously craves what it knew (drunkenness) and what it did not know (normal childhood and adolescent experiences). Because she spent so much of her early childhood in an alcoholic fog, Karen missed many of the normal developmental tasks associated with those years. Not surprisingly, she has trouble with issues related to her sexuality and body image. She has problems in all her relationships, and despite being married, Karen dates other men; she frequently finds herself in date rape situations. In therapy, Karen is working through these more primitive levels of development as she moves through the encapsulated states that were frozen during childhood.

During childhood, Karen's self-memory system was partially disengaged from her cognitive system and from the outside world. She thus saw herself as isolated and alone. Despite making good grades and winning many academic awards in high school and college, she never related to these considerable accomplishments and skills. In her words, it was "as if it were somebody else doing these things." Karen remains in a chronic state of ambivalence because her cognitive and self-memory systems have never been properly introduced.

Clues about the neurobiological mechanisms related to the self-cognitive split that characterizes dissociation can be found in the research on epileptic patients and patients who have suffered callosal resections, cerebral vascular accidents, or amnesia as a result of accidents, injuries, and diseases. Consider Jackson's classic example of Dr. Z., an epileptic physician who suffered a petit mal seizure while he was in the process of examining a patient.[27] The petit mal seizure continued for many minutes. Although Dr. Z. had no subsequent memory of having done so, he managed to diagnose the patient's pneumonia and even wrote the diagnosis into the patient's chart.[27] Dr. Z.'s experience provides an example of a person's cognitive system functioning independently, without the self-system being aware of its deliberate aims and goals.

The nature and location of a disease or injury determines which system is or is not engaged. Dr. Z., for example, functioned at a high cognitive level while examining his patient. Aphasic stroke patients, on the other hand, may be severely impaired cognitively even though their self-memory system is intact and functional. Natasha, a 48-year-old professor of art history, suffered a left hemispheric cerebral vascular accident (CVA), which resulted in severe aphasia and right-sided hemiplegia. Although her self-memory system remained intact, her intellect was severely impaired. A year after her stroke, I worked with Natasha 4 days a week using an in-depth, neuropsychodynamic approach designed to innervate areas of brain functioning which could be engaged for rehabilitation purposes. I used an array of sensory stimulation, including music, poetry, and painting, all of which were aimed at reaching her intact self-memory system. Aspects of cognitive function such as language were successfully reintroduced to Natasha via her self-memory system as she responded to the music, poetry, painting, and psychotherapy.

Attention—a primary executive function for directing one's perceptual activities onto implicit and explicit memory tasks—is critical to any discussion of the self-cognitive splitting that characterizes dissociation.[28] After her CVA, Natasha was no longer able to use her cognitive resources and instead focused her attention on her inner world. This is similar to the intense focus on the self that can be seen in severely traumatized or chronically abused patients. Like these traumatized patients, Natasha felt depressed, withdrawn, and ashamed. She was psychologically enervated to the point of becoming delusional and hallucinatory, and over time immersed herself in an increasingly bizarre fantasy and dream life.

Mesulam[29] suggests that the neocortex, thalamus, and brainstem are linked to the modulation of attention and that the neocortex is responsible for the more complex aspects of executive-self regulation. According to Kihlstrom,[3] efficient memory of any experience greatly depends on the amount and quality of cognitive attention devoted to that event. This idea is central to my model of dissociation: I propose that an individual who is being traumatized can devote attention to the self, to the cognitive system, to the external world, or to any simultaneous combination of all three. Attention may shift rapidly from focus to focus as the event unfolds. Attention itself may fragment when attentional demands exceed attentional resources. The trauma victim may become overwhelmed by the attentional and sensory demands of a situation; his or her attention may rapidly shift from the external world, to the self, to the cognitive system, back to the external world, and so on. It is possible, then, for the trauma victim to take in fragmented pieces of visual, auditory, affective, and linguistic information. These random bits of information, which are absorbed while the attention of the trauma victim was shifting from focus to focus, may become encapsulated as isolated memory units. Because the cognitive system was not fully engaged, little meaning-making is possible, and these perceptual memory fragments may remain isolated from each other on parallel lines of information processing.

Because of the neurophysiological agents (opiates) that are released in response to pain, the amount and degree of physical pain and the nature of the trauma victim's injuries may play a critical role in determining attentional focus. External factors relating to the nature of the event also play an important role in directing attentional focus, as do psychodynamic factors, such as the trauma victim's sense of control, competence, and motivation.[7–12] An adult trauma victim may keep herself cognitively focused on the details of the event—however horrific those details may be—if she feels there is a chance for survival or if she feels competent enough to cope with whatever is happening to her. For example, a woman whose car crashes into a tree may turn her cognitive attention to seeking help or tending to the wounds of her children. On the other hand, a Bosnian woman who is sexually assaulted by a group of armed soldiers may dissociate and focus attention on her self as soon as she becomes aware that she can do nothing to stop the rapes. Young children, who often lack the skills to react competently to an emergency, may dissociate more readily during trauma because there is no reason to focus attention on the painful external situation.

The ability to focus cognitive attention on a problem or event may involve some combination of conscious and unconscious control.[3] The ability to focus cognitive attention on a problem or event is a developmentally based skill; attentional skills are linked to cognitive, visual, and neurosensory maturation. The VOR, or vestibulo-orienting reflex,[30] and the OR, or orienting reflex,[28,31] are important mechanisms for regulating cognitive attention. The VOR allows a person to constantly scan the environment for the presence of novelty in the form of new sights and sounds. Novelty thus serves to hook a person's cognitive attention via the VOR; the OR stays active when the brain confirms the fact that the potentially novel sight or sound is in fact a novelty.[28,30,31]

The OR and VOR mechanisms are important to understanding the degree of cognitive attention that will be devoted to a trauma. A sudden trauma such as a car accident or one-time sexual assault will tend to hook a person's cognitive attention by virtue of its novelty. Conversely, repeated sexual abuse will begin to lose its novelty over time.[32] The sexually abused child may thus focus less and less cognitive attention on the abuse as the attacks become more and more routine. Attention in this case remains focused on the self because her orienting mechanisms find nothing novel in the fact that the perpetrator has entered her room in the middle of the night.

Psychodynamically, a trauma in which the victim is rendered totally helpless will inevitably cause attention to be focused on the self. A vivid example of this inner focusing can be seen in the victims of Nazi-run concentratin camps. Holocaust survivor Primo Levi describes how, upon entrance to the concentration camp, the prisoner who spoke Polish or Russian or French had to focus massive amounts of his cognitive attention on learning the rules of concentration camp life and on understanding the commands that were being shouted at him in a foreign language. Physical survival required that the prisoner pay extreme attention to minute details such as the angle at which his pillow was placed on the bunk—a misaligned pillow could provoke a severe beating or death. As the ordeal dragged on, however, the prisoner's hopes for survival inevitably began to diminish. He became aware of the randomness of violence and death within the camp; anyone could be shot or beaten, no matter how carefully he paid attention to his pillow alignment or to the hundred other senseless and constantly changing rules of the camp commanders. External factors, such as lack of adequate nutrition and sleep, also affected the Holocaust victim's ability and motivation to pay cognitive attention to the tasks of survival. Many prisoners became less and less focused on the tasks of survival and more and more focused on the inner world. Intensely focused on the self, the dissociated prisoner felt increasingly isolated, ashamed, hopeless, and withdrawn.[33]

Emotion is an important factor in regulating how and where an individual will focus his attention and thus in determining the degree of cognitive-self dissociation.[34-36] Affect is thus critical to any discussion about trauma and memory. Emotion itself may be viewed as consisting of extremely potent memory units that enter the parallel distributed system, creating tight associations with coincident events. Numerous brain structures are responsible for processing and integrating affect. The neurophysiological basis of emotion centers around the neurohypophyseal hormones and related peptides, which may be mediated by a receptive complex in the ventral hippocampus. The amgydala may play an important role in mediating affect. McGaugh et al.[37,38] suggest that the amgydala could be a locus for the neural changes underlying the memory of affective experiences. This structure may be especially sensitive to trauma events, serving as a gauge for alerting an individual to potential threats in the environments.

Two curious incidents that occurred soon after the April 1995 bombing of the Federal Building in Oklahoma City demonstrate this strong association between trauma, emotion, and memory. Television reporter Bernard Shaw and preacher Bill Graham both referred to President Clinton as "President Kennedy" during television coverage of the crisis. Both men seemed completely unaware of their verbal slips as they spoke into the camera. The feelings of shock, horror, and disbelief that were evoked by the shattered Federal Building were so strong that they evoked unconscious memories in Shaw and Graham of another emotionally horrifying national tragedy—the assassination of President John F. Kennedy (see Bahannon[39] and Pillemer[40]).

I view affect as a component of the self that resides in the self-memory system. Depending upon the degree of cognitive-self dissociation, memories of a trauma can thus include cognitive memories, affective memories, or a combination of both. During conditions of total or near-total dissociation, an individual may be flooded with powerfully negative emotions that she is unable to think about or make cognitive sense of. These emotions are walled off, or encapsulated, within the self-memory system.

Developmentally, this is why severely dissociated patients may have problems in their interpersonal relationships and in other affective areas of their lives.[32] Consider the case of Virginia, a 43-year-old patient who suffered chronic sexual assault by her father during most of her adolescence. Because her dissociation during the incestuous attacks was so complete, the adult Virginia is now filled with powerful and involuntary emotions that she does not yet "know about" or understand. Unable to make meaning of these negative affects, severely dissociated patients like Virginia suffer from somatic expressions of fear, anger, and shame, including heart palpitations, nausea, gastric ulcers, etc. Psychodynamically, because she has had little practice in recognizing, feeling, and interpreting her emotions, Virginia cannot understand the affective needs of other people and has problems with most of her interpersonal relationships. Chronically abused patients like Virgina may suddenly experience waves of affective horror which they cannot make meaning of. Psychiatric expressions of these encapsulated affects can sometimes include the kind of symptoms seen in atypical psychosis.

Encapsulation of Traumatic Memories Along Developmental Domains

My developmental model of trauma and memory considers parallel distributed systems as avenues for memorializing and making meaning of traumatic events within the context of development. Under normal developmental conditions, the human information processing system is an innervated one: it is a dynamic and integrated system that allows fluid and recursive movement among development domains. When trauma is experienced, however, this normally flexible system for processing information is disrupted. Research has shown that even a single traumatic event can disrupt normal information processing. In a study of disaster survivors Wilkinson[41] found that 36% of the victims reported an inability to feel deeply; 34% reported apathy, and 29% had feelings of detachment. Valent[42] reported that survivors of a fire in Australia felt dazed or stunned, and Feinstein and Spiegel[43] found that 41% of the survivors of an ambush in Namibia showed diminished interest in normal activities and 24% still felt detached 1 week after the attack. Madakasira and O'Brien[44] studied 116 victims of a tornado 5 months after it ripped through their North Carolina community. Fifty-nine percent of the victims fulfilled criteria for posttraumatic stress disorder (PTSD). Symptoms included intrusive thinking, recurrent dreaming, psychic numbing, cognitive disruption, and impaired memory and concentration.

Developmental features play an important role in the formation of these symptoms. In a study of children and adults exposed to a school shooting, Schwarz and Kowalski[45] found that children more frequently suffered from avoidance symptoms than did adults, including losing interest in significant activities, feeling detached from others, and having a restricted range of affect. Avoidance symptoms in adults were associated more strongly with the recall of intense sensory experiences, such as smelling or touching the victim's blood. The authors suggest that the adults' more mature neuropsychological, cognitive, and affective capabilities may have enabled them to better resist the formation of symptoms.

Noam[17] proposes the concept of overassimilation, in which particular experiences, even under normal conditions, resist integration to higher-order systems. Overassimilation is the process of incorporating an experience into a lower-level structure even though higher levels already exist. The products of these overassimilations are called *encapsulations*. I believe that the psyche has the ability to incorporate traumatic experiences into different levels of development, metabolizing them into higher- and lower-levels and systems.[46] Models of information-processing including PDP systems and the Boolean Hypercube,[47] will be discussed later in this chapter, and will provide a theoretical framework for describing the encapsulation process along developmental domains.

Under conditions of prolonged childhood trauma, aspects of the abuse victim's normal development are dissociated from the whole; they are split off from higher and lower levels of development. These fractured units become frozen, or encapsulated, along the seven developmental domains listed above, creating rigid boundaries that defend the trauma victim against the psychic pain of further assault. The encapsulated unit is thus isolated from the developmental whole without the benefit of future learning. Higher stages of human development embrace earlier periods of development, even under conditions of severe trauma; there are thus an infinite number of possible biological, psychological, and psychosocial interconnections from early to late stages of development and from late to early stages. Implicit knowledge about a trauma can exist in multiple, parallel systems. Encapsulated traumatic memories can therefore express themselves through myriad linguistic, motor, behavioral, affective, and cognitive behaviors. A young child who cannot verbalize her trauma may enact it over and over in her play, for example (see Terr[8–10]).

Every trauma does not necessarily cause material to be encapsulated. Material related to the trauma may remain available to implicit and explicit memory, and may be "metabolized" fairly easily into the system. Traumatic events are encapsulated when the victim does not have the ability to metabolize the trauma in a meaningful way; a child who has been abused sexually over time, for example, is likely to dissociate and to form multiple encapsulations along developmental domains.[32] Children do not have the ability to cope with the sensory, affective, and symbolic components of a sexual assault. The material in this case may become less available to verbal memory as the victim dissociates from the repeated attacks. A trauma victim may retain more verbal memories of a sudden, one-time trauma such as a car accident. Because of the speed and unexpectedness of this kind of trauma, there is little time to defend against the horror of it. Depending on attentional resources, the victim in the case of a single, unexpected traumatic event may encapsulate some sensory and affective fragments of the trauma, but the cognitive, psychological, and parallel information processing systems are able to metabolize these fragments more successfully than in the case of repeated trauma occurring during critical developmental periods. In the case of a car accident, the victim almost always receives a great deal of posttrauma care and support from family, friends, and medical personnel. Victims of chronic childhood abuse, however, suffer extensive trauma without the normally soothing and protective external objects that help young children to develop trust in the world.[36] This kind of repeated trauma tears away at normal development, moving the victim away from the external world and toward self-preservation and internal vigilance. Abuse victims create their own internal environment based on a lack of trust with the outside world. Because severe trauma separates self-memory from the cognitive system, meaning cannot be made of the experience. With no possibility for making meaning of events in the external world, the victim remains focused internally, creating a cycle for dissociation that can continue into adulthood. Memories have a mitosis-like quality in that they can split into other memories; each remembrance of a traumatic event may mutate as the trauma victim replays it in her hand, perpetuating an endless cycle of memory distortion and mutation.

Consider the situation of Virginia, the 43-year-old woman who was sexually abused by her father during adolescence. Virginia represents an example of a child whose self-memory system for many years was almost wholly dissociated from her cognitive system. Virginia entered therapy with me suffering from intermittent attacks of right hemiparesis and right ptosis to her eye and lip. An extensive neurological work-up could find no medical explanation for her physical symptoms. Although she was able to function in her professional career at a high cognitive level, Virginia's speech in therapy was limited for many months to one-word answers, nonsequiturs, and verbal slips. These utterances can be understood as expressions of traumatic encapsulations in the linguistic domain: during the incestuous attacks, Virginia tried not to utter a sound or make cognitive meaning of the words her father was saying. She also tried not to move a muscle and held all of her limbs as rigidly as possible.

Virginia's self-memory system, unable to absorb the full affective and semantic horror of being repeatedly abused by her father, had no choice but to separate itself from her cognitive and linguistic systems. Because her cognitive system was disengaged, Virginia's sensorimotor responses to the incest (i.e., holding herself as stiffly as possible during the attacks) were directly incorporated into her self-memory system, emerging many years later as paralysis. The very strategy that helped to protect the adolescent Virginia from psychic pain during the long years of abuse—separating her self-memory system from her motor and linguistic systems—disrupted her development by blocking communication among the various developmental domains. Not surprisingly, this severe disruption has led to numerous professional and relationship problems during Virginia's adulthood. She sometimes becomes paralyzed at work and falls to the floor, unable to speak. Keep in mind that the incest began during Virginia's adolescent years, a time when normal developmental tasks include learning about relationships and coming to terms with body image and sexuality. During adolescence, Virginia was unable to focus on these important developmental tasks; she had submerged herself (her self-memory system) in a deep and dark inner world filled with depression, horror, and omnipotent fantasies.

Therapy with Virginia has involved teaching her how to think about her inner experiences and move toward integrating the levels of development that were disrupted during the years the abuse took place. Therapists who work with trauma victims like Virginia need to keep in mind that expressions of encapsulated developmental material may shift, slide, and change as the trauma victim moves through the various developmental stages that were missed during childhood or when encapsulated memories are brought to consciousness during the therapeutic process.[9–11] Patients in treatment may regress to lower levels of lability and mood, and display considerable ambivalence during the course of therapy.

Recent studies in the field of motor movement have led to an interdisciplinary theory of human development called *the new synthesis*,[48] a model for developmental change which pivots around the dynamic and causal relationships between neural growth and development and the child's sensorimotor explorations and selections. (A full discussion of this new synthesis is beyond the scope of this chapter. See for example, Edelman's[49] and Sporns and Edelman's theory[50] of neuronal group selection). Pulling together information from neurobiology, movement science, and perceptual psychology, Thelen[48] discusses the implications of this new developmental synthesis to therapy:

> Knowing when systems are in transition is important because [the] theory predicts that interventions can only be effective when the system has sufficient flexibility to explore and select new solutions. . . . [T]he therapist needs to know the history of the system in all

its richness and complexity, its current dynamics, and how the interventions can disrupt the stability of the current dynamics to allow new and better solutions to emerge. (p. 94)

In the same way that Thelen is working to develop an interdisciplinary theory of motor development, I believe that understanding how trauma is memorialized across developmental domains requires an interdisciplinary synthesis of the following areas: the neurophysiology of information processing; parallel distribution systems; the self-memory system; and the process of placing therapy in a developmental context. Let me note at this point that memory is more than neurochemical processes taking place in the brain. Memory is individual and beautifully human, and a full understanding of its role in trauma also requires us to draw from disciplines as diverse as philosophy, history, language, myth, religion, literature, and art. As Jeremy Campbell notes in his book about information theory, *Grammatical Man:*[51]

> Like the information system of language, memory can be explained in part by abstract rules which underlie it, but only in part. . . . The passage from the abstractions of structure to the rich products of the mind in its encounters with the world is never simple, seldom direct, and always reflects the uniqueness of the event, the richness of context and meaning, and the peculiarities of the human psyche in action, because that, for better or worse, is the way we are. (p. 229)

My model of the self-memory system, by providing a mechanism for exploring the meaning making aspects of trauma, was designed to allow for discussion of these individual aspects of trauma and memory. I argue that the human, experiential plane must be incorporated into any and all theories of memory. I thus include in this chapter an analysis of the writings and memoirs of Holocaust victims.[1,22–26] From the perspective of my developmental model, the initial encapsulation of Jewish memory of the Holocaust was normal, healthy, instinctual, and necessary. Child survivors of the Nazi Holocaust, unable at first to articulate their experiences, roamed from town to town, organizing and participating in bizarre theatrical productions that emphasized strange, acrobatic-like movements and grotesque plots. These children also drew pictures and wrote fragments of poetry. Many adult survivors of the Holocaust cut themselves off from the external world and surrounded themselves with the silence of deep social isolation. In the first few years, adult survivors limited the telling of their trauma to poetry, journal writing, and personal memoirs.[22] Many years had to pass before encapsulated memories of the Holocaust began to loosen on both the personal and the social levels and before the full horrors of that time could be fully expressed in literature and art. Holocaust scholar Lawrence Langer notes that recent books about the Holocaust have focused on a single theme: that of memory. Langer[25] speculates that perhaps ''we have finally begun to enter the second stage of Holocaust response, moving from what we know of the event, (the province of historians), to how to remember it, which shifts the responsibility to our own imaginations and what we are prepared to admit there'' (p. 13).

The metaphors and symbolic representations found in the recent Holocaust writings about memory contain vivid metaphors for the encapsulation process. Time and again, Holocaust survivors talk about the splitting of the self in response to the atrocities they suffered.[1,22–26] My hope in this chapter is to push current thinking about trauma and memory beyond the clinical and the neurophysiological realm. Dissociation is a natural process that provides protection against the pain of atrocity. As Holocaust survivor Aharon Appelfeld[22] writes,

> . . . [O]ne took refuge in silence. If you read the many collections of testimony written about the Holocaust, you would immediately see that they are actually repressions, meant to put events in proper chronological order. They are neither introspection nor anything resembling introspection, but rather the careful weaving together of many external facts in order to unveil the inner truth. The survivor himself was the first, in the weakness of his own hand and in the denial of his own experience, to create the strong plural voice of the memorist, which is nothing but externalization upon externalization, so that what is within will never be revealed. (p. 14)

The ultimate goal of this chapter is to define memory as dynamically connected to all areas of human existence, and trauma as having historical, moral, and political dimensions.

Parallel Distributed Systems for Memory: A Developmental Perspective

Kihlstrom[3] describes a model of unconscious information-processing along a network of richly interconnected subsystems which include memory, language, congition, motor movements, and affect. Subcortical structures, i.e., the hippocampus, amgydala, hypothalamus, and reticular activating systems, which include the temporal, parietal, and occipital lobes, are in parallel and reciprocal relationship to each other, coordinating developmental domains. Remembering takes place in this parallel distributed system—a normally flexible system that consists of a large number of simple but massively interconnected processing units.[2–5] Information processing takes place through activation among the units, which on the biochemical level is driven by the release of neuromodulators that form a memory trace for an object or event. The experience itself helps to determine if a certain memory trace will be strong or weak: the neuromodulators that are released in response to each experience have strengthening or weakening effects, depending on the amount and type secreted (see Chapter 3). Animal research shows that several hormones, termed stress-response neuromodulators,[52,53] enhance memory consolidation and encourage the formation of conditioned responses that are highly resistant to extinction. Blockage of these hormones, which include ACTH, ACTH fragments, vasopressin, epinephrine and norepinephrine, interferes with memory consolidation and leads to the formation of easily extinguished conditioned responses.

McGaugh et al.[37,38] suggest that evolution has endowed mammals with a memory storage system that aids survival by providing a means to record the importance of an experience via hormonal response to the event.

Existing connections among information processing units (the individual's developmental integrity) influence future patterns for processing, introducing the possibility of additions, omissions, and distortions. How an event is stored in memory depends on the strengths of the connections among the units: the connections from one active unit will strengthen, while the connections from an active to an inactive unit will tend to weaken.[2,4,5,37,38,52,53] Remembering occurs when some aspect of an event re-arises as sensory or affective input, thus activating some of the units that previously participated in the representation of the episode. This activation may, in turn, activate other units via the already established connections.

The parallel distributed processing model is a plausible model to account for how traumatic events and feelings can be sequestered off, or dissociated, from memory. The PDP model illustrates how tangled and muddled memory can become: there are multiple pathways for integrating experiences and corresponding affects within declarative, semantic, and procedural memory systems. It is thus likely that all aspects of memory functioning are subject to some amount of distortion, or to recall, retrieval, and recognition problems.[2–5]

A field of mathematics known as *chaos theory*[47,51,54,55] is providing increasingly sophisticated models for explaining memory and other human information systems such as language, DNA coding, and artificial intelligence. Information theory pivots around the idea that the laws of physics and biology are based on chance but never on accident. Jeremy Campbell[51] explains this new science: "Forces of chance and of anti-chance coexist in a complementary relationship. The random element is called entropy, the agent of chaos, which tends to mix up the unmixed, to destroy meaning. The non random element is information, which exploits the uncertainty in the entropy principle to generate new structures, to inform the world in novel ways" (p. 192).

Applying chaos theory to memory, Campbell[51] notes that there may be more than a thousand billion synapses in the human brain. Thus the sheer number of components pushes the human memory system towards chaos, or entropy: "The effect of the synapse is to introduce a further element of uncertainty into a fundamentally uncertain system" (p. 191).

Campbell states that at least three events may trigger neurochemical release across a synapse to a receiving neuron. The first event, a message from the outside, is certain and predictable. A second occurrence, the spontaneous firing of a neuron, may or may not be random. A third event, the release of neurochemicals across a synapse for no particular reason, is totally random. Thus the mechanism for passing information throughout the brain is a "mixture of the predictable and the unpredictable, a property shared by many information systems which occur in nature"[51] (p. 192).

I believe that information theory, especially concepts related to chaos and predictability, has much to add to any model about trauma and memory. On the neurophysiological level, trauma adds a further element of unpredictability to memory storage and recall. Trauma increases the possibility of memory distortion by disrupting neurochemical release and by triggering morphological changes in the brain (see chapter 3; also see Mazure,[11] Charney,[56] Southwick,[57] van der Kolk,[58,59] and Cotman[60]). Trauma is absorbed by the creation of alternate and more complex parallel processing systems, a process that is similar to reactive synaptogenesis.[60] Neuronal systems are remodeled: sprouting replaces previously effective synapses with newer, less effective ones. Previously established connections for making meaning may be lost or weakened. On the personal level, trauma disrupts the self-memory system, thus mixing up the victim's previous efforts at meaning-making by shattering assumptions about safety, security, the nature of good and evil, etc. In the case of long-term trauma, such as war or childhood neglect and abuse, the neurobiological effects of starvation, chronic head injury, chemical poisoning, illness, and sexually transmitted diseases must also be taken into account. This is why the developmental model is so important to the treatment of trauma victims.

The PDP model demonstrates how individual pieces of a traumatic memory may remain sequestered from preexisting, meaning-making connections: bits or units of information remain encapsulated in time and place, although they may be enlivened under certain environmentally triggered conditions.[2–5,61] These encapsulations can be compared to individual animation celluloids projected at fast speeds to create what seems like a moving image. Each encapsulated unit represents one frame of the animated "film." Specific perceptual, motor, and sensory stimuli may awaken the affective linkages to these memories. Jack, a patient, was 8 years old when the car in which he was riding was hit from behind, which caused the gas tank to burst into flames on impact. At the time of the accident, the highway had been enveloped in a dense white fog that resembled smoke. Jack suffered severe burns to his face and torso and also witnessed his cousin and uncle being engulfed by flames. The uncle died at the scene. Jack underwent many months of painful reconstructive surgery and physical rehabilitation. Several years after the accident, Jack was sitting in the dentist's chair when he saw a puff of steam come out of his mouth. Jack not only instantly recalled the accident, he experienced affective waves of horror as he recalled the foggy highway and the memory of his uncle's head spewing smoke as it burst into flames like a torch.

In some cases, these individual memories of a traumatic event remain sequestered from meaning-making networks in the brain. Against a backdrop of the individual's developmental conditions, Schwarz and Kowalski[45] suggest that one-time traumatic disaster experiences can become rooted as psychobiological configurations termed *malignant memories*. These memories tie affective, cognitive, and arousal functions in toxic configurations that continue to torment disaster victims and chronically disrupt normal development. In his study of children who witnessed a parental murder, Malmquist[62] described a boy who was haunted by the image of his mother's casket being closed for the final time. As the image played itself over and over, the boy found it hard to pay attention at school, eventually experiencing problems in most areas of his life.

Because it was sequestered from existing meaning-making networks,[61] this single-track memory prevented the boy from making meaning of his loss. The memory was sequestered from all of his other ideas and thoughts, playing itself over and over like a phonographic needle caught in a groove.

The PDP system for information processing may be best represented through a computer graphic representation of a four-dimensional Boolean hypercube.[47] The fourth dimension is time. The hypercube is connected by parallel lines on all sides of the cube formation. It is possible to imagine the flow of information by placing pieces of information in time, place, and state on the parallel lines. The system works fairly smoothly under normal developmental conditions. Under trauma conditions, however, information flow can reverse itself. One or many pieces of information may become encapsulated along the routes, blocking or rerouting information flow. Circuitous, less effective, routes may develop. The encapsulation may remain isolated in time and place on the hypercube or it may communicate with other pieces of information. Similar to an optokinetic experience, the shape of an experience, idea, memory, or perception may shift suddenly, reshaping itself as another perceptual activity, thought, impression, or state of mind.

Minsky[61] suggests a graphic model for brain communication that links eight small cubes into a 64-agent super cube. By connecting eight of these supercubes, and repeating this supercube-on-supercube pattern ten times, Minsky created a model for the brain that includes over a billion agents for communication. Linking each agent to 30 others allows any agent to communicate with any other agent in only six steps.

I believe that developmental systems for language, memory, affect, cognition, and self-representation operate in parallel and contain billions of units of information along multiple pathways.[46] The incorporation of time into the Boolean cube provides an extremely rich model for human development, as earlier stages of development may encompass later developmental stages on the cube, and vice versa. Encapsulations may contain incomplete bits of an individual's identity, personality, and neurophysiological functions; they are split off from and remain unavailable to higher and lower levels of development.

The inclusion of time also allows for a deeper understanding of the human experience of trauma. Holocaust scholar Lawrence Langer, in *Admitting the Holocaust*[25] discusses time and memory in a chapter entitled ''Memory's Time: Chronology and Duration in Holocaust Testimonies.'' While a full discussion of his ideas is beyond the scope of this chapter, Langer's work is invaluable to any clinician attempting to understand the social, political, and philosophical dimensions of trauma and memory. Langer proposes the term *durational time* to describe victims' memories of the Holocaust. Durational time, according to Langer,[25] is a time

> which exists *this side* of the forgotten, not to be dredged from memory because it is always, has always been there—an always-present past that in testimony becomes a presented past. . . . The duration of Holocaust time, which is a constantly *re-*

experienced time, threatens the chronology of experienced time. It leaps out of the chronology, establishing its own momentum, or fixation. Testimony may *appear* chronological to the auditor or audience, but the narrator who is a mental witness rather than a temporal one is "out of time" as she tells her story. (p. 15)

REM Sleep, Language, and Memory: Developmental Considerations for Trauma

Structurally, there is a close relationship between those areas of the brain containing emotional memories and those involved in REM sleep.[35,36] Dreams help to solidify relations between affect and memories, thereby helping to establish the unconscious emotional temperaments of individuals. My model of dissociation provides new perspectives for understanding the dreams of traumatized patients. Viewed on the four-dimensional hypercube, dreaming is where the cognitive and self-memory systems may slide together like fast-moving geometric planes. When dreaming, the dissociated patient is forced to experience the coming together of the cognitive and self-memory systems, if only for brief instances of dream time. Encapsulated material pours into the self-memory system, which has no way to protect itself, no place to run. There is no choice: the dreamer can do nothing but dream.

Overwhelmed with negative affect, the dreamer's self-memory tries to make meaning through its images and symbolic representations. These images may become more and more frightening as the cognitive system continues to slide against the self-memory system. Recall the passage of Holocaust victim Charlotte Delbo, whose heart pounds uncontrollably when she dreams about Auschwitz. The nightmare becomes more and more horrific, and eventually she cries out in the darkness and wakes up. She feels drained and exhausted. The released memories linger for days, tormenting her. "It takes days for everything to get back to normal, for everything to get shoved back inside memory, and for the skin of memory to mend itself. I become myself again, the person you know, who can talk to you about Auschwitz without exhibiting or registering any anxiety or emotion"[1] (p. 78).

In some cases of severe trauma or chronic abuse, dissociation may be so complete and encapsulations may be so rigid that the cognitive and self-memory systems may not come together at all, even in dreams. Encapsulations are so rigid in these traumatized patients that the two systems cannot communicate at all during REM sleep. Dreams may still occur, but they will consist of fragments—isolated and meaningless images—and encapsulated packets of emotions such as fear, apprehension, and shame. The dreamer may remember nothing but dream fragments upon awakening. Some dissociated patients thus cannot distinguish dreams from actual experiences in their waking life. They report in therapy their perceptions as "being in a fog, or distant, or behind a veil or a screen"; this is because they are unable to employ their cognitive skills to differentiate the various states of wakefulness, dreaming, and fantasy. This illustrates the depth to which trauma affects psychic life: many dissociated patients abhor dreaming. For nontraumatized people, dreaming is a routine if not enjoyable experience that helps them to make meaning of their daily lives by bringing together their cognitive and self-memory systems. They are thus able to memorialize aspects of their lives during REM sleep without fear of being overwhelmed emotionally.

Viewed another way, this time from the perspective of information theory,[47,51,54,55] REM sleep serves to push the dreamer's information systems simultaneously towards randomness and nonrandomness. The wild and erratic nature of dreams pushes the system toward chaos, or randomness. But the symbolic, or meaning-making, aspect of dreaming pushes the system in the opposite direction, in the direction of nonrandomness. Therapists must recognize this dual nature of dreaming as they probe the self-memory system of traumatized patients. The traumatized person may have multiple and fragmented encapsulations of the trauma, a situation which tends to push his or her dreams and fantasies toward a more disorganized state. The struggle to make meaning of these isolated memory fragments, if unsuccessful during REM sleep, may continue into the individual's waking state in the form of dream-like fantasies and hallucinations; the resulting trance-like state is a manifestation of the self-memory's drive to simultaneously push toxic material away from itself and to make symbolic and representational meaning of it.

Dreams provide a way to measure progress over the course of therapy. As encapsulations loosen or become more permeable in both the self-memory and cognitive memory systems, the dreamer's symbols and representations provide important information about developmental gains and regressions (see Terr[8–10]). The therapist can also analyze the degree to which a dream is dissociated, that is, to what degree the cognitive and self-memory systems are in touch with each other and how well they are working together to make meaning of experiences. Compare from this developmental perspective the following two dreams of Karen C., the patient who spent most of her childhood in an alcoholic fog.

In the first dream, Karen found herself in a parade with a group of children wearing masks and costumes. A giant rabbit was leading the parade. After meandering for a while, the parade came to a rope that sectioned off an area of land; the rabbit lifted the rope and let only Karen crawl through. Karen then found herself on a bridge, where she noticed the body of a child who had jumped off the bridge. Several adults were caring for the hurt child and although Karen was curious she did not feel overly worried about the child. Karen jumped onto a bicycle and crossed the bridge. As she reached the other side, the dream ended.

This dream occurred after 1 year in therapy and represents the progression of the therapy across developmental plateaus, which include themes of separation and attachment, self-objects, trust, safety, and self-cohesiveness. Karen was the only child in the parade to pass through the rope and cross the bridge to the other side. This crossing-over represents her willingness to move through these developmental domains and her increasing abilities to take psychological risks by utilizing the support within the transferential relationship. Developmentally, Karen is still a child in this dream. The dream includes several forms of play, including dressing in costumes, marching in a parade, and riding a bicycle.

The rabbit in the dream is reminiscent of the Easter Bunny and may represent renewal and resurrection, a chance for a new life—symbols which point to her willingness to grow and progress. Although the dream alludes to suicidality through the image of the child who jumped off the bridge, it may represent a transition to a broader sense of autonomy within the therapeutic process. The hurt child was being cared for by concerned others and symbolizes Karen's ability to care for herself and to allow herself to be nurtured by others.

I view this dream as primarily a dream of the self-memory system: it is preverbal, rich in color and visual images, and highly symbolic. In this dream, Karen's self-memory system was still highly dissociated from her cognitive system, for meaning-making in this dream occurred on a symbolic, preverbal plane.

Three months later, Karen had a dream in which the process of integration, or reassociation, had begun: her self and cognitive systems came together to create a richly verbal dream in which Karen and her father had an in-depth conversation about their relationship. In this dream, Karen found herself in a room in her childhood home. Her father (who was deceased at the time of the dream) appeared in the room. Karen began preparing for bed and before she knew what had happened she found herself in bed with her father. Her father rolled over and began to make sexual advances. When Karen asked him what he was doing, the father began to cry. They conversed for a long while, and Karen's father admitted that he had some "bad habits" that included doing bad things to her. Karen instructed her father not to tell anyone about the bad things, especially not her mother. Karen then left the room and a stranger approached her in the hallway. The stranger led her to a window and told her to look outside. Karen looked out the window and saw her father hanging upside down. The stranger handed Karen a note which asks, "Where is Karen?"

When viewed in comparison with Karen's first dream, her second dream represents the beginning stages of the reassociation process. Karen's cognitive system, which was engaged by the verbal dialogue with her father and by the process of reading and reflecting upon the written words in the note, was becoming integrated with important self-memories from her childhood. This cognitive engagement pushed Karen to begin the process of advanced meaning-making in terms of her relationship with her father. The fact that Karen and her father had a conversation in the dream represents her commitment to working out conflicts and concerns in their relationship. Because the second dream is more integrated (less dissociated), it is able to contain material that is more developmentally advanced than the material in the first dream. Without divulging specifics of our therapeutic dialogue, the dream's content alludes to specific developmental issues in her life that relate to forging relationships, to complexity of self, self-objects, and their representations.

Although it is not clear whether Karen's father actually did abuse her, the dream demonstrates a willingness to explore the good and bad aspects of her relationship to him. Even if he did not actually abuse her, the dream makes clear that Karen feels he turned her life upside down. Evidence that Karen wants to "find herself" is found in the note which asks, "Where is Karen?" The level of the therapeutic transference has deepened, allowing for exploration of deeper self-memories. A metaphor for the transference process can be seen in the progression across the two dreams from preverbal levels of expression to more sophisticated linguistic skills that include reading and writing. In fact, the transferential relationship is the vehicle that moves a patient's self-memory system, allowing it to become more integrated with the cognitive system. The level of transference taking place in therapy is further represented in the symbology of the second dream: The question "Where is Karen?" can be interpreted to mean "Where is Karen's self?" Therapy is moving toward deeper issues related to trauma and self-memory, including the question of whether she experienced incest or other forms of sexual abuse during her childhood.

For adult dreamers, dream symbols may shift and change, becoming increasingly sophisticated and abstract, as the dreamer progresses through therapy. Interpreting the dreams of traumatized children may be more difficult than interpreting the dreams of traumatized adults. In her work with traumatized children, Terr has found that the ability to remember, verbalize, and understand the dream progresses along developmental lines.[8–10] She writes:

> New life circumstances add to the dream, as do new internal wishes. The modified dream carries a traumatized nucleus with a changeable orbit . . . occasionally, as the years go by, a repeated dream will take on enough deeply disguised symbolism, wish gratification, and modification with recent content that it no longer seems, at first glance, to be a repeated or traumatic dream at all. Under careful scrutiny, however, such a deeply disguised dream will often reveal its origins as traumatic. One good way to understand these heavily camouflaged dreams is to listen to the child's thoughts in 'association' to the dream. Another way is to plug in what you already know about the child's experience to the dream symbolism and see if it works.[9] (p. 211–212)

Terr believes that a certain level of cognitive and emotional maturation is required at the time of a trauma for children to remember nightmares or understand the symbolic content of dreams. Chronically abused children who struggle to keep the abuse secret often dream repeated terror dreams that they cannot remember or verbalize. These children may cry out in the middle of the night, and experience bedtime fright and fear of the dark.[8–10]

The ability to verbalize is crucial to understanding dream content. In her study of documented trauma in preschool children, Terr[10] found that 28 to 36 months of age is the cut-off time for when children can store and express some verbal memory of a traumatic event. A child's verbal expression of a traumatic event may reflect his or her developmental benchmarks at the time of the event. As children grow, their attempts to make meaning of their trauma are "reworked" as they pass through various developmental phases. Memories of a traumatic event may also be collapsed into memories of subsequent life experiences. Children may add to or subtract from their verbal memories or make substitutions of partial verbal remembrances. Children who form weak or no verbal memories of an event may encapsulate the trauma in prelinguistic and sensorimotor domains. Children may also recapitulate the trauma in their play or reenact it behaviorally.[10] Some of the children who survived the Ash Wednesday fire in Australia played obsessively with fire trucks in the months following the fire.[42]

A Linguistic Theory for Memory and Trauma

Language is critical to any discussion about trauma, memory, and emotion. My model sees language, syntax, and grammar as informational units on the hypercube. As informational units, words are extremely flexible and plastic. A single word can carry many definitions and layers of meaning. Over time, these definitions shift, change, and overlap in response to cultural and personal needs. As informational units, words also have the capacity to carry and convey affect. Some words by nature tend to have more emotion embedded into their dictionary definition than others (compare highly laden words such as "love," "thirst," "cancer," and "tornado" to "cat," "stone," "hat," and "street"). Central to my theory of dissociation is the idea that each word in an individual's native vocabulary holds many layers of personal (self), cognitive, and emotional meaning for that individual. These cognitive and emotional meanings shift, change, and intensify as a person moves through development. I propose that under conditions of severe trauma and abuse, words themselves can be split in half—their cognitive (dictionary) meanings are cleaved from their emotional and personal meanings. Charlotte Delbo[1] discusses how her experiences in the Nazi camps forced her to split the word "thirst" into its affective and literal meanings. Words that have been cleaved in this way may move in opposite directions on the hypercube: the emotional meaning of a word may become fixed on the self-memory system, while the dictionary or literal meaning of a word remains available to the cognitive system. Manifestations of this linguistic splitting can be seen in the flat and toneless speech of some dissociated patients. Cognitively, their words make dictionary sense, but they may carry little or no affective or personal meaning.

Discussions about this phenomenon of word splitting occurs in the writings of Holocaust victims.[1,24,25] As Charlotte Delbo explains in *Days and Memories,* it is simply impossible for the word "thirst" to convey the intensity of the desire for water she experienced in the concentration camps. After suffering week upon week the parched lips and swollen tongue of such terrible thirst, Delbo was forced to split the word into its cognitive and emotional meaning. This was a conscious process that allowed her to continue with the activities of daily life after the war. For Delbo, the word "thirst" must remain forever cleaved; this cleavage of the word for thirst is a way to keep the memories of her suffering from overwhelming her each time she feels the kind of normal thirst that signals it is time to sit down and drink a cup of tea. She writes, "someone who has been tortured by thirst for weeks on end could never again say, 'I'm thirsty. How about a cup of tea.' This word has . . . been split in two. Thirst has been turned into a word for commonplace use. But if I dream about the thirst I suffered in Birkenau, I once again see the person I was, haggard, half-crazed, near to collapse; I physically feel the real thirst and it is an atrocious nightmare . . ."[1] (p. 4).

Many words—perhaps entire languages—were torn in half by the Holocaust. Holocaust survivor Nelly Sachs reiterates this theme in her poem "Peoples of the Earth." Sachs understands that it is difficult to make meaning of events when the victims do not have the full power of their native language behind them. Sachs thus pleads with humankind: "do not destroy the universe of words/let not the knife of hatred lacerate/ the sound born together with the first breath."[63]

Holocaust scholar Lawrence Langer sees this splitting of words as a metaphor for the splitting of the self: "These tributes to the wounded self serve also as dirges to the wounded word. . . . She [the poet Nelly Sachs] picks through the rubble of the Holocaust to rescue separate words that may have survived the disaster, while sadly confessing that their place in the moral architecture of language will never be the same"[24] (p. 556–557).

Langer is correct when he includes morality in his discussion of the Holocaust. Although further exploration of his ideas is beyond the scope of the chapter, future research should include this kind of moral-linguistic analysis of trauma and memory (see, for example, the chapter "Aharon Appelfeld and the Language of Sinister Silence" in *Admitting the Holocaust*[25]. The prevailing zeitgeist has a profound effect on the intersubjectivity of language, culture, morals, and individual development and self-memory. To what extent does a horror like the Holocaust destroy language and memory—on both a personal and cultural level—and how does this destruction of language and memory affect our ability to make meaning of the violence and genocide that have characterized the twentieth century?

Development of the Self-Memory System

Future research on the development of the self-memory system will further our understanding of dissociative mechanisms for coping with trauma. Because it is so deeply concerned with meaning-making, I believe that the self-memory system is a driving force behind development through all phases of the life cycle. It is a holding tank for an individual's ambitions, goals, desires, and sense of accomplishment.

A biological metaphor for the self-memory system is the human immunological system. The immune system, like self-memory, is a noncognitive survival system which has the capacity to memorialize itself—to know the self from the nonself—and to evaluate the degree of threat of an invasive agent or event. A healthy immune system has the ability to fight off most invasive bacteria and viruses, most of the time. A healthy self-memory system, likewise, has the capacity to ward off the minor insults and threats of daily living. And similar to the immune system, the self-memory system has the capacity to be totally overwhelmed by an external threat.

Clark[64] compares the immune system with the brain itself, describing the immune system as a kind of chemical extension of the brain that flows through the bloodstream, and noting that the two systems have the ability to communicate with each other and with the outside world. This deep and mutual engagement between the immune and cognitive systems, and the engagement of the two systems with the outside world, are crucial for physical survival. Each system is thus by necessity fluent in its own language and in the language of the other.

In the same way that the cognitive and immune systems are deeply engaged with each other, the cognitive memory and self-memory systems are deeply and mutually engaged. I believe that this mutual engagement begins at birth and is necessary for human survival. Key to understanding the early development of the self-memory system is understanding the development of other kinds of memory in infants and children. Further research should explore the ways in which the self-memory and cognitive memory systems interact during various developmental stages.

All memory in fact begins earlier in development than previously thought. Researchers have identified memory traces as being laid down from infancy. Rovee-Collier[65] found that infants as young as 2 to 3 months form enduring memories of past experiences. Lacking verbal ability, infants employ a motoric response to tell us about an event they remembered. Greco et al.[66,67] found that infants as young as 3 months may respond by analogy, and Baillargeon[68] found evidence of object permanence in 6-month-olds. Pillemer and While[69] found that a 10-month-old has a functional memory system; past events in the baby's life are evoked by feelings, locations, or other people and are expressed through behaviors and emotions. Ceci and Bruck[70] found that recognition memory is accurate in preschool children and that they can remember as much as adults when verbal recall is not emphasized.

As Stern[71] says, the infant is never in an autistic phase of development, but is involved from the first moments on in a reciprocal relationship with a loving caregiver. Severe early insult to the self-memory system can cause severe developmental arrest, even physical death. In his classic study of foundling home infants, Spitz[72] found that one-third of the babies died in their first year despite good food and meticulous medical care. An even higher number suffered impairments to their physical development: their muscles atrophied and their motor skills stagnated. Unable to engage in an early relationship with a caregiver, these babies languished and died (see also Gardner[73]).

Research into how children withstand the amputation of a limb provides some clues into the processes by which the self and cognitive systems communicate with each other over time.[74,75] Earle[75] has found that children who undergo limb amputations (because of cancer) before age 2 are able to more easily accept the mutilation into their body image than are adults, who suffer from phantom pains and who mourn deeply for the lost limb.[75] It is possible that the self-memory of children under the age of 2 does not contain full sensory, somatic, and aesthetic awareness of their separate body parts. Dissociation between the self and cognitive systems—if it occurred at all during the surgical trauma—may have been brief, allowing these young children to more easily reassociate their self and cognitive memories. Their linguistic and cognitive abilities were just beginning to develop, so these very young children did not understand the functional, aesthetic, and physical ramifications of their cancer or the loss of their limb. The loss of the limb was not in conflict with what they already knew about the self. Only when the loss creates a conflict with self-memory does pathogenesis have an opportunity to affect development.

The level of support was critical for these young amputation patients, as soothing of them by their parents, nurses, and other caretakers may have helped to keep them from dissociating for extended periods of time. Surprisingly, Earle found that those early adolescents who are rapidly undergoing other bodily changes were more able to integrate a limb amputation into their body image than were adults or children in the latency period. Earle speculates that teenagers undergoing the rapid and uncontrollable body changes related to puberty may be more willing to incorporate yet another change to their body image.[75] Self-memory at this time by necessity may be more plastic or flexible, allowing for easier integration of the trauma of an amputation.

For a child to flourish requires that his or her self-memory system be engaged from birth to its fullest capacity. In fact, I believe that the best nurturance of a child occurs when a parent is able to pass on healthy and meaningful aspects of the parent's own self-memory. The very act of parenting may in fact prime the pump of self-memory, allowing aspects of the early self to flow into consciousness as the parent searches for ways to communicate with the child. Louise Erdrich, a Native American novelist and poet, describes how she remembered a deep and long-forgotten memory as she attempted to calm her newborn daughter:

> There is a dance that appears out of nowhere, steps we don't know we know until we are using them to calm our baby. This dance is something we learned in our sleep, from our own hearts, from our own parents, going back and forth through all our ancestors. Men and women do the same dance, and acquire it without a thought. Graceful, eccentric, this wavelike sway is a skilled graciousness of the entire body. Parents possess and lose it after the first fleeting months, but that's all right because already it has been passed on—the knowledge lodged deep within the comforted baby.[20] (p. 54)

Later in her journal, Erdrich writes about how the loving gazes between herself and her baby may have something to do with the creation of the baby's "self." Erdich notes that the Ojibwa word for mirror, *wabimujichagwan*, means "looking at your soul," an idea that conveys the importance of the loving visual exchanges that occur between parent and child. She writes: "If it is true that we are mirrors to our infants and that looking forms the boundaries of the self, then perhaps we are also helping to form a spiritual soul self during these concentrated love gazes during which time stops, the air dims, the earth cools, and a sense of deep rightness takes hold of our being"[20] (p. 135).

Each self-memory system organizes life events differently. All that enters the body and mind is registered—however briefly—and is contained within the self-memory system. This process is similar to the formation of a shoreline as it is influenced by the continuous pounding of the surf. Each wave formation makes its own impression in the sand, weaving over and turning under previous currents of water which moments earlier left their own marks and etchings on the shore. From time to time, violent storms whip the waves into a pounding foam. Through repeated cycles of high and low tides, all manner of shells, sea plants, driftwood, and rocks are swept to the apron of the surf, revealing the contents of the ocean like revealing the contents of the unconscious self. With repeated pounding, the shore continuously takes on a new formation, which represents the visual and symbolic representation of the self as it has been influenced by all external and internal events.

Childhood Sexual Abuse: A Developmental Perspective

In the following section, I use the example of child sexual abuse to illustrate how the encapsulation of long-term trauma hinges on developmental features, and how development in turn can be disrupted by abuse. This discussion also explores how the self-memory system may be affected by sexual abuse and how psychosocial pressures, such as a family's efforts to hide the abuse, may affect the encapsulation process by encouraging the victim to actively deny or distort her memories of the trauma.

Recent studies have explored the relationship of trauma, including sexual abuse, to measures of neurophysiological functioning.[11,12,56–59,76–79] This research expands the PDP developmental model by linking psychological and developmental states with biological mechanisms. For example, it appears that sexual abuse can disrupt the hormonal systems of victims. Putnam and Trickett found that sexually abused girls may have hormonal levels that are associated with high levels of sexual and aggressive behavior.[77,78] Other research has found a higher than expected incidence of precocious puberty in sexually abused girls.[76]

Bremner et al.[80] (see also Chapter 3 in this volume) found an average 8% decrease in the volume of the right hippocampus of 26 Vietnam combat veterans. As they note, these alterations in brain morphology may be consistent with the kinds of deficits in explicit memory functioning that are seen in posttraumatic stress disorder patients. In the case of sexual abuse, physiological and psychosocial responses may work hand in hand to exacerbate the developmental problems of its victims. Abnormal hormonal responses,[77,78] coupled with the possible changes in brain morphology described by Bremner et al.,[80] are some of the neurophysiological disruptions these children may face. It is important for the therapist to consider how these abnormal hormonal levels may compound the psychosocial problems of a sexual abuse victim. Clearly, a hormonally induced precocious puberty may further disrupt the psychosocial, affective, and interpersonal development of sexually abused girls by creating numerous problems at home and at school. These children, for example, may be subject to teasing and suggestive remarks by adults and their peers. This in turn could lead to self re-proach and poor body image as well as learning problems due to attention deficits at school.[12,32,77,78]

Sexual abuse has profound effects on the developing personality of the vic-tim.[6–10,12,32,77,78,81] A history of sexual abuse may in fact be linked to malevolent expectations in subsequent relationships.[82] Severe developmental problems can occur surprisingly early in sexually abused children. Sherkow[83] described the behavior of a child named Tina who had likely been sexually abused by her father. Tina was unable to sleep in her own bed and could not tolerate a moment's separation from her mother. She purposely defecated and urinated all around the house. Tina's play and motor move-ments were filled with sexually explicit gestures, and she was obsessed with the idea that men were staring at her. Tina was 2 and three-quarters years old at the time of this behavior. It is interesting to note that Tina's precocious expressions of her sexual abuse (the explicit motor movements) were coupled with behaviors (such as the purposeful defecating) that expressed her current developmental issues around toilet training.

I believe that Tina's obscene gestures represent expressions of the sexual abuse that were incorporated directly into her self-memory. A recent study[84] on 11-month-old babies has shown that symbolic gestures may be incorporated into a child's memory even if the child is at a preverbal level of language development. A group of children 11 months of age was exposed daily to eight spoken words (e.g., ''kitty'') while another group of babies was exposed to eight symbolic gestures (e.g., flapping the arms for ''bird''). The researchers found that symbolic gesturing is a highly effective way for parents or other adults to communicate with young babies. Babies in the gesturing group learned a higher number of words. The addition of symbolic gestures to the babies repertoire increased their overall vocabularies. Thus, the ability to understand and communicate by using symbolic representation in the form of gestures is present before verbal communication takes place.

The researchers in this study, of course, used symbolic gesturing to positively influ-ence children's preverbal language development. In Tina's case, however, her father's obscene posturing was a powerfully negative use of symbolic gesturing. Gestural aspects of the sexual abuse were directly incorporated into Tina's self-memory. It is important to consider how the incorporation of obscene gestures into a child's self-memory system may affect her future development. An abused child's use of explicit gestures may further exacerbate her developmental problems, as she may be ostracized from other children, scolded by adults, or otherwise suffer from assaults on her self-esteem.

Research has shown that the age at which a child is sexually abused influences her ability to recall, verbalize, and make meaning of the experience. For example, Herman and Schatzow,[85] in their study of female outpatients who had been sexually abused as children, found a strong association between the degree of reported amnesia and the age at which the abuse first occurred. Women who reported no memory deficits were those women whose abuse had begun in or continued through adolescence. Mild-to-moderate memory deficits were usually associated with abuse that began in latency and ended by early adolescence. Marked memory deficits were associated with abuse that began early in childhood. These researchers also found that a period of prior amnesia was associated with more violent abuse.[85]

Duration of the abuse is also a factor in the ability to remember. Terr[8–10] believes that repeated trauma during childhood is more likely to result in dissociation than a one-time traumatic event. In a study of adult women with documented histories of childhood sexual abuse, Williams[81] found that sexual abuse is more likely to be remembered at any age when the abuser is a stranger. Molestation by a stranger is more likely to be easily remembered because of its novelty or because it is more likely to be discussed with family members than would ongoing abuse by a family member.[81]

From the perspective of my developmental model, abuse by a family member is a deeper assault on the self-memory system, thus increasing the likelihood of dissociation. The greater the need to protect the self, the greater are the chances that a child will dissociate.[32,86] Under conditions of complete dissociation, it may be impossible to ever remember what happened, since it is not possible to have an explicit memory of something that was never taken in through the cognitive system.

Williams also found that abuse by a family member or another person close to the victim is more likely to evoke feelings of fear, guilt, conflict, and betrayal, which may lead to confusion about the experience and subsequent difficulty in remembering and making meaning of it. Also, other members of the family may try to hide or ignore the abuse, actions which communicate to the child that she should make an effort to forget the episode.[81]

I believe that ongoing sexual abuse by a parent or close care giver is one of the deepest possible assaults to a child's self-memory system. A child's need to be soothed and held is strong; but sexual abuse serves the diabolical function of partially meeting the child's desire for parental attention and love while simultaneously attacking the child's physical and moral being. Aspects of the abuse, such as cuddling or stroking, may be experienced as pleasurable or soothing.[32] Yet the child senses something is morally wrong. The resulting guilt can permeate the abused child's self-memory system. Her self-memory fills with shame, humiliation, and reproach. Whereas they may have a strong sense of right and wrong, young children do not have the cognitive or psychosocial skills to make more than limited moral sense of the abuse. All of us know that sexuality has the power to access the core of any individual's interiority. In sexual abuse, the child's self-boundaries are repeatedly weakened or perforated; the self has been accessed by a malevolent sexual force during a time in development when the child does not have the cognitive, moral, psychological, sensorimotor, or neurohormonal abilities to make meaning of the event. The self-memory system walls itself off in an effort to contain the shame, guilt, and humiliation. Sequestering itself through full or partial dissociation from the cognitive system, the self-memory system may fill with malignant representations, narcissism, and omnipotent fantasies.

Developmentally, the situation of a child who experiences a one-time trauma is different from that of a child living under conditions of severe and chronic abuse. Because it may cause neuronal systems to be remodeled over and over again, chronic trauma, including ongoing abuse, may adversely affect a child's ability to learn by impeding the formation of effective meaning-making networks. Early childhood educators have long known that learning and neuronal growth are best enhanced by an enriched environment that includes a variety of developmentally appropriate activities and materials. Remedial programs such as Head Start attempt to provide underprivileged preschoolers with a super-enriched learning environment that includes music, art, writing, and drama. Chronic childhood trauma creates what I term a *disenriching* environment for all aspects of development, including learning. In the case of chronic sexual abuse, for example, meaning-making itself is impossible; young children simply do not have the physical, sensory, cognitive, or moral capacity to make sense of sexual contact with an adult. When chronic abuse occurs, this kind of disenriched environment for development can be present even in those homes that are filled to the brim with books, music, and art.

It is important to remember that children who are subjected to sexual abuse may also be subjected to other kinds of chronic trauma. This is especially true under severe conditions such as war or imprisonment. Rosemary, a patient, was hospitalized for severe anorexia nervosa when she was 16 years old. Rosemary was born inside a Mexican prison camp while her mother was serving a sentence for drug smuggling. Her history as an imprisoned child included sexual abuse as well as numerous other traumas which occurred on a daily basis from the moment of her birth. Rosemary was sold for sexual favors by her mother and used as a bartering chip for food and other amenities. She remained in the prison until early adolescence, when she and her mother were released by Mexican authorities and allowed to return to the United States. This horror story was confirmed by her mother and other authorities at the time of her admission into the hospital.

Both Rosemary's cognitive and self-memory systems had incorporated real and fantasized memories of trauma, which were expressed as numerous encapsulations in the sensory, motor, cognitive, affective, and psychodynamic domains. Rosemary was severely depressed, and exhibited psychotic mentation and major distortions in body image and boundary articulation. She suffered the full range of PTSD symptoms, including flashbacks and hallucinations. Because of the extent and duration of Rosemary's dissociation during childhood, she had no words to cognitively link affect and meaning-making efforts; she offered few words in therapy and mostly gestured to signal her basic needs. In therapy, we were left with many disjointed fragments, a swirling mélange of isolated images, sensations, emotions, and ideas.

Rosemary represents one of the most severe cases of ongoing childhood trauma that I have seen. I believe that Rosemary did not "witness" many of the atrocities that were perpetrated against her during childhood. Instead, she utilized dissociation to completely disengage her self-memory system from her cognitive system. Many of the traumas were in fact cognitively bypassed (not witnessed) rather than being forgotten through repression. This accounts for the fragmentary nature of her ideas, thoughts, and feelings.

Freud[87] discussed the concept of negation in relation to repression: "[T]he content of a repressed image or idea can make its way into consciousness on condition that it is negated" (p. 235). Negation, according to Freud, is an intellectual judgment task that requires "taking cognizance" of whatever is repressed in order to affirm or negate its content. The cognitive system is subject to this process. Self-memory, however, as the nonlinguistic meaning-making system, is always operative. In this context, then, repression is the energy that wards off or pushes away unwanted thoughts, images, ideas, events, behaviors, and feelings from the self-memory system. Because this pushing away was constant in Rosemary's case, an integrated self-memory system was impossible. Rosemary had multiple encapsulations along all developmental domains. Dissociation itself became a part of her self-memory and was necessary for physical survival in the environment. In this context, then, I define *dissociation* as an impairment to mentation, whereas I define *repression* as a defense of the psyche.

Conclusions

My model is different from the other theories of memory presented in this book. Self-memory is a noncognitive system which affects all levels of human development and interaction. It is the bedrock of knowing about the self, a vault for containing nontraumatic as well as traumatic memories. A metaphor from Ancient Egypt is relevant here. When Howard Carter and Lord Carnavon opened the burial chamber of King Tutankhamen in the Nile Valley, they found among the priceless treasures a well-preserved clay statuette. The excavators had just enough time to take photographs of the statuette before it collapsed without a sound and turned to dust before their eyes.[88] After thousand years of preservation in the dark and airless tomb, the statuette turned into dust after a moment's exposure to the hot Egyptian sun.

Not unlike the burial vault which held the clay statuette, the mind preserves an image and contains it (encapsulates it) in the vault of self-memory. When analytic therapists and attorneys reach into the minds of their patients, they unearth many artifacts from the vault of self-memory. Some forms of memory are whole and explicit in content, while others are affected by time, the unconscious, affect, and psychodynamic and developmental influences. When we precipitously or without warning ask patients to recall, reflect, reconstruct, and restore traumatic memories to their original form, we risk the possibility of distorting the memory, and its related affect, images, symbols, and representations. When we bring memories into consciousness following years of dissociation we also risk the possibility that patients will not be able to make meaning of them. These memories will have turned to dust, much like the Egyptian statuette brought into direct sunlight after years of entombment.

This section of this book reviewed the historical importance of repression, reparation, and other psychodynamic principles for trauma and analysis. My theory of self-memory provides another perspective and model for therapists as they attempt to help their patients to reassociate memories and find meaning from traumatic experiences. I firmly believe that the drive to reassociate the self-memory and the cognitive systems is innate and instinctual. During trauma, material is dissociated and fragmented, often taking on psychotic and unreal proportions. It is the task of the self-memory system to reassociate the traumatic experiences into a meaningful story. Aspects of memories, including isolated fragments as well as personal myths and fantasies, become the patient's personal story. It is incorporating that story into self-memory that allows healing to take place. Claudia Brenner, who was wounded by a gunman because she is a lesbian, writes about the experience in her book, *Eight Bullets:*[89]

> The more I told the story of the shooting, the less power it had over me, and the more my sense of safety grew. I told it and cried about it so many times that it eventually began to heal into a memory. As a memory, it could be integrated into my regular world. I began to make sense of the shooting as part of my life, my "self story." Integration did not mean that I was in less pain but I did feel less split off from myself. The shooting was not compartmentalized in my thoughts, isolated from the rest of my life. It was becoming a memory that was interwoven with everything else in my world, and that world was being transformed into a place where it was not inconceivable that I could be shot. (p. 159)

Making sense of all our memories—the pleasurable ones as well as the traumatic ones—is a basic human drive. The right to self-memory is a basic human right. An atrocity like the Nazi-induced Holocaust robs its victims of this basic human right, the right to a personal and ancestral story. As Holocaust poet Dan Pagis[90] writes in his poem, "Footprints":

> *Without any right to remember.*
> *What else was there?*

References

1. Delbo C: Days and Memories. (La mémoire et les jours). R Lamont (Trans.). Marlboro, Vt: Marlboro Press, 1990.
2. Hinton GE, Anderson JA: Parallel Models of Associative Memory. Hillsdale, NJ: Erlbaum, 1981.
3. Kihlstrom JF: The cognitive unconscious. Science 1987; 237:1145–1451.
4. McClelland JL: Constructive memory and memory distortion: a parallel-distributed processing approach. *In* DL Schacter, JT Coyle, GD Fischbach, MM Mesulam, LE Sullivan (Eds.),

How Minds, Brains and Societies Reconstruct the Past. Cambridge, MA: Harvard University Press, 1995, pp. 69–90.

5. Rumelhart DE, McClelland JL, PDP Research Group: Parallel Distributed Processing: Explorations in the Microstructures of Cognition, 2 vols. Cambridge, MA: MIT Press, 1986.

6. Benedek E, Schetky D: Patterns in validating allegations of sexual abuse, part 1: factors affecting perception and recall of events. J Am Acad Child Adolesc Psychiatry 1987; 26:912–915.

7. Sivan A: Preschool child development: Implications for investigation of child abuse allegations. Child Abuse Negl 1991; 15:485–493.

8. Terr L: Child trauma: an outline and overview. Am J Psychiatry 1991; 148:10–20.

9. Terr L: Too Scared to Cry. New York: Basic Books, 1990.

10. Terr L: What happened to early memories of trauma? A study of 20 children under age 5 at the time of documented trauma events. J Am Acad Child Adolesc Psychiatry 1988; 27:96–104.

11. Mazure CM (ed.): Stress and Psychiatric disorders. Washington, D.C.: American Psychiatric Press, 1994.

12. Cole PM, Putnam FW: Effects of incest on self and social functioning: a developmental psychopathology perspective. Consult Clin Psychol 1992; 60:174–184.

13. Epstein S: The implications of cognitive-experiential self theory for research and social psychology and personality. Theory Soc Behav 1985; 15:283–310.

14. Epstein S: Integration of the cognitive and the psychodynamic unconsciousness. Am Psychol 1994; 49:709–724.

15. Epstein S: The self-concept revisited, or a theory of a theory. Am Psychol 1973; 29:404–416.

16. Kohut H: The Restoration of the Self. New York: International University Press, 1977.

17. Noam G: The self, adult development, and the theory of biography and transformation. In D Lapsley, FC Power (Eds.), Self, Ego and Identity—Integrative Approaches. New York: Springer-Verlag, 1988, pp. 4–29.

18. Wolf E: Treating the Self. New York: Guilford Press, 1988.

19. Frischholz, EJ: The Relationship Between Dissociation, Hypnosis, and Child Abuse and Development of Multiple Personality. Childhood and Descendants. Washington, D.C.: American Psychiatric Press, 1985.

20. Erdrich L: The Blue Jay's Dance: A Birth Year. New York: Harper Collins, 1995.

21. Levin P: Assessing post-traumatic stress disorder with the Rorschach projective technique. In JP Wilson, B Raphael (Eds.), International Handbook of Traumatic Stress Syndrome. New York: Plenum Press, 1993, pp. 189–200.

22. Appelfeld A: Beyond Despair: Three Lectures and a Conversation with Philip Roth. New York: Fromm International, 1994.

23. Langer L: Holocaust Testimonies. The Ruins of Memory. New Haven: Yale University Press, 1991.

24. Langer L: Art from the Ashes: A Holocaust Anthology. New York: Oxford University Press, 1995.

25. Langer L: Admitting the Holocaust. New York: Oxford University Press, 1995.

26. Wiesel E: Memoirs. All Rivers Run to the Sea. New York: Knopf, 1995.

27. Jackson JH: On a particular variety of epilepsy (intellectual aura): one case with symptoms of organic brain disease. Brain 1888; 11:179–207.

28. Kahneman D, Treisman A: Changing views of attention and automaticity. In R Parasuraman, DR Davies (Eds.), Varieties of Attention. Orlando, FL: Academic Press, 1984, pp. 29–57.

29. Mesulam M: Principles of Behavioral Neurology. Philadelphia: Davis, 1985.

30. Churchland PS: Neurophilosophy. Cambridge, MA: MIT Press, 1986.
31. Rohrbaugh JW: The orienting reflex. *In* R Parasuraman, DR Davies, (Eds.), Varieties of Attention. Orlando, FL: Academic Press, 1984, pp. 273–287.
32. Herman J: Trauma and Recovery. New York: Basic Books, 1992.
33. Levi P: The Drowned and the Saved (I Sommersi i slavati). R Rosenthal (trans.). New York: Simon and Schuster, 1986.
34. Basch MF: The concept of affects: a re-examination. J Am Psychoanal Assoc 1976; 24:759–777.
35. LeDoux JE: Emotion as memory: in search of systems and synapses. Ann N Y Acad Sci 1993; 702:149–157.
36. LeDoux, JE: Memory vs. emotional memory in the brain. *In* P Ekman, R Davidson (Eds.), The Nature of Emotion. New York: Oxford University Press, 1994, pp. 311–312.
37. McGaugh JL: Significance and remembrance: the role of the neuromodulatory systems. Psychol Sci 1990; 1:15–25.
38. McGaugh JL, Introini-Collison IB, Cahill L: Involvement of the amygdala in neuromodulatory influences on memory storage. *In* JT Aggleton (Ed.), The Amygdala. New York: Wiley-Liss, 1992, pp. 431–451.
39. Bahannon JN: Flashbulb memories for the Space Shuttle disaster. A tale of two theories. Cognition 1988; 29:179–196.
40. Pillemer DB: Flashbulb memories of the assassination attempt on President Reagan. Cognition 1984; 16:63–80.
41. Wilkinson CB: Aftermath of a disaster: the collapse of the Hyatt Regency Hotel skywalk. Am J Psychiatry 1983; 140:1134–1139.
42. Valent P: The Ash Wednesday brush fires in Victoria. Med J Aust 1984; 141/5:291–300.
43. Feinstein A, Spiegel D: Post-traumatic stress disorder: a descriptive study supporting DSM-III R criteria. Am J Psychiatry 1989; 146:665–666.
44. Madakasira S, O'Brien K: Acute post-traumatic stress disorder in victims of natural disaster. J Nerv Ment Dis 1987; 175:286–290.
45. Schwarz E, Kowalski JM: Malignant memories: PTSD in children and adults after a school shooting. J Am Acad Child Psychiatry 1991; 30:936–944.
46. Elin MR: A developmental model for trauma. *In* L Cohen, J Berzoff, MR Elin (Eds.), DID: Theoretical and Treatment Controversies. Northvale, NJ: Jason Aronson, 1995, pp. 223–259.
47. Kauffman S: At Home in the Universe: The Search for Laws of Self Organization. New York: Oxford University Press, 1995.
48. Thelen E: Motor development: a new synthesis. Am Psychol 1995; 50:79–95.
49. Edelman GM: Neural Darwinism. New York: Basic Books, 1987.
50. Sporns O, Edelman GM: Solving Bernstein's problem: a proposal for the development of coordinated movement by selection. Child Dev 1993; 64:960–981.
51. Campbell J: Grammatical Man. New York: Simon and Schuster, 1982.
52. Gold PE, van Buskirk R: Facilitation of time: dependent memory processes with post-trial epinephrine injections. Behav Biol 1975; 13:145–153.
53. Gold PE, van Buskirk R: Post-training brain norepinephrine concentration: correlation with retention performance of avoidance training with peripheral epinephrine modulation of memory processing. Behav Biol 1978; 23:509–526.
54. Coveney P, Highland R: The Search for Order in a Chaotic World. New York: Fawcett Columbine, 1995.
55. Gleick J: Chaos: Making a New Science. New York: Viking, 1987.

56. Charney DS, Deutch AY, Krystal JH, Southwick SM, Davis M: Psychobiologic mechanisms of post-traumatic stress disorder. Arch Gen Psychiatry 1993; 50:294–299.
57. Southwick SM, Krystal JH, Morgan A, Johnson D, Nagy L, Nicolaou A, Heninger G, Charney D: Abnormal noradrenergic function in post-traumatic stress disorder. Arch Gen Psychiatry 1993; 50:226–274.
58. van der Kolk BA: The body keeps score: memory and the evolving psychobiology of post-traumatic stress. Harvard Rev Psychiatry 1994; 1:253–265.
59. van der Kolk BA, Greenberg M, Boyd H, Krystal J: Inescapable shock, neurotransmitters and addiction to trauma: toward a psychobiology of post-traumatic stress. Biol Psychiatry 1985; 20:314–325.
60. Cotman CP, Nieto-Sampedro M, Harris EW: Synapsis replacement in the adult nervous system of vertebrates. Physiolog Rev 1981; 61:684–784.
61. Minsky M: The Society of Mind. New York: Simon and Schuster, 1986.
62. Malmquist C: Children who witness parental murder: post-traumatic aspects. J Am Acad Child Psychiatry 1986; 3:320–325.
63. Sachs N: O the Chimneys. Mead M, Mead R, Hamburger M (Trans.). New York: Farrar, Straus, and Giroux, 1967.
64. Clark W: At War Within: The Double-edged Sword of Immunity. New York: Oxford University Press, 1995.
65. Rovee-Collier C: The memory system of prelinguistic infants. Ann N Y Acad Sci 1991; 608:517–536.
66. Greco C, Hayne H, Rovee-Collier C: Role of function reminding and variability in categorization by three-month-old infants. J Exp Psychol Learning Mem Cogn 1990; 16:617–633.
67. Greco C, Hanyne H, Griesler P, Early L: Ontogeny of early event memory: II. Encoding and retrieval by 2- and 3-month-olds. Infant Behav Dev 1986; 9:441–460.
68. Baillargeon R: Representing the existence and location of hidden objects: object permanence in 6 and 8 month olds. Cognition 1986; 23:21–24.
69. Pillemer DD, White SH: Childhood events recalled by children and adults. Adv Child Dev Behav 1989; 21:297–340.
70. Ceci S, Bruck M: Suggestibility of the child witness: A historical review and synthesis. Psychol Bull 1993; 13:3403–3439.
71. Stern D: The Interpersonal World of the Infant. A View from Psychoanalysis and Developmental Psychology. New York: Basic Books, 1985.
72. Spitz RA: Hospitalization: an inquiry into the genesis of psychiatric conditions in early childhood. Psychoanal Study Child 1:53–74.
73. Gardner L: Deprivation dwarfism. In W Greenough (Ed.), The Nature and Nurture of Behavior. San Francisco: William Freeman, 1973, pp. 101–107.
74. Kolb LC: The Psychology of the Amputee. Collected Papers of the Mayo Clinic 1952; 44:586–591.
75. Earle E: Effects of mutilating surgery on children and adolescents. Psychoanal Study Child 1979; 34:527–546.
76. Herman-Giddens ME, Sandler AD, Friedman NE: Sexual precocity in girls; an association with sexual abuse. Am J Dis Children 1988; 142:431–433.
77. Putnam F, Trickett P: Child sexual abuse: a model of chronic trauma. Psychiatry 1993; 56:82–95.
78. Trickett P, Putnam F: Impact of child sexual abuse on females: toward a developmental psychological integration. Psychol Sci 1993; 4:81–87.
79. Eth S, Pynoos R: Posttraumatic Stress Disorders in Children. Washington, D.C.: American Psychiatric Press, 1985.

80. Bremner D, Randall P, Scott T, Bronen R, Seibyl J, Southwick SM, Delaney R, McCarthy G, Charney D, Innis R: MRI-based measurement of hippocampal volume in patients with combat related post-traumatic stress disorder. Am J Psychiatry 1995; 152:973–981.
81. Williams L: Adult memories of childhood abuse. J Consult Clin Psychol 1994; 62:1167–1176.
82. Westen D, Klepser J, Ruffins S, Silverman M, Lifton N, Boekamp J: Object relations in childhood and adolescence: the development of working representations. J Consult Clin Psychol 1991; 59:400–409.
83. Sherkow SP: Evaluation and diagnosis of sexual abuse of little girls. J Am Psychol Assoc 1990; 38:347–369.
84. Acredolo L, Goodwyn S: Symbolic gesturing in normal infants. Child Dev 1988; 59:450–466.
85. Herman J, Schatzow E: Recovery and verification of memories of childhood sexual trauma. Psychoanal Psychol 1987; 4:1–14.
86. Cohen L, Berzoff J, Elin M (Eds.): DID: Theoretical and Treatment Controversies. Northvale, NJ: Jason Aronson, 1995.
87. Freud S: On Negation. Int J Psychoanal 1925; 19:235.
88. Reik T: Listening with the Third Ear. New York, Farrar, Strauss and Giroux, 1949.
89. Brenner C: Eight Bullets. Ithaca, NY: Firebrand Books, 1995.
90. Pagis D: Footprints. *In* Points of Departure. S Mitchell (Trans.). Jewish Publication Society, 1981, New York.

THE MEMORY OF TRAUMA

8

Memory and Posttraumatic Stress Disorder

JULIA A. GOLIER
RACHEL YEHUDA
STEVEN SOUTHWICK

This chapter will focus on the memories of those who have endured traumatic events as adults, particularly those who suffer from posttraumatic stress disorder (PTSD). PTSD is a relatively new diagnostic category that incorporates symptoms resulting from exposure to life-threatening events. Many of these symptoms are related to memory. For example, the re-experiencing symptom cluster is defined by the persistence of traumatic memories in forms that are distressing and sometimes distorted, such as intrusive thoughts, nightmares, or dissociative flashbacks. Paradoxically, in addition to persistent and intrusive memories, survivors often complain of an inability to recall important aspects of their traumatic experience, a phenomenon formerly called "psychogenic amnesia." Additionally, individuals with PTSD also suffer from other symptoms related to memory such as poor concentration and impaired attention.

Whereas a substantial proportion of trauma survivors are symptomatic in the immediate aftermath of a trauma, only a subset develops PTSD. Therefore, the literature on memory impairments in PTSD will not apply to all trauma survivors. However, studying this symptomatic subset may further our understanding of traumatic memories and how they are processed. The memory alterations in PTSD may reflect phenomena that are unique or that are similar to, but more exaggerated than, phenomena experienced by trauma survivors who do not develop PTSD. The goals of this chapter are to summarize existing knowledge about the relationship between trauma and memory in survivors who do and do not develop PTSD.

The Phenomenology of Memory Disturbances in PTSD

Individuals at risk for developing PTSD are those who have undergone a severe, traumatic event. In DSM-IV, a traumatic event is defined as one in which the individual has experienced, witnessed, or been confronted with an event or events that involved actual or threatened death, or serious injury, or threat to the physical integrity of the self or others.[1] In order to meet criteria for PTSD, the individual must experience a host of symptoms from the three symptom clusters: re-experiencing, avoidance, and arousal. The full criteria are met if these symptoms persist for at least one month and cause clinically significant impairment. Those symptoms that directly or indirectly relate to memory will be described below, with an emphasis on their relationship to the inciting traumatic event.

Reliving and Re-experiencing

Traumatic events seem to leave indelible memory traces. Some individuals find significant meaning in "not forgetting" their trauma. For example, a war veteran may consciously or unconsciously believe that by actively remembering combat experiences he is paying tribute to a fellow soldier. A Holocaust victim may view remembering as a way to bear witness to the tragedy and brutality of Nazi Germany. But for some trauma victims there may be little or no personal meaning or moral obligation in their persistent remembering; despite their best efforts, they continue to relive the trauma simply because they cannot forget it. The trauma has left an impression that repeatedly intrudes into consciousness. Attempts to suppress or block memories are often unsuccessful. The traumatic recollection can appear in the waking state as intrusive thoughts, illusions or hallucinations, or in the dream state, as horrifying nightmares. These phenomena, classified as the *cluster B* symptoms in DSM-IV, are referred to as the re-experiencing symptoms of PTSD. The re-experiencing symptoms are uncommonly vivid and may remain so for the lifetime of the individual. Most individuals suffering from PTSD find these re-experiencing symptoms highly distressing and even tormenting—so much so, that they frequently come to treatment wanting "to forget."

Reliving experiences differ from the normal recall of traumatic memory in several ways, one of which is their intrusiveness. The frequency with which the memories are evoked, the intensity of the accompanying pain and arousal, and the persistence of them over time all contribute to the subjective sense of intrusiveness. Additionally, although the remembered event should seem familiar, the form the memory takes may make it seem strange or foreign. This is particularly likely if the memory occurs as an illusion or a fragmented image, such as a dismembered body, an assailant's face, a victim's cry. Out of context, these perceptions seem senseless to the patient, who may fear she or he is "going crazy." Once evoked, the memory is often played over and over again. The inability to contain a memory once it has been recalled, or to suppress or control it, reinforces a feeling of helplessness. Rather than fade over time, the negative feelings associated with the original trauma may remain bound to the memory and may be compounded by distress over the persistence of the memories themselves.

In some cases, the remembering experiences are not perceived as memories but as if the trauma were being relived. A description of a reliving experience can be found in *Dispatches,* a memoir written by Michael Herr, who was a war correspondent in Vietnam.[2]

> During my first month back I woke up one night and knew that my living room was full of dead Marines. It actually happened three or four times, after a dream I was having those nights (the kind of dream one never had in Vietnam), and that first time it wasn't just some holding dread left by the dream, I knew they were there, so that after I'd turned on the light by my bed and smoked a cigarette I lay there for a moment thinking that I'd have to go out soon and cover them.

This passage illustrates the clarity and certainty that accompany reliving experiences, qualities which contribute to their being perceived as current reality. Visual images often predominate in flashbacks, but smells, sounds, and tastes can be incorporated as well. An array of emotions present during the initial traumatization may accompany the images, including fear, rage, excitement, or helplessness. During a flashback a patient may not only feel but also act as if the event were recurring. He or she may duck for cover or act violently in perceived self-defense. Similarly, nightmares may be accompanied by behaviors related to a specific traumatic event. Companions will report that the patient thrashes, screams, or makes verbal references during a nightmare as he or she appears to relive aspects of the trauma. Profuse sweating and autonomic arousal may accompany nightmares that can be so disturbing that the victim dreads going back to sleep for fear of having another nightmare.

Traumatic memories are often recalled with extreme clarity and perceived as highly accurate. Such an experience is described by Oliver Lyttelton, a WW I veteran.[3]

> Fear and its milder brothers, dread and anticipation, first soften the tablets of memory, so that impressions which they bring are clearly and deeply cut, and when time cools them off the impressions are fixed like the grooves of a gramophone record, and remain with you as long as your faculties. I have been surprised how accurate my memory has proved about times and places where I was frightened.

Although it is often assumed by patient and clinician that the content of the re-experiencing phenomena reflects events as they actually happened, this is not easily demonstrated. However, as will be discussed later in Eyewitness Memory, one's confidence in a memory does not always correspond to its accuracy. Indeed the vividness of traumatic memories and the intensity of the accompanying arousal that makes them seem indelible and immutable may also contribute to the process whereby remembered events are misinterpreted as current reality. Very commonly patients report ''I remember it like it was yesterday,'' suggesting a loss of distinction between the recent and the remote past. Sometimes the temporal boundary is lost altogether; the experience and the memory seem one and the same. For example Vietnam veterans with PTSD frequently say "For a minute I was back in Nam.'' In this instance it is as if internally-generated images of remote events are briefly perceived as external events happening in the here and now. The reliving and re-experiencing symptoms, though derived from seemingly indelible and immutable traumatic memories, may arise from a blurring of the distinction between an accurate memory and an emotionally evocative image related to traumatization.

Avoidance and Emotional Numbing

The *cluster C* symptoms of PTSD are defined by the persistent avoidance of stimuli associated with the trauma and a numbing of general responsiveness which was not present before the trauma. Several of the individual symptoms of this cluster are specific to having been traumatized: (*1*) efforts to avoid thoughts, feelings, or conversations associated with the trauma, (*2*) efforts to avoid activities, places, or people which arouse recollections of the trauma, and (*3*) an inability to remember an important aspect of the trauma. The last was formerly called "psychogenic amnesia.''

At first glance, it appears paradoxical that an individual would be distressed by both repeatedly remembering an event and by forgetting important aspects of it. The "amnesia'' associated with PTSD causes distress because the patient is aware that he or she has lost information. In this sense, the "amnesia'' is partial and differs from classic accounts in which the patient is unaware that information has been forgotten. The "amnesia'' associated with PTSD may be the result of several processes. If some aspects of the trauma were never encoded, then the memory was always incomplete and the amnesia represents a gap. A failure to encode could result from selective attentional processing. During states of extreme arousal the most salient details are preferentially attended to (a process that will be described in more detail in Naturalistic Studies in Nonclinical Samples). If this process occurs at the time of the trauma the resulting memory may be fragmented. Psychogenic amnesia may also involve the active suppression or repression of memories that are too painful to think about. This explanation is in keeping with the mechanism posited for the other "avoidant'' symptoms, that is, that the individual engages in behavioral or cognitive efforts to avoid remembering the trauma. Another possibility is that traumatic memories are processed in the same ways as other memories and the inability to remember aspects of the trauma is a result of "normal forgetting.'' The persistence of some memories and loss of others may result from a differential rate of decay. That PTSD patients complain both of excessive forgetting and remembering suggests that it is not only the memory but the distortion of memory and the inability to control it which are distressing for trauma survivors.

Behavioral and cognitive avoidance allows survivors to partially regulate their affect and adapt to having been traumatized. For example, survivors of assault may make elaborate efforts to avoid places reminiscent of the assault. Combat veterans may avoid war movies and war memorials. Vietnam veterans may strenuously avoid areas where they are likely to encounter Asians for fear of being reminded of "the enemy." Avoidant symptoms also can interfere with treatment-seeking, as some survivors fear discussing and being reminded of their traumatic experiences. Avoidance also can extend beyond obvious reminders of the trauma, and into a more generalized withdrawal from intimate contacts and meaningful activity. This expansion of avoidance beyond obvious reminders of the trauma is captured by the remaining symptoms in *cluster C:* markedly diminished interest or participation in significant activities, feeling of detachment or estrangement from others, restricted range of affect, and a sense of a foreshortened future. Although avoidant symptoms may seem adaptive in the short-term, if they progress and persist, significant social and functional impairment ensues. In the most severe cases, the person detaches from work, family, and friends, believing, it seems, that this will keep him or her out of harm's way. Instead they are often angry and isolated, living a highly restricted existence, consumed by the past.

Hyperarousal

Unlike the cluster B or C symptoms, none of the *cluster D* symptoms, the hyperarousal symptoms, are specific to having been traumatized, although reminders of the trauma may provoke or exacerbate them. They hyperarousal symptoms include difficulty falling or staying asleep, irritability or outbursts of anger, difficulty concentrating, hypervigilance, and exaggerated startle response.

The symptoms of increased arousal may be viewed as indirectly related to memory for traumatic events. Immediately preceding and during the event, traumatized individuals generally report feeling alert, aroused, terrified, and in many cases, overwhelmed. After the trauma they often find themselves in a chronic state of arousal. For example, combat veterans frequently talk of sleeping with "one eye open" or constantly scanning the environment for possible dangers. Many report chronically feeling "on guard" even when no apparent threat exists. Some individuals routinely find themselves sitting with their back to the wall and avoiding crowds where it is not possible to monitor innumerable potential sources of threat. To protect themselves and their families, they may establish rituals related to safety, such as multiple nightly checks of locks in their home. They are easily startled by loud or unexpected noises. The Fourth of July, with its explosion of fireworks, is known to be an especially unpleasant holiday for combat veterans who often search in vain for safe, quiet havens.

Poor sleep, hypervigilance, and exaggerated startle do not exclusively accompany or follow specific memories of a past trauma; for some, these symptoms are present much of the time. The individual chronically appears to be living with a "memory" of threat or danger that persists often outside of the individual's conscious awareness. The mind and body seem to respond as if a threat or danger is still present even years after having survived. Thus, following a severe trauma, some individuals subjectively begin to view the world as a consistently dangerous and unpreditable place.

Eyewitness Memory

As just described, trauma survivors can be overwhelmed by both repetitive intrusive recollections and a distressing inability to remember some details of a trauma. In order to fully understand how traumatic memories are processed, it is useful to know exactly what transpired. However, attempts to know for certain what happened during a traumatic event or any life event will be hampered by the imperfection of memory itself. These limitations are delineated in *The Drowned and the Saved* by Primo Levi[4]— writer, chemist, and survivor of Auschwitz.

> The memories which lie within us are not carved in stone; not only do they tend to become erased as the years go by, but often they change, or even grow, by incorporating extraneous features. Judges know this very well: almost never do two eyewitnesses of the same event describe it in the same way and with the same words, even if the event is recent and if neither of them has a personal interest in distorting it. This scant reliability of our memories will be satisfactorily explained only when we know in what language, in what alphabet they are written, on what surface, and with what pen: to this day we are still far from this goal. (p. 23)

This "scant reliability" of memory is an inherent obstacle in the evaluation of traumatic memories as well as a subject of study itself. The effect of emotion and arousal on the reliability of memory is germane to the study of eyewitness memory and traumatic memory. The literature on emotion and memory will be reviewed in detail elsewhere in this volume; however, experimental and naturalistic studies relevant to the fate of traumatic memories will be reviewed below.

Experimental Studies

Laboratory-based studies have attempted to delineate the effects of emotion and arousal on the accuracy of memory. An important direction of research on emotion and memory began with Easterbrook's hypothesis that arousal leads to a "narrowing of attention."[5] One methodologic approach has been to compare the memories of two groups of witnesses who watch scenes that are identical, with the exception that arousing or violent elements have been incorporated into one of the conditions. Using this approach, several studies have found that arousal decreases the overall accuracy of memories. In one study, subjects watched a film of a bank robbery. The two versions of the film were identical except that the ending of one was violent. The group that watched the violent version had poorer memory for the film than the group that watched the neutral version. Importantly, the differences in memory concerned details occurring early in the scene, details that were identical in both versions.[6] In a separate study, the accuracy of subjects' testimony after viewing a videotape of a mugging was assessed. Those who watched the violent version had less accurate recall than those who watched the nonviolent version.[7] In addition to accuracy, the subjects' confidence in their own testimony was measured. In the group that viewed the nonviolent version, confidence was related to accuracy for details, such as identification of the perpetrator. However, for those who watched the violent version, there was no significant relationship between confidence and accuracy. Other investigators also have reported a lack of relationship between accuracy and confidence in memory recall.[8,9] In one study an inverse relationship was found; that is, the more confident the subject, the less likely he or she was to have accurate recall.[10]

The above laboratory studies suggest that arousal may decrease the accuracy of detailed memory over even a short retention interval. But is this effect of arousal general or selective? It is possible that reduced accuracy for some details is the price paid for increased attention to others. This possibility is suggested by the phenomena of "weapon focussing"; some victims can provide elaborate detail for critical aspects of the trauma, such as the weapon used, but little detail for other aspects. Several studies provide empiric evidence for weapon focussing. In one study, eye movements were monitored while subjects watched one of two versions of a videotaped bank scene. The duration and number of eye fixations were greater for a gun pointed at a cashier than for the comparison item, a check, in the neutral version. In addition to focussing on the weapon, upon subsequent testing, subjects in the weapon condition had poorer memory for the overall scene than did those in the neutral condition.[11] In a similar study, subjects were exposed to a staged scene; and while the event was staged, a fear-arousing stimulus, a syringe carried by an assistant, was introduced. The subjects in the emotionally arousing scene could provide significant details about the syringe, but compared with those who witnessed the neutral version of the scene, they were less able to recognize the assistant in a lineup.[12] These studies suggest that attention to central details is heightened in arousing situations, perhaps at the cost of attention to peripheral details. If this process operates at the time of a trauma, it may underlie the fragmentation of memories, during which some aspects are overremembered and other aspects seem inexplicably inaccessible.

Naturalistic Studies in Nonclinical Samples

It is not clear whether the results of laboratory simulation studies can be generalized to real-life events or traumas. Although the laboratory studies may induce physiological arousal, this is only one aspect of the emotional response to trauma, which commonly includes terror and helplessness and may cause marked dissociation. However, these studies do provide an important framework for understanding naturalistic studies of memory for violence or trauma. There are many methodological difficulties in attempting to examine the accuracy of eyewitness memory in naturalistic settings where the precise details of an event cannot be known. One approach has been to collect information from multiple witnesses and compare individual accounts to the composite account. Another approach is to study what happens to eyewitness memories over time by comparing recall after the event to delayed recall of the event. Such an approach does not measure the accuracy of memories, but rather, their stability over time.

One of the first naturalistic studies of eyewitness memory described the types of details crime victims provide to police about their assailants.[13] Included among the subjects were two homicide victims who provided reports before they died. The completeness of the memories rather than their accuracy was addressed by this study. With respect to the type of details remembered, the majority could recall physical characteristics that defined the perpetrator, such as sex, build, complexion, age; they were less likely to recall details like hair or eye color. Crime reports were also compared as a function of the type of crime and the degree of injury. Robbery victims provided more detail than survivors of rape or assault. Uninjured victims provided more information than injured victims. To the extent that a crime report is a measure of memory for a trauma, these findings that victims of more serious crimes could provide less information are consistent with the notion that trauma interferes with the formation of detailed memories.

In another naturalistic study the recall of 13 eyewitnesses of a crime was studied in which a store was robbed, the owner wounded and the thief murdered.[14] The initial accounts given to the police, both free accounts and responses to questions, were recorded verbatim and compared to interviews conducted for research purposes 4–5 months later. Overall, the accuracy for details central to the crime was high. There was little decay in memory over the interval, except for memory of colors, and for some witnesses, estimates of age and height. To assess the effect of arousal on recall, self-reports of stress at the time of the crime were obtained. Witnesses with the highest levels of reported stress had an average accuracy of 93% for detail at the initial report and 88% at follow-up, rates which were slightly higher than those who did not report being stressed. Consistent with their self-reports, the stressed group, but not the other group, was symptomatic immediately after the event and had difficulty sleeping. The results suggest that emotional stress does not have a deleterious effect on recall. In fact, it may have enhanced recall. However, interpretation of the effect of traumatic stress on memory is confounded by the fact that those who were most stressed also had greater direct involvement in the incident. In a similar study, witnesses to a post office robbery, both victims and bystanders, were interviewed by researchers after a delay of between 4 and 15 months. The consistency of initial and later reports was high for details central to the crime (e.g., clothing, the weapon), but was not as good for details surrounding the event. Accuracy was higher for victims than for bystanders. The enhanced accuracy of the victims cannot be clearly attributed to the effect of stress, however, as the victims' self-reported ratings of stress were no greater than those of the bystanders. Therefore, while both studies found that those more closely involved in a crime have more accurate memory than bystanders, it is not clear that this enhancement is due to stress and arousal per se, as opposed to other factors, such as proximity.

The studies cited above measured the accuracy and consistency of traumatic memories over relatively short periods of time. Few naturalistic studies have assessed the fate of traumatic memories over vey long periods of time. The occasion to do so arose when a case against DeRijke, a Kapo accused of Nazi crimes in a Dutch prison, was reopened in 1984 and the veracity of eyewitness accounts some 40 years after the fact was called into question.[15] Data was collected from 72 surviving witnesses of the Dutch prison, some of whom had initially provided testimony between 1942 and 1947 after leaving the prison. On the whole, witnesses agreed about basic facts and provided complementary accounts of the types of punishments and brutalities suffered in the prison. Although the majority remembered DeRijke, several survivors didn't recognize a picture of him or recall his name, despite evidence that they had been repeatedly tortured by him. By comparing accounts provided decades apart, this study investigated not only the fate of memories of what had been routine violence for these survivors but also memory of unique traumatic events. Several witnesses forgot unique details. One recalled witnessing a murder but misattributed the murder to the victim rather than the perpetrator. Two had forgotten about murders they had previously reported witnessing. One of the two, when confronted with the inconsistency, denied having ever made the report. This naturalistic study demonstrates that on the whole, traumatic memories can be accurate and stable over very long retention intervals. However, the notable exceptions demonstrate that even the most horrific of experiences are not immune to forgetting or distortion.

Eyewitness Memory and PTSD

Several questions arise about whether the fate of traumatic memories differs in those with PTSD from other trauma survivors. One question is whether patients with PTSD are more likely to remember details of their trauma. A second question is whether the memories are more likely to be accurate or distorted. And if they are distorted, is it in a way that magnifies or minimizes the trauma?

There has been little overlap between the eyewitness memory literature and the PTSD literature. Only recently have studies begun to systematically examine the question of whether PTSD affects the accuracy of memories and if so, how. The first was a longitudinal study of Australian firefighters exposed to devastating brush fires. Recall of the event was recorded 4 months after exposure and again at 11 months.[16] A major difference in the retrospective recall of the traumatic event was found between those who did develop PTSD and those who did not. Among those with chronic PTSD, recall of personal injury did not change during this interval. In sharp contrast, among those without PTSD, only 43% (13 of 30) of those who had reported injuries at 4 months reported them when asked again at 11 months. The significant reduction of reporting of exposure to disaster in the group without PTSD suggests that traumatic memories are better retained or more accessible in those with PTSD. A limitation of this study is the absence of information at a time point earlier than 4 months. However, if symptoms are related to recall, this raises the question of whether survivors are "better off" not remembering their traumatic events. It may be that decreased accessibility to or retention of painful memories has a protective effect which fosters adaptation. A provocative study of dream recall is consistent with this possibility. Dream recall was measured in a sleep laboratory in Holocaust survivors and controls who had not been traumatized. It was found that well-adapted Holocaust survivors had decreased dream recall compared with both controls and poorly adapted survivors.[17] Dream recall is not directly comparable to conscious recollection, but to the extent that positive adaptation is associated with forgetting; this compels us to reexamine the nature of psychogenic amnesia. The study of firefighters suggests that amnesia may actually be greater in those who do not go on to develop PTSD. This provides further support to the notion that the symptom of psychogenic amnesia in PTSD may be less about forgetting than about the distress forgetting causes. That aspects of the trauma have been forgotten may simply be highlighted in PTSD patients who feel besieged by so many other remembered aspects of the trauma.

In another study of PTSD and eyewitness memory, witnesses to a shooting were questioned at two points in time following the event.[18] All subjects changed their report of the events in some way. However, those who developed PTSD symptoms tended to have distortions which magnified their perceptions of and emotional reactions to the shooting, including their assessment of the potential threat to life. In another study, the self-reported combat exposure of Desert Storm veterans was measured 1 month and then again 2 years after returning from the war. There were many instances of inconsistent recall for events that were highly traumatic and objective in nature. Further, with an increase in trauma-related symptoms over time, there tended to be an amplification of memory for traumatic events.[19] Thus both studies suggest that PTSD patients may be more likely to distort memories of the traumatic event in a malignant direction.

These studies raise the question of what effect symptoms, such as frequent re-evocations, have on the accuracy of the memory for the inciting event. Within the limitations of the small number of naturalistic studies cited above, it may be that posttraumatic stress disorder increases the likelihood that a survivor recalls having been traumatized but at the same time increases the likelihood that the memories become distorted. Much evidence suggests that for a given memory there are multiple individual components which are stored separately and activated simultaneously. This is in contrast to a model in which memories are relatively fixed and are either retrieved intact or not retrieved at all. Different elements may be evoked at different times; extraneous material may be evoked as well and incorporated into the memory. The replaying of traumatic memories may strengthen the memory, while the sheer number of repetitions may simultaneously increase the likelihood extraneous elements become incorporated. If such a process occurs, it is conceivable that PTSD patients, victims of trauma and their memories, could come to perceive themselves as victims of traumas even more horrific than those initially sustained.

Memory and PTSD: Neuropsychological Findings

Memory for Traumatic Stimuli

The nature of traumatic memories has been discussed above. Given that there are differences among traumatic memories in PTSD and non-PTSD survivors, it is reasonable to examine whether the differences can be accounted for by neuropsychological abnormalities. The neuropsychological studies that have examined this question can be broadly grouped into two categories: those that use trauma-related stimuli and those that use neutral stimuli.

A series of experiments has clearly demonstrated that patients with PTSD process information relevant to their trauma differently from other types of information by using a modified version of the Stroop Word–Color Interference Task. To understand the significance of these findings it is first necessary to understand the original experiments conducted by Stroop in 1935 and the ways in which the task has been modified (for a review, see MacLeod 1991).[20]

The stimuli used in the original experiments by Stroop were five words and their matching ink colors: *red, blue, green, brown* and *purple*. The stimulus cards were designed so that the words were printed in incongruent colors (for example, the word *yellow* printed in red ink). In the first part of the study, subjects were asked to read the words aloud. In the second part they were asked to *name the ink color* of the printed words. The subjects did not take any longer to read the words printed in incongruent colors than to read words printed in black ink; they did take longer to name the color of the incongruent words than to name the color of solid-color squares. The interference from the incongruent words on color-naming is called *Stroop interference*.[20]

There is an extensive body of research exploring Stroop interference. Delays in color-naming are thought to be caused by interference from words that stimulate involuntary semantic activation, and distract the subject from the task.[20] Studies examining whether the meaning of the printed word (i.e., the ''irrelevant'' verbal stimuli) affects interference have shown that color-related words and words with great emotional meaning are particularly likely to interfere with color-naming.[20]

The Stroop Interference Test has been used to test the hypothesis that subjects with PTSD have an attentional bias toward traumatic stimuli. The first of these studies was conducted on rape victims with PTSD, whose responses were compared with those of rape victims without PTSD and nontraumatized comparison subjects.[21] The color-naming latency (the time between stimulus presentation and the color-naming response) was recorded for words of four different categories: (*1*) trauma-specific threat words (e.g., *assault, attack, V.D.*), (*2*) general threat words (e.g., *coffin, death, tumor*), (*3*) neutral words, and (*4*) nonwords. Rape victims with PTSD took significantly longer to color-name threat-specific words from the other three categories. Neither the rape victims without PTSD nor the nontraumatized comparison group differed in their response latencies to the four categories of words. Similarly, in a separate study, rape victims with PTSD, but not those without PTSD or nontraumatized controls, took longer to color-name highly threatening words (e.g., *rape*) compared with moderately threatening (e.g., *crime*), positive, or neutral words.[22] The interference from highly threatening words correlated with intrusive symptoms, but not with avoidant symptoms of PTSD, which suggests that the information-processing abnormality responsible for the Stroop interference may underlie the mechanisms of intrusive thoughts.

That trauma-related words cause Stroop interference in PTSD patients has also been demonstrated in combat veterans.[23,24] Vietnam veterans with PTSD and Vietnam veterans without PTSD were asked to color-name words from four different categories, one of which were trauma-related words (e.g., *bodybags, firefight*).[23] Veterans with PTSD, but not the controls, showed Stroop interference for the combat-related words; the groups did not differ in the color-naming latency to the other three word categories. Interference did not correlate with severity of combat exposure but did correlate with severity of PTSD symptoms, which suggests that interference is related to PTSD rather than to trauma per se.

The consistency of these results highlights several points. In all of the above studies, Stroop test results differed between trauma survivors with PTSD and those without PTSD. This suggests that selective processing is a feature of the disorder itself, rather than a nonspecific sequelae of trauma per se. Supporting this notion is the finding that interference is not associated with the severity of trauma, but rather with the degree of PTSD symptomatology.[22,23] The interference was found in groups of PTSD subjects whose traumas differed in type, severity, and duration. These results show that PTSD patients have a specific bias in information-processing for traumatic stimuli. Rapid completion of the color-naming task involves ignoring the "irrelevant verbal stimuli." For subjects with PTSD, when the irrelevant verbal stimulus is also a reminder of their trauma, it is difficult to ignore. The interference from trauma-related stimuli parallels the experience of intrusive cognition in PTSD patients who are easily stimulated by trauma-related cues. It has been hypothesized that traumatic memories are more accessible to conscious recall in patients with PTSD than in other control populations. The Stroop findings are consistent with the notion that traumatic memories are stored in a primed or partially activated state in PTSD patients, which may account for their involuntary intrusion into awareness and their rapid activation in the presence of reminders.[24]

Another information-processing study raised the question of whether PTSD subjects have not only enhanced memory for trauma-related stimuli but also diminished recall for stimuli unrelated to trauma. Subjects were presented with four different types of words: combat words, positive words, neutral words, and social threat words.[25] For the cued-recall portion of the test, subjects were asked to complete three-letter word stems with the missing letters from words that had previously been presented. Both PTSD patients and controls recalled more combat words than other categories of words. To test for a relative bias toward recall of combat words, the number of neutral words recalled was subtracted from the number of words recalled in each of the three other categories (positive, combat, social threat). The PTSD patients remembered more combat words relative to neutral words than did veterans without PTSD. In other words, they showed a relative but not an absolute bias for remembering trauma-related words. As noted by the authors, a relative bias can result from a bias toward remembering trauma words, a bias against remembering neutral or positive words, or both. The results of this study suggest that there may be a bidirectional alteration in memory with enhanced memory for trauma and decreased memory for other stimuli. Data presented in the next section provides some supportive evidence for a deficit in declarative memory for nontraumatic material.

The cued-recall task discussed above tests explicit memory or conscious memory. However, traumatized patients may continue to ''remember'' the trauma in unconscious ways, such as through reenactment or hypervigilance. Therefore, implicit memory for trauma—that is, memory which does not require intentional recollection of the event—was tested as well. Implicit memory was tested by asking subjects to complete three-letter word stems with the first word that comes to mind. PTSD subjects, but not controls, were more likely to complete the stems with combat words than with the other categories of words, confirming that PTSD patients exhibit an implicit memory bias for combat words as well.[25]

At a minimum, these data supplement the clinical impression and other empiric data that traumatic material is represented differently in PTSD patients. Importantly, the bias toward trauma-related material was demonstrated not only for conscious memory but also for unconscious memory. As such, these studies have delineated information-processing abnormalities that may help to explain some of the phenomena of PTSD, such as intrusive thoughts or nightmares. Furthermore the data raise the question of whether the heightened memory for trauma occurs against a background of impaired memory for neutral material, a question which will be further explored below.

Memory for Nontraumatic Stimuli

Several recent studies have demonstrated cognitive impairments in individuals with PTSD that are unrelated to traumatic material. One of the first studies that used formal neuropsychological testing to study traumatized veterans was conducted with WW II veterans some 40 years after the war. Compared to combat veterans, former POWs had impairments in multiple subsets of the Wechsler Adult Intelligence Scale-Revised and the Wechsler Memory Scale.[26] This was an important study in demonstrating the magnitude of cognitive impairment in POWs. The POWs had been exposed to more severe and sustained psychological trauma than the combat veterans and the POWs had a significantly higher rate of PTSD, which raises the question of whether trauma or its sequelae cause cognitive decline. However, the POW group was also more likely to have had head trauma or malnutrition, which likely contributed to the differences. Subsequent studies have attempted to tease apart these factors.

In one study, Vietnam combat veterans with PTSD were found to have significant short- and long-term memory deficits on standard neuropsychological testing as compared with normal controls.[27] The PTSD patients had poorer immediate and delayed recall on the verbal component of the Wechsler Memory Scale and poorer scores on the Selective Reminding Test (they scored lower on all subcomponents of the test, including total recall, long-term retrieval, long-term storage, and consistent long-term retrieval). Importantly, the groups did not differ in important variables that could affect performance, namely, number of years of substance abuse, education, IQ, and not having significant head trauma. This study suggests not only that there may be deficits in memory and attention for nontraumatic stimuli, but also that the deficits may be diffuse and occur at multiple levels of information processing.

Another important question about the cognitive deficits seen in PTSD is whether they are unique or are comparable to the deficits seen in other psychiatric patients. To examine this question Gil et al. compared PTSD patients with a comparison psychiatric group and a normal control group. Twelve Israeli PTSD patients were studied who had been exposed to a range of traumas, including terrorist attacks, car accidents, and attacks while in the army.[28] No significant differences were found between PTSD patients and other psychiatric patients with affective or anxiety disorders who had a similar degree of psychopathology as the PTSD patients, and no history of trauma. The patient groups were balanced in terms of demographics, IQ, and subjective complaints of poor concentration, and they did not differ in any array of verbal and nonverbal memory tests and attention tests. Therefore, while the PTSD patients' performance was impaired, it was comparable in nature and magnitude to that of other nonpsychotic patients.

In contrast, multiple cognitive abnormalities were found in the PTSD group, compared with the normal controls. Importantly, though, the PTSD patients had a significantly lower IQ than the control group (88.1 ± 11.4 vs. 108.1 ± 8.8), which the authors suggest represents a decline from their baseline. Given such a discrepancy in IQ it is unclear whether the diffuse impairments in memory and attention reflect a mismatching of patients and controls or are so significant as to lead to intellectual decline. If the findings represent a true intellectual decline, this is especially remarkable, since patients with identifiable risk factors for organic deficits were excluded (head trauma, alcohol or substance abuse, psychosurgery, electroconvulsive therapy).

In contrast, there are some studies which do not provide support for cognitive impairments. For example, in one study, Vietnam veterans with PTSD ($N = 22$) completed a full neuropsychological battery as part of routine inpatient care and the results were compared to age-scaled norms.[29] On the whole, the group performed in the average range. They did not differ from established norms on the Trail-Making Test, the Serial Digit Learning Test, the Temporal Orientation Test, and the Stroop Color and Word Test. On the Wechsler Adult Intelligence Scale (WAIS) they performed less well on the Digit Span and the Digit Symbol Tests, tests that are susceptible to the effects of anxiety. In another study of Vietnam veterans, neuropsychological testing was performed in tandem with neurological soft signs and EEGs.[30] Medication-free combat veterans with posttraumatic stress disorder were compared to non-PTSD combat controls. The veterans were compared on the Wechsler Memory Scale, the Denman Memory test, the Trail-Making test, the Wisconsin Card Sorting Test, and the Wechsler Adult Intelligence Scale. The PTSD and non-PTSD groups did not differ on these neuropsychological tests. The lack of difference is particularly striking since the PTSD group had more neurological soft-sign abnormalities. In another study of Vietnam veterans with PTSD, multiple cognitive deficits were not found, but circumscribed deficits were.[31] Combat veterans with PTSD were compared with normal controls of equivalent IQ and education. The groups did not differ in initial attention, immediate memory, or cumulative learning on the California Verbal Learning Test, a test of multiserial learning. However, the PTSD patients exhibited a significant amount of retroactive interference; that is, shortly after learning new material they were less able to recall previously learned information. This deficit persisted, thereby decreasing long-term recall of the same previously learned material.

Overall, then, the existing literature provides consistent evidence for information-processing abnormalities involving traumatic material and provocative but inconsistent evidence for abnormalities of neutral material in patients with PTSD. Furthermore, because the above studies were conducted many years after the identified trauma, it is not clear which factors account for the findings. Additional research is clearly needed to better characterize the extent, nature, and course of the deficits.

Potential etiologies for information-processing abnormalities are as diverse as the biological and psychological theories that have been proposed to explain the emergence of PTSD following traumatization. Information regarding the onset of the abnormalities and their course may help elucidate whether the etiologic factors are pretraumatic, peritraumatic, or posttraumatic. Pretraumatic factors could include both preexisting cognitive deficits or predisposing neuropsychological sensitivities. Individuals may have circumscribed or global cognitive deficits prior to being traumatized. When cognitive testing is performed years later, after the trauma, the detected abnormality in information processing would then likely reflect these preexisting deficits as well as both peri- and posttraumatic factors. Clearly, additional prospective studies of at-risk populations (e.g., soldiers, police, firefighters) are needed to determine whether pretraumatic differences in factors such as attention, memory, arousal, cognitive function, hypnotizability, anxiety, or capacity to form images might predict who does and who does not develop PTSD and memory disturbances following trauma.

There are also peritraumatic factors that could affect memory function. The most obvious source for later deficits is the physical trauma that may accompany psychological trauma. Head trauma, malnutrition, hypoxia, and infectious diseases can all have long-term sequelae. Severe stress and psychological trauma itself also cause a whole host of biological changes in the peritraumatic period. There are multiple possible psychic responses to trauma, such as dissociation and denial, which can affect traumatic memory. Fear-conditioning and other learning experiences may contribute to changes in learning and memory. Posttraumatic factors include a multitude of biological abnormalities that have been described in PTSD in the sympathetic nervous system and the hypothalamic pituitary axis, as well as the development of comorbid conditions, such as substance abuse or depression.

Conclusion

In summary, alterations in memory are at the very core of posttraumatic stress disorder. The memory alterations are numerous and diverse. Patients experience these abnormalities through re-experiencing and reliving the trauma, forgetting some aspects of the trauma, being intensely distressed by reminders of the trauma, and having difficulty concentrating. Importantly, the memory alterations seen in PTSD are not seen in all trauma survivors. Patients with PTSD differ from other trauma survivors in their recall of the traumatic event, in the ways in which memory for the event is altered, and in the ways they continue to process information related to victimization. The extent of these memory alterations remains to be elucidated, as there is evidence that a broad range of cognitive functions may be affected. This discussion highlights the profound and myriad effects that severe trauma can exert on memory years after the inciting event. Given the differences between PTSD and non-PTSD survivors, however, the abnormalities seen in PTSD should not be considered synonymous with the effect of trauma on memory. Further research on the onset, course, and magnitude of the memory and attention impairments in PTSD have important implications for understanding the pathophysiology of this frequently disabling disorder.

References

1. Diagnostic and Statistical Manual of Mental Disorders, 4th Ed. (DSM-IV). Washington, DC: American Psychiatric Association, 1994.
2. Herr M: Dispatches. New York: Knopf, 1977.
3. Lyttelton O: From peace to war: A study in contrasts. *In* Fussell P, The Great War in Modern Memory. New York and London: Oxford University Press, 1975, p. 191.
4. Levi P: The Drowned and the Saved. New York: Summit Books, 1988.
5. Easterbrook JA: The effect of emotion on cue utilization and the organization of behavior. Psychol Rev 1959; 66:183–201.

6. Loftus E, Burns T: Mental shock can produce retrograde amnesia. Memory Cogn 1982; 10:318–323.
7. Clifford B, Hollin C: Effects of the type of incident and the number of perpetrators on eyewitness memory. J Appl Psychol 1981; 66:364–370.
8. Clifford B, Scott J: Individual and situational factors in eyewitness identification. J Appl Psychol 1978; 63:352–359.
9. Yarmey AD: The Psychology of Eyewitness Memory. New York: Free Press, 1979.
10. Loftus E: Eyewitness Testimony. Cambridge, MA: Harvard University Press, 1979.
11. Loftus E, Loftus G, Messo J: Some facts about "weapon focus." Law Hum Behav 1987; 11:55–62.
12. Kramer T, Buckhout R, Eugenio P: Weapon focus, arousal and eyewitness memory: attention must be paid. Law Hum Behav 1990; 14:167–184.
13. Kuehn L: Looking down a gun barrel: person perception and violent crime. Percept Motor Skills 1974; 39:1156–1164.
14. Yuille JC, Cutshall JL: A case study of eyewitness memory for a crime. J Appl Psychol 1986; 71:291–301.
15. Wagenaar WA, Groeneweg J: The memory of concentration camp survivors. Appl Cogn Psychol 1990; 4:77–87.
16. McFarlane AC: The longitudinal course of posttraumatic morbidity: the range of outcomes and their predictors. J Nerv Ment Dis 1988; 176:30–39.
17. Kaminer J, Lavie P: Sleep and dreaming in Holocaust survivors: dramatic decrease in dream recall in well-adjusted survivors. J Nerv Ment Dis 1991; 179:664–669.
18. Schwarz ED, Kowalski JM, McNally RJ: Malignant memories: post-traumatic changes in memory in adults after a school shooting. J Traumatic Stress 1993; 6:545–553.
19. Southwick SM, Morgan CA, Nicolaou AI, Charney DS: Consistency of memory for traumatic events. 1996, manuscript.
20. MacLeod CM: Half a century of research on the Stroop effect: an integrative review. Psychol Bull 1991; 109:163–203.
21. Foa EB, Feske U, Murdock TB, Kozak MJ, McCarthy PR: Processing of threat-related information in rape victims. J Abnorm Psychol 1991; 100:156–162.
22. Cassiday KL, McNally RJ, Zeitlin SB: Cognitive processing of trauma cues in rape victims with post-traumatic stress disorder. Cogn Ther Res 1992; 16:283–295.
23. McNally RJ, English GE, Lipke HJ: Assessment of intrusive cognition in PTSD: use of the modified Stroop paradigm. J Traumatic Stress 1993; 6:33–38.
24. McNally RJ, Kaspi SP, Riemann BC, Zeitlin SB: Selective processing of threat cues in posttraumatic stress disorder. J Abnorm Psychol 1990; 99:398–402.
25. Zeitlin SB, McNally RJ: Implicit and explicit memory bias for threat in post-traumatic stress disorder. Behav Res Ther 1991; 29:451–457.
26. Sutker PB, Winstead DK, Galina ZH, Allain AN: Cognitive deficits and psychopathology among former prisoners of war and combat veterans of the Korean conflict. Am J Psychiatry 1991; 148:67–72.
27. Bremner JD, Scott TM, Delaney RC, Southwick SM, Mason JW, Johnson DR, Innis RB, McCarthy G, Charney DS: Deficits in short-term memory in posttraumatic stress disorder. Am J Psychiatry 1993; 150:1015–1019.
28. Gil T, Calec A, Greenberg D, et al: Cognitive functioning in posttraumatic stress disorder. J Traumatic Stress 1990; 1:29–45.
29. Dalton JE, Pederson SL, Blom BE, Besyner: Neuropsychological screening for Vietnam veterans with PTSD. VA Practitioner 1986; 3:37–47.

30. Gurvits TV, Lasko NB, Schachter SC, Kuhne AA, Orr SP, Pitman RK: Neurological status of Vietnam veterans with chronic posttraumatic stress disorder. J Neuropsychiatry Clin Neurosci 1993; 5:183–188.

31. Yehuda R, Keefe RSE, Harvey PD, Levengood RA, Gerber DK, Geni J, Siever LJ: Learning and memory in combat veterans with posttraumatic stress disorder. Am J Psychiatry 1995; 152:137–139.

9

Traumatic Memories

BESSEL A. VAN DER KOLK

Trauma, by definition, is the result of exposure to an inescapably stressful event that overwhelms people's coping mechanisms. This makes the study of traumatic memories a special challenge, since it simply is impossible to present laboratory subjects with the sort of life-threatening stimuli that may give rise to the sensory reexperiences (in the form of flashbacks and nightmares) that are characteristic of postraumatic stress disorder (PTSD). When Roger Pitman (personal communication, 1994) showed normal college students a movie depicting actual executions, even this failed to provoke the sorts of intrusive memories that we see in PTSD. This raises the critical question whether tests using normal subjects exposed to videotaped stresses in the laboratory bear any relevance to the study of how people process traumatic events.

Since the latter part of the nineteenth century there have been numerous descriptions of the ways in which traumatic memories are fundamentally different from the memories of ordinary experience. This started with the explorations of the Frenchman Jean Martin Charcot, the founder of the scientific discipline of neurology, into the nature of "hysteria," which he thought had its origins in psychological trauma. He called traumatic memories the "parasites of the mind."[1] The psychiatric literature of the past century is filled with reports of traumatized people losing all memory for a traumatic event, and subsequently retrieving it in a dissociated state of mind. For example, the accounts of "shell-shock" in World War I are replete with case reports of soldiers who became amnestic for their traumas, which they later relived in the form of nightmares, flashbacks, and behavioral reenactments. E. E. Southard's book *Shellshock and Neuro-*

Parts of this chapter were previously published in van der Kolk BA, Fisler R: Dissociation and the fragmentary nature of traumatic memory. Journal of Traumatic Stress 1995:7:505–526. Reprinted with permission.

psychiatry[2] alone has 23 such detailed case reports. The novelist Pat Barker,[3,4] who in recent years has made the treatment of shell-shocked soldiers in World War I a central theme in her novels, has given poignant descriptions of traumatic memories in her accounts of the treatment of the war neuroses of the poets Siegfried Sassoon and Wilfred Owens by the British psychiatrist W. R. H. Rivers in Craiglockart Hospital. These literary descriptions of the ways traumatized individuals process their memories can be very helpful for professionals who are not in a position to conduct detailed interviews with trauma patients, and who want to gain familiarity with how people reexperience traumatic memories in dissociated states of mind. While novelists are generally better equipped to provide us with such descriptions, the clinical accounts of trauma cases by Janet,[5,6] Kardiner,[7] C. S. Myers,[8] and Lenore Terr[9] sometimes approximate the eloquence and poignancy of the descriptions by novelists. During the past half century psychiatrists and psychologists have largely abandoned detailed case descriptions in favor of enumeration of the relationships between certain symptoms and any number of other variables. This method allows for findings that can be replicated by other scientists in studies of similar design, but it tends to lose the richness of the descriptions of the subjective human experience.

During the past few years, the issue of the delayed retrieval of memories for childhood abuse has become a topic of intense public debate. Interestingly, the issue of delayed recall was not particularly controversial when Charcot (1887) and Janet[10] first described this phenomenon following traumatic life experiences, or when Southard,[2] Myers,[8] and Kardiner[7] gave detailed descriptions of it in their books on combat neuroses. Nor did it create a stir when, after the evacuation from Dunkirk during the Second World War Sargeant and Slater[11] reported that 144 of a thousand consecutive admissions to a field hospital had amnesia for their trauma, or when van de Kolk noted it in Vietnam combat veterans[12,13] and in a survivor of the Cocoanut Grove nightclub fire.[14] As long as men were found to suffer from delayed recall of atrocities committed either by a clearly identifiable enemy, or by themselves, this issue was accepted and incorporated in the canon of the profession (as exemplified by its acceptance in the *Diagnostic and Statistical Manual* (DSM) both under the rubric of *PTSD* and under *dissociative amnesia*). However, when the same memory problems started to be documented in girls and women in the context of domestic abuse, this stirred up an intense public debate, and when female victims started to seek justice against their alleged perpetrators, the issue moved from science into politics.[15] Judith Herman[16] has written extensively about the possible causes for this shift.

The passions raised around the issue of ''false memories'' in sexual abuse victims has prompted some people to ignore the previously collected data about how trauma affects memory and abandon customary scientific restraint. On the one hand, many clinicians seem to have suspended their capacity for doubt and skepticism by uncritically accepting as true all stories of sexual or ''satanic ritual'' abuse in their patients, and many laboratory researchers have overstepped the bounds of their scientific findings by dismissing the relevance of a century of clinical observation on the battlefield, in emergency rooms, and on psychiatric wards. Laboratory experiments of ordinary events have been indiscriminately applied to extraordinary experiences that simply cannot be replicated in a laboratory. The issue of ''false memories'' has become so heated that a leading laboratory researcher on memory distortion simply decided to omit from her own book, *The Myth of Repressed Memory*,[17] not only the numerous clinical studies that have documented this phenomenon, but also her own study that contradicted that ''repression'' is a myth. Prior to the publication of that book, she and her colleagues had documented that 19% of a sample of sexually abused women at some time in their lives had lost all memory of their abuse, and that another 22% had large gaps in their memory.[18]

The ''false memory debate,'' which appears to be primarily a product of the adversarial environment of the court room, is an example of how the method of polarized legal argument may do science a disservice by paying selective attention to only one or the other side of arguments, rather than focusing on the complexity of the issues involved. The adversarial legal environment is devoted to defending the accused; allegiance to truth is not its primary task.[19] During the past few years, under the influence of forensic considerations, rather than clinical realities, hardly any article mentions the fact that traumatic memories are fundamentally different from memories of ordinary experiences. The ferocity of the 'debate' also seems to be responsible for the omission in the press, and in the courtroom, of serious discussions about the nature and extent of therapeutic influence and patient suggestibility. While it is possible for confused or frightened people (confused because of emotional and physical immaturity or organic and psychiatric illnesses, or frightened because their very lives depend on their interrogators, such as occurs to people in states of captivity) to be susceptible to suggestion,[20,21] there have been no published experiments of successful ''implantations'' of the sort of vivid flashbacks that are characteristic of the memories of people who suffer from posttraumatic stress disorder (PTSD).

The Study of Traumatic Memories

The study of traumatic memories questions four basic notions about the nature of memory that have been shown to occur in the laboratory studies of scientists who look at memories of ordinary events: (*1*) that memory is flexible and integrated with other life experiences, (*2*) that memory generally is present in consciousness in a continuous and uninterrupted fashion, (*3*) that memory always disintegrates in accuracy over time, and (*4*) that memory is primarily declarative, i.e., that people generally can articulate what they know in words and symbols. A century of study of traumatic memories shows that (*1*) they generally remain unaffected by other life experiences,[5,6,12] (*2*) they may return, triggered by reminders, at any time during a person's life with a vividness as if the subject is having the experience all over again,[22] and (*3*) these memories are primarily sensory and emotional;[23] they frequently leave victims in a state of speechless terror, in which they may be unable to precisely articulate what they are feeling and thinking.[14,24,25]

Abram Kardiner[7] opened the door for understanding the reason that traumatic memories are different from memories of everyday events. He called the "traumatic neuroses" "*physioneuroses*" psychological problems rooted in biological dysregulation that resulted in an enduring hypervigilance to continuing threat. In recent years, research, such as on hypothalamic–pituitary–adrenal axis abnormalities,[26] has convincingly demonstrated that PTSD has its own distinct neurobiology. Overwhelming social experiences can become indelibly etched in people's memory and set up a cascade of disturbances that can permanently alter their capacity to regulate their biological systems. This biological dysregulation, in turn, affects how people think, feel, and act. While everyday stress evokes homeostatic mechanisms that lead to self-conservation and resource reallocation (e.g., Selye),[27] PTSD involves a unique combination of learned conditioning, problems modulating arousal, and shattered meaning propositions. This complexity is best understood as the co-occurrence of several interlocking pathogenic processes including (*a*) an alternation of neurobiological processes affecting stimulus discrimination (expressed as increased arousal and decreased attention), (*b*) the acquisition of conditioned fear responses to trauma-related stimuli, and (*c*) altered cognitive schemata and social apprehension.[28]

Without the option of inflicting actual trauma in the laboratory, there are limited options for the exploration of traumatic memories. These include collecting retrospective reports from traumatized individuals, observations of individuals as they develop their psychological problems subsequent to a traumatic event, and provoking, then studying, traumatic memories and flashbacks in people with PTSD. Surprisingly, since the early part of this century, there have been very few published studies that systematically explore the nature of traumatic memories based on detailed patient reports. Provocation studies of traumatic memories in the laboratory have examined psychophysiologic responses to visual or auditory stimuli (e.g., Pitman et al.,[29] and Rauch et al.[30]), and biological agents have been shown to promote access to trauma-related memories as well.[31,32]

Comparison of Memories of Stressful Events and of Trauma

Contemporary memory research has demonstrated the complexity of memory systems, with many components and functions that operate outside of conscious awareness, and which seem to operate with a relative degree of independence from each other. *Declarative memory* (also known as *explicit memory*) refers to conscious awareness of facts or events that have happened to the individual.[33] This form of memory functioning is seriously affected by lesions of the frontal lobe and of the hippocampus, which also have been implicated in the neurobiology of PTSD.[34,35] *Nondeclarative memory (im-*

plicit or *procedural memory*) refers to memories of skills and habits, emotional responses, reflexive actions, and classically conditioned responses. Each of these implicit memory systems is associated with particular areas in the central nervous system.[36]

At least since 1889, when Janet[10] first wrote about the relationship between trauma and memory, it has been widely accepted that what is now called declarative, or explicit, memory is an active and constructive process. What a person remembers depends on existing mental schemata: once an event or a particular bit of information is integrated into existing mental schemes, it is no longer available as a separate, immutable entity, but is liable to be altered by associated experiences, demand characteristics, and emotional state at the time of recall.[6,10] As Schachtel[37] defined it: ''Memory as a function of the living personality can be understood as a capacity for the organization and reconstruction of past experiences and impressions in the service of present needs, fears, and interests'' (p. 3).

However, accuracy of memory is affected by how emotionally arousing the experience is for the individual. Personally highly significant events generally are unusually accurate, and tend to remain stable over time.[38–41] Evolution favors the consolidation of personally relevant information. For example, Yuille and Cutshall[42] interviewed 13 out of 22 witnesses to a murder 4–5 months after the event. All witnesses had provided information to the police within two days after the murder. These witnesses were found to have very accurate recall, with little apparent decline over time. The authors concluded that emotional memories of such shocking events are ''detailed, accurate and persistent''[42] (p. 181). They suggested that witnessing real ''traumas'' leads to ''quantitatively different memories than innocuous laboratory events.''

Researchers also have studied the accuracy of memories for less personal, but culturally significant events, such as the murder of President Kennedy and the space shuttle *Challenger*. Brown and Kulik[43] first called memories for such events *''flashbulb memories.''* Whereas people report that these experiences are etched accurately in their minds, research has shown that those memories are subject to some distortion and disintegration over time. For example, Neisser and Harsch[44] found that people changed their recollections of the space shuttle Challenger disaster considerably after a number of years. However, typical for much academic memory research, no attention was paid to the personal significance of this event for the affected individuals. Clinical observations of people who suffer from PTSD suggest that there are important differences between flashbulb memories for more distant events and the intrusive memories characteristic of PTSD. As of early 1995, we could find no scientific literature addressing changes in intrusive recollections of traumatic events in patients suffering from PTSD.

The Apparent Uniqueness of Traumatic Memories

The *Diagnostic and Statistical Manual* definition of PTSD[45] recognizes that trauma can lead to extremes of retention and forgetting: terrifying experiences often are remembered with extreme vividness, but the DSM IV also includes includes amnesia among the diagnostic criteria for PTSD. Elsewhere, it also includes a separate diagnostic entity of *Dissociative Amnesia*. Clinical experience teaches us that traumatized individuals often suffer from a combination of vivid recall for some elements of the trauma, and amnesias for others. While memories of ordinary events disintegrate in clarity over time, some aspects of traumatic events appear to get fixed in the mind and to remain unaltered by the passage of time or by the intervention of subsequent experience. For example, in our studies of posttraumatic nightmares, subjects claimed that they saw the same traumatic scenes over and over again, without modification, over a 15-year period.[12] For the past century, many students of trauma have noted that the imprints of traumatic experiences seem to be qualitatively different from memories of ordinary events. Starting with Janet, accounts of the memories of traumatized patients con sistently mention that emotional and perceptual elements tend to be more prominent than declarative components (e.g., Grinker and Spiegel,[46] Kardiner,[7] and Terr[9]). Schacter[47] has referred to the descriptions of traumatic memories by Janet as examples of implicit memory. These recurrent observations about the nature of traumatic memories have given rise to the notion that traumatic memories may be encoded differently than memories for ordinary events, perhaps via alterations in attentional focusing, perhaps because extreme emotional arousal interferes with hippocampal memory functions.[10,34,39,48–52]

Amnesias and Delayed Recall

Trauma can affect a wide variety of memory functions. For convenience sake, we will categorize these into four different sets of functional disturbances: traumatic amnesia, global memory impairment, dissociative processes, and the sensorimotor organization of traumatic memories.

Traumatic Amnesia

While the vivid intrusions of traumatic images and sensations are the most dramatic expressions of PTSD, the loss or absence of recollections for traumatic experiences is also well documented. Amnesias for some or all aspects of the trauma have been noted in a wide variety of traumatized patients, starting with reports by Janet.[10] More recently, amnesia after natural disasters and accidents, with later return of memories for all or parts of the trauma, has been noted.[53,54] Amnesias, often with delayed recall, also have been reported in numerous other studies of combat soldiers.[2,7,12,13,24,46,55–65] For example, Sargeant and Slater[11] observed the presence of significant amnesia in 144 out of 1,000 consecutively admitted combat soldiers to the Sutton Emergency Hospital during the Second World War. Amnesia also has been documented in victims of kidnapping, torture, and concentration camp experiences,[66–68] in victims of physical and sexual abuse,[18,69–72] and in people who have committed murder.[73] A recent general population study by Elliot and Briere[74] reported complete or partial traumatic amnesia after virtually every form of traumatic experience, with childhood sexual abuse, witnessing murder or suicide of a family member, and combat exposure yielding the highest rates. Hispanics had three times the rates of amnesia following trauma than did Caucasians; there was no relationship between gender or socioeconomic class and the rate of amnesia, and an equal percentage of people in the never-in-therapy group and the group who had received therapy reported episodes of total amnesia for a range of traumatic experiences (about 15% overall).

Traumatic amnesias tend to be age and dose related: the younger the age at the time of the trauma, and the more prolonged the traumatic event, the greater the likelihood of significant amnesia.[69,70,72,75] The best available study on amnesia in victims with documented histories of sexual abuse was conducted by Linda Meyer Williams,[71,72] who reinterviewed a sample of 129 subjects who had been examined for sexual abuse experiences an average of 17 years before. Of these subjects, only 80 (62%) could recall the index sexual abuse which had brought them to the attention of the study. Even among the girls who had been between 7 and 15 years old at the time of the abuse, 30% reported no recall of the incident. Of the subjects who now remembered the index abuse, 16% reported having had total amnesia at some time in their lives. Amnesia was related to age, degree of force used in the sexual abuse, and weak maternal support. If anything, memories of the subjects who reported total amnesia some time in the past were somewhat more accurate than the memories of the subjects who claimed they always remembered. However, the subjects who at some time had forgotten the abuse experienced a greater degree of subjective uncertainty about the accuracy of their recollections.[72] The memories of all subjects in this study in essence reflected what had been reported 17 years before.

Amnesia for these traumatic events may last for hours, weeks, or years. Generally, recall is triggered by exposure to sensory or affective stimuli that match sensory or affective elements associated with the trauma. It is generally accepted that the memory system is made up of networks of related information; activation of one aspect facilitates the recall of associated memories.[76,77] Affect seems to be a critical cue for the retrieval of information along these associative pathways. This means that the affective valence of any particular experience plays a major role in determining what cognitive schemes will be activated. In this regard, it is relevant that many people with trauma histories, such as rape, spouse battering, and child abuse, seem to function quite well as long as feelings related to traumatic memories are not stirred up. However, under particular conditions, they may feel or act as if they were traumatized all over again. Fear is not the only trigger for such recall; any affect related to a particular traumatic experience may serve as a cue for the retrieval of trauma-related sensations, including longing, intimacy, and sexual arousal.

Global Memory Impairment

While amnesias following adult trauma have been well documented, the mechanisms for such memory impairment remains insufficiently understood. This issue is even more complicated when it concerns childhood trauma, since children have fewer mental capacities to construct a coherent narrative out of traumatic events. More research is needed to explore the consistent clinical observation that adults who were chronically traumatized as children suffer from generalized impairment of memories for both cultural and autobiographical events. It is likely that the combination of autobiographical memory gaps and continued reliance on dissociation makes it very hard for these patients to reconstruct a precise account of either their past or their current reality.[78] The combination of lack of autobiographical memory, or continued dissociation, and of meaning schemas that include victimization, helplessness, and betrayal, is likely to make these individuals vulnerable to suggestion and to the construction of explanations for their trauma-related affects that may bear little relationship to the actual realities of their lives.

Trauma and Dissociation

Dissociation refers to a compartmentalization of experience: elements of the experience are not integrated into a unitary whole, but are stored in memory as isolated fragments consisting of sensory perceptions or affective states.[6,79,80] However, the word *dissociation* is currently used to describe four distinct, but interrelated phenomena: (*1*) the sensory and emotional fragmentation of experience, as measured by the Traumatic Memory Inventory (see below); (*2*) depersonalization and derealization at the moment of the trauma (peritraumatic dissociation), as measured by the Peritraumatic Dissociation Experiences Questionnaire (PDEQ);[81] (*3*) ongoing depersonalization and ''spacing out'' in everyday life, as measured by the Dissociative Experiences Scale;[82] and (*4*) containing the traumatic memories within distinct ego-states (dissociative disorder), as measured by the Dissociative Disorders Interview Scale[83] or the SCID-D.[84] The precise interrelationships among these various phenomena remain to be spelled out. Not all people who have vivid sensory intrusions of traumatic events also experience depersonalization, whereas only a small proportion of people who have both of these experiences will go on to chronically dissociate, or to develop a full-blown dissociative disorder.

The British psychiatrist C. S. Meyers[8] described the issue of dissociation in traumatized soldiers as follows: ''The recent emotional experiences of the individual have the upper hand and determine his conduct: the normal has been replaced by what we may call the 'emotional' personality. Gradually or suddenly an 'apparently normal' personality returns—normal save for the lack of all memory of events directly connected with the shock [i.e., trauma], normal save for the manifestation of other ('somatic') hysteric disorders indicative of mental dissociation'' (p. 67). Contemporary research has shown that "spacing out" at the moment of the trauma (peritraumatic dissociation) is a significant long-term predictor for the ultimate development of PTSD.[81,85,86] Bremner et al.[35] found that Vietnam veterans with PTSD reported having experienced higher levels of dissociative symptoms during combat than men who did not develop PTSD. Koopman, Classen, and Spiegel[87] found that dissociative symptoms early in the course of a natural disaster predicted PTSD symptoms 7 months later. A prospective study of 51 injured trauma survivors in Israel[88] found that peritraumatic dissociation was the strongest predictor of PTSD at 6-month follow-up, explaining 30% of the variance in PTSD symptoms over and above the effects of gender, education, age, event severity, and the intrusion, avoidance, anxiety, and depression symptoms that followed the event.

Christianson[89] has described how, when people feel threatened, they experience a significant narrowing of consciousness, and remain focused on the central perceptual details. As people are being traumatized, this narrowing of consciousness sometimes evolves into amnesia for parts of the event, or for the entire experience. Students of traumatized individuals have repeatedly noted that during conditions of high arousal, explicit memory may fail. The individual is left in a state of speechless terror in which he or she lacks words to describe what has happened.[54] However, whereas traumatized individuals may be unable to give a coherent narrative of the incident, there may be no interference with implicit memory; they may "know" the emotional valence of a stimulus and be aware of associated perceptions, without being able to articulate the reasons for feeling or behaving in a particular way.

More than 80 years ago, Janet observed: "Forgetting the event which precipitated the emotion . . . has frequently been found to accompany intense emotional experiences in the form of continuous and retrograde amnesia"[90] (p. 1607). He claimed that when people experience intense emotions, memories cannot be transformed into a neutral narrative: a person is "unable to make the recital which we call narrative memory, and yet he remains confronted by [the] difficult situation"[91] (p. 660). This results in "a phobia of memory"[91] (p. 661) that prevents the integration ("synthesis") of traumatic events and splits off the traumatic memories from ordinary consciousness. Janet claimed that the memory traces of the trauma linger as what he called "unconscious fixed ideas" that cannot be "liquidated" as long as they have not been translated into a personal narrative. Failure to organize the memory into a narrative leads to the intrusion of elements of the trauma into consciousness as terrifying perceptions, obsessional preoccupations, and as somatic reexperiences, such as anxiety reactions.[6,90]

Similar observations have been made by other clinicians treating traumatized individuals. For example, in 1945 Grinker and Spiegel noted that some combat soldiers developed excessive emotionality under stress, which they thought to be responsible for the development of a permanent disorder: "Fear and anger in small doses are stimulating and alert the ego, increasing efficacy. But, when stimulated by repeated psychological trauma the intensity of the emotion heightens until a point is reached at which the ego loses its effectiveness and may become altogether crippled.''[46] (p. 82). Grinker and Spiegel described traumatic amnesias in these soldiers, which were accompanied by confusion, mutism, and stupor. Kardiner, in *The Traumatic Neuroses of War*,[7] noted that when patients develop amnesia for the trauma, it tends to generalize to a large variety of symptomatic expressions: ''[t]he subject acts as if the original traumatic situation were still in existence and engages in protective devices which failed on the original occasion'' (p. 82). Kardiner noted that fixation occurs in dissociative fugue states. Triggered by a sensory stimulus, a patient might lash out, employing language suggestive of his trying to defend himself during a military assault. He noted that many such patients, while riding a subway train that entered a tunnel, had flashbacks to being back in the trenches. Kardiner also viewed panic attacks and hysterical paralyses as the reexperiencing of fragments of the trauma. Piaget[92] claimed that dissociation occurs when an active failure of semantic memory leads to the organization of memory on somatosensory or iconic levels. He pointed out: ''It is precisely because there is no immediate accommodation that there is complete dissociation of the inner activity from the external world. As the external world is solely represented by images, it is assimilated without resistance (i.e., unattached to other memories) to the unconscious ego''.

The realization of the role of dissociation in the processing of traumatic memories was revived for contemporary psychiatry when Horowitz[93] described an ''acute catastrophic stress reaction'' in civilian trauma victims, which was characterized by panic, cognitive disorganization, disorientation, and dissociation. Such dissociative processing of traumatic experience complicates the capacity to communicate about the trauma. In some people the memories of trauma may have no verbal (explicit) component at all; the memory may be entirely organized on an implict or perceptual level, without an accompanying narrative about what happened. Recent symptom-provocation neuroimaging studies of people with PTSD support that clinical observation. During the provocation of traumatic memories there was decreased activation of Broca's area, the part of the CNS most centrally involved in the transformation of subjective experience into speech. Simultaneously, the areas in the right hemisphere that are thought to process intense emotions and visual images had significantly increased activation.[30]

People who have learned to cope with trauma by dissociating are vulnerable to continuing to do so in response to minor stresses. The repeated use of dissociation as a way of coping with stress interferes with the capacity to fully attend to life's challenges. The severity of ongoing dissociative processes (often measured with the Dissociative Experiences Scale [DES])[82] has been correlated with a large variety of psychopathological conditions that are thought to be associated with histories of trauma and neglect: severity of sexual abuse in adolescents,[94] somatization,[95] bulimia,[96] self-mutilation,[97] and borderline personality disorder.[98] The most extreme example of this ongoing dissociation occurs in people who suffer from dissociative identity disorder (multiple personality disorder), who have the highest DES scores of all populations studied and in whom separate identities seem to contain the memories related to different traumatic incidents.[99]

The Perceptual Organization of Traumatic Experience

Numerous authors on trauma, for example Janet,[5,10] Kardiner,[7] and Terr,[9] have observed that trauma is organized in memory at sensorimotor and affective levels. Having listened to the narratives of traumatic experiences from hundreds of traumatized children and adults over the past 20 years, my colleagues and I frequently have heard both adults and children describe how traumatic experiences initially are organized without semantic representations. Clinical experience and our reading of a century of observations by clinicians dealing with a variety of traumatized populations led us to postulate that "memories" of the trauma tend to, at least initially, be experienced primarily as fragments of the sensory components of the event: as visual images, olfactory, auditory, or kinesthetic sensations, or intense waves of feelings (which patients usually claim to be representations of elements of the original traumatic event). What is intriguing is that patients consistently claim that their perceptions are exact representations of sensations at the time of the trauma. For example, when Southwick and his group injected yohimbine into Vietnam veterans with PTSD, half of their subjects reported flashbacks that they claimed to be "just like it was" [in Vietnam].[32]

In order to examine the retrieval of traumatic memories in a systematic way, we designed a structured interview, the Traumatic Memory Inventory (TMI), which inquires about sensory, affective, and narrative ways of remembering, about triggers for unbidden recollections of traumatic memories, and about ways of mastering unwanted intrusions of traumatic memories in subjects' lives. We now have conducted two studies[23,100] in which people first traumatized as adults, and 32 subjects first traumatized as children were interviewed with the Traumatic Antecedents Questionnaire (self-rating version) (TAQ[S]), a 78-item questionnaire to identify exposure to traumatic life events,[96,97] as well as the Traumatic Memory Inventory.[23]

The TMI is a 60-item structured interview that systematically collects data about the circumstances and means of memory retrieval of a target traumatic memory and a target memory of a personally highly emotionally significant, but nontraumatic, event. The TMI interview inquires about (*1*) the nature of the trauma(s)/events(s); (*2*) its duration; (*3*) whether the subject has always been aware that the trauma/event happened, and if not, when and where she/he became conscious of it; (*4*) circumstances under which the subject first experienced intrusive memories, and circumstances under which they occur presently; and (*5*) sensory modalities in which memories were experienced. Such sensory modalities include (*a*) a story, (*b*) an image (what did you see?), (*c*) sounds (what did you hear?), (*d*) a smell (what did you smell?), (*e*) feelings in one's body (what did you feel? where?), and (*f*) emotions (what did you feel, what was it like?). These data were collected for three time periods: initially, while subject was most bothered by the memory, and currently. The TMI interview also asked about (*6*) the nature of flashbacks; (*7*) the nature of nightmares; (*8*) precipitants of flashbacks and nightmares; (*9*) ways of mastering intrusive recollections (e.g., by eating, working, taking drugs or alcohol, cleaning, etc.); and (*10*) whether confirmation of the event was available through court or hospital records, direct witnesses, or other means. All information was collected first for the traumatic event, then for the nontraumatic event. Twenty-seven of the 36 subjects with childhood trauma (75%) reported confirmation of their childhood trauma from a mother, sibling, or other source who knew about the abuse, from court or hospital records, or from confessions or convictions of the perpetrator(s).

All subjects, regardless of when they were traumatized, reported that initially they failed to be able to construct a narrative for the traumatic event. All subjects, regardless of age at which the first trauma occurred, reported that they initially ''remembered'' the trauma in the form of somatosensory or emotional flashback experiences. At the peak of their intrusive recollections all sensory modalities were enhanced, and a narrative memory started to emerge. Currently, since most subjects continue to have PTSD, the majority continue to experience their trauma in sensorimotor modes, but 89% also are able to narrate a satisfactory story about what happened to them. In the second study, in which we compared the memory retrieval process in traumatized adults with those of adults who had been traumatized as children, we found no significant differences between these two groups in regards to their sensorimotor organization of traumatic memory, with the sole exception that the adults tended to retrieve their memories more frequently as auditory flashbacks. This can be easily understood by the information that many of the traumatized adults had been in serious automobile accidents, which tend to have a significant auditory component, while those who had been traumatized as children more often remembered their traumas as smells, something that can be easily understood by the fact that many of their traumas were sexual in nature.

Our studies showed that there are critical differences between the ways people experience traumatic memories versus other memories of significant personal but non-traumatic events. They also support the idea that it is the very nature of traumatic memory to be dissociated and to be initially stored as sensory fragments without a coherent semantic component. All of the subjects in our study claimed that they only came to develop a narrative of their trauma over time. Five of the subjects who claimed to have been abused as children were, even as adults, unable to tell a complete narrative of what had happened to them. They merely had fragmentary memories that supported other people's stories, and their own intuitive feelings, that they had been abused.

All these subjects, regardless of the age at which the trauma occurred, claimed that they initially ''remembered'' the trauma in the form of somatosensory flashback experiences. These flashbacks occurred in a variety of modalities: visual, olfactory, affective, auditory and kinesthetic, but initially these sensory modalities did not occur together. As the trauma came into consciousness with greater intensity, more sensory modalities came into awareness. Initially, the traumatic experiences were not condensed into a narrative. It appears that as people become aware of more and more elements of the traumatic experience, they construct a narrative that ''explains'' what happened to them. This transcription of the intrusive sensory elements of the trauma into a personal narrative does not necessarily have a one-to-one correspondence with what actually happened. This process of weaving a narrative out of the disparate sensory elements of an experience is probably not dissimilar from how people construct a narrative under ordinary conditions. However, when people have day-to-day, nontraumatic experiences, the sensory elements of the experience are not registered separately in consciousness, but are automatically integrated into the personal narrative.

This study supports Piaget's notion that when memories cannot be integrated on a semantic/linguistic level, they tend to be organized more primitively as visual images or somatic sensations. Even after considerable periods of time, and even after acquiring a personal narrative for the traumatic experience, most subjects reported that these experiences continued to come back as sensory perceptions and as affective states. The persistence of intrusive sensations related to the trauma after the construction of a narrative contradicts the notion that learning to put the traumatic experience into words will reliably help abolish the occurrence of flashbacks.

Conclusions

When people receive common or nontraumatic sensory input, they generally are able to synthesize this incoming information into narrative form, without conscious awareness of the processes that translate sensory impressions into a personal story. Our research shows that, conversely, traumatic experiences in people with PTSD are initially imprinted as sensations or feeling states that are not immediately transcribed into personal narratives. This failure of information processing on a symbolic level following trauma is at the very core of the pathology of PTSD.[13]

Recently, we collaborated in a neuroimaging symptom-provocation study of some of the subjects who were part of the memory study referred to above. When these subjects experienced flashbacks in the laboratory, there was significantly increased activity in the areas in the right hemisphere that are associated with the processing of emotional experiences, as well as in the right visual association cortex. At the same time, there was significantly decreased activity in Broca's area, in the left hemisphere.[30] These findings are in line with the results of our study: that traumatic "memories" per se consist of emotional and sensory states, with little verbal representation. In other work we have hypothesized that, under conditions of extreme stress, the hippocampally based memory categorization system fails, leaving memories to be stored as affective and perceptual states.[34] This hypothesis proposes that excessive arousal at the moment of the trauma interferes with the effective memory processing of the experience. The resulting speechless terror leaves memory traces that may remain unmodified by the passage of time, and by further experience.

A century of observations of traumatized individuals indicates that there are clear distinctions between traumatic and ordinary memory. Traumatic memory initially consists of images, sensations, affective, and behavioral states that do not seem to change over time. As people develop a narrative about what has happened to them, these narratives tend to coexist with these sensory reliving experiences which are highly state-dependent and cannot be evoked at will. In contrast, narrative (explicit, or declarative) memory is semantic and symbolic, it is social, and it can be adapted to the needs of both the narrator and the listener and can be expanded or contracted, according to social demands.

The question of whether the sensory perceptions reported by our subjects are accurate representations of the sensory imprints at the time of the trauma is intriguing. The study of flashbulb memories has shown that the relationship between emotionality, vividness, and confidence is very complex, and does not necessarily reflect accuracy. While it is possible that these imprints are, in fact, reflections of the sensations experienced at the moment of the trauma, an alternative explanation is that increased activity of the amygdala at the moment of recall may be responsible for the subjective assignment of accuracy and personal significance. Once these sensations are transcribed into a personal narrative, they would presumably be subject to the laws that govern explicit memory: to become a socially communicable story that is subject to condensation, embellishment, and contamination. Thus, while trauma may leave indelible sensory and affective imprints, once these are incorporated into a personal narrative, this semantic memory, like all explicit memory, is likely to be subject to varying degrees of distortion.

There clearly is a need for further studies of dissociative processes and their relationship to the development and maintenance of PTSD. However, in the process of trying to gain a deeper understanding of traumatic memories, great caution should be exercised against making careless generalizations that infer how traumatic memories are stored and retrieved from laboratory experiments involving less overwhelming experiences.

References

1. Charcot JM: Leçons sur les Maladies du Système Nerveux Faites à La Salpetriere (Lessons on the Illnesses of the Nervous System Held at the Salpetriere) Tome III. Paris: Progres Medical en A. Delahaye & Lecrosnie, 1887.
2. Southard EE: Shell-shock and Other Neuropsychiatric Problems. Boston: WW Leonard, 1919.
3. Barker P: Regeneration. New York: Viking, 1991.
4. Barker P: The Eye in the Door. New York: Viking, 1993.
5. Janet P: L'amnesie continue. Rev Gen Sci 1893; 4:167–179.
6. van der Kolk BA, van der Hart O: The intrusive past: the flexibility of memory and the engraving of trauma. Am Imago 1991; 48(4):425–454.
7. Kardiner A: The Traumatic Neuroses of War. New York: Hoeber, 1941.
8. Myers CS: Shell Shock in France 1914–18. Cambridge: Cambridge University Press, 1940.
9. Terr L: Unchained Memories. New York: Basic Books, 1993.
10. Janet P: L'automatisme psychologique. Paris: Alcan, 1889.
11. Sargeant W, Slater E: Amnesic syndromes in war. Proc R Soc Med 1941; 34:757–764.

12. van der Kolk BA, Blitz R, Burr WA, Hartmann E: Nightmares and trauma: life-long and traumatic nightmares in veterans. Am J Psychiatry 1984; 141:187–190.
13. van der Kolk BA, Ducey CP: The psychological processing of traumatic experience: Rorschach patterns in PTSD. J Traumatic Stress 1989; 2:259–274.
14. van der Kolk BA: Psychological Trauma. Washington DC: American Psychiatric Press, 1987.
15. van der Kolk BA, McFarlane AC (Eds.): Traumatic Stress: Effects of Overwhelming Experiences on Mind, Body, and Society. New York: Guilford Press, 1996.
16. Herman JL: Trauma and Recovery. New York: Basic Books, 1992.
17. Loftus EF: The Myth of Repressed Memory. New York: St. Martin Press, 1994.
18. Loftus EF, Polensky S, Fullilove MT: Memories of childhood sexual abuse: remembering and repressing. Psychol Women Q 1994; 18:67–84.
19. McFarlane AC, van der Kolk BA: Conclusion and future directions. In BA van der Kolk, AC McFarlane, L Weisaeth (Eds.), Traumatic Stress: Effects of Overwhelming Stress on Mind, Body and Society. New York: Guilford, 1996, pp. 559–575.
20. Gudjohnsson GH: The Psychology of Interrogations, Confessions and Testimony. New York: Wiley, 1992.
21. Brown D, Sheflin A, Hammond C: Memory, Trauma Treatment and the Law. Hillsdale NJ: Erlbaum. In press.
22. Elliot DM, Fox B: Delayed recall of child abuse memories: prevalence and triggers to memory recall. Paper presented at the annual meeting of the International Society of Traumatic Stress Studies. Chicago IL, November 1994.
23. van der Kolk BA, Fisler RA: Dissociation and the fragmentary nature of traumatic memories: overview and exploratory study. J Traumatic Stress 1995; 8:505–526.
24. Rivers WHR: The repression of war experience. Lancet 1918; 173–177.
25. Blank AS: The unconscious flashback to the war in Viet Nam veterans: clinical mystery, legal defense, and community problem. In SM Sonnenberg, AS Blank, JA Talbott (Eds.), The Trauma of War: Stress and Recovery in Viet Nam Veterans. Washington DC: American Psychiatric Press, 1985, pp. 293–308.
26. Yehuda R, Giller EL, Southwick SM, Lowy MT, Mason JW: Hypothalmic-pituitary-adrenal dysfunction in posttraumatic stress disorder. Biol Psychiatry 191; 30:1031–1048.
27. Selye H: The Stress of Life. New York: McGraw-Hill, 1956.
28. Shalev AY: Stress versus traumatic stress: from acute homeostatic reactions to chronic psychopathology. In AC McFarlane, BA van der Kolk, L Weisaeth (Eds.), Traumatic Stress: Effects of Overwhelming Experience on Mind, Body, and Society. New York: Guilford Press, 1996, pp. 77–101.
29. Pitman RK, Orr SP, Forgue DF, deJong J, Clairborn JM: Psychophysiologic assessment of posttraumatic stress disorder imagery in Vietnam combat veterans. Arch Gen Psychiatry 1987; 17:970–975.
30. Rauch S, van der Kolk BA, Fisler R, Orr SP, Alpert NM, Savage CR, Fischman AJ, Jenike MA, Pitman RK: PET imagery: positron emission scans of traumatic imagery in PTSD patients. Arch Gen Psychiatry 1996; 53:380–387.
31. Rainey JM, Aleem A, Ortiz A, Yaragani V, Pohl R, Berchow R: Laboratory procedure for the inducement of flashbacks. Am J Psychiatry 1987; 144:1317–1319.
32. Southwick SM, Krystal JH, Morgan A, Johnson D, Nagy L, Nicolaou A, Henninger GR, Charney DS: Abnormal noradrenergic function in posttraumatic stress disorder. Arch Gen Psychiatry 1993; 50:266–274.
33. Squire LR, Zola Morgan S: The medial temporal lobe memory system. Science 1991; 153:2380–2386.

34. van der Kolk BA: The body keeps the score: memory and the evolving psychobiology of posttraumatic stress. Harvard Rev Psychiatry 1994; 1:253–265.
35. Bremner JD, Randall P, Scott TM, Bronen RA, Seibyl JP, Southwick SM, Delaney RC, McCarthy G, Charney DS, Innis RB: MRI-based measures of hippocampal volume in patients with PTSD. Am J Psychiatry 1995; 152:973–981.
36. Squire LR: Declarative and nondeclarative memory: multiple brain systems supporting learning and memory. *In* DL Schacter, E Tulving (Eds.), Memory Systems. Cambridge MA: MIT Press, 1994, pp. 203–231.
37. Schachtel EG: On memory and childhood amnesia. Psychiatry 1947; 10:1–26.
38. Bohannon JN: Flashbulb memories for the Space Shuttle disaster: a tale of two theories. Cognition 1988; 29:179–196.
39. Christianson SA: Emotional stress and eyewitness memory: a critical review. Psychol Bull 1992; 112:284–309.
40. Pillemer DB: Flashbulb memories of the assassination attempt on president Reagan. Cognition 1984; 16:63–80.
41. Yuille JC, Cutshall JL: A case study of eyewitness memory of a crime. J Appl Psychol 1986; 71:318–323.
42. Yuille JC, Cutshall JL: Analysis of the statements of victims, witnesses and suspects. *In* JC Yuille (Ed.), Credibility Assessment. Dordecht: Klewer Academic Publishers, 1989.
43. Brown R, Kulik J: Flashbulb memories. Cognition 1977; 5:73–99.
44. Neisser U, Harsch N: Phantom flashbulbs: false recollections of hearing the news about Challenger. *In* E Winograd, U Neisser (Eds.), Affect and Accuracy in Recall: Studies of "Flashbulb Memories." Cambridge: Cambridge University Press, 1992, pp. 9–31.
45. American Psychiatric Association: Diagnostic and Statistical Manual of Mental Disorders (4th ed.). Washington DC: American Psychiatric Association, 1994.
46. Grinker RR, Spiegel JP: Men Under Stress. Philadelphia: Blakiston, 1945.
47. Schacter DL: Implicit memory: history and current status. J Exp Psychol Learn Mem Cogn 1987; 13:510–518.
48. Heuer F, Rausberg D: Emotion, arousal, and memory for detail. *In* SA Christianson (Ed.), The Handbook of Emotion and Memory. Hillsdale NJ: Erlbaum, 1992, pp. 151–180.
49. LeDoux JE: Emotion as memory: in search of systems and synapses. Ann NY Acad Sci 1993; 702:149–157.
50. McGaugh JL, Introini-Collison IB, Cahill LF, Castellano C, Dalmaz C, Parent MB, Williams CL: Affect, neuromodulatory systems, and memory storage: role of the amygdala. Behav Brain Res 1993; 58(1–2):81–90.
51. Nilsson LG, Archer T: Biological aspects of memory and emotion: affect and cognition. *In* SA Christianson (Ed.), Handbook of Emotion and Memory. Hillsdale NJ: Erlbaum, 1992, pp. 289–306.
52. Pitman RK, Orr S, Shalev A: Once bitten twice shy: beyond the conditioning model of PTSD. Biol Psychiatry 1993; 33:145–146.
53. Madakasira S, O'Brian K: Acute postraumatic stress disorder in victims of a natural disaster. J Nerv Ment Dis 1987; 175:286–290.
54. van der Kolk BA, Kadish W: Amnesia, dissociation, and the return of the repressed. *In* BA van der Kolk (Ed.), Psychological Trauma. Washington DC: American Psychiatric Press, 1987, pp. 173–190.
55. Myers CS: A contribution to the study of shell-shock. Lancet 1915; January:316–320.
56. Oppenheim R: L'amnesia traumatique chez les blessés. Progr Med 1917; 189–199.
57. Gregor: Granatenkontusion mit ausgedehntem amnestichen Defekt. Munch Med 1915; 62:1055.

58. Babinski J: Discussion de la conduite à tenir vis-à-vis des blessures du crane-par P Marie. Rev Neurol 1916; 29:464.
59. Schlesinger H: Fall von hochgradiger retrograder Amnesie nach Gehirnverletzung. Wien Med Wochnschr 1915; 49:1815.
60. Archibald HC, Tuddenham RD: Persistent stress reaction after combat. Arch Gen Psychiatry 1956; 12:475–481.
61. Hendin H, Haas AP, Singer P: The reliving experience in Vietnam veterans with postraumatic stress disorder. Compr Psychiatry 1984; 25:165–173.
62. Kubie LS: Manual of emergency treatment for acute war neuroses. War Med 1943; 4:582–599.
63. Sonnenberg SM, Blank AS, Talbott JA: The Trauma of War: Stress and Recovery in Vietnam Veterans. Washington, DC: American Psychiatric Press, 1985.
64. Thom DA, Fenton N: Amnesias in war cases. Am J Insanity 1920; 76:437–448.
65. van der Kolk BA, Roth S, Pelcovitz D: Complex PTSD: Results of the PTSD Field Trials for DSM IV. Washington DC: American Psychiatric Association, 1993.
66. Goldfeld AE, Mollica RF, Pesavento BH, Faraone SV: The physical and psychological sequalae of torture: symptomology and diagnosis. JAMA 1988; 259:2725–2729.
67. Kinzie JD: Posttraumatic effects and their treatment among Southeast Asian refugees. *In* JP Wilson, B Raphael (Eds.), International Handbook of Traumatic Stress Syndromes. New York: Plenum Press, 1993, 311–319.
68. Niederland WG: Clinical observations on the ''survivor syndrome.'' Int J Psychoanal 1968; 49:313–315.
69. Briere J, Conte J: Self-reported amnesia for abuse in adults molested as children. J Traumatic Stress 1993; 6(1):21–31.
70. Herman JE, Shatzow E: Recovery and verification of memories of childhood sexual trauma. Psychoanal Psychol 1987; 4:1–14.
71. Williams LM: Adult memories of childhood abuse. J Consult Clin Psychol 1994; 62(6):1167–1176.
72. Williams LM: Recovered memories of abuse in women with documented child sexual victimization histories. J Traumatic Stress 1995; 8:649–676.
73. Schacter DL: Amnesia and crime: how much do we really know? Am Psychol 1986; 41(3):286–295.
74. Elliot DM, Briere J: Posttraumatic stress associated with delayed recall of sexual abuse: a general population study. J Traumatic Stress 1995; 8(4):629–648.
75. van der Kolk BA, Roth S, Pelcovitz D: Complex PTSD: Results of the PTSD Field Trials for DSM IV. Washington DC: American Psychiatric Association, 1993.
76. Collins AM, Loftus EF: A spreading activation theory of semantic processing. Psychol Bull 1975; 82:407–428.
77. Leichtman MD, Ceci S, Ornstein PA: The influence of affect on memory: mechanism and development. *In* SA Christianson (Ed.), Handbook of Emotion and Memory. Hillsdale NJ: Erlbaum, 1992, pp. 181-199.
78. Cole P, Putnam FW: Effect of incest on self and social functioning: a developmental psychopathology perspective. J Consult Clin Psychol 1992; 60:174–184.
79. Nemiah JC: Early concepts of trauma, dissociation and the unconscious: their history and current implications. *In* D Bremner, C Marmar (Eds.), Trauma, Memory and Dissociation. Washington DC: American Psychiatric Press, 1996, in press.
80. van der Kolk BA, van der Hart O: Pierre Janet and the breakdown of adaptation in psychological trauma. Am J Psychiatry 1989; 146:1530–1540.

81. Marmar CR, Weiss DS, Schlenger WE, Fairbank JA, Jordan K, Kulka RA, Hough RL: Peritraumatic dissociation and post-traumatic stress in male Vietnam theater veterans. Am J Psychiatry 1994; 151:902–907.
82. Bernstein EM, Putnam F: Development, reliability, and validity of a dissociation scale. J Nerv Ment Dis 1986; 174(12):727–735.
83. Ross CA, Heber S, Norton GR, Anderson D, Anderson G, Barchet P: The dissociative disorders interview schedule. Dissociation 1989; 2:169–189.
84. Steinberg M, Rounsaville B, Cicchetti D: Detection of dissociative disorders in psychiatric patients by a screening instrument and a structured diagnostic interview. Am J Psychiatry 1991; 148:1050–1054.
85. Holen A: A Long-term Outcome Study of Survivors from Disaster. Oslo: University of Oslo Press, 1990.
86. Spiegel D: Dissociation and trauma. *In* American Psychiatric Press Annual Review of Psychiatry, vol 10. Edited by Tasman A, Goldfinger SM. Washington DC: American Psychiatric Press, 1991, pp. 261–276.
87. Koopman C, Classen C, Spiegel D: Predictors of posttraumatic stress symptoms among survivors of the Oakland/Berkeley, California firestorm. Am J Psychiatry 1994; 151:888–894.
88. Shalev AY, Orr SP, Pitman RK: Psychophysiologic assessment of traumatic imagery in Israeli civilian patients with posttraumatic stress disorder. Am J Psychiatry 1993; 150:620–624.
89. Christianson SA: The relationship between induced emotional arousal and amnesia. Scand J Psychol 1984; 25:147–160.
90. Janet P: Les Nervoses. Paris: Flammarion, 1909.
91. Janet P: Psychological Healing, Vols 1–2. New York: Macmillan, 1925. (Original published as Les Medications Psychologiques, Vols 1–3. Paris: Alcan, 1919).
92. Piaget J: Play, Dreams, and Imitation in Childhood. New York: Longmans, Green, 1962.
93. Horowitz MJ: Stress Response Syndromes. New York: Aronson, 1978.
94. Sanders B, Giolas MH: Dissociation and childhood trauma in psychologically disturbed adolescents. Am J Psychiatry 1991; 148(1):50–54.
95. Saxe GN, Chinman G, Berkowitz R, Hall K, Lieberg G, Schwartz J, van der Kolk BA: Somatization in patients with dissociative disorders. Am J Psychiatry 1994; 151:1329–1335.
96. Demitrack MA, Putnam FW, Brewerton TD, Brandt HA, Gold PW: Relation of clinical variables to dissociative phenomena in eating disorders. Am J Psychiatry 1990; 147:1184–1188.
97. van der Kolk BA, Perry JC, Herman JL: Childhood origins of self-destructive behavior. Am J Psychiatry 1991; 148:1665–1671.
98. Herman JL, Perry JC, van der Kolk BA: Childhood trauma in borderline personality disorder. Am J Psychiatry 1989; 146:490–495.
99. Putnam FW: Diagnosis and Treatment of Multiple Personality Disorder. New York: Guilford, 1989.
100. van der Kolk BA, The psychobiology of traumatic memory: implications from recent neuroimaging studies. Ann NY Acad Sci 1997, In press.

10

Continuous Memory, Amnesia, and Delayed Recall of Childhood Trauma: A Clinical Typology

MARY R. HARVEY
JUDITH L. HERMAN

The phenomenon of delayed recall of traumatic childhood events has recently drawn the attention of the popular media, clinical practitioners, and academic investigators. Because a number of states now allow victims of childhood abuse to file charges once they have achieved majority age,[1,2] or have acquired new memories of childhood events,[3,4] some perpetrators who were once beyond the reach of the law have been convicted or held liable for crimes committed in the distant past. Successful prosecution of a few highly publicized court cases has prompted defense attorneys and some academic investigators to question the accuracy, authenticity, and forensic legitimacy of child abuse claims brought forward by adult complainants. Loftus, for example, speculates that most, if not all, delayed memories of childhood trauma are confabulations, implanted in the minds of suggestible patients by naive or unscrupulous psychotherapists.[5] Ofshe and Watters posit a virtual epidemic of fictitious claims of childhood abuse, supposedly resulting from intense pressures placed on vulnerable patients by practitioners whom they label "recovered memory therapists."[6] These authors, in particular, bolster their speculations with demeaning characterizations of psychotherapy patients and practitioners. Whatever research may ultimately reveal about the accuracy of traumatic recall and the authenticity of adult memories of childhood trauma, these polemics go far beyond the reach of available data and cast a chill on serious scientific dialogue.[7,8,9]

The confabulation hypothesis has two major flaws. First, and most importantly, it

Parts of this chapter were adapted with permission from Harvey MR, Herman JL: Amnesia, partial amnesia and delayed recall among adult survivors of childhood trauma. Consciousness and Cognition 1994; 3:295–306.

disregards the evidence from documented cases in which the reports of adults who remembered childhood abuse after a period of amnesia have been confirmed by admission of the perpetrator.[10,11] Secondly, it fails to explain how an individual might be induced (by a psychotherapist or anyone else) to reconcile the contradiction between newly acquired, wholly fictitious memories of childhood trauma and prior (presumably more accurate) memories of happy family life. There is no empirical evidence that psychotherapists have the degree of suggestive power that would ordinarily be required to produce this remarkable effect. Indeed, there is no empirical evidence that psychotherapists play any role whatsoever in the majority of cases of delayed recall.

Clinicians do, however, see many patients reporting histories of psychological trauma. We propose that a more appropriate point of departure for the study of traumatic memory is to be found in careful and respectful attention to the large existing body of relevant clinical data. Memory disturbances have been described in many traumatized populations, including disaster and accident victims, combat veterans, and concentration camp survivors.[12,13] Indeed, amnesia is recognized as one of the cardinal symptoms of posttraumatic stress disorder.[14] Reports of childhood abuse are relatively common in the clinical presentations of adult psychotherapy patients. For example, Andrews et al., in a survey of 810 British psychologists, found that 92% had seen at least one patient reporting childhood sexual abuse in the previous year.[15] Dissociative symptoms, including amnesia, have been particularly noted in many clinical studies of adult survivors of childhood abuse.[16–19]

Nine retrospective studies, employing varying methodologies, have specifically addressed the question of memory continuity in adult survivors of childhood abuse. Six are studies of patients in treatment,[20–25] and three are community studies.[26,27,28] All studies find a spectrum of memory disturbances, with some subjects reporting continuous memory of their childhood abuse and some reporting a period of partial or complete amnesia. The proportion of subjects reporting a period of complete amnesia ranges from 19% to 59%, with most studies reporting between 20% and 50%.

In addition to the clinical studies, two community studies have focused on subjects whose recall of childhood abuse could be independently corroborated. Grassian and Holtzen surveyed 42 men and women who had been victims of sexual abuse by a parish priest; of these subjects, 47% reported a period in which they had no memory of the abuse.[28] The perpetrator, who acknowledged molesting numerous children over the course of many years, was ultimately convicted of his crimes. In a prospective study of 129 women with documented histories of childhood sexual abuse, Williams reported that 38% failed to recall the incidents described in their medical records.[29] An additional 16% described a previous period of amnesia followed by delayed recall of the abuse.[30] Subjects reporting amnesia and delayed recall did not differ from those with continuous memory in the accuracy of their reports. This study, which far surpasses the retrospective clinical literature in sophistication of research design and methodology, nevertheless produces results that are quite consistent with previous clinical reports.

Several clinical studies have also addressed the issue of corroboration of patient accounts of childhood trauma. Herman and Schatzow found that a majority (74%) of 53 outpatients reporting histories of childhood sexual abuse also reported obtaining confirming evidence from independent sources. Patients with delayed recall did not differ from those with continuous memory in their ability to obtain confirmation.[20] In a study of female adolescent patients, Westen et al. obtained independent confirmation in all 14 cases where childhood sexual abuse was reported.[31] Coons, in a chart review of inpatients with dissociative disorders, reported collateral information confirming the patients' accounts of childhood abuse in 20 out of 21 cases (95%).[32] And Silk et al. obtained independent confirmation of patients' reports of childhood sexual abuse from family interviews in 8 or 11 cases (73%).[33] These consistent results indicate that patients' retrospective reports of childhood trauma are generally credible and present no unusual problems with verification. The presumption that patients in psychotherapy might be particularly prone to confabulate a trauma history is not borne out by these data.

A Clinical Typology of Traumatic Recall

Each year the client population served by The Cambridge Hospital Victims of Violence Program includes approximately 50 adults who report at least one instance of sexual or physical abuse before age 18. It is our impression that the majority of these patients do not enter psychotherapy solely or even primarily to acquire new memories of a suspected abuse history, but for help in understanding and managing the distress associated with memories already acquired. Some are hoping to contain a flood of intrusive and unwelcome remembrances; some are wanting to understand better the psychological impact of histories that are at least partially recalled; and some are wanting to give context, comprehensibility, and meaning to a bizarre and troubling assortment of fragmentary images that they do not know how to interpret. Most bring into psychotherapy a combination of long-remembered and more recently recalled material.

Amnesia following psychological trauma is not a simple, all-or-none phenomenon, but a complex and continuous one. In a previous paper, we have outlined a typology that attempts to capture the in vivo complexity of traumatic memory.[34] Among our patients, three general patterns of traumatic remembrance can be identified: (1) relatively continuous and complete recall of childhood abuse experiences coupled with changing interpretations (delayed understanding) of these experiences, (2) partial amnesia for abuse events, accompanied by a mixture of delayed recall and delayed understanding, and (3) delayed recall following a period of profound and pervasive amnesia.

Patients in the first category report largely intact and continuous remembrance of their abuse experiences. Some, but not all, also report a much delayed understanding of their early experiences: a belated awareness of the abusive nature of these experiences and a lifting not of the amnesia but of the veil of denial and minimization that enabled them to preserve secrecy. It appears that many patients who find themselves rethinking and reinterpreting a long-remembered past do so as a result of specific developmental or relational events. The majority of patients seen in our program fall into this category.

Patients in the second category present with a mixture of newly recalled and continuously remembered events and a mixture of delayed recall and delayed understanding. These patients generally report partial amnesia for particular time periods, or focal amnesia for specific traumatic events. Contemporary precipitants to delayed recall also include developmental challenges and relational events. The content of newly recalled material often leads to a review and rethinking of the remembered past and then ushers in new interpretations and delayed understanding of an abusive past.

The third category describes patients who recover memories of childhood abuse after a period of global amnesia. This is the type of patient of concern to critics. However, in our experience, these patients do not conform in any way to the pejorative stereotype of a person with a confabulated complaint. None of these patients has taken legal action against an offender. Most are less interested in uncovering additional memories than in understanding and containing the press of recently acquired memories. All report severe and repeated sexual and physical abuse, beginning in early childhood and continuing into early adolescence. Many report amnesia not only for the abuse that occurred, but also for whole eras of development and whole categories of experience. Many have symptoms characteristic of a dissociative disorder.

Adult Remembrances of Childhood Trauma: Three Case Vignettes

In the current debate about the veracity of delayed recall of childhood trauma, the positive remembrances of one family member have often been cited as evidence of the inaccuracy of negative remembrances held by another. Our clinical typology of memory may account for some of these discrepancies in recall. It is quite possible that even within the same family, individuals may differ in the characteristics of their recall. The following composite vignettes, each drawn from the clinical case materials of several adult patients treated in our clinic, illustrate differences in recall among three siblings in the same family.

Vignette Number 1: Continuous Recall, Delayed Understanding

Amy is a 35-year-old married mother of three children. She is the oldest daughter of a minister in a small suburban community. She recalls her father as a perfectionist and a strict disciplinarian who was extremely concerned about appearances. She recalls her mother as a semi-invalid who was preoccupied with her health and often spent days in bed. From the age of 10, when her mother was hospitalized for a protracted period with complications of a pregnancy, Amy recalls performing household duties such as cooking, cleaning, and looking after her younger siblings. She also recalls that at that time her father began molesting her. He told her that if she ever disclosed the incest her mother would die. The abuse continued until she ran away with a boyfriend at age 17.

Amy states that she has never forgotten the abuse; rather, she has made a conscious effort to avoid thinking about it, and she has never told her husband about it. She does not believe in "dwelling on the past." Recently, however, she has been troubled by vivid, intrusive memories in which she feels almost as though she is reliving the abuse. She is also constantly afraid that someone will molest her 4-year-old daughter. She has developed an aversion to sex, and this has caused difficulties in her marriage. Her anxiety has become intolerable following a recent holiday visit to her parents' home. Distressed by these symptoms, she makes a decision to seek psychotherapy.

Therapy focuses initially on symptom management and an assessment of Amy's current situation. It becomes apparent that she is in a stable relationship with a supportive partner and her children are doing well. She has many unresolved feelings, however, about the past. She is troubled not only by her own memories, but also by her guilt feelings over the fate of the siblings she left behind when she excaped from her family. She is aware that her father regularly whipped both her brothers, Bobby and Chuck, and often locked them in their rooms for long periods without food or water. She now considers this treatment abusive. She is also concerned that he may have molested her sister Diane, who was only four when she left home. All of her siblings have had problems. Bobby has a history of alcoholism. Chuck died at age 21 of a self-inflicted gunshot wound which was officially ruled to be an accident. Diane is a withdrawn, reclusive person who has never left the family home.

As a result of her psychotherapy, Amy makes a decision to disclose the incest to her husband, who responds sympathetically. After much deliberation, the couple decide that Amy's parents cannot be allowed to spend any time alone with their children, and that holiday visits should be curtailed. They send a letter explaining their decision to Amy's parents. They also send copies of their letter to Amy's two surviving siblings. The disclosure precipitates a family crisis. Amy's parents vehemently deny her allegation of incest and insist that Amy's therapist is to blame for instigating a false accusation.

Vignette Number 2: Partial Amnesia, Delayed Recall, and Delayed Understanding

Bobby, age 30, is single and works as an emergency medical technician. Growing up, he was considered the family "troublemaker." At age 7 he set fire to his father's study; at 14 he was sent to boarding school, where he performed well academically but was expelled for alcohol and drug abuse. At age 17 he enlisted in the military, where, in spite of continued heavy drinking, he again performed well. He spent most of the next decade overseas and had little contact with the family. A year ago he began a serious relationship, and recently his girlfriend confronted him about his alcoholism. Because he does not want to lose her, he is making his first serious effort to stop drinking. He has been sober for 4 months. During this time he has been extremely irritable, his chronic insomnia has worsened, and he has had frequent nightmares.

Amy's disclosure causes Bobby a great deal of distress. He has always remembered the severe beatings he received, and he also recalls resenting the fact that Amy received special attention and was never beaten. Though he has not thought about it in a long time, he now recalls that Amy was often alone with their father, and that several times he was severely punished for intruding upon them. For the first time, he remembers hearing noises in the study, peeking through the door, and seeing his father lying on top of Amy. He does not know how old he was when this happened, but he thinks that he set the fire soon afterwards. Mostly he remembers his feelings of agitation, nausea, and fear. After recovering this memory, he spends the night drinking. Alarmed, his girlfriend persuades him to seek professional help.

Psychotherapy focuses on supporting Bobby's fragile sobriety. He is encouraged to attend meetings of Alcoholics Anonymous and to develop a relationship with a sponsor. Antidepressant medication proves helpful in attenuating his insomnia and nightmares. After a period of stabilization, he is able to explore the significance of his new memory. He now feels he understands why his father favored Amy and scapegoated him. He calls Amy to tell her he believes her.

Vignette Number 3: Profound Amnesia and Delayed Recall

Diane, age 22, has always been considered the "good girl" and the "quiet one" in the family. She keeps house for her parents and nurses her mother, whose medical condition has deteriorated over the years. She has few friends, and her very limited social life revolves around her father's church. She takes her parents' side in the conflict that follows Amy's disclosure; she also indignantly denies Amy's suggestion that she herself might have been abused.

Six months after the disclosure crisis, Diane is found unconscious at home and brought to the hospital, where she is found to have taken a potentially lethal overdose of her mother's medications. When she regains consciousness in intensive care, she states that she has no recall of the suicide attempt. She is also unable to account for the numerous healed cigarette burns found on her arms, thighs, breasts and abdomen. She is transferred to an inpatient pscyhiatric unit where she is frequently observed cowering in a corner of her room. When approached during these episodes, she becomes extremely frightened and speaks in a childlike voice, saying "Please don't make me do it." She does not recall these episodes in her normal state of consciousness. In response to probing questions regarding the recent family crisis, she becomes rigid, stares, and whispers "I can't tell, I promised not to tell." During the course of the hospitalization, after being assured repeatedly that she is now safe and will be protected, Diane recovers fragmentary memories of oral and vaginal rape by her father. These memories are experienced predominantly as smells, choking sensations, and burning sensations in her vagina. She also remembers the sound of his breathing and the threatening tone of his voice. There is no sense of time or sequence of events; she has the impression that the abuse started when she was very small. After awhile she learned to "go away" by staring at a crack on the ceiling in her father's study. Things were better once she could "go away" because she didn't feel any pain and it all seemed like a dream.

Diane is emotionally overwhelmed by her memories. At times she doubts their reality. At these times she berates herself furiously for being disloyal to her father and feels an intense desire to hurt and punish herself. Psychotherapy focuses on helping Diane manage the intense feelings associated with her memories without resort to self-destructive behavior or "going away." She gradually realizes that her extraordinary ability to dissociate, while it may have protected her when she was a child, is no longer useful to her as an adult. On the contrary, her dissociative coping style is now contributing to her social isolation and maintaining her subjection to her father. Group treatment is recommended to build social support and relieve feelings of shame, guilt, and self-blame. The goal of group treatment is promotion of safety and self-care in the present; active exploration of traumatic memories will not be encouraged until Diane's self-destructive behaviors and dissociative symptoms are under better control.

Although the content of Diane's traumatic childhood memories are not the current focus of therapy, issues of personal autonomy are central to her treatment. Careful attention to her day-to-day interactions with her father reveals a current pattern of physically intrusive and controlling behavior on his part. For example, he does not respect her privacy in the bedroom or bathroom. Both group and individual therapy will explore the emotional dilemma inherent in Diane's dependent attachment to a domineering father, and will foster the gradual development of strategies of emancipation.

Discussion

The clinical cases from which these vignettes were compiled suggest that adult survivors of childhood trauma arrive at their remembrances in a number of ways. They differ from one another on many dimensions, including the age at which the remembered events first occurred, the frequency, duration, chronicity and degree of violence and violation which attended these events, the type of relationship they had or may still have with the perpetrator, the social or ecological context in which the abuse occurred and in which protection was or was not afforded, and in the recency, clarity, and confidence with which they are able to recall the abuse. Most are able to confirm salient aspects of their histories even though they are unable to recall other, perhaps equally salient, features of those same histories.

The case vignettes presented here illustrate not only the type of traumatic remembering that is witnessed in clinical settings, but also the kind of issues that typically prevail in clinical work with trauma survivors. Most patients who enter psychotherapy for help in dealing with a traumatic past do so because of what they do remember, and not because of what they do not. Many enter psychotherapy after years of silence and secrecy, not after years of amnesia. They are hoping to better understand the impact of a long-remembered past. Others, like Amy in Vignette Number 1, may find themselves newly preoccupied with long-remembered events and feel stunned by their extreme emotional reactions to new understandings of these events. They enter therapy for help in managing their distress, for assistance in absorbing their new understandings, and, sometimes, for help in resolving the issue of family disclosure. Still others, like Bobby in Vignette Number 2 and Diane in Vignette Number 3, have acquired new memories that are deeply troubling. While these new memories may indeed become a focus of psychotherapy, psychotherapy is not the source of the memories. When clinicians work with trauma survivors who are experiencing distress as a result of traumatic re-membrances, the work typically involves the containment of runaway affect and help with stabilization of functioning, not an archaeological search for more in the way of traumatic recall. Contrary to the caricature of "recovered memory therapy," the aim of clinical exploration of the traumatic past is neither to uncover more and more horror, nor to assign blame and responsibility for adult life to others, but rather to help the adult survivor name and assign meaning and comprehensibility to the past, to facilitate the integration of traumatic remembrance into an ongoing personal narrative, and to help the patient grieve the past and be freed of it.

From our vantage point, characterizations of "false" versus "true" memory fail to capture the complexity of traumatic remembrance that is regularly witnessed in clinical settings. Neither these vignettes nor the patients whose experiences contributed to them fit such descriptions. Instead, the most apt characterization of the adult survivor is a person who arrives at adulthood with some, but not all, memories of the abuse intact, and who at some point in time begins to confront and rethink the past, blending new memories with earlier ones, new assessments with alternative ones, gradually con-structing a meaningful and largely verifiable personal history: a history that is patently "true" though never complete and never wholly accurate in all detail. The process of discovering one's history is not an all-or-none event, but rather unfolds in a relational and developmental context accompanied by marked emotional and symptomatic changes. The veracity of the history does not hang on the accurate and detailed recall of specific events. The development of a complete narrative often includes a search for confirmation of facts and verification in the remembrances of others; however, the timing and circumstances of this verification process are idiosyncratic and highly vari-able.

Clinical observation suggests that memories of childhood victimization—and rein-terpretations of childhood events not originally understood as abusive—may resurface unexpectedly when life cycle changes introduce new relational demands. The adult survivor may begin to recall a history of childhood trauma upon entering or ending an intimate relationship, for example. Memories may start to break through in the form of flashbacks or nightmares when the survivor gets involved in a sexual relationship, marries, or has a child. Delayed recall may occur when another victim of the same perpetrator discloses the abuse or when an aging perpetrator falls ill and expects his victim to care for him.

Clinicians familiar with traumatic disorders emphasize the role of memory retrieval in a multidimensional recovery process and the danger inherent in premature or poorly paced traumatic recall.[35-39] To date, however, neither the phenomenon of delayed recall of traumatic memories nor specific approaches to memory work with trauma survivors have been subjected to systematic study. Required catalysts for these investigations are inquiries into the psychological mechanisms, biochemical mediators, and neurological substrata of delayed recall, on the one hand, and on the other, conceptualizations of normal and traumatic memory that can facilitate inquiry by basic researcher and clinical investigator.

The questions raised by the phenomenon of delayed recall and the varied clinical presentations of patients who report distressing memories of childhood trauma are many and compelling. Clinical observation is a reasonable and valid starting point for the scientific exploration of these issues. An adequate theory of human memory cannot ignore or dismiss clinical observations. On the contrary, a science of memory must be able to account for the aberrations of memory and consciousness repeatedly witnessed by ethical, reliable, and observant clinicians. Similarly, effective treatment of these phenomena can and must be informed by basic research. Future advances in scientific understanding are most likely to develop from the mutually respectful collaboration of clinicians and basic memory researchers.

References

1. Washington Rev. Code Ann, Sec. 4 16.340 (1989 Suppl).
2. *Lofft v. Lofft,* Case # 617151, Superior Court of the State of California, 1989.
3. *Riley v. Presnell,* 409 Mass. 239 (1991).
4. *Munsey v. Kellett,* Middlesex (Massachusetts) Superior Court, Civil Action 91-5984, 1992.
5. Loftus E: The reality of repressed memories. Am Psychol 1993; 48(5):518–537.
6. Ofshe RJ, Watters E: Making monsters. Society 1993; 30:4–16.
7. Herman JL: Crime and memory. Bull Am Acad Psychiatry Law 1995; 23:5–17.
8. Appelbaum PS, Zoltek-Jick R: Psychotherapists' duties to third parties: *Ramona* and beyond. Am J Psychiatry 1996; 153:457–465.
9. Bowman CG, Mertz E: A dangerous direction: legal intervention in sexual abuse survivor therapy. Harvard Law Rev 1996; 109:555–639.
10. Coakley T: Porter pleads guilty to assaults as priest, admits molesting 28 youths in the 1960s. Boston Globe, Oct. 5, 1993, p. B16.
11. Sjainberg NM: Recovering a repressed memory and representational shift in an adolescent. J Am Psychoanal Assoc 1993; 42:711–727.
12. van der Kolk BA: The body keeps the score: memory and the evolving psychobiology of posttraumatic stress. Harvard Rev Psychiatry 1994; 1:253–265.

13. van der Kolk BA: Trauma and memory. *In* BA van der Kolk, A McFarlane, L Weisaeth (Eds.), Traumatic Stress. New York: Guilford Press, 1996, pp. 279–302.
14. American Psychiatric Association: Diagnostic and Statistical Manual of Mental Disorders (4th ed.). Washington, DC: American Psychiatric Press, 1994.
15. Andrews B, Morton J, Bekeriaan DA, Brewin C, Davies GM, Mollon P: The recovery of memories in clinical practice: experiences and beliefs of British Psychological Society practitioners. The Psychologist 1995; May:209–214.
16. Putnam FW: Dissociation as a response to extreme trauma. *In* RP Kluft (Ed.), Childhood Antecedents of Multiple Personality Disorder. Washington, DC: American Psychiatric Press, 1985.
17. Goodwin J: Sexual Abuse: Incest Victims and Their Families. Chicago: Year Book Medical, 1989.
18. Briere J, Runtz M: Childhood sexual abuse: long term sequelae and implications for psychological assessment. J Interpers Violence 1993; 8(3):312–330.
19. Chu JA, Dill DL: Dissociative symptoms in relation to childhood physical and sexual abuse. Am J Psychiatry 1990; 147:887–892.
20. Herman JL, Schatzow E: Recovery and verification of memories of childhood sexual trauma. Psychoanal Psychol 1987; 4(1):1–4.
21. Briere J, Conte J: Self-reported amnesia for abuse in adults molested as Children. J Traumatic Stress 1993; 6:21–31.
22. Cameron C: Women survivors confronting their abusers: issues, decisions, and outcomes. J Child Sex Abuse 1994; 3:7–35.
23. Gold SN, Hughes D, Hohnecker L: Degrees of repression of sexual abuse memories. Am Psychol 1994; 49:441.
24. Loftus E, Polonsky S, Thompson-Fullilove M: Memories of childhood sexual abuse: remembering and repressing. Psychol Women Q 1994; 18:67–84.
25. Roesler TA, Wind TW: Telling the secret: adult women describe their disclosures of incest. J Interpers Violence 1994; 9:327–338.
26. Feldman-Summers S, Pope KS: The experience of ''forgetting'' childhood abuse: a national survey of psychologists. J Consult Clin Psychol 1994; 62:1–4.
27. Elliot DM, Briere J: Posttraumatic stress associated with delayed recall of sexual abuse: a general population study. J Traumatic Stress 1995; 8:629–648.
28. Grassian S, Holtzen D: Memory of sexual abuse by a parish priest. Paper presented at Trauma and Memory: An International Research Conference, Portsmouth, NH, July 1996.
29. Williams LM: Recall of childhood trauma: a retrospective study of women's memories of child sexual abuse. J Consult Clin Psychol 1994; 62:1167–1176.
30. Williams LM: Recovered memories of abuse in women with documented child sexual abuse victimization histories. J Traumatic Stress 1995; 8:649–673.
31. Westen D, Ludolph P, Misle B, Ruffins S, Block J: Physical and sexual abuse in adolescent girls with borderline personality disorder. Am J Orthopsychiatry 1990; 60:55–66.
32. Coons PM: Confirmation of childhood abuse in child and adolescent cases of multiple personality disorder and dissociative disorder not otherwise specified. J Nerv Ment Dis 1994; 182:461–464.
33. Silk KR, Lee S, Hill EM, Lohr NE: Borderline personality disorder symptoms and severity of sexual abuse. Am J Psychiatry 1995; 152:1059–1064.
34. Harvey MR, Herman JL: Amnesia, partial amnesia and delayed recall among adult survivors of childhood trauma. Consciousness Cogn 1994; 3:295–306.
35. Herman JL: Trauma and Recovery. New York: Basic Books, 1992.

36. Lebowitz L, Harvey M, Herman JL: A stage by dimension model of recovery from sexual trauma. J Interpers Violence 1992; 8(3):378–391.
37. van der Hart O, Steele K, Boon S, Brown P: The treatment of traumatic memories: synthesis, realization and integration. Dissociation 1993; 6:162–180.
38. Brown D: Pseudomemories: the standard of science and the standard of care in trauma treatment. Am J Clin Hypn 1995; 37:1–24.
39. Harvey MR: Principles of practice with remembering adults. *In* A Tishelman, C Newberger, E Newberger (Eds.), Trauma and Memory. Cambridge, MA: Harvard University Press (in press).

11

Traumatic Experiences: The Early Organization of Memory in School-age Children and Adolescents

ROBERT S. PYNOOS
ALAN M. STEINBERG
LISA ARONSON

There are two trends currently working to unduly restrict discussions of traumatic memories. Recent judicial controversies concerning ''repressed memories,'' ''delayed memories'' and ''false memory syndromes'' in adults, as well as a number of sensationalized legal cases involving allegations of sexual abuse by preschool children, have resulted in social polarization over the veracity of presumed traumatic memories among adults and the reliability of young children's recall of traumatic experiences.[1-4] At the same time, there have been efforts to conceptualize traumatic memories in neurobiological terms as involving an extreme consolidation of memory due to danger or fear-induced, augmented stimulation of endogenous stress hormones.[5,6] Such terms as *malignant memories* and *super memories* suggest that traumatic memories are virtually fixed and indelible. Both the vehement polarization of opinion and the biological reductionism profoundly underrepresent the extraordinary complexity of traumatic experiences and the extreme activity of children's minds in the experience and remembering of traumatic events. This chapter will present clinical and research material gathered from traumatized children and adolescents to elucidate this contention.

Throughout our discussion of children's memory of traumatic experiences, we will take both a functional and developmental approach. By *functional,* we refer to how such experiences contribute to a child's evolving schematization of the world, especially of threat, danger, security, safety, risk, injury, loss, protection, and intervention. By *developmental,* we refer to maturational and experiential processes that govern the

The authors gratefully acknowledge support from the Bing Fund and the John D. and Catherine T. MacArthur Foundation.

mental representation of external and internal dangers. These include a progressive capacity for the metacognition of emotions, acquisition of cognitive competencies, and plasticity and consolidation of neuroanatomical structures within memory systems of the brain.[7]

The material for this chapter is largely derived from over a decade of clinical experience and research findings of the UCLA Trauma Psychiatry Program. The Program has extensive experience in the evaluation and treatment of children and adolescents exposed to extreme intrafamilial, interpersonal and community violence, war, catastrophic natural and man-made disaster, serious accidental injury, and life-threatening physical illness and life-endangering medical procedures. Our observations have consistently indicated that a number of essential considerations must be taken into account in discussing remembrances of traumatic experiences.

These considerations include (*1*) traumatic situations involve a convergence of external and internal dangers; (*2*) traumatic experiences are *extremely* complex; (*3*) the organization of memory and strategies of recall of traumatic experiences differ as children focus on different memory anchor points and their meaning, forming an elaborate memory network; (*4*) intervention fantasies, which occur during and after the traumatic experience are invariably associated in memory schematization of the experience; (*5*) cognitive, affective, social, and neurophysiological development play a role in the appraisal of external and internal threats and in the processing and remembering of traumatic eperiences; (*6*) the process of remembering traumatic experiences may engage self-protective mental efforts to "weaken" certain traumatic details or moments; (*7*) children's traumatic narratives typically rely on co-construction with parents or other adult caretakers, or siblings and peers; and (*8*) new information, further experience, and maturity can lead to reschematization of the mental representation of a traumatic situation through revised appraisals, new attributions of meaning to aspects of the experience, and new considerations regarding intervention.

The Convergence of Internal and External Dangers

The complexity of traumatic situations is in part due to what we have previously termed the "tripartite etiology of posttraumatic stress reactions,"[8] which includes (*1*) objective and subjective features of traumatic experiences, (*2*) proximal secondary stresses and adversities, and (*3*) proximal traumatic reminders. In his analysis of a traumatic situation, Freud insisted that it is one in which "external and internal, real and instinctual dangers converge."[9] According to Freud, traumatic situations include the appraisal and response to *both* external and internal dangers. Such a conceptualization of traumatic stress fits well with current DSM-IV criteria for posttraumatic stress disorder. Criterion A requires that a traumatic event involve objective features (such as direct life-threat to self or other and witnessing of injury or death), as well as subjective features of terror, horror, and helplessness.

Children's subjective traumatic experiences can be strongly associated with the severity of posttrauma distress.[10,11] In our 1994 Northridge earthquake study, we found that, in addition to objective features such as being trapped or injured, specific subjective experiences during the earthquake, including fear of dying, feeling one's heart beating fast, and feeling very upset about how one acted during the earthquake, were highly predictive of overall severity of PTSD symptoms at 5 months. Subjective experiences, such as guilt over acts of omission or commission perceived to have endangered others, have also been found to strongly predict ongoing distress.[12-14] The generation of other negative emotions, for example, shame and rage, can have a similar impact.[15]

The experience of internal threat includes a sense of inability to tolerate the affective responses and physiological reactions—not only their valence but also the rate of their acceleration—as well as a sense of catastrophic personal consequence. The latter includes both dire external and phase-specific psychodynamic threats. In addition, internal threats arise from attributions of meaning to specific features or details of the traumatic situation and the aftermath that provoke intense concerns over immediate and future developmental consequences. Trauma not only activates conflicts from the immediate developmental period or recruits earlier conflicts but often reevokes conscious and unconscious material specific to prior traumatic experiences that provide special significance to portions of the current situation and its aftermath.

The experience of external and internal threat is influenced by subjective appraisals and the adequacy of efforts to address the situation and manage the internal responses. These appraisals and efforts at coping vary with developmental and experiential maturation. For example, from childhood through adolescence, there is a developmental progression in the evolution of self and object representations that mediates the degree of reliance on self, parents, adult caretakers, siblings, peers, and agents of social institutions in regard to the estimation of danger, of the capacity to regulate or tolerate extreme negative emotions and psychophysiological responses, and of the efficacy and agency of protective action. The internal responses include not only the autonomic or affective reactions but also the emerging attribution of symbolic meaning and psychosexual interpretation.

The Complexity of Traumatic Experiences

Case Study

A 6-year-old boy survived a life-threatening automobile accident in which his mother suffered irreversible brain damage that led to her death. He and his mother were returning home from a special outing when, from the back seat passenger side, the boy saw a speeding car heading directly at his side of the car. He instantaneously became afraid, felt his heart beating and yelled ''Mommy'' in an effort to warn her. From her side of the car, she was unaware of the oncoming vehicle and did not react. He immediately thought about taking defensive action, imagining undoing his seat belt, diving over the front seat to the brake pedal, and applying the brake with his hand to stop the car before the other car collided with them. As the other car hit his side of the car, he was terrified by the terrible noise of the impact, of the shattering of glass and the explosion-like noise of a tire bursting. He watched as his mother's head hit the driver's side window and recoiled, with blood then gushing from her mouth and covering her face. For a moment he was not sure if she was vomiting or bleeding, and felt an intense negative reaction to the thought of vomiting, which reminded him of how much he hated to vomit when he was sick. At first, after the collision, he did not think about whether he had been injured or about his own safety, but was preoccupied with concerns about his mother. In fear over her condition, he screamed out "Mommy." When she did not respond, he began to shake uncontrollably and to feel extremely cold. He tried to move toward her, but could not because his seat belt remained fastened. He then realized that he did not know how to release it and recalled momentarily his mother's last protective action of having put him in it just before the accident occurred. His attention then turned to himself, as he now noticed that his nose was bleeding and his head hurt. He could not tell how badly he was hurt. His focus shifted from wanting to help his mother to desperately wishing for her to be able to help him. At this moment of extreme helplessness, he felt trapped and became panicked. Later, as he was being helped out of the car, he saw rescue workers cutting the driver's side door in order to remove his mother from the vehicle. He was glad that she was being rescued, especially because he became aware of a gasoline-fueled fire beginning to surround the car. An arriving rescue helicopter moved the air as it landed nearby, fanning the flames. He felt a renewed sense of impending danger, frightened by the thought of the fire rapidly catching up to him, imagining being electrocuted as if in a lightening storm. He saw his mother lifted into the helicopter, just after which he was transported to a hospital by ambulance. When he arrived at the hospital, he wanted his mother but was told he could not go see her because she was badly hurt and that the doctors were trying to help her. He intensely wished that they would be able to save her. He was relieved to see his father in the emergency room, but at once felt afraid by the father's facial expression of sadness that indicated to him a sense of impending loss of his mother. He was phycially examined in the ER and released. He never saw his mother alive again.

Our studies among traumatized children have included relatively large-scale traumatic events and extreme situations of interpersonal violence in which the major objective features of children's traumatic experiences were well-defined and known. We have consistently found that the experience of a child during a traumatic situation involves complex sensory, physiological, affective and cognitive processing of multiple moments with differing vantage points of concern. Table 11-1 summarizes our observations regarding the complexity of traumatic experiences, which have been described in more detail elsewhere.[8]

Table 11-1. The Complexity of Traumatic Experiences

Context
Circumstances, affective state, cognitive preoccupations and developmental concerns

Multiple Traumatic Moments (even within a relatively circumscribed situation)
Moment-to-moment perceptual, kinesthetic, and somatic registration

Ongoing appraisal of external and internal threats

Continuous efforts to address situation in behavior, thought, and fantasy

Continuous efforts to manage physiological and emotional reactions

Changes in Foci of Attention or Concern
Attention drawn away from own safety out of concern for danger or injury to other

Moment of estrangement from others when immediate threat or injury to self

Sudden preoccupation with concerns about severity of injury, rescue, or repair after injury to self or other

Inhibition of wishes to intervene or suppression of retaliatory impulses from fear of provoking counter-retaliatory behavior

Radical Shift in Attention or Concern When Physical Integrity Is Violated
Attention directed towards fears/fantasies about nature/extent of psychic/physical harm

Engagement of self-protective mechanisms to meet internal threats and pain (including ''dissociative'' physiological responses and fantasies)

Efforts to invoke or disclaim affiliative needs/desires in order to mitigate fear or ward off sense of active participation

Additional Traumatic Moments After Cessation of Violence or Threat
Efforts to seek outside help, e.g., police, paramedics

Efforts to aid injured or dead family members or friends

Experiences during acute medical or surgical care

Acute separations from significant others, including injured or dead family members or peers

Additional Dimensions to Traumatic Experiences
Worry about safety of significant others whose well-being is unknown

Reactivation of previous danger/fears/anxieties from prior experience

Acute grief reactions to witnessing death or destruction even while threat to self continues

Disturbances in Evolving Developmental Expectations Regarding Danger
Failure of alarm reactions to elicit effective intervention[16]

Failure of social referencing to appraise danger[17]

Failure of protective shield to prevent harm

Inability to resist coercive violation[18]

Betrayal of basic affiliative assumptions

Failure of catastrophic emotions to protect against harm[19]

Disruption of belief in socially modulated world

Struggle over surrender to unavoidable moment of danger[16]

Radical shifts in self-object representations, for example, when parent or child acts cowardly, ineffectually, or heroically

The registration and appraisal of both objective and subjective threats may include distortions, misperceptions, and estimates of danger that either minimize or exaggerate the actual extent of threat or harm. We would emphasize that *dissociation* should not be used as an all inclusive term to describe a child's overall response to a traumatic situation, as such responses are most often particularly directed at specific traumatic moments within a broader traumatic circumstance or situation. When there is actual violation of the physical or psychological integrity of the child, the child is more likely to invoke what are commonly referred to as *dissociative mechanisms*. Such mechanisms include efforts to down-regulate physiological autonomic arousal[20] or pain, and engagement in fantasies that allow the child to feel a physical distancing from what is happening and to feel it is not happening to him or her. These mechanisms also serve to decrease a sense of active participation and to manage shame or guilt.[21]

The Role of Memory Markers in Episodic Memory of Trauma

Our studies of the recounting of traumatic experiences by school-aged children within the first hours, days, weeks, and months of a traumatic situation confirm earlier formulations regarding the recall of episodic, autobiographical memory as a reconstruction, rather than as a reproduction of the event.[22] We found that, in unassisted recall, children's narratives were shortened, with certain features becoming central, apparently serving as anchor points for remembering. Some details were emphasized while others were omitted. The younger the child, the more likely the memory marker was confined to a central action, for example, when injurious harm occurred.[23]

In our studies of children exposed to a sniper attack on a school playground, we identified a variety of memory anchor points that guided children's unassisted reconstruction and recounting of their experience.[23] Such memory anchor points included location in relation to the violence; perceptual experiences; cues of distress; sight of victims, injury, or blood; physiological responses; worst moments; location and actions of adults; worry about a sibling; hearing the news that a child had been killed; reunion with parents and parental reaction; guilt over acts of omission or commission believed to have caused harm; and reminders of previous life experience.

Two central findings have emerged from this study. First, in remembering life-threatening situations, children's memory is not organized as a single episode. Rather, spatial and temporal descriptions and relationships, affective and cognitive responses, and sets of perceptions differed across memory anchor points. Consequently, the organization of memory and strategy of recall differed as children focused on different memory anchor points and their meaning. For example, when an 8-year-old boy focused on his own experiences of life-threat, he began with his first misappraisal of gunshots as car backfires until he saw another child hit by a bullet, his terror, his protective actions and wishes for outside intervention, and his reaching a location out of the line of fire. However, when he turned his attention to his worry about his younger brother, he began and ended his narrative with a different temporal sequence. He began with his thoughts about his brother's whereabouts and safety, even as he himself was being fired upon. These thoughts included fantasies of harm, his renewed thoughts about his brother after the boy reached a safe location, his sense of responsibility for looking after his brother to and from school, his courageous efforts to search for him (which placed the boy in additional danger), and finally, his responses to their reunion which occurred hours later at home.

Especially important memory anchor points are significant interactive moments, which include not only the moment of harm or protective intervention but also charged affective and verbal exchanges with and between others. When a previous life experience is recalled in association with a portion of the experience, there may be a deviation in the account, with a side-narrative that emphasizes certain details and dangers, and that takes on special meaning attributions.

A second finding from the sniper attack study was that memory anchor points are associated with imagined or intended interventions that become inextricably part of the memory network associated with the experience. These interventions include contemplated actions that occur both during the episode and in the immediate aftermath. They represent complex mental activities, which are influenced by maturity, gender, and life experience, that demonstrate a developmental hierarchy in children's efforts to address the convergence of external and internal threats.[24]

Self-Protective Mechanisms in Remembering and Recounting Traumatic Experiences: Weakened Versions

It is a common misconception to characterize the mental representation of traumatic situations as if it existed as a photographic reproduction, or to assume that any distortions in these representations signify error in memory storage rather than modifications introduced during recall. As Freud suggested, the mind looks for ways to "weaken the version" of the traumatic situation in order to be able to mobilize effective intervention fantasies to offset a full admission of traumatic helplessness. Our research has investigated five basic parameters that are commonly modified in producing a "weakened version" in the mental representation of the objective features of a threatening or injurious situation. These are: (*1*) proximity to the violence; (*2*) lethality of the instrument; (*3*) intentionality; (*4*) object of the violence; and (*5*) seriousness of the injury. The manner of weakening of the version may be quite subtle and not readily identifiable. We discovered this when, over a decade ago, we examined the transcripts of the acute trauma narrative of the children exposed to the deadly sniper attack on their school playground. Distortions, omissions, reframing of aspects of the experience, and spatial or temporal misrepresentations of threat appeared to reflect early efforts to minimize the objective threat and to regulate emotional distress during recall.[23] Children may recount in detail other fearful moments in order to screen a memory of a more horrifying moment[24] or introduce premonitions.[25]

Detailed examination of these children's unassisted recall revealed that children who had the greatest proximity to the fatal violence and were in the direct line of gunfire introduced significant spatial misrepresentations of their own life-threat. For example, they placed the murdered child at a further distance from themselves than had been the case or they recalled themselves as being in safer locations than their most dangerous locations during the event. However, when the children walked the school yard with the interviewer, there was no error in positioning themselves accurately in terms of locations and proximity to the dead girl. Conversely, nontraumatized children who were not on the playground, especially those who had not even been at school that day, appeared to be able to increase their sense of proximity to the violence. For example, several of these students reported having come that day to the school and having viewed the blood on the playground, when indeed, the area had been cordoned off by the police until the following day.

Bjork and Richardson-Klavehn[26] have summarized the laboratory evidence to support how memory disturbances may reflect specific modifications that occur during recall. Children may be especially susceptible to these modifications during recall because of their immaturity in affective regulation and their difficulty in tolerating a renewed awareness of the traumatic helplessness that they experienced.

Intervention Fantasies

As an outgrowth of our finding about the invariable incorporation of intervention fantasies within the memory network associated with a traumatic experience, we began to investigate the phenomenology and evolution of these fantasy accompaniments to experience and memory. We sought to characterize their type and their developmental and experiential determinants. They represent mental efforts to contend with or counter traumatic helplessness and injurious outcome or loss. We have described five categories of intervention fantasies.[24] These include fantasies to (*1*) alter the precipitating events; (*2*) to interrupt the traumatic action; (*3*) to reverse the lethal or injurious consequences; (*4*) to gain safe retaliation; and (*5*) to prevent future trauma.

Our clinical and research observations regarding the formation and evolution of intervention thoughts and fantasies have confirmed that (*1*) during a traumatic situation, different intervention fantasies are associated with the changing appraisal of the danger and estimation of protective action; (*2*) as a result, each of the memory anchor points is linked to specific intervention fantasies and concerns; (*3*) intervention fantasies are directed at addressing both external dangers, inherent in the objective features of the traumatic moments, and the internal dangers which emanate from the subjective distress and developmental concerns; (*4*) remembering or recounting a traumatic situation reengages these intervention fantasies; (5) intervention fantasies, as expressed verbally, in play, reenactment behavior, or transference, indicate ongoing efforts to address traumatic helplessness and serve as a precursor to the clinical exploration and reconstruction of unaddressed traumatic moments; and (6) among younger children, there is a tendency for intervention thoughts as intended actions to be spoken of in an initial traumatic narrative as if they had occurred. In effect, we are taking issue with an approach to traumatic memories at any age that construes their mental representation as "facts" and "feelings," without due consideration to the accompanying appraisals, protective efforts, and intervention fantasies.

The following clinical case example provides an illustration of the intimate link between emerging intervention fantasies and their reference to aspects of the traumatic experience over the course of the clinical reconstruction of the trauma narrative. The example captures the progression toward the worst traumatic moments and most intense negative affects.

Case Study

A 5-year-old boy had been viciously attacked by a dog while playing alone in front of his home. Alerted to the attack, the mother rushed out, grabbed her son, lifting him away from the dog. The dog remained poised to attack her until neighbors used metal garbage can lids to fend him off. During the attack, the dogs teeth pierced the boy's skull, inflicting injuries that later required extensive neurosurgery. While recovering from the neurosurgery, a pet therapist employed by the pediatric unit, attempted to desensitize the boy to dogs by bringing a dog to his hospital room. Despite his outward manner of cooperation, in his hypervigilant state, the boy could not yet discriminate among dogs, and he now linked hospital settings with a traumatic expectation about the reappearance of the attacking dog. The boy insisted that his mother bring his play suit of armor to the hospital. At the beginning of psychotherapy, 3 months after the attack, the dog was still impounded but had not yet been destroyed. The boy was required to wear a football helmet until new bone formed over the open area of his skull.

At the time of the first psychotherapy session, the therapist knew from the parents that the boy had expressed his conviction that he would never be able to outrun an attacking dog. He knew he was coming to see a doctor who talked to children and let them play with toys in the office. The first session intervention fantasies referred to the context under which the dog attacked—that the boy had been playing out of sight of his mother, and that the dog had been unrestrained and without his owner. Soon after entering the psychotherapy office and insisting that his mother stay, the boy tied string to the door knob and jammed chairs against the door to protect against the entry of a dog that he imagined could unexpectedly enter the room and attack him at any time. These interventions also reflected the child's need to ensure certain safeguards before he would permit himself any play activity.

We have often observed in the earliest stage of work with an acutely traumatized child that the trauma narrative, intervention fantasies, and reenactment behavior may initially move past the worst traumatic moments to the time of rescue and assistance. This manner of recall often represents a dual effort to approach the trauma narrative from a posttrauma safe vantage point and expresses transference wishes or concerns regarding the helping role of the psychotherapist. In this boy's case, this effort was complicated by a previous traumatic experience in which he had choked on a coin while in the care of a baby-sitter, and had been taken to the hospital accompanied only by paramedics. During the next session, he played that he was in a toy ambulance, alone, gagging, while the ambulance accelerated to a dangerous speed. In observing his play, the mother, who attended this session, helpfully reminded her son of this earlier experience. He then immediately described a discrete moment of intense panic when being placed in the ambulance after the dog attack; he feared that his mother would not accompany him to the hospital.

It is common for children to suppress concern for themselves in their overwhelming concern for their parents during the course of an event and in the order of recounting the traumatic moments. In the next session, the boy permitted his mother to be outside the room, but then frequently checked on her welfare, fearing that she was in danger of being attacked by a dog that had followed them to the hospital, now that she was outside the protected haven of the psychotherapy room. This coincided with a pattern of traumatic reenactment, where he would require his mother to pick him up high when going out into the hallway from the office. This behavior included the intervention fantasy of his mother carrying him high enough so that a dog could not attack him. However, the checking behavior also referred to the moment when he became scared for his mother after she had separated him from the dog and now faced possible attack herself from the menacing dog.

After identifying his empathic arousal over his mother's safety from attack, he began to address his own life-threatening experience. Identification with the aggressor, as clarified by Anna Freud,[27] is a form of intervention fantasy in which children protectively align themselves with the aggressor in order not to be an object of attack. Acutely traumatized children will often engage this intervention in therapy by having the therapist become the object of attack in traumatic play, while the child tries to communicate the frightening acceleration of physiological arousal, affective intensity, and internal and external dangers that he or she had experienced.

The boy then played at attacking the therapist like a dog, growling, drooling all over her, mouthing her while saying he was chewing her like a dog bone, and jumping at her repeatedly, trying to create a frightening sense of surprise. At the same time, he accused the therapist of peeing and pooping in her pants. In remembering the experience, he not only addressed the surprise, terror, and helplessness he felt at the external danger, but also the internal danger, describing how upset he had been to lose bladder control and wet his pants during the dog's attack. He had been so proud during the past year of becoming toilet trained and without accident. Furthermore, he elaborated on how scared he was at the dog biting his buttocks and his terror that next his penis would be bitten by the dog.

The subsequent series of intervention fantasies were directed at the experience of feeling like he was the dog's prey. Having concluded that he could not outrun the dog, and having demonstrated the viciousness and determination of the attacking dog in the previous sessions, he now engaged in fantasies of hiding and playing possum. Perry et al.[20] have suggested that such protective behaviors are related to efforts to down-regulate the autonomic arousal that can be associated with remembering the experience. The boy next began to hide in the office. He would willingly let an imagined dog into the office, while he sat in a box and ducked down so that the dog would be unable to find him. After endless searching, the dog would give up the hunt and go away, exclaiming, "Nothing here to eat. I'm going now."

The next sessions illustrated how, when physical injury has occurred, especially with ongoing physical vulnerability or disability, a different set of intervention fantasies will be entertained that melds the original fantasies of protection with ongoing concerns over future harm. At this time, when he no longer was required to wear the protective helmet, he chose as his favorite toy a stuffed turtle he found in the office. He would launch it from a shelf and have it land on its feet or back, while remarking with relief that the shell did not break. He then would have the turtle join him in the box that he had chosen as a protected area. These fantasies initiated his approaching of his sense of physical vulnerability that his skull bone could be bitten through and his ongoing concerns that this area of his skull remains more vulnerable. The boy became more active in addressing his symptomatic difficulties and took the turtle, now endowed with protective powers, home to help him sleep better and ward off his traumatic nightmares.

The progressive reconstruction of his traumatic experience, including the content of his evolving intervention fantasies, was now diverted by the mother's insistence on getting a family dog. Although seeing him safe with the puppy gave her repeated temporary relief from her intrusive recollections of the attack, the boy experienced renewed fears of attack and moments of intense physiological arousal. The intervention fantasies at this stage now addressed an admixture of elements of the original experience and current concerns. For example, he became preoccupied with how to climb the ladder to his slide to get away, if necessary, from the puppy. Only after the puppy had been housed at his grandparents for a number of weeks did the boy resume the progression towards addressing the worst moments of his traumatic experience.

During these weeks, he progressed toward recounting the actual experience of the dog's attack, first by creating a scenario to successfully appease the dog or keep him at bay, and then by imagining ways to take revenge commensurate with the forms of violence he experienced, and finally to rid himself of the threat once and for all. For example, he would hide in the office, without any need for a safe box or turtle, and direct the therapist to act like a hungry, maniacal dog. From behind the chair where he hid, he cautiously offered the dog some food from a slightly exposed hand, and directed the therapist (as dog) to act satiated, calm and grateful. Following this intervention play, he was able to recapture and describe his experience of the uncontrollable, ferocious aggression of the dog during the attack and to talk about how intolerable it felt not to know when it would end, being utterly helpless in the face of such viciousness.

Then followed a series of sessions in which he entertained various forms of revenge fantasies, each of which addressed different aspects of his experience, culminating in one that, for the first time, reflected his worst moment during the attack. In many of the revenge fantasies, the dog was made to experience the traumatic helplessness the boy experienced, including that from both the external and internal dangers. For example, he pretended to pee on the dog's face, both to ward off the dog and to do to the dog what had been most shameful to him. In so doing, he spoke more fully about the extent of his shame and fear that his newly gained competency would be lost to him forever, resulting in accidents at school, a renewed need for diapers, and relentless teasing by peers. Next he played at sneaking up on the dog, jumping on him, and biting him all over. This set of revenge fantasies led the boy for the first time to approach in recall what it felt like to have the dog jump up, knock him over and penetrate his skin and his skull with his teeth.

Lastly, he decapitated dolls in the office, with the fantasy of doing the same to the dog. Now, he expressed his worst fear during the attack, that when the dog took hold of his head, it felt like the dog was shaking it so violently that it would be torn off. These sessions initiated a process in which he regained a more age-appropriate sense of self-efficacy in the face of danger and more cognitive capacity to discriminate among dogs.

Selected Developmental Issues in Children's Traumatic Memories

We would like to bring attention to five selected areas related to the early processing, memory networking, and remembrance of children's traumatic experiences. First, particular developing memory systems and neurophysiologic structures subserve the overall evolving schematization of real dangers. Second, the registration, processing, and recall of specific traumatic moments are influenced by a variety of maturing developmental factors. Third, the construction of a trauma narrative requires a maturing capacity to integrate many traumatic moments into a complex, coherent representation of the traumatic situation. Fourth, the biology of acute traumatic memories permits a prolonged period of reappraisal and reframing that allows adult influence on children's schematization of danger and protective action. Fifth, the child's construction of a trauma narrative and schematization depends both on maturation of strategies of recall and on assistance from parents and caretakers in co-construction.

The following three examples illustrate the relevance of evolving memory systems and neurophysiological structures. Perry et al.[20] have pointed out how early physical or severe psychological insults and traumatic experiences can alter the manner and rate of maturation of different brain structures, thereby permanently altering their relative influence in appraising and responding to danger, including physiological, cognitive, emotional and behavioral responses.

Nadel[7] has specifically discussed the importance of the differential rates of maturation of the hippocampus and the amygdala to the schematization of danger in childhood. He suggests that these two brain structures subserve two separate but interrelated functions. The hippocampus participates in establishing a spatiotemporal context to experience while the amygdala assists in providing affective valence and significance to incoming sensory and affective experience. As he notes, the hippocampus does not fully mature in its function for the first several years of life, so that the response to danger is dominated by alarm and enhanced fear reactions to sensory/affective material. With maturation of the hippocampus, these reactions are better mediated by appropriate contextual discrimination. He has proposed that this developmental maturation accounts for a relative change in symptoms from alarm reactions to panic, to phobia, to posttraumatic stress symptoms, from infancy through late childhood.

Finally, Pynoos[28] has proposed that there is a relationship between the neurophysiological maturation of the startle mechanism and the evolving content of intervention fantasies. During early childhood, there is an immaturity in the capacity to inhibit the startle reflex. In contrast to older children, where presentation of a prestimulus warning to a startle stimulus leads to startle inhibition, preschool children may exhibit a facilitation of the startle response.[29] This early lack of inhibitory modulation of the startle promotes avoidant or escape behavior and corresponds to a developmental stage characterized by conscious thoughts of turning away from danger and seeking out external protection and intervention. Acquisition of inhibitory modulation of the startle, which occurs at approximately 8 years of age, corresponds to a developmental stage in which children actively begin to entertain conscious thoughts and fantasies of personally addressing, disarming, or directly harming the source of danger. They begin to construct intervention fantasies that anticipate dangerous situations to prevent or avert danger. By early adolescence, when inhibitory modulation of the startle reflex is consolidated, thoughts or fantasies of intervention are typically accompanied by decisions to intervene directly, even during the course of a traumatic situation.

The experience and recall of traumatic moments are influenced by the differential manner over the course of development in which sensory information is registered, processed, and recalled; by the maturation of the capacity for a metacognition of emotions; and by the way in which external and internal dangers are apprehended, signified, and tolerated. For example, the registration and processing of sensory information varies developmentally according to the type of sensory input and the relative prominence of sensory, kinesthetic, and somatic experience during the traumatic situation. Even young children may register the smell of gunfire during a violent event with very little processing and accurately discriminate its smell among others in recall. This is perhaps related to the underlying neuroanatomy of olfaction.[30] Visual information, however, which utilizes a "visual-spatial pad"[31] to represent distance and location of a threat, requires a more mature ability to estimate and discriminate. Because temporal registration in young children appears to require accurate spatial serialization of an event,[32] they may be vulnerable to temporal errors in recalling the sequence of events.

The ability to process and reflect in the trauma narrative negative affective experiences depends on the maturing capacity for what has been termed *the metacognition of emotions.*[33] Traumatic experiences often challenge the child emotionally by eliciting two or more concurrent or successive emotions, for example, fear, sadness, excitement, or rage, within a short period of time. The lack of an ability to differentiate among concurrent emotions may interfere with the preschool child's reconstruction of the experience, either by requiring the assignment of concurrent emotions to different portions of the experience or the omission of a competing emotion. Increasing capacity to make affective discriminations, especially among negative emotions,[34] permits the more mature child to distinguish among complex traumatic moments.

The nature, mental representation, and remembrance of external and internal threats are strongly influenced by developmental and experiential factors. For example, a young child may focus on, and well remember, the facial expression of an approaching assailant, which serves as a measure of his malevolence, or the cries of distress of a family member. However, when attention shifts to internal threats, for example, once penetrated, injured, or physically coerced, the young child may not have sufficiently mature ego observational capacities to register, locate, and monitor moment-to-moment sensations, feelings, and thoughts.

The capacity to integrate the multiple traumatic moments into a complex and coherent memory representation and trauma narrative relies on the ability to regulate stimulus completion and affect, and on maturing cognitive analytic and synthetic functions. For example, the neuroprocessing system of the amygdala, hippocampus, and cortical feedback is said to tend toward stimulus completion,[35] whereby one sensory, affective, or cognitive reminder tends to elicit the full range of associated stimuli, affects, and meanings. As Freud[9] first proposed, young children are vulnerable to suppression, repression, lack of integration, and fragmentation of frightening memories in an effort to interrupt stimulus completion. In latency, the combined maturation in cortical inhibitory control,[36] and capacities for increased contextual discrimination and affective tolerance, reduces the defensive engagement of these protective mechanisms.

The role of development cannot be fully understood without an appreciation of the evolutionary significance of the special biology of memory formation that appears to be associated with traumatic situations. In terms of remembrance, traumatic experiences initiate neurohormonal responses that appear to enhance and extend the period of reappraisal and assignment of "personal consequentiality."[5,37] From an evolutionary perspective, this period of reappraisal can facilitate a more accurate discrimination of potential dangers. This "re-working" memory may incorporate other forms of mental modificaion that mediate the adaptational response, including evolving intervention contingencies, not only acutely but also over time. At the same time, an aspect of the underlying biology of the traumatic experience, and schematization of the extreme nature of a danger and its personal consequentiality, seem similar to the model of one-trial aversion learning, making specific aspects of the traumatic memory more resistant to modification or extinction.[38–40]

From a developmental point of view, this extended period of consolidation of memory has the function of permitting adults with more experience, through co-construction, to influence the valence of what is placed in memory, to alter the spatial–contextual definition of the danger, and to integrate other, more constructive responses to the danger into memory. Co-construction can assist a child in clarifying details of the traumatic experience, its context and meaning, and in addressing cognitive confusions. Alternatively, adult caretakers may introduce prohibitions, misleading explanations, misattributions, or biased attributions of accountability, or invoke a covert conspiracy of silence.[41–43] Of special note, co-construction can address "pathogenic beliefs"[44] that emerge out of the child's inaccuracies and misattributions of accountability or psychosexual conflicts, or it can impart them through misinformation or suggestion.

Laboratory studies of young children's memory have demonstrated that it is often immaturity in their strategy of recall, rather than any deficit in memory retention, that accounts for difficulties in memory tasks.[45] When children have initial difficulty in recall, it is often because they do not have an adequate retrieval strategy or do not recognize the need for one. Lack of integration of traumatic moments, which may appear to be fragmentation of the memory, in young children may be due to the immaturity of their cognitive processing and strategy of recall, as well as to their reliance on contextual cues. These strategies of recall also depend on an evolving capacity for autobiographical episodic memory.[46,47] This maturation of autobiographical memory corresponds with a developmental progression in initial intervention fantasies. Typically, preschool children confine their intervention thoughts to the immediate moments when threat or injury had occurred; the school-age child will entertain intervention thoughts encompassing the day of the traumatic situation; and adolescents will often consider intervention or protective actions over a much longer time period.

Other studies have demonstrated that techniques of assisted recall can improve children's accurate recollections of stressful situations.[48] These techniques need not provide new information or suggestions. In our study of the sniper attack, for example, when we directed children to go over their school yard experience in "slow motion," they were able to fill in gaps, sequence events more correctly, add details, and elaborate on their emotional responses, appraisals, and thoughts about protective action.[23]

Saywitz et al.[49] have demonstrated that memory-jogging techniques, based on the premises that memory-jogging features should overlap with memory and that there may be several retrieval paths or cues to a memory for an event, significantly increased 7- to 11-year-old children's recall. Assisted recall interview techniques can be particularly important in this age-group,[50] given the complexity of a traumatic experience, the multitude of memory anchor points and their association with different traumatic moments, and the different nature of the organization of episodic memory that may be associated with each memory anchor point.

Perhaps least considered in prior literature is the role of the acute consultation interview in providing a strategy of recall for the child, and how that strategy may also become part of the child's memory network.[23] It has been our consistent observation that the manner in which the child is assisted in both remembrance and reconstruction of a trauma narrative becomes incorporated as part of any ongoing memory processing. In general, our findings are consistent with the complex social-motivational model of memory proposed by Saywitz and Moan-Hardie.[51]

Conclusion

An adequate characterization of acute traumatic memory in childhood requires a functional and developmental approach which includes consideration of objective and subjective features of multiple traumatic moments and accompanying intervention fantasies and their evolution over time, and ongoing efforts to "weaken the version." Recall of the experience is influenced by a variety of biological, cognitive, affective, and social developmental processes, by additional motivational and social factors associated with the recall setting, and by co-construction of the trauma narrative. We hope this clinical research approach contributes to a scientific understanding of the complex nature of traumatic memories in childhood, to the advancement of clinical work with acutely traumatized children, and to a more informed societal debate over children's trauma narratives and recollections in forensic settings.

References

1. Boodman SG: Advocacy group for "aggrieved" parents fight back. Washington Post 1994; April 12, p. 15.
2. Grant L: Tricks of memory: a new group concerned about child sex abuse is taking up the fight against the doctrine of false memory syndrome. Guardian 1994; April 25, pp. T008–T009.
3. Pendergrast M: Victims of Memory: Incest Accusations and Shattered Lives. Hinesburg VT: Upper Access, 1995.
4. Ceci SJ, Bruck M: Suggestibility of the child witness: a historical review and synthesis. Psychol Bull 1993; 113:403–439.
5. McGaugh JL: Significance and remembrance: the role of neuromodulatory systems. Psychol Sci 1990; 1:15–25.
6. Pitman RK: Posttraumatic stress disorder, hormones, and memory. Biol Psychiatry 1989; 26:221–223.
7. Nadel L: Multiple memory systems—What and why. J Cogn Sci 1992; 4:179–188.
8. Pynoos RS, Steinberg AM, Wraith R: A developmental model of childhood traumatic stress.

In D Cicchetti, D Cohen (Eds.), Manual of Developmental Psychopathology, Vol. 2. Risk, Disorder and Adaptation. New York: John Wiley, 1995, pp. 72–95.

9. Freud S: Inhibitions, symptoms and anxiety. *In* J Strachey (Ed. and Trans.), The Standard Edition of the Complete Psychological Works of Sigmund Freud, Vol. 20. London: Hogarth Press, 1959, pp. 87–156. (Original work published 1926)

10. Yule W, Bolton D, Udwin O: Objective and subjective predictors of PTSD in adolescence. Paper presented at the World Conference of the International Society for Traumatic Stress Studies, Amsterdam, June 1992.

11. Schwartz ED, Kowalski JM: Malignant memories: PTSD in children and adults after a school shooting. J Am Acad Child Adolesc Psychiatry 1991; 30:936–944.

12. Pynoos RS, Goenjian A, Tashjian M, Karakashian M, Manjikian R, Manoukian G, Steinberg AM, Fairbanks LA: Posttraumatic stress reactions in children after the 1988 earthquake in Armenia. Br J Psychiatry 1993; 163:239–247.

13. Pynoos RS, Steinberg AM, Goenjian A: Traumatic stress in childhood and adolescence: recent developments and current controversies. *In* BA van der Kolk, A MacFarlane (Eds.), Traumatic Stress: The Effects of Overwhelming Experience on Mind, Body and Society. New York: Guilford, 1996, pp. 331–358.

14. Yule W, Williams R: Posttraumatic stress reactions in children. J Traumatic Stress 1990; 3:279–295.

15. Lansky MR: Fathers Who Fail: Shame and Psychopathology in the Family System. Hillsdale NJ: Analytic Press, 1992.

16. Krystal H: Integration and self-healing in post-traumatic states: a ten year retrospective. Am Imago 1991; 48:93–117.

17. Emde R: Positive emotions for psychoanalytic theory: surprises from infancy research and new directions. J Am Psychoanal Assoc 1991; 39:5–44.

18. Murray HA: Explorations in Personality. London and New York: Oxford University Press, 1938.

19. Rangell L: Castration. J Am Psychoanal Assoc 1991; 39:3–23.

20. Perry BD, Pollard RA, Blakley TL, Baker WL, Vigilante D: Childhood trauma, the neurobiology of adaptation and ''use-dependent'' development of the brain: how ''states'' become ''traits.'' Infant Ment Health J 1995; 16:271–291.

21. Rose DS: A model for psychodynamic psychotherapy with the rape victim. Psychotherapy 1991; 28:85–95.

22. Bartlett A: Remembering. Cambridge: Cambridge University Press, 1932.

23. Pynoos RS, Nader K: Children's memory and proximity to violence. J Am Acad Child Adolesc Psychiatry 1989; 28:236–241.

24. Pynoos RS, Nader K: Issues in the treatment of posttraumatic stress in children and adolescents. *In* JP Wilson, B Raphael (Eds.), The International Handbook of Traumatic Stress Syndromes. New York: Plenum Press, 1993, pp. 535–549.

25. Terr L: Childhood traumas: an outline and overview. Am J Psychiatry 1991; 148:10–20.

26. Bjork RA, Richardson-Klavehn A: On the puzzling relationship between environmental context and human memory. *In* Current Issues in Cognitive Processes: The Tulane Flowertree Symposium on Cognition. Hillsdale NJ: Erlbaum, 1989, pp. 313–344.

27. Freud A: Identification with the aggressor. *In* The Writings of Anna Freud, Vol. 2. The Ego and the Mechanisms of Defense (Rev. ed.). New York: International University Press, 1966, pp. 109–121.

28. Pynoos RS: The traumatic moment revisited: toward a developmental psychoanalytic model of internal and external dangers. Paper presented at the Los Angeles Psychoanalytic Society and Institute, March 1995.

29. Ornitz EM: Developmental aspects of neurophysiology. *In* M Lewis (Ed.), Child and Adolescent Psychiatry: A Comprehensive Textbook. Baltimore MD: Williams & Wilkins, 1991, pp. 38–51.

30. Buck L, Axel R: A novel multigene family may encode odorant receptors: a molecular basis for odor recognition. Cell 1991; 65:175–187.

31. Baddeley AD: Memory theory and memory therapy. *In* B Wilson, N Moffat (Eds.), Clinical Management of Memory Problems. London: Aspen, 1984, pp. 5–27.

32. Baddeley AD: Psychology of Memory. New York: Basic Books, 1976.

33. Saarni C, Harris PL: Children's Understanding of Emotion. Cambridge: Cambridge Universtiy Press, 1991.

34. Parens H: A view of the development of hostility in early life. J Am Psychoanal Assoc 1991; 39:75–108.

35. Rolls ET: Functions of neuronal networks in the hippocampus and neocortex in memory. *In* J Byrne, W. Berry (Eds.), Neural Models of Plasticity: Experimental and Theoretical Approaches. San Diego: Academic Press, 1989, pp. 240–265.

36. Shapiro T, Perry R: Latency revisited. Psychoanal Study Child 1976; 31:79–105.

37. Conway MA: Emotion and memory. Science 1993; 261:369–370.

38. Garcia J, Lasiter PS, Bermudez-Rattoni F, Deems A: A general theory of aversion learning. Ann NY Acad Sci 1986; 43:8–21.

39. Yehuda R, Antelman SM: Criteria for evaluating animal models of posttraumatic stress disorder. Biol Psychiatry 1993; 33:479–486.

40. van der Kolk BA: The intrusive past: flexibility of memory and the engraving of trauma. Am Imago 1991; 4:425–454.

41. Bowlby J: On knowing what you aren't supposed to know and feeling what you are not supposed to feel. Can J Psychiatry 1979; 24:403–408.

42. Cain A, Fast I: Children's disturbed reactions to parent suicide: distortion and guilt, communication and identification. *In* A Cain (Ed.), Survivors of Suicide. Springfield IL: C.C. Thomas, 1972, pp. 93–111.

43. Kestenberg JS: How children remember and parents forget. Int J Psychoanal Psychother 1972; 1:103–123.

44. Weis M: The centrality of adaptation. Contemp Psychoanal 1990; 26:660–676.

45. Johnson MK, Foley MA: Differentiating fact from fantasy: the reliability of children's memory. J Soc Issues 1984; 40:33–50.

46. Fivush R: Developmental perspectives on autobiographical recall. *In* GS Goodman, B Bottoms (Eds.), Child Victims, Child Witnesses. New York: Guilford, 1993, pp. 1–24.

47. Nelson K: The psychological and social origins of autobiographical memory. Psychol Sci 1993; 4:7–14.

48. Saywitz K, Goodman G, Nicholas E, Moan S: Children's memories of a physical examination involving genital touch: implications for reports sexual abuse. J Consult Clin Psychol 1991; 59:682–691.

49. Saywitz K, Geiselman RE, Bornstein GK: Effects of cognitive interviewing and practice on children's recall performance. J Appl Psychol 1992; 77:744–756.

50. Lamb ME, Sternberg KJ, Esplin PW: Factors influencing the reliability and validity of statements made by young victims of sexual maltreatment. J Appl Dev Psychol 1994; 15:255–280.

51. Saywitz KJ, Moan-Hardie S: Reducing the potential for distortion of childhood memories. Consciousness Cogn 1994; 3:408–425.

IV

TRAUMA AND MEMORY: EVALUATION AND TREATMENT

12

Psychoanalysis, Reconstruction, and the Recovery of Memory

HOWARD B. LEVINE

Over the course of treatment, when the details of forgotten events do not emerge spontaneously in the mind of the patient, they may be inferred by the analyst and interpreted to the patient as possibly having occured. We call these inferences of what seems plausible or what might have been, *constructions* or, when referring to past events, reconstructions. The aim of reconstructions is either to stimulate the recall of the forgotten past or to substitute for important memories that may never be recaptured. In the latter instance, it is the conviction which the analyst and patient assign to the reconstruction that fills in the blanks in a narrative account of the patient's life and in the development of the patient's neurosis that is decisive for the treatment. As noted by Freud,[1] "if the analysis is carried out correctly, we produce in [the patient] an assured conviction of the truth of the construction which achieves the same therapeutic result as a recaptured memory."

The reconstruction or recovery of forgotten (repressed) memories of significant, often traumatic events that date from a patient's infancy and childhood has always occupied a role in the clinical practice of psychoanalysis. What has varied at different stages in the evolution of psychoanalytic theory, however, is the degree to which reconstruction or recovery of childhood memory was seen as a therapeutic factor and central preoccupation for psychoanalytic technique. In the first two periods of Freud's thought, from his earliest experiments with the treatment of neuroses (1887–1897) through the period of the topographic theory (1900–1920), the lifting of repression via reconstruction or recall was the singular aim of psychoanalytic treatment. With the introduction of the structural theory, however, the goal of psychoanalytic technique began to shift away from a single-minded focus on making the unconscious conscious toward the analytic exploration of the motivations for and purposes served by resistance and transference. As a result of this shift in emphasis, the reconstruction and recovery of forgotten childhood memories came to occupy a less central position in analytic technique than did the broader task of analyzing unconscious fantasies and conflicts. By the 1960s–70s, the developments and preoccupations of ego psychology had so influenced the practice of psychoanalysis in the United States that Greenacre[2] lamented the loss of interest in reconstruction as a component of analytic technique and regretted the inability of more recently trained analysts to teach its subtleties to subsequent generations of clinicians.

Our current climate, in which questions concerning the emotional consequences and therapeutic remediation of childhood trauma—especially childhood sexual abuse and incest—have come to assume such prominence and immediacy, compels us to reexamine the possibilities and place of recollection and reconstruction in analytic therapy. In particular, therapists and patients have felt sorely challenged by instances in which one or the other has suspected childhood sexual abuse or incest, but memories or other data confirming these events have not been forthcoming. Under such circumstances, questions of the validity and methodology of reconstruction, with all of its attendant possibilities of unwitting therapist suggestion contributing to "false memory syndrome," have taken on a sense of great importance and even therapeutic urgency.

In the chapter that follows, I will review the evolving role and significance of reconstruction and recall as therapeutic factors in psychoanalytic therapy in the light of the evolution that has taken place in the psychoanalytic theories of mental functioning, neurosogenesis, and therapy. With this historical review as background, I will then present a contemporary psychoanalytic perspective on the problem of memory and discuss some epistemological difficulties in ascertaining the truth value of reconstructions and memories and the technical dilemma that these present for the patient and therapist.

Trauma, Abreaction, and the Seduction Theory

When Freud began the clinical research that led to the publication of *Studies in Hysteria*,[3] the recovery of memory occupied a central role in his therapeutic method. At that point in the development of his ideas, Freud's theory of pathogenesis held that, because of their shocking, unpleasant, or morally repugnant nature, certain thoughts, feelings, or experiences were repudiated by the neurotic to such an extent that they were isolated from "the dominant mass of ideas" that constituted the rest of the patient's "ego" (psyche). Since the repudiated thoughts, feelings, and experiences were relatively disconnected from and unintegrated into the main portions of the neurotic's mind, they remained inaccessible to consciousness during normal states of awareness. As a result, the "emotional charge" which Freud assumed that they carried could not be modulated or discharged by the mind's usual means of doing so.

A central assumption in Freud's theory of mental functioning at this point in time was that the human mind regulated the flow of psychic energy controlling affective discharge processes. He believed that under normal circumstances, this regulation was mediated by the direct discharge (expression) of affect or by indirect discharge via processes of *association* with similar or related thoughts. Following a physical analogy with the pain caused by an enlarging abscess, Freud proposed that the undischargable psychic energy associated with repressed (forgotten) and dissociated thoughts, experiences, and feelings exerted a persistent force or pressure in the patient's mind. If not relieved by adequate discharge, this pressure would continue to build until it spilled over into the somatic realm and "erupted" in the production of symptoms. Thus, Freud assumed that neurotic symptoms were symbolic equivalents of repressed or dissociated thoughts, experiences or feelings—"hysterics suffer from reminiscences"[3]—and functionally were the result of the neurotic's failure to adequately discharge psychic energy via the modulation and expression of affect.

Freud's theory of treatment at this stage of his work followed accordingly. It depended heavily on hypnotic and other suggestive techniques that attempted to force the patient into recalling—and hence, reconnecting—all that had once been isolated from consciousness. Once this occurred, Freud believed that the psychic dam would be breached and the previously loculated energies would escape in a cathartic flood of feelings, thoughts, and memories that he felt would be therapeutic. This process of emotional outpouring was called *abreaction*.

In what many observers now believe to be a circular fashion, Freud reasoned that if patients suffered from the consequences of undischarged psychic energy, then abreaction and recollection were appropriate goals of treatment. And if abreaction and recollection led to relief of symptoms, then pathogenesis must therefore be associated with a loculation and isolation within the mind of undischargable energy associated with unacceptable thoughts, experiences, and feelings. These assumptions fit well with early experiments in which hypnosis was used to temporarily reproduce or dispel the symptoms of hysteria and with the clinical results obtained with Freud's technique of pressing on his patients' foreheads in order to help them to recall what had previously been repressed or dissociated from consciousness. The term Freud chose to describe the structural condition of the neurotic's "ego," in which two or more relatively separate complexes of mental contents existed within the mind was one that was already familiar to his contemporaries from the work of Janet and others: *splitting of consciousness*.

As part of this initial theory, Freud felt that it was important to address the reasons why his patients were motivated to repress or dissociate the thoughts, feelings, and memories that were causing their symptoms. When he was still working in close collaboration with Joseph Breuer, Freud felt that two possible conditions could be obtained. In one condition, the thoughts, feelings, and experiences that were responsible for the neurotic symptoms were repressed and dissociated, because they were unacceptable or repugnant to the patient. That is, their exclusion from consciousness was in the service of protecting the individual from unpleasant thoughts and feelings that would produce some degree of conscious psychic conflict or distress; hence the name, *defense hysteria*.

In the other condition, certain mental contents wound up being repressed or dissociated, because they occurred at moments when normal consciousness was thought to be "weakened." These states, which Breuer felt approximated the condition of the mind in an hypnotic trance, were called *hypnoid states*. While Janet believed such states to be hereditarily determined, a constitutionally derived structual weakness of the mind, Breuer hypothesized that times of febrile illness or semiconsciousness, such as the periods immediately around awakening or falling sleep, were moments in which the mechanisms of consciousness—and therefore, the mind—were naturally weakened. As a result of this "weakness," experiences that occurred during such times were more likely to be dissociated or forgotten.[4] Instances of what Freud and Breuer called *passive* or *hypnoid hysteria* were reported in *Studies in Hysteria*[3]. However, their importance and even their possible existence were soon overshadowed by Freud's interest in and "discoveries" about the etiological roots of hysterical symptoms that were produced in the service of defense.[a]

As Freud delved more closely into his patients' pasts, he began to encounter stories of childhood sexual seductions that appeared to be causally connected to the development of their neurotic symptoms. Ultimately, he erroneously[6,7] concluded that *an actual seduction prior to puberty was the root of every neurotic illness*. This theory, known today as *the seduction theory*, went through a number of alterations before it was finally discarded.[8] In each of its variations, what remained constant was Freud's belief that behind *every* nuerosis was a childhood sexual seduction.

In the metaphoric language of Freud's first theory of neurosogenesis, the thoughts and feelings attending the events of a childhood seduction were repugnant and therefore had to be repressed or dissociated. When these were separated from the main portion of the mind, "the dominant mass of ideas," the child's consciousness was "split" and weakened. Once an idea or memory was removed from consciousness, it was thought to function like a magnet, attracting to itself any subsequent thoughts, feelings, or experiences that would imply or require the acceptance of what was already repudiated. In this way, the presence of a repressed or dissociated "complex" made the mind of the neurotic more susceptible to subsequent acts of repression and dissociation, when later unpleasant or repugnant thoughts, feelings, and experiences came along. The more thoughts, feelings, and experiences underwent repression and dissociation, the weaker was the child's consciousness and the greater the child's tendency to repress or dissociate subsequent thoughts, feelings, and experiences.

Freud believed that the repressed or dissociated thoughts, feelings, and experiences linked to childhood seductions remained sequestered in the psyche of the child until

---

a. In his introduction to *Studies in Hysteria*,[3] Strachey notes (p. xxii) that it was Breuer who originated the term *hypnoid states,* and that Freud, in a footnote to the Dora case,[5] later dissociated himself from this hypothesis.

they were reawakened by the normal developmental processes of adolescence. Then, the inevitable stirring of sexual feelings that is so much a part of adolescent development somehow dynamically activated the experiences of the childhood seduction and transformed them into trauma. As Freud[9] said, ''It is not the experiences themselves which act traumatically but their revival as a *memory* after the subject has entered on sexual maturity.''[b]

There are two problems that immediately present themselves in regard to Freud's seduction theory. While ingenious as a first formulation, the theory of mental functioning in which it is embedded is too simplistic and no longer tenable, compared with our current models of the mind. Far more goes into the complex forces that eventuate in pathogenesis than this first model allows. The second, more important objection is that without access to the clinical data upon which Freud formulated his seduction hypothesis, we do not know the extent to which his patients *reported* histories of childhood sexual seductions, as opposed to the extent to which Freud *reconstructed* these histories from the symptoms, dreams, associations, and behavior of his neurotic patients (e.g., ''given your symptoms, it is likely that such-and-such must have happened''). Without such data, it is impossible for us to judge the validity of Freud's initial conclusions.

The resulting dilemma, which confronts us as students of the history of psychoanalysis, is also, of course, quite familiar to us as clinicians. It is not unusual for us to find ourselves perplexed by the uncertain data of a clinical case and our own responses to the material as we attempt to determine whether or not sexual abuse or another form of significant, but not yet recollected childhood trauma has occured. The urgency and bewilderment of our position may be made all the more complicated by the current politicized climate of accusation and counter-accusation regarding ''false memory syndrome'' versus ''denial of trauma.''

In any evaluation of the seduction hypothesis, it is important to note that Freud developed this theory before he formulated the concept of *transference*. As a result, he could not have been fully sensitive to the impact on his patients of their unconscious childhood wishes or the influence of his relationship with them upon their current fantasies produced in treatment. His clinical method at the time was forceful, positive, and determined. If relevant memories were not spontaneously forthcoming, he resorted to hypnosis, to pressing on a patient's forehead in order to stimulate feelings, thoughts, and memories, or to verbal insistence that something relevant *will* come to mind. He would not take no for an answer.

Freud's technique at this period of time attempted to bypass resistance, rather than investigate the motivation for its being employed. In the current light of our sensitivity to the impact of the analyst's actual behavior on the unfolding and development of the transference[10] and our understanding of the intersubjective nature of the analytic pro-

---

b. This process of ''deferred action'' is often referred to in contemporary psychoanalytic accounts by its German or French equivalents as *Nachtraglichkeit* or *aprés coup*.

cess,[11,12] we would now wonder if Freud's clinical methods did not lend themselves to the unwitting creation of conditions in which patients would inadvertently feel overstimulated and intruded upon. To the extent that such feelings were induced, patients would be more likely to either comply with Freud's forceful demands and suggestions or experience them as overwhelming and seductive in their own right.

Contemporary psychoanalysts are familiar with the kinds of fantasies that such forceful and intrusive interventions may stimulate in patients, especially those who were sexually abused as children. As I have noted elsewhere:

> From the perspective of current knowledge, it would not be too far afield to surmise that such forceful intrusions were, in at least some instances, countertransference enactments in which a childhood sexual trauma was symbolically being repeated. Thus, it remains quite unclear how much Freud's reconstructions were based on observations of what we would now view as erotized transference phenomena, how often these transferences reflected childhood fantasies as opposed to actual childhood seductions or sexual trauma, or the extent to which Freud recognized the possibility that his analysands' transferences may have colored their reports of earlier childhood events."[13]

In reviewing the evolution and evidentiary basis of Freud's seduction theory, Schimek[14] comes to a similar conclusion.

Ultimately, Freud himself came to recognize the limitations of this early theory. Though self-analysis and broadening clinical experience, he realized that as important as actual childhood seductions had been in the etiology of some neuroses, they could never be implicated as the *universal* agent in neurosogenesis. The resulting crisis in his thinking ultimately led Freud to his theory of infantile sexuality, an appreciation of the central importance of unconscious fantasy in human mental life and to the birth of psychoanalysis as we know it today.

Years later, in his "Autobiographical Study,"[15] Freud described this momentous change in his views as follows:

> I was at last obliged to recognize that these scenes of seduction had never taken place, and that they were only phantasies which my patients had made up, *or which I myself had perhaps forced on them.* . . . When I had pulled myself together, I was able to draw the right conclusions from my discovery: . . . I had in fact stumbled for the first time upon the *Oedipus complex.* . . . Moreover, *seduction during childhood retained a certain share, though a humbler one, in the aetiology of neuroses.* (italics added)

Infantile Sexuality and the Topographic Theory

When Freud replaced the seduction theory, he did so with a view of neurosis that emphasized its origins in the conflicts that followed from the development and press of *instincts* in emotional life. Of particular interest to Freud were the sexual instincts, which he called the *libido.* These, he felt, were constitutionally determined and present from birth ("infantile sexuality"). They developed spontaneously from the beginnings of life along a preordained path, passing through oral, anal, and genital phases. Although Freud assumed that in their "pure" state, the sexual instincts were "quantities of excitation" and therefore unconscious, their energy could be connected to various ideas—"derivatives"—and thereby raised to consciousness or gratified in action in a displaced or symbolic fashion.[16,17]

Each of the libidinal phases described by Freud was thought to be associated with phase-specific desires and fantasies that were reflected in symbolic form in dreams, children's play, "the psychopathology of everyday life," and neurotic symptoms. In regard to the latter, Freud believed that at least one meaning of a neurotic symptom was the (symbolic) "representation" or "realization" of a wishful fantasy with a repressed, infantile sexual content.[18] Successful development required that the child's mind mediate between the press of instinctually determined, infantile sexual desires and the dangers and limitations of reality. The latter evoked a response from the "ego instincts," which functioned in the service of "self preservation." The *Oedipus complex,* which Freud mentioned so prominently in his autobiographical account of his renunciation of the seduction theory and which assumed a central place in his theory of human development, was the name that Freud gave to the intense feelings of love and incestuous sexual desire (usually for the parent of the opposite sex) and murderous rivalry (usually towards the parent of the same sex) that each child invariably experienced during ages 3–6.

A more thorough explication of the development of Freud's theory of the instincts is beyond the scope of this chapter. In order to appreciate the role of recollection and reconstruction in Freud's theory of therapeutic action and technique during this period, however, it is important to note two components of his theory that are relevant to our present study: (*a*) the relationship between actual events, instinctual conflicts, and the production of symptoms and (*b*) the designation of consciousness and unconsciousness as structural properties of the mind.

In coming "to regard neurosis as a conflict of instincts rather than a conflict of disagreeable and incompatible ideas concerning the self,"[19] Freud de-emphasized, but did not totally abandon, the role of sexual seduction, actual trauma, and external reality in the etiology of neurosis. What critics such as Masson[20] have failed to appreciate is that although Freud's predominant interest shifted from the psychic consequences of actual events and *material reality* to that of fantasies and *psychic reality,* he never abandoned the recognition that external reality was important in the ultimate shaping of neurotic symptoms or that childhood sexual seductions, trauma, and incest were responsible for the production of *some* neuroses. For example, in his *Introductory Lectures on Psychoanalysis,* Freud wrote: "Phantasies of being seduced are of particular interest because so often they are not phantasies but real memories"[21] and, "[t]he childhood experiences constructed or remembered in analysis are sometimes indisputably false and sometimes equally certainly correct, and in most cases compounded of truth and falsehood."[22] In subsequent writings he noted: "Actual seduction is common enough''[23] and, ''[t]he object of sexual seduction may direct her later sexual life so as to provoke entirely similar acts.''[24]

Thus, while Freud abandoned the belief that a childhood sexual experience was the root of every neurotic symptom, he continued to believe that actual, external events played a role, albeit a lesser one, in the production of neurosis. What also changed were his views of the mechanisms through which actual events operated upon the emotions. In Freud's new theory, conflicts between internally derived, instinctual forces were inevitable parts of the human condition. Neurotic conflict was conceptualized as the consequence of the individual's internal strivings, rather than the result of excessive excitation which originated in the external world. Fixations of the libido to unconscious infantile wishes led to conflicts between fantasy (derived from infantile sexual instincts) and reality (as perceived by the ''ego instincts'' of self-preservation). Because neurotics could not let themselves have what they desired, they remained frustrated. It is this frustration of repressed, infantile sexual desires that Freud believed ultimately led to the development of neurotic symptoms.

Trauma, then, came to be defined in terms of instinctual conflict and the impact of that conflict on the psyche and emotions of the developing child. Where real events retained a potentially neurosogenic impact was in their influence as a contributing cause of instinctual conflict and fixation. For example, it was the premature exposure to adult sexual activity (''the primal scene''), that Freud suggested was responsible for the production of the Wolf Man's neurosis.[25] In Freud's formulation, primal scene exposure led to overstimulation and fixation to incestuous desires directed toward unavailable love objects. This condition led to frustration, defensive measures (repression), and intensified instinctual pressure. The resultant ''damming up'' of large quantities of libido pressed inexorably and unsuccessfully for discharge and gratification and ultimately became converted into anxiety and other neurotic symptoms.

According to Freud's theory in this phase of his thinking, the mind was structurally divided into two main compartments: those thoughts, feelings, and memories which were capable of being thought of without much effort (the conscious and preconscious portions of the mind), and those that could not be directly thought of at all (the unconscious), with an internal ''censor'' regulating movement of mental contents between the two. As noted in his earlier writings,[17,26,27] Freud believed that elements of the unconscious appeared in symbolic form in such phenomena as dreams, day dreams, jokes, parapraxes, and neurotic symptoms. It was Freud's metaphoric spatial division of the mind according to the quality of consciousness that earned this model the name, *the topographic theory*.

In terms of a strategy for and theory of therapy, once again, the problem of neurosis was thought to lay with silent build-up of mental energies (unsatisfied libido) whose press for relief through discharge was doomed to failure, because their very presence remained beyond the individual's awareness. Freud believed that the therapeutic solution to the problem of neurosis lay in making the neurotic aware of the unknown desires (instinctual wishes) and the conflicts in which they had become enmeshed. Hence, his therapeutic strategy emphasized informing patients ("interpretation") of those contents of their mind (derivatives of infantile sexual wishes and the conflicts to which they had given rise) that they had repressed. In a famous clinical dictum, Freud summed up the aim of analytic therapy as "making the unconscious conscious."[17] Thus, during the period of the topographic theory, *the lifting of repression,* i.e., the reconstruction and recollection of the past, remained the central goal and principle therapeutic factor in psychoanalytic treatment.

Ego Psychology and the Structural Theory

As a result of clinical observations regarding aggression, narcissism, and unconscious guilt, Freud felt it necessary once more to revise his theory of the etiology of neurosis and the organization of the mind.[28,29] In his final theory—called *the structural theory,* because it divided the psyche into the three familiar categories (structures) of id, ego, and super ego—Freud elevated aggression to the status of an instinct, making it co-equal to sexuality, reduced consciousness/unconsciousness to an attribute of various psychic contents rather than a structurally defining property of the mind, and revised his views about the origins of anxiety and its function in relation to defense.

Freud's reconceptualization of anxiety as an adaptive, control process of the ego, rather than a transformation of libido, is of crucial importance to the contemporary analytic theory of therapy and our current understanding of the place of reconstruction and recall in analytic technique. According to the structural theory, the well-functioning ego was constantly unconsciously scanning the environment, anticipating the potential consequences of proposed actions (especially in relation to the gratification of instinctually derived wishes) and using small quantities of unconscious anxiety as a signal of impending danger to which it responded with a variety of defensive measures.

These defensive measures, the "mechanisms of defense,"[30] went far beyond repression to include such now familiar processes as isolation of effect, rationalization, intellectualization, splitting, projection, identification, denial, etc. Unlike repression, which in the topographic theory was synonymous with defense, the operation of these defense mechanisms did not necessarily involve the removal of mental contents from consciousness. Rather, they operated by means other than forgetting, such as the splitting off of affect from ideational content, the minimizing of feelings associated with an idea, or the removal of ideas and affects from contextual significance. Given this broadened concept of defense, the goals of the analyst's interventions would now extend beyond that of assisting the return to consciousness of what formerly been repressed. In the hierarchy of analytic technique, the lifting of the repression barrier by recollection and reconstruction would have to cede pride of place to strengthening the ego and facilitating its development through the analysis of unconscious conflicts.

The introduction of the structural theory ushered in the era of *ego psychology.*

Neurosis, which Freud now defined as the product of intrapsychic conflict between and within the major structures of the mind, increasingly came to be understood in terms of "psychic reality"—i.e., personal meanings and subjective interpretations of perceptions that were influenced by unconscious conflicts and fantasies that blended with the objective facts of material reality—rather than the mechanics of psychic energy transfer. ("In the world of the neuroses, it is psychical reality which is the decisive kind."[31]) The topographic theory's concerns with instinctual fixations was expanded to include arrests in ego development. These were marked in the clinical setting by excessive reliance on maladaptive, infantile defensive operations and infantile interpretations of reality. Technically, clinical emphasis and priority were increasingly given to the exploration and elucidation of the unconscious, defensive activities of the ego, especially as they related to the patient's experience of and relationship with the therapist (transference). Resistances in therapy were no longer simply to be overcome, they were to be analyzed (explored). And the analysis of resistance in the transference became the central focus of the analytic task.

As a result of these and other changes, a small but significant shift took place in the therapeutic aim of analysis with regard to the recovery of memory. Reconstruction and recall were de-emphasized as therapeutic ends in and of themselves, and were replaced by the exploration and analysis of unconscious conflict and conflict-determined subjective experiences and meanings.[32] The preoccupation with discovering the actual historical facts of past experience, which had occupied so prominent a place in the analytic therapeutic enterprise, was progressively supplanted by the demonstration of the ways in which current phenomena—symptoms, transference reactions, and character traits—reflected past conflicts and the fantasies and experiences from which they derived; by the "working through" of unconscious meanings, conflicts, and fantasies; and by the strengthening and integration of the ego and facilitation of ego development via the resolution of unconscious conflicts. Making the unconscious conscious was replaced by a new dictum: "Where id was, there ego shall be."[28]

The new emphasis on stengthening the ego rather than remembering the past extended to the treatment of the consequences of traumatic experiences, such as childhood sexual abuse and incest. Technical priority was given to the exploration and understanding of the conscious and unconscious meanings of the past experience and to the systematic analysis and working through of the sequelae of traumatic experiences and the unconscious conflicts that they produced. The concept of what was to be reconstructed in treatment shifted away from the discrete, specific, events of the trauma to include fantasies and affects associated with the trauma, childhood object relationships, dynamically meaningful patterns of experience, unrelated repressed fantasies that had become condensed and connected to the traumatic experiences, etc. Ultimately, "the unconscious fantasy elaboration and the structural developmental impact of a particular experience or set of experiences became more important that the actual history."[33]

The Nature of Memory

The developments of ego psychology also led analysts to become increasingly suspicious of the elusive—and illusory—nature of memory. In a naturalistic observation of preschool children, Kris[32] demonstrated how past and present context, subsequent development, and conflicts operating at the time of registration and attempted recall influenced the "facts" of what children were able to remember (see also Freud[34] and Levine[35,36]). Kris' work was seminal in establishing that memories of formative events are altered in the course of development as they become absorbed into significant patterns of character and defense. It is the latter that are more likely to be relived in the transference and hence reconstructed in the treatment than are the discrete events from which they may be constituted. Consequently, rather than viewing memory as the pristine imprint of an objective experience, contemporary analysts are more likely to regard it as a construction, one that is subject to unconscious dynamic influences that favor screening and distortions, repression or recall. In this sense, memories are now understood to be amalgamations of both *historical truth* and *narrative truth*—of what actually happened and the subjective interpretations, fantasies and contextual determinants surrounding an occurance and its recall.

Recognizing these changes is crucial for any contemporary understanding of the psychoanalytic approach to the consequences of childhood trauma. They emphasize the extent to which trauma, in the psychoanalytic sense, is seen as a *psychological* event that reflects the ways in which a given individual subjectively experiences and tries to make sense out of whatever it is that has happened to them. Individual experience always contains irreducibly subjective elements that affect the ways in which actual events are felt, understood, and remembered.[12,37] The objective facts of an event do not fully determine how that event will be felt or understood by a child or remembered by that child when he or she becomes an adult. Nor will they alone determine the specific ways in which the resulting experience will feel or function as a trauma. It is the subjective, psychic representation of events that will determine the child's experience and continue to operate within the mind of the child, affecting and being affected by subsequent events and emotional development. Hence, Freud's comment that in terms of the neuroses, it is *psychic reality* that is decisive[17] and Dowling's observation that in so far as trauma is a psychological experience, it is an experience of *meaning*.[38]

These assertions do not mean that the actuality of what did or did not happen was of no consequence. Clearly it is, and many analysts, beginning with Freud, have called attention to the importance of actual events in the formation of neurosis. Greenacre, for example, described how *actual* traumatic childhood experience could powerfully reinforce drive or developmentally based infantile fantasies, impacting on further development and creating conflicts and fixations that were harder to remove in treatment than those that resulted from predominantly intrapsychic origins (fantasy) alone.[39] Loewenstein also pointed out the significant differences that can exist between the consequences of actual traumatic events, as opposed to those produced by unconscious, instinctually derived conflicts.[40]

Thus, while it is true that psychoanalytic interest in psychic reality resulted in a period in which the impact of actual events was relatively de-emphasized in the analytic literature,[13] it would be incorrect to infer from the writings of the ego psychologists that analysts disregarded patients' reports of what they remembered as ''mere fantasy'' or assumed that these reports held no truth value. Rather, observations, such as those made by Kris,[32] served as a reminder that the determinants of all memories include subjective, intrapsychically determined components, and context and developmentally derived influences that must always be allowed for, even though they may never be fully or adequately delineated. This fact introduces into any discussion regarding recollection and reconstruction an important note of caution about the extraordinary complexities involved in determining the historical truth value of the significant experiences of early childhood.

Psychic Reality and Historical Reality

In considering the complex relationship between psychic reality and historical reality, it is important to remember that the actual events, whatever thay were, are fixed and immutable. They happened and can never be undone. But how they registered, were interpreted, preserved, altered over time, and are retrieved from the mind of the subject as ''memory''—the unconscious meanings, conflicts, and fantasies to which they have given rise and with which they have become entangled; the symptomatic, developmental, and characterological antecedents and consequences—these are what constitute the realm of *psychic reality,* in which the psychological dimension of trauma is defined and operates and in which treatment must take place.

Unlike the external world, in which events are fixed and objective, this inner world is one of subjective, shifting facts and feelings that change with time, context, development, regression, and subsequent experiences. As important as the actual, objective events of the traumatogenic experience are, they are only a part of what makes up the patient's experience. As Arlow notes: ''In the mind of the young child, perception and fantasy are inextricably intertwined and what remains dynamically active, as either memory or fantasy, is an amalgam of what was wished for and what was experienced.''[41]

Analysts cannot, therefore, presume to understand a patient's experience solely on the basis of the objective facts of what actually happened. Moreover, the objective facts of the traumatic events are not what are dynamically operable in the patient's mind or in the treatment situation and therefore not what analysts are after in their work with patients. Potentially traumatic events contribute to unconscious fantasies and conflicts, and it is the exploration of these fantasies and conflicts and their psychological sequelae, not the recollection or reconstruction of the repressed, actual events by themselves, that is of therapeutic value. Boesky writes: "Only the painstaking understanding of the relation between real events, fantasies, conflicts and defenses of the patient as these conflicts are ramified through developmental changes and as they are meaningfully evoked in the arena of resistance and transference will ultimately help the patient."[42]

The predicament that confronts patients who were traumatized in childhood—and their therapists—is that those events have left psychological scars and deformations that have affected their emotional development and deformed their inner worlds.[43] The difficulties encountered in their transferences and in the other kinds of intimate relationships that they form attest to this.[13,35] The psychological consequences of childhood trauma take on a life of their own within the individual and produce and contribute to still further difficulties, distortions, unconscious conflicts, pathological fantasies, etc. It is all of this and not simply the uncovering of the events of a discrete trauma that must be addressed in therapy in a long and careful process of exploration, analysis, and working through. For this reason, *the reconstruction, recovery, and disclosure of memories are not in themselves sufficient for therapy.*[c]

In many instances, however, recovery and disclosure of repressed or otherwise hidden memories do play a crucial role in the course of treatment—not as a therapeutic end in themselves, but as a starting point for the building of trust in the therapeutic relationship and for understanding (reconstruction) of the impact of those events on the emotional life and development of the patient. As attested to in the recent literature,[44–48] the relief that can follow from the recollection or reconstruction of past childhood sexual trauma can be dramatic and is often essential for the *beginning* engagement of a therapeutic process. On the other hand, cases such as the one reported by Raphling,[49] where a patient who was not sexually abused in childhood wished to discover a history of childhood sexual abuse for defensive reasons, and those cited as part of the recent furor concerning "false memories"[50] created by the combination of overzealous therapists and suggestible patients, indicate the perils of memory and the reconstructive process.

Validation of Trauma and Validation of Truth: Reconstruction and the Problem of Suggestion

The technical problem confronting therapists of steering a course between the extremes of being open to recognizing and accepting the possibility of childhood sexual abuse and incest on the one hand, and not implanting the idea of childhood trauma as a suggestion in the mind of a patient on the other, is a complex one, indeed. Unfortunately, there is little in the patient's symptomatic or characterological presentation that can be reliably used as an invariable indicator of childhood sexual abuse. As I have written elsewhere:[43]

---

c. Davies and Frawley [44] come to a similar conclusion.

Despite claims to the contrary in the self-help literature, neither specific symptom clusters nor character formations offer a reliable basis for establishing the diagnosis of prior childhood sexual trauma or incest. If one *must* point to a presumptive indicator of the existence of previous childhood sexual abuse, the most reliable candidate is the nature and quality of the therapeutic relationship (transference and countertransference) that is lived out between patient and analyst. But . . . given all the pitfalls and subjectivities that this relationship is subject to, as a diagnostic tool, it is an equivocal instrument, at best.

For example, the patient's attitude towards the analyst or the treatment may reflect a repetition of one or another affect or attribute connected to the abuse or to the major participants in the abusive transaction, e.g., abused child, abusive adult, unprotecting parent, unconsciously consenting adult, etc. Alternatively, the patient's attitude towards the analyst or treatment may reflect a reversal or defense against that affect or attribute. Thus, the dominant quality of relationship that may be experienced by the patient or, as is often the case, lived out in the transference and/or countertransference may involve either patient or analyst in the reciprocal roles of abuser and abused, hurt child and unprotecting caretaker, hurt child and idealized protecting caretaker, sinful child and punishing superego, etc.

The actual forms that these relationships may take are as varied and idiosyncratic as individual human experience. Thus, some patients may feel that the treatment is too painful, overstimulating, or intrusive, or they may submit to the rigors of analysis with a depressed and masochistic sense of hopeless resignation. Others may complain that the analyst is failing to adequately regulate their feelings or protect them from harm. Still others will suspect that the analyst is being dishonest, flirtatious, vicariously stimulated, seductive, or corrupt. Or patients will entertain their own fantasies of or make demands for physical or sexual contact with the analyst, or for special arrangements regarding hours or fees that seek to bend or violate the usual rules and boundaries and place them in a special relationship to the analyst. Whereas any of these developments in the transference may contribute to the analyst's suspicion that a patient may have a past history of childhood sexual abuse, they are not, unfortunately, necessary or sufficient in and of themselves to establish the diagnosis.

In trying to sort out fantasy from reality, analysts and their patients have repeatedly come up against the fact that there are no reliable psychological markers in either participant that will allow them to unfailingly distinguish true recollections or reconstructions from false ones. And since, as Blum notes, "reconstruction [and, indeed, all analytic exploration] deals with the creation as well as the re-creation of the past, [a past] which is altered in the process of being reconstructed [and recollected],"[51] the very material upon which analyst and patient must rely, is continually being influenced, changed, and restructured by the act of engaging in the work of analysis. In such a situation, which is compounded by the extraordinary pressures to know the truth that can be mobilized in the analytic treatment of these patients,[36] the possibilities for inadvertent suggestion are legion.

Here it is worth noting an important distinction between analytic therapies and those therapies that are more specifically aimed at the recovery of past traumatic memories and the empowering of the patient to act in the present to rectify the wrongs of the past. Too often, some nonanalytic treatments, sometimes called *trauma* or *recovered memory therapies,* begin with the therapist's presupposition that certain symptoms, such as anorexia or fears of sexual intimacy, are de facto proof of childhood sexual abuse or incest. Patients may also be told, directly or indirectly, by their therapists that their failure to recognize these "facts" are further proof of prior sexual abuse, which is now contributing to their being "in denial." Moreover, the therapeutic goal of these therapists may include the wish not only to help patients recover past memories but to help them confront their past abusers in the service of healing or to advocate for their patients' attempts to obtain apologies, admissions of guilt, financial compensation, or other forms of redress for past grievances.

These nonanalytic assumptions and techniques may prove therapeutically useful in instances where the patient has, in fact, been sexually traumatized in childhood. They may also, however, offer symptomatic relief to some patients who have not been sexually abused, by providing them an opportunity to reorganize their selves around a new identity as "trauma victim" that is sanctioned and supported by a needed, valued, and often idealized, therapist.

A trade-off of this kind, of incorrect reconstruction (false memory) in return for symptomatic relief, might not be unacceptable to some patients or therapists, were it not for the social and legal consequences that often follow in its wake. The issue is enormously complex, highly sensitive, and has become politicized in a way that often goes beyond scientific inquiry and the safeguarding of our patients' well-being. While it cannot be further elaborated upon in the present chapter, the possibility of its occurring should be carefully borne in mind.

Analytic therapies are, of course, also subject to the danger that the analyst may unwittingly contribute to the inculcation of false memories. However, certain features inherent in the analyst's technical stance and integral to the analyst's working attitude contribute towards protecting the patient against incorrect reconstructions. To begin with, analysts attempt, as much as possible, to avoid prejudging the meaning or genesis of any given symptom. While they inevitably bring certain basic assumptions into the treatment setting, such as the importance of unconscious forces in human emotional life and the expectation of finding the consequences of unresolved conflicts that reflect universal stages of emotional development, analysts attempt to make no preconceived judgments about how these conflicts and consequences will appear in the life of any given patient. Nor do they have preconcieved ideas about which outcomes will prove most desired or therapeutic for a given patient.

Ideally, the only "action" that the analyst's position favors in regard to the patient's life is that of maintaining a committment to analyze. That is, to explore their conflicts and reflect upon the meanings and motivations of their experience. The patient's life decisions are obviously important to the patient and reflect various unconscious motivations and conflicts. However, they should not be predetermined by analytic theory or the analyst's beliefs about what constitutes the "good life." They are left, instead, to the patient out of respect for the patient's freedom of choice and autonomy. Since the latter is always potentially subject to being undermined by the transference feelings that are aroused and intensified by the analytic situation, the analysis of the transference, particularly as it has been conceptualized in contemporary analytic theory of technique, becomes the most important safegard to the patient's autonomy.

In more traditional formulations, transference, by which we mean the attribution of feelings, thoughts, and attitudes to a contemporary figure in the patient's life that are more appropriately related to past important figures, was conceptualized as a projection of the patient's inner world onto the figure of the analyst. That is, transference was assumed to be entirely the product of the mind of the patient. In more contemporary views, the transference is expected also to contain a contribution from the actuality of the analyst's relationship to the patient around which the patient's projections may be organized. What this implies in terms of technique is that the analyst must be committed to try to explore the consequences of the impact of the analyst's participation in the analytic relationship on the patient's experience of that relationship.

In order to better understand this view, it is useful to begin with a description of the psychoanalytic situation offered by Gill:[52]

> It is a situation in which, however they temporarily stray from it, analyst and patient both remain committed to the idea that the proximal goal [of their relationship] is to understand the relationship, not only to engage in it, while the distal goal is to understand the patient's psychopathology in the light of the patient's development. (p. 116)

"Understanding the analytic relationship" implies inquiry rather than action, a continual search for the ways in which the patient's expectations about the analyst's views, beliefs, and desires and the actuality of the analyst's views, beliefs, and desires are impacting upon and influencing the thoughts and feelings of the patient. Thus, for example, within the limits of human fallability and if all is working well, the possible effects on the patient of an analyst's belief that a patient was sexually abused in childhood, or a patient's assumption that their analyst held such a belief, would be explored as part of the ongoing work of the analysis. And part of that exploration would include an examination of any elements of the patient's need or wish to conform to their analyst's wishes about what might be found in the treatment.

As noted above, one important goal of such exploration is to build into the analyst's stance and technique a respect for and encouragement of the patient's autonomy. Another is to provide a safeguard against patient compliance and unwitting analyst suggestion. This shift in the analyst's attitude about transference also reflects the development of a less authoritarian position on the part of the analyst in regard to knowing the "truth" of the patient's experience.

In considering the various forces in the treatment situation that can move patient and analyst away from an optimal position of analytic contemplation and inquiry, I have written elsewhere[36] that

[o]ur most appropriate position in regard to reconstruction of the unknown past is that of using our skills, knowledge and experience *to suggest what is plausible as psychic reality* rather than what is veridically true. Thus, to a patient who suspects that he was sexually traumatized in childhood, I might acknowledge that particular symptoms and fantasies are consistent with those reported by others who were more certain of having experienced childhood sexual abuse. Or, to a doubting patient, I might point out that she now seems to have lost the conviction of her own memory that she held with such certainty yesterday and wonder with her what this change might mean. In either case, I would be attempting to support the patients' attempts to think, reflect and inquire about the nature and meaning of their experience, particularly their experience with me in the treatment, rather than assuming an implicitly omniscient stance of "validating their experience" or telling them "the truth" of what happened to them in the past. In addition, as with any intervention made by the analyst, including the intervention of not saying anything, I would subsequently be watching and wondering what the impact and effect of my behavior was upon the patient and his or her sense of me, the transference and the treatment relationship.

In that same paper I also noted the following.

Adopting this stance in the treatment might appear to run counter to the view advocated by some authors that the analyst must "bear witness" to the reality of the patient's childhood injury; that the failure to do so only repeats the compounding of trauma at the hands of those who may have turned away from recognizing, acknowledging and taking steps to protect the child from further abuse. I do not believe this to necessarily be the case. To begin with, I am not proposing that we disbelieve our patients when they relate memories of childhood sexual trauma. Rather, I am saying that our position as analysts does not give us a special purchase on knowing "the truth" of what did or didn't happen in either direction. We have no more reason to assume that we can know when our patient's surmises or memories are fantasies than we can to asume that we can, without error, successfully reconstruct what they cannot yet remember. As I have discussed elsewhere,[35] too great an emphasis on the discovery of "what happened" may reflect the analyst's unconscious enactment of and identification with the patient's confusion and wish for certainty or the enactment of a wish held by patient and/or analyst for a grandiose, omniscient parent figure.[36]

In the view that I am proposing, the analyst's reconstruction is not a description of what was. Rather, it is offered as a conjecture of what might have been. Like any other interpretation, it is not necessarily true or false, but simply something more for the patient to consider. And like any other interpretation, it is another instance of potential analyst-derived influence that patient and analyst must reflect upon and explore for its possible impact on the emotional life of the patient.

The problem of validation, of ascertaining the historical, truth value of past events, particularly when the putative childhood trauma is reconstructed—i.e., *suggested*—by the analyst rather than remembered by the patient, is as old as psychoanalysis itself. The fact that hysterical symptoms could be induced or temporarily relieved by hypnosis led many critics of Freud's early work to claim that the therapeutic effects of psychoanalysis were simply another form of hypnotic suggestion based on the patient's idealized view of the physican/analyst. While the specter of "suggestion" in the first phase of Freud's work referred predominantly to suggestion as a therapeutic factor in the removal of symptoms, it later took on the added meaning of the patient's compliantly accepting an incorrect interpretation and clinging to this new belief for defensive purposes. In such instances, suggestion may be conceptualized as operating in a manner analogous to an "inexact interpretation"[53] to produce an iatrogenically induced or reinforced defensive position.

Throughout his life, Freud argued strenuously and repeatedly against the charge that the therapeutic results of psychoanalysis amounted to nothing more than suggestion. His formulation of the transference and recommendations on technique,[54] particularly in regard to the importance of transference analysis and the analyst's neutrality within the treatment, were attempts to account for and reduce the impact of the patient's view of the analyst on the part of the therapeutic process and as safeguards against the introduction of unintended suggestion on the part of the analyst.

It is surprising, then, and uncharacteristic of Freud, that when he raised the problem of validation in *Constructions In Analysis*,[55] he seemed to treat it so lightly and to dismiss its potential dangers:

> [T]he question arises of what guarantee we have while we are working on these constructions that we are not making mistakes and risking the success of the treatment by putting forward some construction that is incorrect. . . . [W]e may lend our ear to some comforting information that is afforded by analytic experience. For we learn from it that no damage is done if, for once in a way, we make a mistake and offer the patient a wrong construction as the probable historical truth. A waste of time is, of course, involved, . . . but a single mistake of the sort can do no harm. What in fact occurs in such an event is rather that the patient remains as though he were untouched by what has been said. . . . (p. 261)

In a recent article entitled "Memories of Childhood Sexual Abuse," Brenneis[56] offers a sobering discussion of the problems surrounding suggestion and validation of reconstructions and memories. He notes that the literature on the treatment of adults who were sexually abused as children contains two contending paradigms. In one, which he calls the *belief paradigm*, the analyst's belief in the possible or actual occurrence of a childhood sexual experience is a precondition for the emergence of repressed or dissociated memories. Many authors [44–48] have noted the importance to patients of the analyst or therapist not turning a blind eye to the possibility of childhood sexual abuse or incest. To do so may replicate the real or imagined attitude of one or both parents in the childhood situation and destroy the development of hope and trust in the therapeutic relationship that are such a crucial preliminary foundation upon which further therapeutic progress can be built.

In the other paradigm, the *suggestion paradigm*, the analyst's belief in the existence and ultimate accessibility of repressed memories of early trauma or the zealous expectation that such memories will be found contributes to the creation of a treatment situation which heightens the possibility that such memories will be suggested rather than truly discovered. Even under the best of circumstances, patients may become unconsciously eager to satisfy their analysts by fulfilling their wishes in regard to what they imagine their analysts want them to find. They may seek out explanations that will place blame for their difficulties upon those that they are angry with, or they may seek to relieve themselves of guilt or personal responsibility for the difficulties in their lives by placing causal responsibility for their emotional difficulties outside of their personal control. They also seek relief from uncertainty, doubt, and confusion by too quickly accepting the closure offered by an incorrect reconstruction, or may be pressured by popular political views or societally derived expectations into uncritically and prematurely concluding that certain symptoms are de facto evidence of prior sexual abuse.

The dilemma is perplexing. On the one hand, as Brennais[57] notes, "If one does not believe, no memory can be tolerated; and if one does believe, whatever memory appears is suspect."[57] On the other hand, "[v]ivid, affectively charged and apparently genuine presentations of repressed memory do not guarantee authenticity. Similarly, even directly expressed belief and blatant suggestive question do not conclusively invalidate authenticity. *We cannot, as yet, discriminate false from genuine recovered memory either on the basis of process or presentation*"[57] (italics added).

Conclusion

Where then do we stand? Do all patients, or patients of a particular kind, such as those who have experienced early childhood trauma or sexual abuse, require reconstruction of the forgotten or dissociated past? Do particular forms of data, such as dreams, transference manifestations, nonverbal behaviors, or screen memories especially lend themselves to the reconstructive process, or does that process rest more generally on the totality of the analytic process?

Despite all that has been written about reconstruction and the lifting of repression, psychoanalysis is unable to offer more than the most general statements concerning the technique of reconstruction or the explanation of how and why recovered memories appear when they do. What is even more crucial is that we do not yet know with any degree of certainty the extent to which remembering, as opposed to just suspecting, the occurrence and details of past traumatic events is necessary to a successful treatment outcome. The absence of criteria that specify techniques for facilitating the appearance of previously missing memories, or for informing us as to just exactly how particular data, such as screen memories or dreams, might be used in the process of reconstruction, is a problem, especially when attempting to devise guidelines for student therapists, or when responding to unfriendly critics who charge that the hard-won insights of analytic treatment are merely the results of iatrogenic suggestion.

Given what we know about the importance of comprehensiveness and coherence in the personal understanding of one's past and the contributions of the past to one's present character, it is safe to assume that reconstruction and recall will occupy important roles in the process of working through issues related to past conflicts and trauma. What is still uncertain in any given clinical instance is just how far back in time or how completely that process must be taken in order to achieve a "good enough" therapeutic result. We must await a more specific researching of our combined clinical experience before we know the extent to which patients may improve without the actual recapture of memory. From our clinical experience to date, however, what we do know is that neither the therapist's reconstruction nor the patient's actual recall are, in and of themselves, sufficient to relieve the distress and heal the wounds caused by childhood sexual trauma. As I have tried to emphasize, any achievement of effective therapeutic results will depend upon a process of exploration and analysis of the myriad ways in which actual (traumatic) experiences have interacted with and influenced developmental trends to produce the unconscious conflicts and fantasies that underlie neurotic symptoms and characterological traits and defenses.

In describing the potentially positive value of reconstruction in analytic therapy, a value that applies equally to the recall of the forgotten past, Arlow notes that "[r]econstruction, like any other interpretation, is a dynamic instrument. It demonstrates how the past influences the present and leads to a deepening of insight. . . . [I]t integrates and synthesizes various trends of the material . . . and serves as the base for the elaboration of the patient's unconscious fantasies, facilitating the emergence of additional material, thematically associated or consonant with the nature of the reconstruction. In effect, it does what any good interpretation does."[58]

The trauma produced by childhood sexual abuse and incest is long term and far reaching, subjective as well as objective, psychological and developmental as well as physical. The unconscious fantasies and conflicts produced by childhood sexual trauma can lead to difficulties in emotional development, object relations, affect tolerance, guilt, assertiveness, and sense of responsibility. In the course of any individual's maturation, the problems produced in each of these areas may acquire a momentum and trajectory of their own and become the source of additional difficulties that require analytic attention in their own right.

This multiplication of pathogenic influence and effect contributes to the complexity of the psychotherapeutic treatment of the consequences of childhood sexual abuse and incest. Such treatment is long and arduous. To expect or believe that therapy will solely or primarily consist of helping patients to remember what they have dissociated or forgotten is to neglect the innumerable advances made in psychoanalytic theory and practice over the past 100 years. Reconstruction and recall of past events can only function as *part* of an analytic treatment process. To be successful, the latter must extend far beyond the search for the actuality of the past, beyond the uncovering or inferring of who did what to whom, to include analytic exploration of the many unconscious fantasies, conflicts, and fixations that underlie neurotic symptoms, ego weaknesses, and character traits and deformations.

References

1. Freud S: Constructions in analysis. *In* J Strachey (Ed. and Trans.), The Standard Edition of the Complete Psychological Works of Sigmund Freud, Vol. 23. London: Hogarth Press, 1964, pp. 265–266. (Original work published 1937).
2. Greenacre P: A historical sketch of the use and disuse of reconstruction. Psychoanal Study Child 1980; 35:35–40.
3. Freud S: Studies in Hysteria. *In* J. Strachey (Ed. and Trans.), Standard Edition, Vol 2. London: Hogarth Press, 1955, pp. 1–311. (Original work published 1895).
4. Yankelovitch D, Barrett W: *Ego and Instinct*. New York: Vintage Books, 1970.
5. Freud S: Fragment of an analysis of a case of hysteria. *In* J. Strachey (Ed. and Trans.), The Standard Edition, Vol 7. London: Hogarth Press, 1955, pp. 3–122. (Original work published 1905).
6. Freud S: Further remarks on the neuropsychoses of defense. *In* J. Strachey (Ed. and Trans.), Standard Edition, Vol. 3. London: Hogarth Press, 1962, pp. 157–185. (Original work published 1896).
7. Freud S: The aetiology of hysteria. *In* J. Strachey (Ed. and Trans.), Standard Edition, Vol. 3. London: Hogarth Press, 1962, pp. 191–221. (Original work published 1896).
8. Garcia EE: Freud's seduction theory. Psychoanal Study Child 1987; 42:443–468.
9. Freud S: Further remarks on the neuropsychoses of defense. *In* J. Strachey (Ed. and Trans.), Standard Edition, Vol. 3. London: Hogarth Press, 1962, p. 164. (Original work published 1896).
10. Gill MM: Psychoanalysis in Transition. A Personal View. Hillsdale, NJ: The Analytic Press, 1994.
11. Natterson JM, Friedman RC: A Primer of Clinical Intersubjectivity. Northvale, NJ: Jason Aronson, 1995.
12. Levine HB: The analyst's participation in the analytic process. Int J Psychoanal 1994; 75:665–676.
13. Levine HB: Introduction. *In* HB Levine (Ed.), Adult Analysis and Childhood Sexual Abuse. Hillsdale, NJ: Analytic Press, 1990, pp. 7–8.
14. Schimek J: Fact and fantasy in the seduction theory: a historical review. J Am Psychoanal Assoc 1987; 35:937–966.
15. Freud S: An autobiographical study. *In* J. Strachey (Ed. and Trans.), Standard Edition, Vol. 20. London: Hogarth Press, 1964, pp. 34–35. (Original work published 1925).
16. Freud S: Instincts and their vicissitudes. *In* J. Strachey (Ed. and Trans.), Standard Edition, Vol. 14. London: Hogarth Press, 1957, pp. 117–140. (Original work published 1915).
17. Freud S: Introductory Lectures on Psychoanalysis. *In* J. Strachey (Ed. and Trans.), Standard Edition, Vols. 15, 16. London: Hogarth Press, 1963, pp. 3–463. (Original work published 1917).
18. Freud S: Fragment of an analysis of a case of hysteria. *In* J. Strachey (Ed. and Trans.), Standard Edition, Vol. 7. London: Hogarth Press, 1955, p. 46. (Original work published 1905).
19. Yankelovitch D, Barrett W: Ego and Instinct. New York: Vintage Books, 1970, p. 35.
20. Masson JM: The Assault on Truth. New York: Farrar, Strauss, Giroux, 1984.
21. Freud S: Introductory Lectures on Psychoanalysis. *In* J. Strachey (Ed. and Trans.), Standard Edition, Vols. 15, 16. London: Hogarth Press, 1963, p. 370. (Original work published 1917).

22. *Ibid.*, p. 367.

23. Freud S: Female sexuality. *In* J. Strachey (Ed. and Trans.), Standard Edition, Vol. 21. London: Hogarth Press, 1961, p. 232. (Original work published 1931).

24. Freud S: Moses and Monotheism. *In* J. Strachey (Ed. and Trans.), Standard Edition, Vol. 22. London: Hogarth Press, 1964, pp. 75–76. (Original work published 1939).

25. Freud S: From the history of an infantile neurosis. *In* J. Strachey (Ed. and Trans.), Standard Edition, Vol. 17. London: Hogarth Press, 1964, pp. 7–122. (Original work published 1918).

26. Freud S: The Psychopathology of Everyday Life. *In* J. Strachey (Ed. and Trans.), Standard Edition, Vol. 6. London: Hogarth Press, 1960, pp. 1–310. (Original work published 1901).

27. Freud S: The Interpretation of Dreams. *In* J. Strachey (Ed. and Trans.), Standard Edition, Vols. 4, 5. London: Hogarth Press, 1953, pp. 1–627. (Original work published 1900).

28. Freud S: The Ego and the Id. *In* J. Strachey (Ed. and Trans.), Standard Edition, Vol. 19. London: Hogarth Press, 1961, pp. 12–66. (Original work published 1923).

29. Freud S: Inhibitions, symptoms and anxiety. *In* J. Strachey (Ed. and Trans.), Standard Edition, Vol. 20. London: Hogarth Press, 1959, pp. 87–127. (Original work published 1926).

30. Freud A: The Ego and the Mechanisms of Defense. New York: International Universities Press, 1936.

31. Freud S: Introductory lectures on psychoanalysis. *In* J. Strachey (Ed. and Trans.), Standard Edition, Vols. 15, 16, pp. 3–463. London: Hogarth Press, 1963, pp. 368.

32. Kris E: The recovery of childhood memories. Psychoanal Study Child 1956; 11:54–88.

33. Blum HP: Reconstruction in Psychoanalysis. Madison, CT: International Universities Press, 1994, p. 139.

34. Freud S: Screen memories. *In* J. Strachey (Ed. and Trans.), Standard Edition, Vol. 3. London: Hogarth Press, 1962, pp. 301–322. (Original work published 1899).

35. Levine HB: Clinical issues in the analysis of adults who were sexually abused as children. *In* HB Levine (Ed.), Adult Analysis and Childhood Sexual Abuse. Hillsdale, NJ: Analytic Press, 1990, pp. 197–218.

36. Levine HB: Difficulties in maintaining an analytic stance in the treatment of adults who were sexually abused as children. Psychoanal Inquiry 1997, in press.

37. Renik O: Analytic interaction: conceptualizing technique in the light of the analyst's irreducible subjectivity. Psychoanal Q 1993; 62:553–571.

38. Dowling S: Discussion of the various contributions. *In* A Rothstein (Ed.), The Reconstruction of Trauma: Its Significance in Clinical Work. Madison, CT: International Universities Press, 1986, pp. 205–217.

39. Greenacre P: Re-evaluation of the process of working through. *In* Emotional Growth. New York: International Universities Press, 1971, pp. 641–650.

40. Loewenstein R: Some thoughts on interpretation in the theory and practice of psychoanalysis. Psychoanal Study Child 1957; 12:127–150.

41. Arlow J: Methodology and reconstruction. Psychoanal Q 1991; 60:539–563, p. 554.

42. Boesky D: Consequences of childhood abuse: fantasy and reality. Paper presented at the American Psychoanalytic Association's Seminar for Clinicians, October 1994, Miami, FL.

43. Levine HB: The consequences of childhood sexual abuse and their implications for psychoanalytic therapy. Paper presented at the American Psychoanalytic Association's Seminar for Clinicians, October 1994, Miami, FL.

44. Davies JM, Frawley MG: Treating the Adult Survivor of Childhood Sexual Abuse. New York: Basic Books, 1994.

45. Herman JL: Trauma and Recovery. New York: Basic Books, 1992.

46. Williams M: Reconstruction of an early seduction and its aftereffects. J Am Psychoanal Assoc 1987; 35:145–163.
47. Scharff JS, Scharff DE: Object Relations Therapy of Physical and Sexual Trauma. Northvale, NJ: Jason Aronson, 1994.
48. Levine HB (ed.): Adult Analysis and Childhood Sexual Abuse. Hillsdale, NJ: Analytic Press, 1990.
49. Raphling DL: A patient who was not sexually abused. J Am Psychoanal Assoc 1994; 42:65–78.
50. Loftus EF: The reality of repressed memories. Am Psychol 1993; 48:518–537.
51. Blum HP: Reconstruction in Psychoanalysis. Madison, CT: International Universities Press, 1994, p. 4.
52. Gill, MM: Psychoanalysis in Transition. A Personal View. Hillsdale NJ: Analytic Press, 1994, p. 116.
53. Glover E: The therapeutic effect of inexact interpretation: a contribution to the theory of suggestion. *In* The Technique of Psychoanalysis. New York: International Universities Press, 1968, pp. 353–366.
54. Freud S: Papers on Technique. *In* J. Strachey (Ed. and Trans.), Standard Edition, Vol. 12. London: Hogarth Press, 1958, pp. 85–174. (Original work published 1911–1915).
55. Freud S: Constructions in analysis. *In* J. Strachey (Ed. and Trans.), Standard Edition, Vol. 23. London: Hogarth Press, 1964, p. 261. (Original work published 1937).
56. Brenneis CB: Memories of childhood sexual abuse. J Am Psychoanal Assoc 1994; 42:1027–1054.
57. *Ibid.*, p. 1049.
58. Arlow J: Methodology and reconstruction. Psychoanal Q 1991; 60:539–563, pp. 561–562.

13

Psychodynamic Therapy for Patients with Early Childhood Trauma

JULIA A. MATTHEWS
JAMES A. CHU

Recent years have seen a dramatic rise in the attention to the psychological and therapeutic issues associated with severe childhood abuse. Mental health professionals have become increasingly aware of the high prevalence of childhood maltreatment, and have recognized the contribution of actual trauma to the development of adult psychopathology.[1-4] In response to this increasing awareness, we are currently witnessing a swing of the pendulum back to a theoretical perspective, reminiscent of Freud's earliest theory of the etiology of hysteria,[5] that places actual external trauma as the central causative factor in many forms of psychiatric illness. In the clinical arena, the acknowledgement of the reality of early traumatic experiences leads to a more empathic formulation of current difficulties and can guide treatment interventions. Taken to an extreme, however, the focus on external childhood trauma can gain such a central position that the diverse insights of psychodynamic psychiatry concerning the complexities of interpersonal relationships and intrapsychic processes are all but disregarded. The result can be a reductionistic and simplistic vision of human suffering that is framed exclusively in terms of victimization.

This chapter presents a contemporary perspective on selected issues regarding psychodynamic psychotherapy for individuals who have suffered severe childhood trauma, with particular attention to the trauma of sexual abuse. In the first section of this chapter

The authors wish to thank Drs. David Bellinger, Axel Hoffer, Ana-Maria Rizzuto, and Robert Pyles for their helpful comments during the preparation of this chapter.

we briefly summarize clinical findings regarding the psychological impact of early trauma (see also Chapters 5, 12, 17, this volume). In the second part of this chapter, we use these observations to discuss some central issues in the evaluation and treatment of adults reporting histories of childhood trauma. Since most studies of childhood sexual abuse have focused on women, we will refer throughout the chapter to female patients. However, it should be understood that young boys are also frequently the victims of sexual abuse, suffer similar psychological consequences, and have comparably complex treatment needs.

Since the concept of psychological trauma, as broadly defined, has always been central to psychodynamic theory, a comprehensive review of this area could encompass the entire history of psychoanalytic thinking. Despite this attention to trauma, however, no clear consensus currently exists regarding central theoretical and clinical issues related to the effects of childhood abuse. Many important questions can be raised about the psychoanalytic understanding of memory and the validity of the concept of repression,[6-10] or the relationship between the mechanisms of repression and dissociation;[11-13] about the relative contributions of remembering, abreaction, and reconstruction in the therapeutic process;[14-18] and about the place of subjective reality versus objective reality in healing.[19-21]

A full discussion of all these issues clearly exceeds the scope of this chapter. We will focus more narrowly on therapeutic work with both existing and so-called recovered memories of childhood trauma, especially memories of sexual abuse. This is a highly controversial topic, with extensive debate over the reliability and validity of traumatic memories, and about the putative role of therapists in the emergence of recovered memories.[8,22-27] This debate has been most intense regarding memories of childhood sexual abuse, with less controversy and emotionality attending other forms of child maltreatment such as physical or emotional abuse, neglect, and nonsexual exploitation. While this selective focus may be explained, in part, by the recent increase in litigations involving alleged sexual abuse, it also reflects the particularly intense horror and denial elicited by this form of abuse. In this way, the controversy is an expression of our common unconscious conflicts regarding sexuality and children and the sexual exploitation of the youngest members of our society.

A Psychodynamic Understanding of the Impact of Abuse

The most basic postulate of psychodynamic theory is that conscious thoughts, feelings, and behaviors are shaped by unconscious mental processes that include instinctual impulses, fantasies, conflicts, and past experiences. There are dynamic tensions within the unconscious itself, and between conscious and unconscious needs. Unconscious impulses or fantasies that are threatening or unacceptable are actively kept out of consciousness. Similarly, threatening or intolerable experiences can be actively excluded from consciousness and voluntary recall. However, these fantasies and experiences, even though unconscious, can profoundly influence conscious thought and overt behavior.

Childhood experiences are particularly important in shaping adult thought and behavior. Early development proceeds through a series of predictable stages, each characterized by specific psychological challenges and achievements. The outcome of each developmental stage influences passage through subsequent stages. A disturbance at one stage may alter subsequent growth, influencing how a later experience is interpreted and integrated. Individual experience is ultimately reflected in psychic structures and functions, including ego capacities and defenses, self-regulatory mechanisms, and concepts of the self and others. In a broad sense, psychic structure can be described as "memorial," revealing past experience through its form and function.[28]

Traumatic experiences in childhood can alter every aspect of psychological functioning. In particular, abuse that is severe and repetitive leaves psychological "scars" that extend beyond the specific domain of the trauma itself.[1-4,20,29-36] Unfortunately, many children and adults seen in clinical settings have suffered multiple abuses rather than a single form, often living in an environment of chronic isolation, helplessness, and terror.[1-4,37] This kind of traumatization, over multiple phases of development, powerfully influences the sense of self and others, and the ability to cope with internal psychological processes and external reality.

The form and content of the internal representation of traumatic experiences depends on the child's developmental stage, cognitive capacities, and preexisting intrapsychic structure when the trauma occurred. Mastery of age-appropriate developmental tasks may be delayed, altered, or derailed. Trauma may also induce regression, forcing the child to revisit conflicts from earlier stages, and hence altering earlier developmental achievements that predate the trauma. Issues from each psychological phase are challenged.[3,4,36] Trauma forms a powerful core for an unconscious organizing "fantasy/memory complex"[18] about the self and world that can dominate and shape all subsequent experiences and relationships. As Kris[38] has noted:

> The material of actual occurrences, of things as they happen, is constantly subjected to the selective scrutiny of memory. . . . Not only were the events loaded with meaning as they occurred, each later stage of the conflict pattern may endow part of the events or their elaboration with added meaning. But these processes are repeated throughout many years of childhood and adolescence and finally integrated into the structure of the personality. They are molded, as it were, into patterns, and it is with these patterns, rather than the events that the analyst deals. (pp. 76–77).

Sexual abuse may be particularly traumatic because of the intrinsic physical and psychological overstimulation, the bodily invasion, the associated betrayals of trust, the confusion of loving and hostile meanings, and the imposed deceit and secrecy. In what Ferenczi[39] eloquently referred to as "confusion of tongues," the child's search for "tenderness" is met by the adult's "passion" and sexual aggression. The child may be compelled to accept the abuse as the price of the relationship, internalizing a confusing mixture of gratifications (e.g., nurturance) and personal violations, which then becomes the expected interpersonal experience.

The capacity to integrate and master traumatic experience is strongly affected by the interpersonal context, including the relationship to the abuser, the degree of external validation of the experience, and the availability of empathic supports.[40,41] Most child sexual abuse occurs repetitively within the extended family and is often symptomatic of substantial family dysfunction, parental psychopathology, failed empathy, neglect, and unmodulated aggression.[20,42,43] Furthermore, the child often encounters external denial or rationalization of the abuse, and "enforced silence,"[44] which magnify the impact of the trauma. As Herman[4] has noted, "[p]sychological trauma is an affliction of the powerless." The child who is living in an abusive situation is captive to the experience, and is emotionally and physically dependent on the abuser(s).[4,20,36,39,43–46] Faced with overwhelming traumatic experience and the failure of external supports, the child has powerful motives to deny, distort, or rationalize the traumatic events in order to maintain needed emotional ties, and to reduce the feelings of helplessness.

The most devastating consequences of early chronic and/or severe abuse are the profound disturbances in the development of the sense of self and of relationships to others.[4,20,34,36,39,42,47–53] These disturbances are commonly manifested in the adult character structure as pathological object relations and deficits of basic trust, reality testing, autonomy, and affect regulation (particularly rage and aggression). When children are victimized, both their internal and external worlds are shattered.[4,36,45,54] The child victim experiences the failure of caregivers to provide basic safety and protection as central to the abuse experience. The experience of neglect or parental absence is a substantial part of the traumatic experience, often of equal significance to the trauma itself.[20,36,55,56] The developing capacities for trust, self-esteem, self-cohesion and self-regulation, which are all based on the internalization of adequate nurturing figures, are all severely impaired by the abuse experience.

Victims of severe childhood abuse almost universally take on the responsibility for the abuse, blaming themselves, and explaining the maltreatment as deserved or even sought. This defensive position serves to protect both the child and abuser from overwhelming rage, and offers the victim the illusion of power and control.[20,46,52,56] The sense of control may be further enhanced through pathological identifications with the abuser. However, in a self-perpetuation of the abuse, the internalized abusive authority sustains the assault on the self in harsh self-criticisms, self-doubt, guilt, and self-hatred.[29,39,42,43,53] Thus, many adults who have been chronically traumatized as children have thoughts, feelings, and behavior that seem irrational, self-defeating, or even self-destructive, but that make sense in the context of early experiences.

The following case illustrates many of these difficulties, and will be referred to and developed later in this chapter.

Case Study

Ms. K entered therapy in her late thirties, several days after she had experienced the sudden and terrifying reemergence of memories and images of repetitive sexual assaults by her brother, 9 years her senior. Over the next several weeks she recalled details of his abuse (from age 3 to 8), as well as rapes and sadistic torture by a group of his adolescent friends. She had no prior recollection of these events, although she had learned several years earlier that one of her older sisters had some unspecified sexual contact with this same brother (which she had assumed occurred in their teens). Ms. K had struggled throughout her entire adult life with periods of depression, self-loathing, shame, and a variety of self-defeating behaviors. She was chronically isolated, a "workaholic," and was aware of a pattern of flight from any relationship that "threatened" to become sexual. She had also struggled since adolescence with complusive fantasies and behavioral reenactments of anal rape, that were simultaneously exciting and intensely shameful. The emerging memories, while extremely painful and overwhelming, seemed to make sense of many confusing aspects of her life. In retrospect, she recognized that many of the memories she previously had about her childhood were inventions created to cover over and deny her traumatic past. When she disclosed the abuse memories to her two older sisters, they each reported similar memories involving their older brother, including corroborating memories of times when they recalled being abused together.

The Role of Dissociation

Severe traumatization, including incest trauma, is overwhelming and intolerable to a child's psyche. Moreover, the child's perceptions are often ignored, minimized, or denied by others, creating a conflict of living in two realities: the abuse reality and the family myth.[4,20,34,47] Faced with intolerable external experience and internal conflict, the child often resorts to internal splitting, with feelings, behaviors, and knowledge related to the abuse being held in separate parts of the psyche. In psychodynamic terms, trauma overwhelms the ego's capacity to cope with the acute experience, or to integrate the traumatic experience into personal identity, consciousness, and memory. Thus, as a general statement, aspects of traumatic experiences may remain "incoherent," i.e., memory, affect, meaning, and fantasy are not integrated into a choherent personal history. Rather, they tend to remain disavowed and dissociated from usual conscious awareness, but may be remembered or reexperienced as isolated fragments. As such, separated from contextual perspective, these fragmented aspects of the traumatic experiences may have a timeless and indelible quality.[13]

The propensity towards dissociation (broadly defined as a disconnection of the perceptual, affective, behavioral, somatic, and memory components of experience) varies with age, but is thought to be greater in young children.[57] With severe abuse, the innate dissociative capacity of children is recruited as a defense against the traumatic experience, and as a means of escape and restorative fantasy. Repetitive abuse may lead to persistent reliance on dissociative defenses into adulthood.[1,3,4,35,58–61] Differentiation of inner and outer reality is disturbed, sometimes resulting in deficient reality testing or the emergence of pathological self-doubt, i.e., confusion about thought (fantasy) and action (experience), mistrust of perceptions, and excessive dependence on external validation—or its opposite, defensive over-certainty and intolerance of alternative perspectives.

One of the most common forms of dissociation in response to early abuse is disconnection of cognition and affect. That is, there is psychological gain in not connecting what happened and how it felt. As Ms. K eloquently expressed it:

> I looked at my feelings as the enemy. I couldn't do anything about the abuse, but if I let my feelings out they'd betray me, so I guess, in a way, having no feeling was equivalent to safety, and feeling was the enemy. . . . It sounds so silly to say it, but the abuse was bad only if you felt bad about it. . . . Trying to control my feelings about it during and after was the only way I could live with it.

In this way, patients become numb and disconnected from their emotional life. The abuse is remembered but described in bland tones that belie the profound emotional significance and actual terror. Or conversely, the affective states of terror, rage, despair, and helplessness may be relived without any awareness of the connection with the underlying abuse. Traumatized patients commonly experience these kinds of intensely dysphoric affects without being able to articulate their source.

Traumatized patients, who have often relied on dissociation and repression to manage intolerable experiences, are also particularly prone to hallucinatory repetitions of the trauma. These repetitions may take the form of flashbacks or traumatic nightmares, which are intense, involuntary, and intrusive.[3,13,17,62] This vivid remembering or "reliving" of the trauma may be experienced as occurring in the present, with the full measure of pain, terror, helplessness, or rage associated with the past experiences. The intensity and the lack of temporal perspective usually make these experiences extremely confusing, overwhelming, and potentially retraumatizing to patients. This presents a difficult challenge to therapists. The goal, as will be discussed later, is to transform these experiences from helpless and passive reexperiencing to active control and mastery in the context of a helping relationship.

Behavioral reenactment of the trauma also occurs in many traumatized persons. "Traumatic play," in which the traumatic experience is literally or symbolically reenacted, appears to be nearly universal in children, and is often seen even in the absence of verbal recall of the event.[2,63] As in the case of Ms. K, unconsciously driven behavioral repetitions of the traumatic experiences often persist into adulthood in both simple and complex recreations of the abusive situation.[13,62,64–66] Freud[64,65] introduced the concept that has come to be known as the *repetition compulsion* to describe this phenomenon, and postulated that it was a form of "remembering in action":

> The patient cannot remember the whole of what is repressed in him, and what he cannot remember may be precisely the essential part of it. . . . . He is obliged to repeat the repressed material as a contemporary experience instead of remembering it as something in the past.[65]

Freud and subsequent writers theorized that these repetitions are ultimately aimed at mastery and integration.[64,65,67]

The concept of repetition of trauma encompasses both circumscribed behaviors, and more complex recreations of interpersonal events, including actual retraumatizations, such as rape. Furthermore, the patient has strong unconscious pressures to repeat the traumatic relationships within the therapy. The dynamics of the early trauma will inevitably be reexperienced in the therapeutic situation, and the therapist must work to understand, contain, and interpret these forms of reexperiencing while providing a context for a new kind of experience. In the treatment of patients with severe trauma, the therapist must be especially alert to the potential for mutual reenactment and actual re-traumatization. Transference repetition (the recreation of early dynamics within the therapeutic relationship) is a universal and central element of psychodynamic psychotherapies.[64,68–70] The recognition and clarification of unconscious repetitions in the therapy yields valuable clues to the patient's history and internalized experience.[28,36,62,67,71] The gradual understanding and working through of old conflicts, behaviors, and fantasies as they reemerge in the transference is generally considered to be the central healing thread of dynamic therapies.[69]

As described here, the effects of childhood trauma can be complex, profound, and self-perpetuating. Descriptive studies have documented the wide range of symptoms associated with severe and chronic early abuse.[1,3,4,33,34] The dissociation that commonly occurs under such conditions leads to the development of adult posttraumatic syndromes,[1,31,37,72,73] characterized by states of hyperarousal, hypervigilence, and intrusive reexperiencing, alternating with states of emotional constriction, numbing, and social withdrawal. Some forms of severe or repetitive trauma are so overwhelming that the child's psyche is pathologically shattered, resulting in partial or complete amnesias,[74–76] or in fragmentation of the child's developing sense of self, and the formation of dissociated self-states (dissociative identity disorder).[35,58–60,77] All of these difficulties frequently coexist with characterologic difficulties that massively impair the ability to sustain relationships, tolerate dysphoric affect, contain impulses, and maintain a stable and positive sense of self. Clinical studies have demonstrated a correlation between early trauma and borderline personality disorder,[50,72,78–80] although some investigators and clinicians have urged the use of other diagnostic labels, such as Herman's *complex posttraumatic syndrome,* because of the pejorative connotations of the borderline diagnosis.[4,81] Whatever terminology is used, it is apparent that many traumatized patients will need to be understood with considerable sophistication, and that their treatment will require both patience and skill. The healing process must occur through the gradual building of coping ability, positive relationships, and sense of self-worth, and the slow process of working through memories, old conflicts, behaviors, and fantasies as they reemerge in the therapy.

Trauma and Memory

Traumatic experience is associated with a variety of disruptions of memory.[2,3,20,27,35,60,74] Enhanced clarity of memory (hypermnesia) has been observed for single-event, circumscribed traumatic experiences, in contrast to partial or complete anmesia in response to repetitive and severe traumatization.[2,63] Amnesia, i.e., the failure of voluntary recall, is common in victims of chronic childhood abuse[2,74–76,82–84] and is discussed elsewhere in this volume. The nature of memory for traumatic events, particularly memory recalled after partial or complete amnesia has been the subject of considerable investigation. The central unresolved question is whether traumatic memory is qualitiatively different from ordinary memory.

Both psychoanalytic and neuropsychological investigators assert that memory is far more complex than the processes available to conscious verbal recall.[71,85–87] There is considerable agreement that consciously accessible memories are not stored as permanent and immutable memory traces awaiting retrieval. While Freud at times postulated the timelessness and permanence of "memory traces," he also recognized, along with many subsequent theorists,[70,71,87–91] the fragility of memory, and the cognitive revision of past experience based on subsequent understandings and defensive modifications. This was expressed well by Loewald:[87] "Insofar as memory (in the sense of memory traces) as a record is passive repetition, conscious remembering can be described as active repetition that, while founded on it, replaces and reorganizes the record in the act of remembering" (p. 94).

In various terminologies, theorists emphasize the "schematic" function of memory, i.e., the formation of "schemata" or "scripts" that represent and synthesize past experience, organize the perception of current experience, and are constantly revised by the assimilation of new information.[71,87,92–95] The psychodynamic perspective asserts that these schemata are constructed (and reconstructed) from the commingling of actual experience and fantasy, and are modified through both conscious and unconscious processes to serve the needs of coherence, defense, and adaptation. The internal representation of actual traumatic experience will always contain (in varying degrees) elements of fantasy, and it is important to understand both the actual and fantasized components of a traumatic experience.[24,34,36,38,47,96–100]

The circumstances and meaning of a traumatic experience strongly affect the need for fantasy. A physical injury sustained in a natural disaster will have different meanings than the same injury at the hands of a rageful parent. Sexual assault by a stranger will have different meanings than sexual seduction by a parent. In both cases, intrafamilial abuse results in the child having an increased need to fantasize about the abuse, e.g., fantasized reasons or circumstances that justify the abuse. Thus, the experience at the time of the actual trauma and the subsequent memory of the traumatic experience are composed of both external and internal constituents. For example, actual threats of death are all too common in childhood abuse; but when an adult patient recalls childhood threats, this may, alternatively or additionally, represent the child's fears of annihilation at the time of the trauma, the child's projected homicidal rage, or the child's fantasied guilt and expectation of punishment. In the past, some psychoanalysts postulated that since it is the "psychic reality" that defines the traumatic experience, the psychological impacts of actual and fantasied trauma are indistinguishable, and that therefore the issues of external "reality" or "truth" are unimportant. This assertion is highly questionable, and neglects the crucial element of actualization, i.e., that *the external trauma makes actual the most feared or dangerous fantasies, replacing the fantasy with a horrible reality.*

Personal memory, the individual's narrative history, is largely verbal. The integration of experience into personal narrative history and consciously available memory may depend on the capacity for language. Preverbal childhood experience, lacking the synthetic and integrative operations of language, is unavailable to this level of organization and cannot be integrated into a personal narrative. However, as Bonanno[71] notes, "[w]hile early memories may be fragmentary or limited in context, they can nevertheless greatly influence perception and behavior in subsequent events by posing constraints on the development and organization of schematic structures" (p. 179). Preverbal childhood experience may persist outside verbal representation, or may subsequently acquire verbal representation and integration into the narrative history, as discussed by Loewald:[101]

> It is often clear that in so-called recovery of a childhood memory we are confronted, not with recall of something forgotten, but with a creative event in which something for the first time can be put into words, and more, that it never had been capable of being put into words because the original experience had taken place on a level of integration which did not render it available for preconscious or conscious integration. (p. 41)

Because traumatic experience overwhelms the individual's coping and integrative functions, the normal mechanisms of coherent conceptual representation fail, forcing a reversion to exclusively nonverbal forms of representation. It has been suggested since the time of Janet[13,38,101,102] that traumatic experience may induce an altered state of consciousness. The internal representation of the trauma is dissociated from normal consciousness and remains unassimilated. Loewald[101] compared the "hypnoid" states of hysteria as studied by Breuer and Freud,[5] to the immature mental state of the child, and suggested that experiences in these states remain segregated and "unabsorbed." Severe trauma, even in adults, may be internalized in nonverbal representations— images, feelings, and sensations without words—that may subsequently be reexperienced as "flashbacks."

The consistent clinical observations over the past century regarding altered memory function following traumatic events have led many to postulate that traumatic memory is distinct from ordinary memory, i.e., that it is nonverbal, non-narrative, and subject to different mechanisms of recall and revision.[13,27,38,66,95,102] It has been proposed that because traumatic memory is not integrated into the ordinary flow of consciousness, it may be less susceptible to normal processes of reconstruction and revision.[13,25,38] However, it is also possible that such dissociated experiences are less easily distinguished from fantasy or dreams, leading to subjective confusion about the reality of the events, and greater primary process elaboration.[18,25,27] Therefore, the dissociation of traumatic events may not necessarily result in greater accuracy of subsequent recall.

There is as yet no accepted theoretical distinction between the concepts or mechanisms of repression and dissociation.[12,13,17,74,103,104] Dissociation was originally conceptualized as a passive process, a result of traumatic induction of an altered state of consciousness.[5,13,17,102] In contrast, Freud postulated an active process, repression, that excluded an aspect of psychic experience from consciousness.[5,13,105,106] This distinction is sometimes captured in simplistic terms by describing repression as "horizontal splitting," in which certain psychic experiences are actively barred from conscious awareness, and describing dissociation as "vertical splitting," in which psychic experiences are segregated into different states of conscious awareness. Dissociation at the time of a trauma may result in traumatic memory that may remain outside of ordinary consciousness.[5,13,38,102] Repression may function secondarily to actively block the emergence of traumatic memories into consciousness.

Ms. K recalled the "moment" in which she rejected her memories of the abuse:

> I think I'd been burying it for awhile, telling myself, "That couldn't have happened, it must be a dream, or imagination," or I was a sick person. . . . I think the moment was a decision to believe that it wasn't real. . . . It resolved a lot of confusion. . . . From the perspective of an 8- or 9-year-old, I had sort of reasoned myself to a clear and unclouded picture of reality.

This is an articulate description of the form of repression in which something that is once "known" (consciously experienced) becomes unavailable to consciousness. When such events are subsequently remembered, they are often experienced as "always known,"[38,64] or as having been simultaneously "known and not known." Remembering (derepression) makes the experience once again available to consciousness for evaluation and integration at a new level of synthesis. In contrast, when dissociated memory is "remembered," it is typically experienced as alien and intrusive, without narrative and without the sense of ownership that derives from cognitive and affective integration.[13,62]

Based on these clinical observations, it is plausible that these two mechanisms, repression and dissociation of traumatic experiences, may represent different psychological (and neurophysiological) processes. Both concepts may be clinically useful in describing memory disruption following trauma. Careful investigation of these processes may lead to further understanding of memory function in trauma, and suggest differential therapeutic interventions.

The Assessment of Trauma Patients

In an initial assessment with traumatized patients, two interrelated areas should be evaluated. First, what is the specific history of childhood trauma that may be contributing to the current difficulties? Second, what are the specific presenting posttraumatic symptoms, and in what specific ways has psychological development been disrupted by the early traumatic experiences? The first question clarifies history and helps in the initial case formulation. The second question assesses current psychological functioning, which then guides the form, pace, and focus of the therapeutic work.

Adult patients with histories of childhood abuse may seek treatment for difficulties related to acknowledged childhood trauma, but they also commonly present with more diffuse symptoms such as chronic depression, low self-esteem, anxiety, panic attacks, self-destructive behaviors, identity disturbance, difficulties in relationships, sexual problems or substance abuse. Comprehensive initial assessment should include direct, open-ended, nonsuggestive inquiries about childhood experiences, including possible areas of maltreatment or abuse. It is important to communicate a willingness to hear the patient's life story and subjective recollections without presupposition or prejudgment. Openness to the possibility of abuse may be a necessary background for the patient to be able to disclose abuse[4,29,30,36,43] (see discussion by Brenneis[23]). Sometimes the patient remembers and reports the early trauma but does not connect it to the present difficulties. Sometimes the history of the early trauma is consciously withheld in the early contacts due to feelings of shame, self-doubt, or mistrust. Sometimes the history of abuse cannot be reported, because it is not consciously available to the patient.

Numerous authors have attempted to identify psychological markers indicative of early trauma which could guide the therapist in further exploration. Herman[45] noted that incest survivors often reported a turbulent adolescence with sexual acting out, a history of rape or abusive relationships, a history of substance abuse, and a history of maternal absence or unavailability. Others[3,34,36,53,56,100,107] have identified a broad constellation of psychological symptoms, evident in the therapeutic interaction, that may be associated with childhood sexual abuse: depressive affect, dissociative episodes, difficulties with trust, panic attacks or other sudden mood shifts, fears (and expectations) of seduction, somatizations, motoric or behavioral enactments, intrusive images, psychotic manifestations, intense self-doubt and impaired reality testing. While many patients with childhood sexual trauma will have some or all of these findings, none of these findings are pathognomonic or exclusive to sexual abuse.[22]

Clinicians should perform a careful assessment of posttraumatic and dissociative symptomatology, as these symptoms are most specifically related to a history of traumatization. In clinical situations where there is a known history of early traumatization, the extent of intrusive and numbing symptomatology and hyperactivation should be noted. In the absence of known abuse, a more sophisticated differential assessment of possible posttraumatic symptoms is necessary. Intrusions of unwanted thoughts and feelings, dysphoria, anxiety, numbing, and chronic hyperarousal may be evidence of a covert presentation of posttraumatic difficulties, but these symptoms also occur in many other psychiatric difficulties. While clinicians need to be sensitive to more covert forms of posttraumatic symptoms, they must carefully avoid the naive stance of seeing all symptoms in the light of trauma-based psychopathology.

Dissociative symptomatology may provide stronger evidence of posttraumatic difficulties. It is uncommon for high levels of depersonalization and derealization to occur in adulthood. In the absence of neurologic dysfunction, these symptoms may suggest posttraumatic sequelae. Clinicians should also carefully determine any evidence of amnesia. Difficulties with current memory may suggest changes in self-states, and an extensive history of amnesia in childhood (e.g., no memory of years in childhood) strongly suggests traumatic amnesia. Abrupt changes in mood and behavior, or a sense of self that is inconsistent over time, may also suggest switches between different self-states. Again, these kinds of difficulties need to be carefully distinguished from symptoms of other disorders.

A recent survey study[108] of experienced therapists in the U.S. and Britain revealed that, in practice, therapists use a wide variety of nonspecific indicators (such as sexual dysfunction, relationship difficulties, low self-esteem or identity issues, depression, or amnesia regarding childhood) to identify patients who may have suffered sexual abuse. A significant minority of therapists felt they could confidently identify patients who had suffered childhood sexual abuse at the time of the initial interview, even when the patient denied this history, and these therapists were more likely to employ specific memory recovery techniques (e.g., hypnosis or age regression), and were more likely to eventually ''uncover'' sexual abuse. However, the majority of all therapists had treated patients who recovered memories of previously unrecalled abuse. The pooled sample of therapists estimated that approximately 15% of women who initially denied childhood sexual abuse subsequently recovered memories of abuse, and even the most technically ''cautious'' therapists reported a significant proportion (7%) of patients who initially denied sexual abuse and later recovered memories of abuse. These data fit with previous studies that consistently confirm a subpopulation of abused patients who report a period in their lives in which they had no conscious recall of the abuse.[75,76,82,84] Nor is this memory recovery restricted to the context of therapies. For example, Ms. K remembered her abuse while home alone, considering her life patterns and her psychological pain, and, as she expressed it, ''fingering the well-worn photographs in my mind.'' Her own questions and associations led to the reemergence of hidden memory.

Like all historical data, a history of abuse must derive from the patient and should not be suggested (or presumed) by the therapist. The patient must be allowed to tell her own story at her own pace. Premature disclosures, in the absence of a trusting and supportive relationship, may simply result in retraumatization, intense shame and guilt, and fear of rejection. Unless these reactions are empathically understood and interpreted, there is a risk of flight from the therapy. Since clear verbal memory of traumatic experience may not be initially available to the patient, the evaluation of abuse history is an ongoing process as trust develops, as defenses and resistances soften, and as the therapy unfolds.[3,4,49,62]

The second major aspect of patient evaluation, which is also ongoing during the treatment, is the assessment of psychological structure and functioning. It is essential that the therapist thoroughly evaluate the patient's ego strengths and weaknesses early in the treatment of traumatized patients. Characterologic difficulties in the following areas should be assessed.

1. Intolerance of intense affect (particularly anger), and the vulnerability to periods of disorganization, fragmentation and dissociation
2. A debased self-concept, with self-blaming and self-hatred, a deficient sense of personal agency, and vulnerability to shame, helplessness, and despair
3. Difficulties with self-object differentiation, and chronic problems in forming and maintaining supportive relationships including the therapeutic relationship
4. A limited range of defenses, characteristically including dissociation, splitting, projection, externalization, denial, somatization, and aggression turned towards the self
5. Maladaptive coping strategies and difficulties with impulse control including self-injury, revictimization, promiscuity, substance abuse, eating disorders, or suicidal behaviors
6. Difficulties with being direct, authentic, and honest, and in being committed to life change.

Patients with histories of severe childhood trauma frequently have significant difficulties in all of these areas, and the early therapy work (which may extend for months or years) must center on basic issues of safety, stabilization, establishing the treatment frame, development of a therapeutic alliance, and the shared formulation of problems and goals. Empowerment of the patient is a fundamental and unifying theme in all these tasks.[4,36,49] It must be accepted that some patients are unable to move beyond these basic issues, and will require long-term supportive therapy with minimum exploration or "uncovering." Insight oriented work with these patients stays focused in the present, on current patterns of experience, feelings, and coping strategies, and is aimed at optimal safety and functioning. Burland & Raskin[100] suggest that the therapist explore the patient's history of repetitions as part of the evaluation. It is a good prognostic sign when the repetitions have served a process of mastery (for example, transforming an abusive situation into an experience of enhanced personal control) rather than simple reactualization (for example, repetitive abusive relationships or rapes in adulthood).

The Goals of Treatment and the Place of Remembering

. . . The life of an individual is determined by his infantile history, his early experiences and conflicts; but everything depends on *how* these early experiences are repeated in the course of life, to what extent they are repeated passively—suffered again . . . —and to what extent they can be taken over in the ego's organizing activity and made over into something new—a recreation of something old as against a duplication of it. In such recreation the old is mastered. (Loewald,[68] p. 89; italics in original)

Psychodynamic psychotherapy relies on the progressive development of affective and cognitive insight about both personal history and the present-day unconscious conflicts and defenses. As these insights are worked through, old schemas are revised, conflicts are resolved, and the patient is freed of unconscious compulsions to repeat. These processes allow the patient to achieve greater autonomy, more mature and adaptive ego functioning, more satisfying relationships, and more life fulfillment.

In discussions of the treatment of traumatized patients, it is common to hear simplistic statements suggesting that the treatment is largely or exclusively organized around the "recovery" of traumatic memory.[8,109] For example, Loftus[8] states that, "the core of treatment, it is widely believed, is to help clients reclaim their traumatic past." While the process of the detailed remembering of the traumatic past, in the context of a supportive relationship, has clear therapeutic value for many patients, this does not imply that remembering is the sole, primary, or sufficient function of the therapy. Even in the treatment of adult rape victims, short-term counseling focused on ventilation, support, education, and reassurance is generally insufficient to relieve posttraumatic symptoms because the victims have "reorganized their personalities around symptoms, conflicts, and defenses activated by the trauma."[54,110] The work of the therapy must go deeper, to help the victim resolve persistent issues of shame, guilt, loss of control, and the intense conflicts about their own aggressive fantasies. Similar strategies apply for child or adolescent victims of a single circumscribed trauma. However, in situations of chronic or severe childhood trauma, the entire psychic structure has been unconsciously organized around the traumatic experience, and the trauma is continuously relived (repeated) in the present day. As Freud stated,[64] " . . . we must treat his illness not as an event of the past, but as a present-day force."

Fortunately, this fact of repeating also provides the means for the treatment to heal. Transference repetitions and the reexperiencing of dissociated behaviors, affects, or perceptions bring the traumatic past into the present of the therapy where they can be gradually verbalized, understood, and integrated. The patient is then able to achieve affective and cognitive understanding of the links between past and present,[38] and between actions and their unconscious meanings.[87]

Effective psychodynamic therapy goes far beyond the process of remembering specific traumatic events. The patient must confront her ambivalence about the "memories," and develop an acceptance of the reality aspects of the abuse. She must also confront the social/familial context that allowed the abuse to occur, and that failed to recognize or intercede. She must achieve an understanding of the blended contributions of reality, fantasy, and revision in the remembered experiences. She must become aware of her own real or fantasied role in the abusive relationship, and resolve the associated feelings of confusion, shame, guilt, and self-hatred. She must gain insight into her internalized representations of both victim and abuser, and the ways she has played *both* roles in her life (and in the therapy). She must come to terms with her own rage and aggression. And she must come to a full realization of the impact of the abuse in her current inner and outer life. In other words, the patient must rework not only the trauma itself but the complex constellation of psychological issues, e.g., identity issues, relational issues, fantasies, conflicts, and compromises, which arise from and are organized around the trauma.

If recovery of traumatic memory is not the primary goal of psychodynamic psychotherapy,[4,36,38,49,61,71,90] what then is the place of remembering (or abreaction) of specific traumatic events? It is clear that controlled abreaction, the full affective and cognitive reexperiencing and verbal sharing of traumatic experience, in the presence of a trusted other, can be an important step in the healing process. In this way, the patient can bear the previously unbearable, and the experience can be incrementally integrated as part of the personal past.[4,17,36,49,60,62] Furthermore, in the telling, the patient has the opportunity to reevaluate the experience in the light of adult understandings. Hence, the trauma undergoes a "narrative revision"[71] leading to a more advanced conceptual understanding. The reclaiming of the past and the development of a coherent life story consolidates a stable sense of identity.

Stages of Treatment

It is generally recognized that treatment of traumatized patients must be structured and paced to allow the therapy to unfold with adequate containment and safety.[3,4,36,49,111,112] Chu[49] has argued against "the erroneous belief system that seems widespread among patients and their therapists . . . that in any situation where childhood abuse is discovered, all efforts should be made to immediately explore and abreact those abusive experiences." This belief arises from the common fantasy that once the trauma is completely remembered, the patient will no longer suffer (a model of therapy which is analogous to removing a foreign body or lancing an abscess). This strategy commonly leads to retraumatization and potentially dangerous disorganization, with little therapeutic gain.

Traumatized patients enter therapy with marked difficulties in basic trust, the conscious and unconscious expectation of abuse in all relationships (including the therapeutic relationship), and the unconscious compulsion to repeat traumatic experiences and relationships.[4,36,49,52,111–113] All authorities agree that the initial focus must be on the development of trust and a workable therapeutic alliance. Trust develops slowly from the experience of the therapist as consistent, nondefensive, forthright, and tolerant. The capacity for trust is further consolidated as the patient gradually develops tolerance for her own aggression, and recognizes that aggression can be managed without victimization of others.[52]

Because of the intense distrust and expectations of abuse, a withholding "classical" analytic stance is contraindicated for many traumatized patients.[36,39,49,55,100,107] The therapeutic situation itself mimics the early situation of abuse, i.e., an intense, emotional, regressive situation, usually maintained in isolation from others (secrecy), with an intrinsic power differential built into the relationship, in which the patient is asked to expose herself to (or even "submit to") the interventions of another. Acknowledgment and interpretation of the patient's fears generally helps to contain these feelings. In the early phase of treatment, the therapist should be relatively supportive, emotionally available and responsive, and should avoid the development of an early intractable negative ("traumatic") transference which may lead to stalemate or premature termination. For example, traumatized patients typically experience extensive silences or even "restrained coolness"[39] as abandonment, neglect, disinterest, or overt hostility, as do many nontraumatized patients, but the traumatized patient may not have the observing ego capacity to recognize the transference elements in these feelings and to maintain a working alliance. Ferenczi[39] characterized the optimal therapeutic attitude:

> The setting free of his critical feelings, the willingness on our part to admit our mistakes and the honest endeavor to avoid them in the future, all these go to create in the patient a confidence in the analyst. *It is this confidence that establishes the contrast between the present and the unbearable traumatogenic past*, the contrast which is absolutely necessary for the patient in order to enable him to re-experience the past no longer as hallucinatory reproduction but as an objective memory. (p. 227, italics in original)

In this phase the therapist functions as an auxiliary ego, offering support and validation of feelings, tolerating and helping to contain outbreaks of intense affects, mediating in areas of internal conflict, and tempering the activity of the patient's harsh archaic superego by the attitudes of tolerance and acceptance. While the patient may feel fragmented or split, the therapist holds and communicates an appreciation of the (potential) integrated self.

The specific tasks of the first stage of the treatment have been well detailed by Chu:[49] (*1*) optimizing self-care and the maintenance of safety (including direct work on self-injurious behavior, substance abuse or revictimization); (*2*) acknowledgment of the trauma and its impact on psychological functioning (without direct exploration); (*3*) maximizing the patient's current functioning and potential sources of self-esteem; (*4*) developing safe forms of affective expression; and (*5*) enhancing the patient's connections to supportive others. All of these tasks support the patient's overall stabilization and foster the development of internal controls and a sense of personal agency. As traumatic material emerges during the early phase of treatment, it must be acknowledged as important and difficult, while refocusing to the immediate tasks of stabilization. Denial or avoidance of the trauma risks enactment of the patient's early experiences of denial or neglect. However, premature validation is equally nontherapeutic because it deprives the patient of the space to resolve doubt and to grapple with her own ambivalence about denial versus acceptance of the painful experience.

Medication may be considered for treatment of concurrent symptoms such as depression, anxiety, or insomnia. It is also often effective to incorporate cognitive and behavioral strategies in this early stage of treatment. Adjunctive hypnotherapy may have a restricted role, with a focus on developing relaxation skills, managing the dissociative experiences, developing self-soothing strategies, etc. Hypnotherapy or other techniques aimed toward uncovering traumatic experience should not be used in the early stages of treatment.

Once patients have established sufficient internal and interpersonal safety to manage the intense work of abreactions and reconstructions of traumatic experiences, the therapy enters the middle phase (although the early work is often revisited many times during the course of the therapy in times of extreme stress). The uncovering and telling of well-guarded "secrets" is painful, frightening, and sometimes disorganizing, and the therapist should assist the patient to establish a pace which is bearable. Since, as noted, sexual trauma frequently occurs in an atmosphere of denial and forced silence, the trauma may be unspoken and "wordless." Dissociated experience and nonverbal memory must gradually attain verbal expression, the translation of enactive or imagistic representation to verbal representation.[71,87] Once again, quoting Ms. K:

> It's just hard to put a lot of things into words . . . like making a translation from one language into another where there just aren't words . . . It's trying to take a non-verbal memory, which most of the time is just a visual clip, but which sometimes has an emotion attached to it . . . or sometimes it's just an emotional clip . . . and trying to shoehorn that emotional feeling or image into words which by definition can't express the experience.

This is an important aspect of the process of reconstruction within the therapy. As Greenacre[97] described it:

> [Reconstruction] consists of a gradual and comprehensive unrolling with the patient of his life experiences which cling together in both direct and derivative memories. These are uncovered in parts of his present activities, dreams, relationships, and interests, and references to them lead to and from his neurotic problems. Free association, dreams, and investigation of screen memories are the most important channels of the work. (p. 38)

Kris[38] and Herman[4] also emphasize that careful and detailed exploration of available memory and associations fosters the gradual reemergence of traumatic memory. Remembering and reconstruction are further facilitated by careful attention to and interpretation of the manifold transference recreations (and partial reenactments) within the therapy. This aspect is particularly emphasized by Davies and Frawley[36]: "It is our contention that the elusively shifting interplay in the transference–countertransference configurations played out between patient and therapist remain the most powerful way to potentiate reemergence of traumatically dissociated experience." Through these complementary processes of mental associations, "lived" transference repetitions, and interpretation, the patient achieves insight into personal history, ultimately leading to a new level of integration and resolution of conflicts.

It should be emphasized that the therapist's part in the therapeutic dialogue is essentially facilitative, through making tentative connections, inquiring about discrepancies or gaps, noting repetitive elements or behaviors, and interpreting transference phenomena. These activities support the patient's efforts to construct a coherent personal history. Reconstruction does not connote pronouncements, but rather a shared process of new understandings which "make sense" of the patient's experience. Typical reconstructions refer to patterns and interrelationships rather than specific events, are qualitative rather than exact, and are aimed at facilitating further associations and memories.[14,28,97] Reconstructions and remembering refer not only to traumatic experience, but to the larger context of childhood relationships and developmental challenges. In this work, it is *never* the therapist's role to suggest or confirm that a patient was sexually abused.

As the middle stage unfolds, the patient must face and come to accept not only what was, but also what wasn't. This is a period of intense mourning, and necessarily involves foregoing the fantasy of ever having either the wished-for childhood or present-day compensation. It also involves a substantial revision of world schemas, which have been built around the experiences of abusers and victims. While this insight offers great potential psychological gain, it also is accompanied by tremendous feelings of loss. Ferenczi[114] described this process:

> In this new traumatic struggle, the patient is no longer alone. Although we cannot offer him everything which he as a child should have had, the mere fact that we can or may be helpful to him gives the necessary impetus towards a new life in which the pages of the unretrievable are closed and where the first step will be made toward acquiescence in what life yet can offer instead of throwing away what may still be put to good use. (p. 234)

The late stage of treatment resembles later stages of any thorough dynamic therapy, with the common tasks of consolidation of new insights, "practicing" new skills in real world situations, developing supportive relationships, letting go of the identity of patient (or victim), and the painful work of termination. This is the stage of "working through," in which new, more adaptive and more flexible psychic structures are formed. Interpersonal group therapies are often incorporated into the treatment at this stage for their focus on building interpersonal skills and consolidating new object relations.

Reconstruction, Recollection, and Truth

The place of analytic reconstruction as a technique has been extensively debated since Freud's early cases.[14,18,28,90,97,115–118] As Schimek[90] has carefully documented, Freud developed his "seduction theory," in which he postulated that very early (repressed) sexual trauma was the pathogenic force in hysteria, based on his own clinical reconstructions of the putative very early traumas (rather than actual recollections of patients). Following this period, as he gradually recognized the importance of childhood sexuality and the important component of fantasy, he rejected the seduction theory as overly simplistic. What he was rejecting was his own uncritical acceptance of *reconstructions* of early traumas as historical fact, not the fact of actual sexual trauma in the lives of many patients or its potential traumatic significance. Throughout his writings he acknowledged the occurrence and destructive effects of actual sexual abuse.[56,90] However, his shift to a predominant focus on intrapsychic conflict and fantasy resulted in a tragic neglect of the role of actual external trauma.[119]

The debate about reconstruction revolves around the issue of historical ''truth.'' Reed[18] gives a well-documented clinical example of a detailed reconstruction of an early traumatic experience (the traumatic death of a younger sibling), demonstrating the shared contributions of objective reality, personal meanings, and fantasies in the final ''fantasy/memory complex.'' The fact of the child's death was, of course, known to the patient, but the unconscious interpretations, fantasies, and associated feelings (such as guilt) were not. She argues, along with others,[14,28,39] that such reconstructions have great therapeutic value, with the potential to free the patient from the ''tyranny'' of the past. However, Reed[18] argues that an important aspect of such reconstruction is the separate clarification of the dual contributions of reality and fantasy:

> . . . one function of reconstruction might be that of differentiating as much as possible the defended registration of a (specified) historical event from the (specified) fantasy elaborated around it. When reconstruction is explicitly attended to, as in recent discussions of childhood sexual abuse, such important distinctions tend to be blurred. A focus on recovering the past rather than on the past as the basis of the system by which an individual has established meaning for himself or herself often predominates. (p. 55, footnote)

Once this work is achieved, the further therapeutic task remains to trace the impact of the reconstructed ''fantasy/memory complex'' on subsequent conflicts and compromises in the patient's life.[18,28,36] Arlow[28] wrote:

> The unforgettable, but unrecallable, events of the past are dynamically embedded in the patient's psychic functioning in the here and now. They become understandable as part of the ego's function and defense. What is reconstructed is not an objective event as viewed by an outside observer. It is the historic dynamism that is reconstructed. Recollection and reconstruction become significant only when they are placed in direct connection with the persistent psychological consequences that ensued. . . . This is different from the idea that a reconstruction is the nearest acceptable substitute for the undoing of amnesia. (p. 555)

One can make entirely parallel statements about the essential need to clarify the separate but interacting contributio... of reality and fantasy in relation to nonreconstructed ''recollection,'' i.e., subjective memory. From the patient's perspective, the acts of remembering and reconstructing serve multiple psychological functions, including both the gaining of insight and the defense against insight. Therefore, no recollection or reconstruction, whether it is asserting trauma or denying trauma, should be accepted uncritically as "historical truth." Ms. K had lived most of her adult life with essentially false (fabricated) memories of her childhood, created under the synergistic pressures from external influences (family) and internal needs to deny the horrible truth. Her childhood situation closely conformed to situations in which "pseudomemory" is created[8,25]: subjective confusion about the events, assertion of misinformation by an authority figure, and high social pressure. In an abusive family, these conditions may meet Brown's[25] criteria of "interrogatory suggestion": ". . . misinformation suggestibility plus a combination of explicit social influence factors (source credibility, systematic rewards and punishments, systematic misleading, and a demand for acceptance)."[25] The point is that suggestibility and malleability of memory can work for or against the recollection of abuse memories.

Inaccurate "memory" of early abuse may result from the combined effects of cognitive limits and the fantasies of childhood. Good[24] has provided a case report in which the patient "remembered" undergoing a traumatic clitoridectomy, which was understood by the child as punishment for sexual exploration. Indeed, she apparently had experienced intense parental prohibitions and threats regarding masturbation, and had then misunderstood an actual procedure (an exam) as the actualization of the threatened castration. Clarification of the actual historical event led to an understanding of the combined contributions of external truama and fantasy, and helped to move the therapy forward. In this case, as in most cases, there is no either/or, true/false dichotomy, but rather a complex interplay of reality and internal construction, actual trauma and fantasy. To recognize a contribution of fantasy does not necessarily negate an essential truth within the memory.

Erroneous memories of abuse may arise through therapeutic suggestion, particularly with overzealous therapists who persistently probe for memories, openly suggest early trauma, or provide uncritical acceptance. Brenneis[23] has eloquently outlined the technical and therapeutic dilemma as a tension between two paradigms, the "paradigm of belief" and the "paradigm of suggestion." The belief paradigm postulates that the therapist's capacity to believe the patient *permits* the emergence of repressed or disguised memories of trauma; memory malleability or distortion is seen as serving the psychic function of defense against intolerable memory. In contrast, the suggestion paradigm asserts that memories of trauma arise from subtle conscious and unconscious suggestions from the therapist, based on the therapist's theoretical assertion that painful memories can be lost to consciousness; memory malleability and distortion then allow the patient to confirm and elaborate the therapist's *expectation*, creating pseudomemories of abuse. As Brenneis[23] notes, "There is no obvious way to differentiate these paradigms on the basis of predictions, for they predict the same outcome, but assigned inverse valence: belief (suggestion) leads to memory (false)."

Memories of sexual abuse, even memories presented with great conviction and affect, may ultimately be shown to be erroneous.[120,121] Memory, like every other human behavior, serves multiple psychological functions. The therapist must hold onto this understanding, and remain open to and curious about the functions of the abuse memories in the patient's psychic structure and in the therapeutic process.[38,67,121–123] In some instances, the "memories" may be largely factitious and serve, for example, to externalize aggression or guilt, to gratify forbidden wishes, to achieve fantasied punishment, or to justify a grandiose sense of entitlement.[120,121,123] In other cases, the traumatic memory may be accurate, but may still serve to screen even more painful traumatic experience.[55,122,123] In some cases, the patient's persistent focus on real past trauma may serve as a resistance in the therapy, for example, by avoiding present conflicts, or by repetitive reliving of traumatic experience without integration or mastery (a recreation of the abusive relationship within the therapy).[38,62,67] Finally, the presentation of traumatic material may be unconsciously directed toward the reenactment in the transference to elicit wished-for rescue and reparation, to confirm expectations of disbelief, to accuse the therapist (in the transference), and so on.[36] The elucidation of such unconscious defensive or enactive functions does not imply that the basic memory is false. But if these other levels go unrecognized and uninterpreted, the therapeutic process may founder.

There are no definite guidelines by which a therapist can measure the "truth" of a patient's recollections. Memories of actual trauma may be presented with either strong conviction or tormenting doubts, intense affects or numbing detachment. The therapist must listen for internal reality but also continually assess the patient's external reality testing, and attend to the internal and interpersonal function of statements about abuse. Credibility is generally increased by the convergence of memories, associative details, and repetitive elements in behaviors and dreams, by historical coherence, by dissociated symptomatic manifestations, by repetitions in the patient's life, and by the emergence of abuse-related transference configurations (the various dynamics of abuser and victim).[4,23,34,36,47,49,53,124] Ultimately, however, coherence provides a necessary but not sufficient indication of truth,[21] and historical truth can only be substantiated by independent corroborative evidence.

Patients almost invariably suffer from marked ambivalence, confusion, and doubt about their memories of abuse. These feelings are a consequence of the horror, the difficulty of accepting that anyone could hurt them in these ways, and the wish to deny. It also reflects the chronic self-doubt, the patient's distrust of her own perceptions, and the impaired reality testing (which were a direct result of the mixed messages and outright denial at the time of the abuse). Patients often pressure the therapist to validate the memories or to say that they "believe" the reported events. It may be helpful to acknowledge generally that terrible things do happen to children, and it is important to take a clear stand that abuse of children is always wrong. However, the therapist is rarely in the position to confirm any aspect of the patient's history, and should not accept the role of arbiter of truth. Authoritarian interpretations disempower the patient, reinforce passivity and compliance, and symbolically repeat the experience of traumatic intrusion. It is more useful to validate the patient's feelings and fears, and to empathically interpret the patient's wish for clarity and resolution of her doubts.[49,123,125] As Ganaway[123] notes,

> [m]aintaining a neutral therapeutic stance on the veracity of uncorroborated trauma memories is one of many ground rules necessary for maintaining a secure therapy frame with this patient population, no less important than other limit and boundary issues. The patient ultimately must reinternalize the insatiable need for external validation . . . finally reaching a level of self-validation that will give her a sense of mastery over what once was a fragmented internal world of interwoven fact, fantasy, and illusion. (p.216)

Therapeutic neutrality goes hand in hand with a position of curiosity, an appreciation of the complexity of the question of "truth," and support for the patient's efforts to discover the truth, both within the therapeutic process and potentially through efforts to obtain corroboration. The therapist demonstrates honesty in the therapeutic relationship, and should validate the patient's realistic perceptions when appropriate. These reality-based interactions support the patient's increasing capacity to trust her own perception and to strive for truth, creating " . . . an *atmosphere of support* and faith in the patient's own ability to adopt a critical attitude in separating fact from fantasy"[25] (italics in original).

Is there a point when a memory of early abuse becomes a "fact" within the therapeutic dialogue? In our experience, patients often do reach a position where they have resolved the internal doubts, are realistically confident of their own histories, have an understanding of the associated fantasies and conflicts, and accept the limits of absolute knowledge. By this time, both patient and therapist can speak of the abuse memories as a part of the past, similar to other memories of childhood experiences or family relations. The memories are well integrated into the self and world schemas, and can be referred to as part of the shared understanding of the patient's life story.

Conclusions

Treatment of severely traumatized patients is arduous and complicated and cannot be reduced to simplistic formulas. Therapists need to appreciate the far-reaching impact of childhood trauma, and understand the special therapeutic challenges that these patients commonly present. While the integration of specific abuse memories is important, the bulk of the therapy revolves around the integration of broader insights regarding the total experience and context of the traumatic events and traumatic relationships. The patient gains understanding and mastery by reworking truamatic experience and trauma-based schemas, as these are manifested in everyday interactions both within and outside of the therapy. Once the trauma is understood and mastered as one part of the personal history, it loses its toxicity.

Given the complexity of influences on memory, combined with the complexity of the therapeutic process, the therapist must be ever mindful of the multiple levels of meanings of any material (or behavior) presented by the patient. As Brenneis[23] has stated, "believe skeptically and doubt empathically." Partly formed ideas, dreams, or fantasies about abuse, are not necessarily evidence of actual abuse. The therapist must maintain an open, accepting, and compassionate stance toward memories of trauma, without either premature validation or disbelief. When patients struggle with what to believe, this struggle should be explored and interpreted in terms of the patient's own uncertainty and ambivalence. Patients need to be helped to carry the burden of their own conflicts and ultimately to find their own resolution.

"Truth" lies with the patient, but not all that the patient says or believes, however psychologically valid, is necessarily "truthful." The therapeutic dialogue should assist the patient in constructing a personal history which is thoughtful and appreciative of the complexity of the individual experience and psychic life. As the past is connected to the present, the patient reclaims her future.

References

1. van der Kolk BA: Psychological Trauma. Washington, DC: American Psychiatric Press, 1987.
2. Terr LC: Childhood traumas: an outline and overview. Am J Psychiatry 1991; 148:10–20.
3. Briere JN: Child Abuse Trauma: Theory and Treatment of the Lasting Effects. Newbury Park, CA: Sage Publications, 1992.
4. Herman JL: Trauma and Recovery. New York: Basic Books, 1992.
5. Breuer J, Freud S: Studies on Hysteria. *In* Strachey J (Ed. and Trans.), The Standard Edition of the Complete Psychological Works of Sigmund Freud, Vol. 2. London: Hogarth Press, 1955, pp. 1–309. (Original work published 1893–1895).
6. Cohen J, Kinston W: Repression theory: a new look at the cornerstone. Int J Psychoanal 1983; 65:411–422.
7. Holmes DS: The evidence for repression: an examination of sixty years of research. *In* JL Singer (Ed.), Repression and Dissociation: Implications for Personality Theory, Psychopathology, and Health. Chicago: The University of Chicago Press, 1990, pp. 85–102.
8. Loftus EF: The reality of repressed memories. Am Psychol 1993; 48:518–537.
9. Pope HG, Hudson JI: Can memories of childhood sexual abuse be repressed? Psychol Med 1995; 25:121–126.
10. Schacter DL: Memory wars. Sci Am 1995; 272:135–139.
11. Kihlstrom JF, Hoyt IP: Repression, dissociation, and hypnosis. *In* JL Singer (Ed.), Repression and Dissociation: Implications for Personality Theory, Psychopathology and Health. Chicago: The University of Chicago Press, 1990, pp. 181–208.
12. Singer JL (Ed.): Repression and Dissociation: Implications for Personality Theory, Psychopathology, and Health. Chicago: University of Chicago Press, 1990.
13. van der Kolk BA, van der Hart O: The intrusive past: the flexibility of memory and the engraving of trauma. Am Imago 1991; 48:425–454.
14. Blum HP: The value of reconstruction in adult psychoanalysis. Int J Psychoanal 1980; 61:39–52.

15. Wetzler S: The historical truth of psychoanalytic reconstructions. Int Rev Psychoanal 1985; 12:187–197.
16. Erdelyi MH: Repression, reconstruction and defense: history and integration of the psychoanalytic and experimental frameworks. *In* JL Singer (Ed.), Repression and Dissociation: Implications for Personality Theory, Psychopathology, and Health. Chicago: The University of Chicago Press, 1990, pp. 1–31.
17. van der Hart O, Brown P: Abreaction re-evaluated. Dissociation 1992; 5:127–140.
18. Reed GS: On the value of explicit reconstruction. Psychoanal Q 1993; 62:52–73.
19. Spence D: Narrative Truth and Historical Truth: Meaning and Interpretation in Psychoanalysis. New York: W.W. Norton, 1984.
20. Shengold L: Soul Murder: The Effects of Childhood Abuse and Deprivation. New York: Fawcett Columbine, 1989.
21. Hanly C: The concept of truth in psychoanalysis. Int J Psychoanal 1990; 71:375–383.
22. Berliner L, Loftus E: Sexual abuse accusations: desperately seeking reconciliation. J Interpers Violence 1992; 7:570–578.
23. Brenneis CB: Belief and suggestion in the recovery of memories of childhood sexual abuse. J Am Psychoanal Assn 1994; 42:1027–1053.
24. Good MI: The reconstruction of early childhood trauma: fantasy, reality, and verification. J Am Psychoanal Assoc 1994; 42:79–101.
25. Brown D: Pseudomemories: the standard of science and the standard of care in trauma treatment. Am J Clin Hypn 1995; 37:1–24.
26. Frankel FH: Discovering new memories in psychotherapy—childhood revisited, fantasy, or both? New Engl J Med 1995; 333:591–594.
27. Chu JA, Matthews J, Frey LM, Ganzel B: The nature of traumatic memories of childhood abuse. Dissociation 1996; in press.
28. Arlow JA: Methodology and reconstruction. Psychoanal Q 1991; 60:539–563.
29. Courtois C: The incest experience and its aftermath. Victimology 1979; 4:337–347.
30. Courtois C: Healing the Incest Wound: Adult Survivors in Therapy. New York: W.W. Norton, 1988.
31. Herman JL, Russell D, Trocki K: Long-term effects of incestuous abuse in childhood. Am J Psychiatry 1986; 143: 1293–1296.
32. Russell DEH: The Secret Trauma: Incest in the Lives of Girls and Women. New York: Basic Books, 1986.
33. Bryer JB, Nelson BA, Miller JB, Krol PA: Childhood physical and sexual abuse as factors in adult psychiatric illness. Am J Psychiatry 1987; 144: 1426–1430.
34. Dewald PA: Effects on an adult of incest in childhood: a case report. J Am Psychoanal Assoc 1989; 37:997–1014.
35. Braun BG: Dissociative disorders as sequelae to incest. *In* RP Kluft (Ed.), Incest-Related Syndromes of Adult Psychopathology. Washington, DC: American Psychiatric Press, 1990, pp. 227–245.
36. Davies JM, Frawley MG: Treating the Adult Survivor of Childhood Sexual Abuse: A Psychoanalytic Perspective. New York: Basic Books, 1994.
37. Davidson J, Smith R: Traumatic experiences in psychiatric outpatients. J Traumatic Stress 1990; 3:459–475.
38. Kris E: The recovery of childhood memories in psychoanalysis. Psychoanal Study Child 1956; 11:54–88.
39. Ferenczi S: Confusion of tongues between the adult and the child. Int J Psychoanal 1949; 30:225–230 (originally published 1933).

40. Conte JR, Schuerman JR: Factors associated with an increased impact of child sexual abuse. Child Abuse Negl 1987; 11:201–211.

41. Romans SE, Martin JL, Anderson JC, O'Shea ML, Mullen PE: Factors that mediate between child sexual abuse and adult psychological outcome. Psychol Med 1995; 25:127–142.

42. Steele BF: Psychoanalysis and the maltreatment of children. J Am Psychoanal Assoc 1994; 42:1001–1025.

43. Swanson L, Biaggio MK: Therapeutic perspectives on father-daughter incest. Am J Psychiatry 1985; 142:667–674.

44. Lister ED: Forced silence: a neglected dimension of trauma. Am J Psychiatry 1982; 139:872–876.

45. Herman JL: Father-Daughter Incest. Cambridge, MA: Harvard University Press, 1981.

46. Summit RC: The child sexual abuse accommodation syndrome. Child Abuse Negl 1983; 7:177–193.

47. Sachs O: Distinction between fantasy and reality elements in memory and reconstruction. Int J Psychoanal 1967; 48:416–423.

48. Krystal H: Trauma and affects. Psychoanal Study Child 1978; 33:81–116.

49. Chu JA: The therapeutic roller coaster: dilemmas in the treatment of childhood abuse survivors. J Psychother Pract Res 1992; 1:351–369.

50. Gunderson JG, Chu JA: Treatment implications of past trauma in borderline personality disorder. Harvard Rev Psychiatry 1993; 1:75–81.

51. Steele BF: Some sequelae of the sexual maltreatment of children. In HB Levine (Ed.), Adult Analysis and Childhood Sexual Abuse. Hillsdale, NJ: Analytic Press, 1990, pp. 21–34.

52. Catherall DR: Aggression and projective identification in the treatment of victims. Psychotherapy 1991; 28:145–149.

53. Bernstein AE: The impact of incest trauma on ego development. In HB Levine (Ed.), Adult Analysis and Childhood Sexual Abuse. Hillsdale, NJ: Analytic Press, 1990, pp. 65–91.

54. Rose DS: "Worse than death": psychodynamics of rape victims and the need for psychotherapy. Am J Psychiatry 1986; 143:817–824.

55. Bigras J: Psychoanalysis as incestuous repetition: some technical considerations. In HB Levine (Ed.), Adult Analysis and Childhood Sexual Abuse. Hillsdale, NJ: The Analytic Press, 1990, pp. 173–196.

56. Levine HB: Clinical issues in the analysis of adults who were sexually abused as children. In HB Levine (Ed.), Adult Analysis and Childhood Sexual Abuse. Hillsdale, NJ: Analytic Press, 1990, pp. 197–218.

57. Spiegel D (Ed.): Dissociative Disorders: A Clinical Review. Lutherville, MD: The Sidran Press, 1993.

58. Chu JA, Dill DL: Dissociative symptoms in relation to childhood physical and sexual abuse. Am J Psychiatry 1990; 149:887–893.

59. Kirby JS, Chu JA, Dill DL: Severity, frequency, and age of onset of physical and sexual abuse as factors in the development of dissociative symptoms. Compr Psychiatry 1993; 34:258–263.

60. Kluft RP (Ed.): Incest-related syndromes of Adult Psychopathology. Washington, DC: American Psychiatric Press, 1990.

61. van der Hart O, Steele K, Boon S, Brown P: The treatment of truamatic memories: synthesis, realization and integration. Dissociation 1993; 6:162–180.

62. Chu JA: The repetition compulsion revisited: reliving dissociated trauma. Psychotherapy 1991; 28:327–332.

63. Terr LC: What happens to early memories of trauma? a study of twenty children under age

five at the time of documented traumatic events. J Am Acad Child Adolesc Psychiatry 1988; 27:96–104.

64. Freud S: Remembering, repeating and working through. *In* J Strachey (Ed. and Trans.), The Standard Edition of the Complete Psychological Works of Sigmund Freud, Vol. 12. London: Hogarth Press, 1958, pp. 145–156. (Originally published 1914).

65. Freud S: Beyond the Pleasure Principle. *In* J Strachey (Ed. and Trans.), Standard Edition, Vol. 18. London: Hogarth Press, 1955, pp. 1–64. (Originally published 1920).

66. Person ES, Klar H: Establishing trauma: the difficulty distinguishing between memories and fantasies. J Am Psychoanal Assoc 1994; 42:1055–1081.

67. Malev M: Use of the repetition compulsion by the ego. Psychoanal Q 1969; 38:52–71.

68. Loewald HW: Some considerations on repetition and repetition compulsion. *In* HW Loewald (Ed.), Papers on psychoanalysis. New Haven, CT: Yale University Press, 1973/1980, pp. 87–101.

69. Roth S: Psychotherapy: The Art of Wooing Nature. Northvale, NJ: Jason Aronson, 1987.

70. Modell AH: Other Times, Other Realities. Cambridge, MA: Harvard University Press, 1990.

71. Bonanno GA: Remembering and psychotherapy. Psychotherapy 1990; 27:175–186.

72. Herman JL, Perry JC, van der Kolk BA: Childhood trauma in borderline personality disorder. Am J Psychiatry 1989; 146:490–495.

73. Horowitz MJ: Stress Response Syndromes (2nd ed.) Northvale, NJ: Jason Aaronson, 1992.

74. Loewenstein RJ: Psychogenic amnesia and psychogenic fugue: a comprehensive review. *In* A Tasman, SM Goldfinger (Eds.), Review of Psychiatry, Vol. 10. Washington, DC: American Psychiatric Press, 1991, pp. 189–222.

75. Briere J, Conte J: Self-reported amnesia for abuse in adults molested as children. J Traumatic Stress 1993; 6:21–31.

76. Herman JL, Shatzow E: Recovery and verification of memories of childhood sexual trauma. Psychoanal Psychol 1987; 4:1–4.

77. Spiegel D: Dissociation and trauma. *In* A Tasman, SM Goldfinger (Eds.), Review of Psychiatry, Vol. 10. Washington, DC: American Psychiatric Press, 1991, pp. 261–275.

78. Goodwin JM, Cheeves K, Connell V: Borderline and other severe symptoms in adult survivors of incestuous abuse. Psychiatric Ann 1990; 20:22–32.

79. Zanarini MC, Gunderson JG, Marino MF: Childhood experiences of borderline patients. Compr Psychiatry 1987; 30:18–25.

80. Ogata SN, Silk KR, Goodrich S, Lohr NE, Westen D, Hill EM: Childhood sexual and physical abuse in adult patients with borderline personality disorder. Am J Psychiatry 1990; 147:1008–1013.

81. Vaillant GE: The beginning of wisdom is never calling a patient borderline. J Psychother Pract Res 1992; 1:117–134.

82. Williams LM: Recall of childhood trauma: a prospective study of women's memories of child sexual abuse. J Consult Clin Psychol 1994; 62:1167–1176.

83. Williams LM: What does it mean to forget child sexual abuse? a reply to Loftus, Garry and Feldman (1994). J Consult Clin Psychol 1994; 62:1182–1186.

84. Loftus EF, Garry M, Feldman J: Forgetting sexual trauma: what does it mean when 38% forget? J Consult Clin Psychol 1994; 62:1177–1181.

85. Squire LR: Memory and the hippocampus: a synthesis from findings with rats, monkeys and humans. Psychol Rev 1992; 99:195–231.

86. Schacter DL: Primary and multiple memory systems: perceptual mechanisms of implicit memory. J Cogn Neurosci 1992; 4:244–256.

87. Loewald HW: Perspectives on memory. Reprinted in HW Loewald (Ed.), Papers on Psychoanalysis. New Haven, CT: Yale University Press, 1976/1980, pp. 148–173.

88. Freud S: The psychopathology of everyday life. *In* J Strachey (Ed. and Trans.), Standard Edition, Vol. 6. London: Hogarth Press, 1960, pp. 1–310. (Originally published 1901).

89. Freud S: From the history of an infantile neurosis. *In* J Stachey (Ed. and Trans.), Standard Edition, Vol. 17. London: Hogarth Press, 1955, pp. 7–122. (Originally published 1918).

90. Schimek JG: Fact and fantasy in the seduction theory: a historical review. J Am Psychoanal Assoc 1987; 35:937–965.

91. Cheshire N, Thoma H: Freud's *Nachträglichkeit* and Strachey's "deferred action": trauma, constructions and the direction of causality. Int Rev Psychoanal 1991; 18:407–427.

92. Tomkins SS: Script theory. *In* J Aronoff, AI Rabin, RA Zucker (Eds.), The Emergence of Personality. New York: Springer, 1987, pp. 147–216.

93. Luborsky L, Barber JP, Diguer L: The meaning of narratives told during therapy: the fruits of a new observational instrument. Psychother Res 1992; 2:277–290.

94. Horowitz MJ: Introduction to Psychodynamics: A New Synthesis. New York: Basic Books, 1988.

95. Horowitz MJ, Reidbord SP: Memory, emotion and response to trauma. *In* S-A Christianson (Ed.), The Handbook of Emotion and Memory. Hillsdale, NJ: Erlbaum, 1992, pp. 343–357.

96. Greenacre P: The prepuberty trauma in girls. Psychoanal Q 1950; 19:298–317.

97. Greenacre P: Reconstruction: its nature and therapeutic value. J Am Psychoanal Assoc 1981; 29:27–46.

98. Arlow JA: Fantasy, memory, and reality testing. Psychoanal Q 1969b; 38:28–51.

99. Panel, Fall Meeting of the American Psychoanalytic Association: The seduction hypothesis. J Am Psychoanal Assoc 1988; 36:759–771.

100. Burland JA, Raskin R: The psychoanalysis of adults who were sexually abused in childhood: a preliminary report from the discussion group of the American Psychoanalytic Association. *In* HB Levine (Ed.), Adult Analysis and Childhood Sexual Abuse. Hillsdale, NJ: Analytic Press, 1990, pp. 35–41.

101. Loewald HW: Hypnoid state, repression, abreaction and recollection. Reprinted in HW Loewald (Ed.), Papers on Psychoanalysis. New Haven, CT: Yale University Press, 1955/1980, pp. 33–42.

102. Janet P: L'Automatisme Psychologique, Paris: Alcan, 1889. (Reprinted Paris: Societe Pierre Janet, 1973.)

103. Perry C, Laurence J-R: Mental processing outside of awareness: the contributions of Freud and Janet. *In* KS Bowers, D Meichenbaum (Eds.), The Unconscious Reconsidered. New York: Wiley, 1984, pp. 9–48.

104. Bower GH: Awareness, the unconscious, and repression: an experimental psychologist's perspective. *In* JL Singer (Ed.), Repression and Dissociation: Implications for Personality Theory, Psychopathology and Health. Chicago: The University of Chicago Press, 1990, pp. 209–231.

105. Freud S: The unconscious. *In* J Strachey (Ed. and Trans.), Standard Edition, Vol. 14. London: Hogarth Press, 1957, pp. 159–215, (Originally published 1915).

106. Freud S: Repression. *In* J Strachey (Ed. and Trans.), Standard Edition, Vol. 14. London: Hogarth Press, 1957, pp. 141–158. (Originally published 1915).

107. Raphling DL: Technical issues of the opening phase. *In* HB Levine (Ed.), Adult Analysis and Childhood Sexual Abuse. Hillsdale, NJ: Analytic Press, 1990, pp. 45–64.

108. Poole DA, Lindsay DS, Memon A, Bull R: Psychotherapy and the recovery of memories of

childhood sexual abuse: U.S. and British practitioners' opinions, practices, and experiences. J Consult Clin Psychol 1995; 63:426–437.

109. Wakefield H, Underwager R: Recovered memories of alleged sexual abuse: lawsuits against parents. Behav Sci Law 1992, 10:483–507.

110. Rose DS: A model for psychodynamic psychotherapy with the rape victim. Psychotherapy 1991; 28:85–95.

111. Kluft RP: Multiple personality disorder. *In* A Tasman, SM Goldfinger (Eds.), Review of Psychiatry, Vol. 10. Washington, DC: American Psychiatric Press, 1991, pp. 161–188.

112. Putnam FW: Diagnosis and Treatment of Multiple Personality Disorder. New York: Guilford Press, 1989.

113. Braun BG: Psychotherapy of the survivor of incest with a dissociative disorder. Psychiatr Clin North Am 1989; 12:307–324.

114. Ferenczi S: Notes and fragments. Int J Psychoanal 1949; 30:231–242 (originally published 1931).

115. Freud S: Construction in analysis. *In* J Strachey (Ed. and Trans.), Standard Edition, Vol. 23. London: Hogarth Press, 1964, pp. 255–269. (Originally published 1937).

116. Greenacre P: A historical sketch of the use and disuse of reconstruction. Psychoanal Study Child 1980; 35:35–40.

117. Friedman L: Reconstruction and the like. Psychoanal Inquiry 1983; 3:189–222.

118. Brenman E: The value of reconstruction in adult psychoanalysis. Int J Psychoanal 1990; 61:53–60.

119. Simon B: "Incest—see under Oedipus complex": the history of an error in psychoanalysis. J Am Psychoanal Assoc 1992; 40:955–988.

120. Shengold L: A variety of narcissistic pathology stemming from parental weakness. Psychoanal Q 1991; 60:86–92.

121. Raphling DL: A patient who was not sexually abused. J Am Psychoanal Assoc 1994; 42:65–78.

122. Glover E: The 'screening' function of traumatic memories. Int J Psychoanal 1929; 10:90–93.

123. Ganaway GK: Historical versus narrative truth: clarifying the role of exogenous trauma in the etiology of MPD and its variants. Dissociation 1989; 2:205–220.

124. Brenneis CB: Can early childhood trauma be reconstructed from dreams? On the relation of dreams to trauma. Psychoanal Psychol 1994; 11:429–447.

125. Chu JA: Ten traps for therapists in the treatment of trauma survivors. Dissociation 1988; 1:24–32.

14

Hypnosis and Hypnotherapy

FRED H. FRANKEL
NICHOLAS A. COVINO

Those who undertake to research the nature and practice of hypnosis along with their clinical colleagues are no strangers to controversy. From long before the Viennese physician Mesmer (1734–1815) promoted the use of magnetism to cure patients of their physical ailments and Sigmund Freud (1856–1939) made the trip to the laboratory of Charcot (1825–1893) to apprentice himself to the famous neurologist, practitioners of hypnosis have been ambivalently held, and their craft has been the target of suspicion and criticism matched only by the overly enthusiastic claims of its champions. Over the years, due to the occasionally dramatic and underexplained amelioration of symptoms with hypnosis and the often theatrical personalities of some practitioners in this area, "the voice of moderation and reason has been rare."[1]

What Is Hypnosis?

Hypnosis has been variously defined as a technique that can facilitate a state of relaxation, focused attention, or imaginative involvement, much like that experienced in a daydream or fantasy state.[2] Whether the results of hypnosis are due principally to the ability of an hypnotic subject to play a role with the intensity of a method actor[3,4] or to enter an altered state of consciousness,[5] or both, reality testing is abandoned[6] in favor of the comfortable production of distortions in perception, mood, and memory.[7]

The psychophysiological effects of hypnosis usually involve changes in heart rate, respiratory rhythm, muscle tension, arterial blood pressure, and oxygen consumption that are similar to those that occur in yoga, biofeedback, relaxation training, zen, and other meditative practices.[8] Neurological changes in patients as measured by EEG seem to involve an increase in alpha and theta rhythms, with some debate as to whether the change is accomplished by the production of the state of relaxation alone or is due to a cerebral trait of those who are more susceptible to hypnosis.[9,10,11] Neurological markers seem to exist in the p300[12,13] and N1 and P1[14] components of the cortical event-related brain potential (ERP). Hypnotized subjects show shifts in amplitude on these measures that coincide with their efforts to restrict peripheral awareness, increase self absorption, and narrow their attention.[15] Some theorists maintain that the hypnotic state is observed by these changes rather than caused by them and that the amplitude seems to differ with type of suggestion.[16] What, precisely, is indexed by these findings is not yet clear.

Subjects in a variety of clinical and experimental studies have been able to utilize hypnosis effectively to alter cognitive and sensory perception in order to control a variety of complaints. A subgroup of patients with disorders associated with the autonomic nervous system (e.g., anxiety, pain, asthma, irritable bowel syndrome, and sleep disorders) have been found to profit from the application of hypnotic techniques. These patients have been able to change behaviors associated with their illness (e.g., change medication usage) and experience a reduction in their ailment with hypnotic interventions. The majority of patients with symptoms that seem to be related to principles of classical or operant conditioning (e.g., phobias, nausea and vomiting, bulimia, and trichotillomania) have been found to possess high levels of hypnotizability that might contribute to the acquisition or maintenance of their disorder.[17–19]

Hypnotizability levels appear to be relatively normally distributed, with some 15% of the population possessing very high levels and about 25% being relatively unresponsive to it.[5] A number of measures exist[20] that involve the presentation of a series of suggestions or challenging items to the hypnotized subject (e.g., hand catalepsy or arm rigidity). Respondents are divided into low, moderately, and highly hypnotizable groups, depending on the number of items passed. Such tests are most commonly employed in laboratory studies rather than in clinical practice, since the failure of more difficult items might discourage moderately or poorly hypnotizable persons from working within their ability. The clinician, on the other hand, usually looks for evidence of hypnotizability in a patient's preference for activities that are congruous with the self-absorbed state of hypnosis (e.g., reading, watching films, running), the use of creative imagination (e.g., design, art, drama) or the presence of clinical problems that are usually associated with hypnotizability (e.g., phobias, multiple personality disorders).[19]

Hypnotized subjects are motivated to change their interpretation of events by the hypnotist's suggestions. While this is a psychological concept as old as the discipline itself, few adequate descriptions and fewer explanations of its mechanism are available to us. Most definitions of the term hypnosis convey the idea that a response to a suggestion is made without critical reflection and that, while the subject is truly free to reject the proposal, some demand characteristic of the situation, quality of the suggestion, or psychological property of the subject begs compliance with it.[21]

In a manner similar to a cognitive-behavioral intervention, a reframed understanding of an event can produce a change in autonomic nervous system activity with the accompanying changes in catecholamine activity and hormonal production. Whether this symptom relief is due to a reversal of the patient's tendency towards sympathetic arousal or the production of a parasympathetic "relaxation response,"[8] a subgroup of patients can control a variety of symptoms with the assistance of their new understanding. Behavioral changes can also be produced by the same altered understanding resulting from the persuasions of psychotherapists and secular and other healers.[22]

An unresolved debate exists between those who feel that hypnosis involves an altered state of consciousness much like that achieved in a daydream or fantasy state[5] and those who assert that it is merely an intense from of role play.[20] The group that adheres to the former position draws its roots from Janet (1859–1947), who described a division of consciousness that occurs in a person's attention, thoughts, affects, memories, and behaviors. In this so-called dissociative state, psychological material is thought to exist on a number of levels of consciousness that may or may not be evident to the subject. Some behaviors, for example, are experienced as having an automatic quality and some emotions can exert an influence on the body without the person seeming to be aware. Memories of traumatic events as well as conflictual emotions can be "filed on separate channels" and "disaggregated" from the subject's conscious experience. The early analytic notions of conversion disorder, the dramatic psychosomatic cures of Charcot, and the early approaches of talking therapies are evidence of this thinking.

Social psychologists believe that the successful subject is willing to adopt the role of an hypnotized person along with its attendant behaviors and expectations. For these theorists, no special state exists, but what is accomplished is seen as the result of the subject's willingness to accept uncritically and to comply with the suggestions of the hypnotist.[20]

Why Is Hypnosis Thought To Facilitate Memory Retrieval?

Perhaps it is the act of forgetting (i.e., a cognitive process that seems to occur outside of the person's active awareness) that is responsible for the link between recovery of memory and hypnosis. Or, it might be the manner in which memories are sometimes recalled in a dramatic moment of insight during psychotherapy. But many lay persons and professionals alike have seen a role for hypnosis in the recovery of memories. Subjects in legal cases, a psychoanalytic understanding of hysteria, some experimental literature, and a number of case reports have also helped to establish the idea that hypnosis can assist with the recall and retrieval of important historical information.

Most clinical hypnotists will tell a story about a person who sought treatment in order to retrieve some object that was misplaced.[1] Inevitably, these lost objects are usually some "valuable gem" or the equivalent. (Obviously, this is an area that defies laboratory or even quasi-experimental research and must rely on the case report for exposure and discussion.) These reports suggest that some barrier, usually a conflictual emotion, is present and interferes with a retrieval cue to create an experience of amnesia. The hypnotist either follows that affect with the patient or might review the events surrounding the loss as an integrative agent who can ''bring to the patient's awareness what was previously unorganized, incomprehensible, invisible, unspeakable and intangible.''[23] In the absence of controlled investigations, only the ''successful'' cases seem to exist in the literature, adding to the lore in this area.

Cognitive flexibility and an ability to use vivid mental imagery are thought to be important influences on memory. Researchers have been impressed with the individual differences displayed by low and highly hypnotizable subjects in their ability to enhance recall by means of visual memory. Those with higher levels of hypnotizability have been found to be better able to form a vivid mental gestalt of a stimulus and to be able to shift recall strategies from only detail-oriented to a more holistic recreation of the image. In turn, investigators postulate that this aids in encoding information and its recall.[24]

In the mid 1970s, a group of school children and their bus driver were abducted by kidnappers and transferred by van to a vault buried in a remote place in California. The driver and several of the children were able to free themselves from the tomb and went to the police. Initially, the driver was understandably anxious and unable to recall more than rough details of the event. When he was treated with hypnosis, he recollected two license numbers, one of which turned out to be almost the exact number of the kidnappers' van. This information led the police to capture the perpetrators.[25] In a similar situation, two youngsters who were raped, transported to Mexico, and released were helped by the police, using hypnosis, to recall the events of the trip. Again, after the application of this technique, one of the girls was able to recall several details that offered important clues to the capture and conviction of the perpetrator.[25]

Much of the clinical and some of the research opinion in this area is informed by a model of memory that implies that information is acquired much like the way a video camera registers it. Proponents of the use of hypnosis to enhance memory largely believe that the special concentration that comes with this relaxed state can be used to access a repressed memory and permit it to emerge into consciousness. In fact, most of the imagery employed by hypnotists in this area involves an invitation to the subject to ''use their memory like a videotape recorder'' to replay an incident and ''as with the videotape, slow down, still or speed up'' the events of interest while the hypnotist offers suggestions and engages in a dialogue with the subject that is designed to facilitate the exploration.[26]

The psychological defense mechanisms of repression, suppression, and dissociation are invoked as the mechanisms that justify this approach. Although not well defined and differentiated, these psychological constructs have in common the relatively successful removal of troublesome thoughts and affects from consciousness. Freud's work on hysteria,[27] along with his early theory building, led him to the supposition that the experience of real traumatic events (usually sexual) was responsible for a person's symptoms. It was the early aim of psychoanalysis to uncover these memories and events and, by means of an emotional abreaction, to permit the subject to resolve them. As Freud's theory evolved into his structural model of the mind with its ideas about intrapsychic conflict, drives, and defenses, only the couch remained as a remnant of his early interest in hypnosis. Where some practitioners of hypnosis use hypnotic techniques to teach patients how to terminate dissociative states and to cope with psychological distress from many sources, there remains an unsubstantiated belief among hypnotists that a well-facilitated trance can "lift the veil of repression" and permit the patient to "revisit" a traumatic event for the purposes of mastering and integrating the memories and affects.

At the heart of the controversy surrounding the use of hypnotic techniques in the area of memory, then, are several issues: the nature of memory; the nature of suggestion and the influence of suggestibility; and an understanding of the concept of psychological defense.

A Review of Some of the Experimental Work

Recall

A number of laboratory experiments have sought to measure the influence of hypnosis on recall. The earliest work in this area included presenting subjects with long lists of vocabulary words or associated pairs of words and, after some passage of time, asking them to recall what was learned.[28] An effort was made to determine the effect of hypnosis on memory by hypnotizing subjects in the learning phase, in the recall phase, or both. Most of these experiments found that hypnosis was no better at facilitating recall than learning in the waking state.[29]

Dywan and Bowers[30] added to these word list experiments by offering a group of high and low hypnotizable subjects a number of line drawings to memorize and recall. For each of 7 days, they asked the subjects to deposit their recollections of the drawings in a drop box. They then divided their group into those who received hypnosis to assist with the recall of the stimulus drawings and those who were motivated to recall without hypnosis. The hypnosis group reported more than twice the number of items as did the controls, including a number of items that were not reported during the baseline condition. The "cost" for the additional information was computed by subtracting the false memories from those accurately recalled to find that the hypnosis group made almost three times as many errors as did the subjects in the other conditions. The authors concluded that the use of hypnosis permitted subjects to relax their caution about what they were willing to report as memory, which resulted in increased production due more to disinhibition than to increased powers of recollection. Alternatively, they posited that a vivid image may feel compelling enough to the subject to promote the report of something, even if it is in error.

In line with criticisms that word list and neutral stimuli experiments lacked meaning and context that might facilitate the recall of stimuli with hypnosis,[31,32] Wagstaff and Maguire[33] presented a videotape of a crime scene taken from a popular television show to a group of undergraduate students who were divided into three groups. The first group was not hypnotized, but the subjects were guided by orienting questions that redirected their attention to their arrival at the experimental site and to the film. They were then asked to complete a multiple-choice questionnaire regarding the details of the video. The second group was hypnotized and offered age-regression suggestions to again view the video prior to completing the questionnaire. The control group was merely offered the same questionnaire. Seven days later, the identical conditions were presented, minus the viewing of the film. When the results were analyzed, the hypnosis group was found to be the least successful at recalling the details, with the guided memory group demonstrating an improvement at the 1-week recall. The authors not only challenged the supermemory claims of other hypnotists, but cautioned that reported gains in the memories of eyewitnesses in forensic situations could be due more to the nonspecific factors of guided imagery and reassurance than to hypnosis alone.

Perhaps, thought Sanders and Simmons,[34] "hypnosis might evoke images that are too vague or subtle to help in recall, but that are substantial enough when reinforced by the same image physically present." To test this idea, they had subjects watch a 20-second film of a robbery in which the perpetrator was dressed in a leather jacket, but the perpetrator's face was visible for only 3 seconds. An experimental group of hypnosis-aided subjects was invited to "replay the incident on an internal mental TV screen, complete with slow down and . . . freeze features." All subjects were invited back 1 week later to view two lineups, one with the thief present without the leather jacket and a second with an impostor wearing the jacket. In contrast to their hypothesis, the investigators found that the hypnotized group made more errors than controls in identifying the thief, due largely to the tendency of these subjects to choose the person wearing the distinctive jacket with confidence. The authors conclude that hypnosis does not seem to enhance eyewitness accuracy, but it can invite a subject to err, based on a tendency to respond with confidence to misleading cues.

In a recent article, Erdelyi[32] argued that some of the reported gains in memory attributed to hypnosis can be better explained by the other aspects of the methodology of the studies. Merely repeating the information, without hypnosis, would contribute something to the subject's ability to recall, as would inviting the person to concentrate on the original task in the absence of hypnosis. These strategies facilitate the emergence of additional cueing strategies or permit subjects to relax their criteria for what is seen as a guess versus a memory. "Hypnotic hypermnesia," he concludes, "is nothing more than hypermnesia."[33]

Implanted Memories

The tendency of hypnotized subjects to bear witness to the veridicality of implanted memories with conviction has been the subject of a number of recent experiments.

Researchers at Concordia University[35] asked a group of hypnotized subjects to revisit an evening during the previous week when, as suggested by the experimenters, their sleep had been disturbed by a loud sound (which had not in fact occurred). Of the group of 27 subjects, 17 were responsive to the suggestion. They then asked those who had "heard" the sound to describe it in some detail. When the hypnosis was terminated, 13 of these subjects persisted in their belief (in contrast to their prehypnosis reports) that some sleep-distrubing sound had indeed occurred. Later, these researchers repeated the study and included measures of hypnotizability along with tests of absorption and of a preference for imagic cognitive style.[36] Again, about 50% of the subjects maintained that their sleep had been distrubed by a sound. Interestingly, further analysis revealed that none of the low-hypnotizable subjects believed that their sleep had been disturbed. The authors concluded that those who find it easy to involve themselves in imaginary thinking may be more likely than those for whom fantasy is an effort to incorporate a pseudomemory into their thinking. Thus, a quality of the person, in addition to the contextual effects (e.g., expectancy), seems to be an important influence on a subject's ability to distort memory.

Other studies have suggested erroneous information to a hypnotized subject in an effort to create pseudomemories. These find that hypnotic susceptibility, the method of testing the memory, and the opportunity to verify the veridicality of a stimulus event are important moderating factors on the degree to which a pseudomemory is maintained. Lynn, Weekes, and Milano[37] found that highly hypnotizable subjects were willing to say that they had heard a telephone ring as well as a staged conversation, which were suggested to them in hypnosis. Low-hypnotizable subjects were not willing to offer such reports. The high hypnotizables retracted their reports when given a forced choice rather than a free-recall opportunity to reply. As in the case of neurological patients who confabulate,[38] a more structured presentation that includes some cues (i.e., forced choice) and the opportunity to check out a pseudomemory seem to reduce the subject's confidence in that pseudomemory/memory. Subjects may maintain a pseudomemory for as long as several weeks,[39] but here too, hypnotizability, the salience of the item recalled (e.g., recall whether an actor wore a mask rather than if he swore), and the assessment method (e.g., free vs. structured recall) were important moderating variables in the commitment to pseudomemory.

It does seem to be the case that experimental subjects can be influenced by hypnotists to believe that they experienced something that was merely suggested to them. The more such an experience differs from their usual life or is vague, novel, or unstructured, the greater their vulnerability to suggestion. Those subjects with greater hypnotic talent seem to be more likely to be victims to this phenomenon, due to their increased ability to picture events with vividness that can be misconstrued as true experience. Most of the authors working in this area caution that those who utilize hypnosis in their work (e.g., in forensic settings) must take extreme care to avoid any semblance of leading questions, and to scrutinize the setting for demand characteristics that could lead especially suggestible subjects to report material in error, but with confidence.

Posthypnotic Amnesia

Subjects can receive instructions from hypnotists to remember something, but also to intentionally forget something. Hypnotic anmesia usually occurs when the hypnotized subject has a number of experiences (e.g., limb catalepsy, gustatory hallucination), then is told by the hypnotist that it will take such effort to recall these experiences that they will prefer to forget them until instructed to remember. When good subjects are invited to repeat (but, not yet instructed to recall) what was experienced in hypnosis, they usually find it difficult to do so. Some sort of ''tip-of-the-tongue'' awareness without words seems to be the normative response, with subjects clearly working hard at trying to remember. However, even this area of hypnosis is not immune to controversy. The ability to recover information that has been experienced but temporarily forgotten seems to some to be a useful model for the study of other suppressed memories.

On one side of the debate are those who feel that subjects experience suggestions for amnesia much as they encounter other important learning experiences.[5,40,41] In posthypnotic amnesia, connections that are usually present among bits of an experience are disrupted and retrieval cues are absent, so that the material is unavailable to recall until recovery is permitted by the hypnotist. Social psychologists,[3,4] by contrast, find a more active role for the subject. These researchers believe that hypnotized persons are actively focused on something else (e.g., the hypnotist's suggestion or playing the role of the good subject) in a way that fills their attention and distracts them from recalling the previous experience.

A considerable amount of attention has been devoted by researchers to understanding the factors that might influence a subject to abandon the suggestion to forget once it is established. Subjects have been found to regain control of memories in the absence of a reversal cue, a phenomenon called *breaching,* when subjected to social pressures such as instructions to be honest, lie detector examination,[42] or influences that affect their response expectancies.[43] Furthermore, when subjects are offered more specific retrieval cues than the general invitation to free recall or are rehypnotized, many more subjects will breach, although similar results can be obtained with relaxation alone.[44] Hypnosis itself does not seem to be a retrieval cue nor a vehicle for the recall of previously unrecalled memories.

Forensic Applications of Hypnosis

Not long ago, the Los Angeles police department initiated a program to train a number of their officers in hypnosis.[45] The motivation for this program came from the officers' experience with the use of hypnosis in facilitating eyewitness testimony. Their strong belief was that, in many cases, useful information was elicited in hypnosis after usual questioning failed. The FBI and other law enforcement agencies have also employed hypnotic procedures in their efforts to obtain evidence from people who have observed events, and some agencies have developed specific protocols for its use. The usual procedure is to invite subjects, who have limited recall of a crime scene or other important experience, to review the circumstances in their mind under hypnosis. Sometimes subjects will attempt to reexperience pertinent emotions or the hypnotist will serve as a coach, as they seek information to add to the investigation.

As with the laboratory experiments on memory, eyewitnesses to crimes are more likely to provide additional information to investigators with the application of hypnosis. However, in the absence of controlled studies, these gains can be best attributed to the efforts of the police and the hypnotist to reassure a subject that no further harm will come from a criminal because of an increase in recall or that embarrassing details might be forgotten when the trance is terminated. The hypnotist's attention to the subject, and/or an increase in associative cues stemming from their creative and unconventional methods of representing the material, might also be factors that influence eyewitnesses to report more information with hypnosis.[46] As in the experimental work on recall, Wagstaff[47] cautions that hypnotized subjects may be unusually influenced by the hypnotic situation to comply and confuse fantasy and reality and give "less accurate information in some circumstances." Indeed, Orne et al.[29,48] write that witnesses have testified in court to seeing characteristics of a perpetrator that were impossible to observe with the naked eye. Other witnesses have recalled with certainty eating food in restaurants that did not have the item in question on the menu. Witnesses have also been led by attorneys to speak with certainty about facts that could not be known to them. The element of certainty facilitated by the hypnotic intervention has then been translated to a convincing performance in court.

In an interesting experiment, Wagstaff and his colleagues[49] showed a videotape of a criminal trial to a group of student subjects who were asked to be "jurors." The subjects believed the trial to be real. They were placed in three groups and told that the witness was initially unable to provide much information to the police, but Group A was told she could remember with the aid of hypnosis; Group B, that she could remember with the assistance of guided imagery; and Group C, that she could not provide additional details at all. An analysis of the three groups revealed that more subjects in the hypnosis group found the defendant to be guilty. The authors concluded that these students were more likely to convict a defendant on the basis of testimony elicited through hypnosis than when no memory aid was reported.

Mindful of the laboratory studies mentioned above, Orne[50] developed a set of guidelines for the use of hypnosis in the forensic context. These guidelines advocated tape recording of all contacts with the subject, including the hypnosis sessions, and suggested that the hypnotic work be done by a qualified person. Furthermore, others should not be present who could inadvertently cue or lead the subject to offer information in any desired direction. Others extend these guidelines to recommend milieu considerations, as well as cases in which this technique should not be employed.[51] Most courts currently will not admit testimony from persons who have utilized hypnosis in the recovery of memory. This *per se exclusion* of hypnotically elicited testimony was first explicated in *State v. Mack*.[52] Here the court found that a witness to a crime who had been hypnotized could not give testimony in the case. Diamond[53] writes that witnesses who have been hypnotized should not be permitted to testify in court because their competence to do so is compromised. Among those who advocate lifting the per se exclusion rule is Scheflin,[54] who would prefer to permit the court to determine the value and circumstances of the testimony on a case-by-case basis. Most states at this time, however, still adhere to the per se exclusion rule.

Psychotherapy

Much of the controversy in the area of psychotherapy has to do with an understanding of the concepts of repression, dissociation, state-dependent learning, imagination, and suggestibility. The important issues relate to the nature of the psychological material that is recalled in psychotherapy, the manner in which it is revealed, and the veridicality of it.

At this point in time, there is no doubt that a large number of people have been the unfortunate victims of traumatic experiences. Whether at the hands of trusted individuals who betrayed their position of authority or resulting from some event of life that overwhelmed the individual, many people have experienced life problems that are extremely painful and that promote a persisting sense of helplessness. As with other disturbing thoughts and emotions, these people seek to banish this awareness from consciousness by means of psychological defenses like repression. Some relief is thus obtained by merely not remembering, yet, for many, these events continue to exert some influence on the person's life.

Some believe that a neurophysiological event (emotional hyperarousal) takes place under conditions of extreme stress[55] and that patients use the psychological defense mechanism of dissociation to "split off" the psychological and even physical pain of the event from conscious awareness. The price to be paid for this protection is the fragmentation of memory which can represent itself in symptoms of amnesia, fugue, numbness, startle responses, and the spontaneous abreactive reliving of the traumatic situation.[55,56] The putative common ground between the dissociation in trauma and that which occurs in hypnosis is the belief that "reliving" the trauma through hypnosis can recreate something of the original neurochemical and psychological conditions. Recalling these can permit emotional abreaction and the integration of memories, feelings, and thoughts related to the original trauma.

Much of the writing in the area of psychotherapy consists of case studies that generally follow the description of Phillips,[56] who reports on three patients who "appeared to have experienced the trauma of child or adolescent sexual abuse, though conclusive evidence is available in only one of the three cases" (p. 186). Using ideomotor signaling to receive information regarding "the abuse" from her patients, she used hypnosis to explore the details of the trauma as well as to teach a variety of coping strategies. Other therapists follow the strategy of first stabilizing a patient with training in coping strategies that facilitate the management of intrusive thoughts and affects before systematically uncovering the traumatic event. This permits the expression and integration of memories, thoughts, and affects and allows them to be brought into the patient's personal and relational world.[57]

In a recent report, Yapko[58] relates the results of a survey of psychotherapists whom he sampled with questionnaires to identify attitudes towards hypnosis and its use in recovery of patient memories. More than 800 psychotherapists, at various stages of training, were sampled. The group averaged 44 years of age with 11 of these in clinical practice. One-half of the sample reported that they use hypnosis in their work and greater than one-third said that they use it to retrieve memories from their patients at least occasionally. Unfortunately, a majority of these practitioners maintained erroneous beliefs about the domain of hypnosis and the accuracy of memories. For example, an alarming number reported beliefs in the ability of hypnosis to access memories of the earliest stages of infancy or even of past lives! They seemed generally to be aware of the research that suggests that people in hypnosis can be influenced to incorporate pseudomemories as true events. However, almost one-fifth of them had knowledge of a psychotherapist colleague who asserted to a patient that some abuse had taken place, despite the absence of corroborating or authenticating data.

The predominant focus of psychotherapists for the past 50 years has been the uncovering of past experiences. The motive for revisiting the past in this setting can be found in the writings of Janet[59] and Freud,[27] who both described a mental mechanism of defense whereby painful affects and events were dismissed from conscious awareness. Although both of these major theorists believed their concepts to be distinguishable, the terms that they introduced, repression (Freud) and dissociation (Janet), have now come to be used almost interchangeably. In fact, in some of his earlier writings, Freud himself failed to make a distinction between the two.

Since the introduction of these concepts over a century ago, the skeptical have questioned the nature of defensive processes and the influences upon them. Like Freud, they have expressed the view that suggestibility might contribute more than a small amount to autobiographical reports, especially in the recall of traumatic events. An historical focus provides a remarkable opportunity for a nurturing and caring relationship to develop between patient and therapist, which can provide some understanding of current symptoms and complaints that are otherwise not comprehensible to the patient. The success of psychotherapy, however, does not necessarily depend upon the accuracy of what is recalled, since the narrative that is constructed need only have personal meaning for patient and therapist. Most therapies rely heavily upon metaphor and other symbolic efforts at meaning making to resolve and integrate important aspects of a person's experience, symptoms, and complaints. Participants on both sides of the relationship will offer that the experience of psychotherapy is often accompanied by distortions of reality by patient and therapist alike! When this material is taken out of the clinical context and transferred to the judicial system or even to the court of public opinion, different rules apply and particular attention must be paid to issues of veridicality.

Although Freud abandoned the "copper of suggestion for the pure gold of psychoanalysis," Janet did not. Janet continued to use this technique to treat patients with conversion disorders and other somatic and psychiatric complaints, and he taught others to do the same. Supporting the use of hypnosis as an aid in uncovering the past is the notion that hypnosis is the equivalent of dissociation; the former is seen as a directed and controlled experience and the latter as uncontrolled and spontaneous. State-dependent learning theory is invoked to augment this viewpoint with the claim that a hypnotically created dissociative state can permit access to traumatic memories and affects formerly dissociated. The hypnotic experience, thus, is viewed as a bridge to the previously dissociated or disconnected painful traumatic memory. While this particular use of hypnosis awaits empirical validation, psychotherapists successfully use hypnotic strategies to assist their patients.

Since it remains primarily a relaxation technique that utilizes focus and concentration, hypnosis can be taught to patients in psychotherapy who wish to distract themselves at times from painful psychological material. Instruction in self-hypnosis can assist the individual to focus actively and become absorbed in more neutral or soothing images in a fashion that permits distressing thoughts to fade from conscious awareness. Patients in hypnosis can be educated as to the narrowness of attention and the manner in which the mind serves as an editor for the brain by selecting what input will be granted attention (e.g., becoming more aware of the pressure and shape of a wristwatch or an article of clothing). Most patients can be taught simple distraction techniques that can serve as coping devices. Some subjects who are prone to experience episodes of dissociation can learn more readily to identify and terminate them.

A number of theoretical factors limit the applicability of hypnosis in recovering memories in psychotherapy. As we have seen earlier, memories are subject to many influences, including cognitive schemas, emotional attitudes, misunderstandings, and misperceptions that prevail both at the time of encoding and at the time of retrieval. When memories are recalled in any setting, they are likely to be colored by these influences. Hypnosis serves as a useful technique in psychotherapy to facilitate the mastery of a variety of feelings. However, the idea that hypnosis is the equivalent of dissociation, because sharply separated mental channels exist during a trance, pushes the metaphor too far. Since hypnosis is governed to a large extent by an invitation to fantasy and imagination, its product is burdened by the high probability that what is recalled contains a substantial amount of illusion. Furthermore, studies find that patient and therapist alike are unable to distinguish fact from fantasy in what emerges with hypnosis.[50]

Summary and Recommendations

At the moment, we are forced to concur with the AMA committee[60] that there does not seem to be any substantial evidence to support the claims that hypnosis can be a dependable instrument in the recovery of true memory. Hypnotized subjects will offer more information in hypnosis, a good deal of which will be in error. This seems to be more likely when the subject is blessed with elevated levels of hypnotizability or when the recall task involves information that is vague, difficult to verify, novel, or emotionally charged.

Hypnotized subjects can be easily led to conclusions by suggestive techniques. These subjects can even come to believe strongly in information that is clearly in error. This is especially true when they are able to picture such information vividly or have a strong emotional attachment to the material. Hypnotizable subjects who can picture with greater vividness and emotional intensity can experience their ''recollections'' as real. It is this emotional intensity, rather than a real experience, that invites confidence in the truth of what is remembered. When knowledge is scarce, or social or contextual pressures exist, people will fill in the gaps even without hypnosis with information that ''feels right'' to them.

Alternative hypotheses seem to exist for a number of the successes that are attributed to hypnotic interventions. Subjects may volunteer additional information because they are more relaxed with hypnosis, reassured by the examiner, or refreshed by a second or third review of the material. Even though hypnotized subjects seem to be able to perform better on visual tasks, their success is judged to relate more to superior encoding than to the use of hypnosis to picture the past. The highly hypnotizable person might well possess a better memory than the person with low hypnotizability, but may not necessarily possess greater accuracy in retrieving past information. Given the propensity of hypnotizable subjects to be misled in hypnosis, alternative techniques such as reassurance, relaxation, and review should be tried before proceeding to hypnosis, especially in cases where primacy is placed on establishing the truth of a recollection.

Absent any controlled studies in the use of hypnosis to retrieve validated memories in psychotherapy, the rules of psychotherapy need to govern our use of hypnosis in this area and we are forced to use the laboratory data that do exist (even though they are not clinical) to offer what guidance can be given in this area. The rules of psychotherapy suggest that dialogue between patient and psychotherapist is meaningful and motivated. What is recalled and presented for discussion is subject to the influence of intrapsychic conflicts, emotional pressures, transference and other distortions, and the limits of the individual to understand these. At times, these recollections will be about the recovery of painful and difficult memories of traumatic events that have not been remembered. At times, the recollections will be a symbolic way to communicate something to the therapist. These recollections should be treated in the context in which they are found and not seen as easily transferable (e.g., to a forensic context).

Although insight-oriented psychotherapy is tolerant of ambiguity and uncertainty, the confrontative nature of the forensic setting cannot be. Allegations of sexual or other abuse that are presented in court must be accurate to be useful. When this information is obtained for the first time through the use of guided imagery or hypnosis, the reactivated memories obtained cannot be relied upon to be valid. Following the laboratory models, they could even be entirely in error, but feel totally accurate to the subject. In the absence of external validation, psychological material regarding sexual or other traumatic abuse should be reserved for the psychotherapist's consulting room rather than the courts. Furthermore, in clinical situations, when it seems that a patient might become involved in a subsequent legal action, many psychotherapists believe that it is best to avoid the use of hypnotic techniques altogether, even for unrelated complaints, so as not to jeopardize the legal case.

Words like "reliving" and "refreshing" ought to be taken only as a metaphor and used with caution. Memory is reconstructive, not reproductive, and can be influenced by many factors. There is no evidence to suggest that the aging brain goes stale and efforts to cue the subject can be helpful (structured or multiple choice), less helpful (free association), or misleading. Memories do not present the original experience without the influence of social factors, perceptual distortion, wishes, fears, and other interpersonal and intrapsychic forces. Hypnosis does not lift a veil of years to reveal the original as if it were a painting. Likewise, what is encoded (subject to perceptual and other distortion) forms the basis of what gets replayed. In memory there are few live performances that are replayed as delivered!

References

1. Crasilneck HB, Hall JA: Clinical Hypnosis: Principles and Application. New York: Grune and Stratton, 1975.
2. Gill MM, Brenman M: Hypnosis and Related States: Psychonanalytic Studies in Regression. New York: International Universities Press, 1959.
3. Sarbin TR: Contributions to role-taking theory: I. hypnotic behavior. Psychol Rev 1950; 57:255–270.
4. Sarbin TR, Coe WC: Hypnosis: Two Social-Psychological Analyses of Influence Communication. New York: Holt Rinehart and Winston, 1972.
5. Hilgard ER: Hypnotic Susceptibility. New York: Harcourt Brace and World, 1965.
6. Shor RE: Three dimensions of hypnotic depth. Int J Clin Exp Hypn 1962; 10:23–28.
7. Orne MT: The nature of hypnosis: artifact and essence. J Abnorm Soc Psychol 1959; 58:277–299.
8. Benson H: The Relaxation Response. New York, William Morrow, 1975.
9. London P, Hart JT, Leibovitz MP: EEG alpha rhythms and susceptibility to hypnosis. Nature 1967; 219:71–72.
10. Morgan AH, MacDonald H, Hilgard ER: EEG alpha: lateral asymmetry related to task, and hypnotizability. Psychophysiology 1974; 11:275–282.
11. Crawford H, Gruzelier J: A midstream view of the neuropsychophysiology of hypnosis: recent research and future direction. In E Fromm, M Nash (Eds.), Contemporary Hypnosis Research. New York: Guilford Press, 1992.
12. Barabasz AF, Gregson RA: Antarctic wintering-over, suggestion and transient olfactory stimulation: EEG evoked potential and electrodermal responses. Biol Psychol 1979; 9:285–295.

13. Spiegel D, Cutcomb S, Ren C, Pribram K: Hypnotic hallucination alters evoked potentials. J Abnorm Psychol 1985; 94:249–255.

14. Schwyer DM, Allen JJ: Attention-related electroencephalographic and event-related potential predictors of responsiveness to suggested posthypnotic amnesia. Int J Clin Exp Hypn 1995; 48:295–315.

15. Tellegen A, Atkinson G: Openness to absorbing and self-altering experiences (''absorption''), a trait related to hypnotic susceptibility. J Abnorm Psychol 1974; 83:268–277.

16. Spiegel D, Barabasz AF: Effects of hypnotic instructions on P300 event-related-potential amplitudes: research and clinical implication. Am J Clin Hypn 1988; 31:11–17.

17. Covino NA, Frankel FH: Hypnosis and relaxation in the medically ill. Psychother Psychosom 1993; 60:75–90.

18. Covino NA, Jimerson DC, Wolfe BE, Franko DL, Frankel FH: Hypnotizability, dissociation and bulimia nervosa. J Abnorm Psychol 1994; 103:455–459.

19. Frankel FH, Orne MT: Hypnotizability and phobic behavior. Arch Gen Psychiatry 1976; 33:1259–1261.

20. Barber TX, Spanos NP, Chaves JF: Hypnotism: Imagination and Human Potentialities. New York: Pergammon Press, 1974.

21. Gheorghiu VA, Netter P, Eysenck HJ, Rosenthal R: Suggestion and Suggestibility: Theory and Research. New York: Springer-Verlag, 1989.

22. Frank JD: Persuasion and Healing: A Comparative Study of Psychotherapy. New York: Schocken Books, 1961.

23. Kluft RP: On the use of hypnosis to find lost objects: a case report of a tandem hypnotic technique. Am J Clin Hypn 1987; 29:242–248.

24. Crawford HJ, Allen SN: Enhanced visual memory during hypnosis as mediated by hypnotic responsiveness and cognitive strategies. J Exp Psychol Gen 1983; 112:662–685.

25. Kroger WS, Douce RG: Hypnosis in criminal investigation. Int J Clin Exp Hypn 1979; 27:358–374.

26. Reiser M, Nielson M: Investigative hypnosis: a developing specialty. Am J Clin Hypn 1980; 23:75–84.

27. Freud S: The aetiology of hysteria. In JE Strachey (Ed. and Trans.), The Standard Edition of The Complete Psychological Works of Sigmund Freud. Vol. 3. London: Hogarth Press, 1962, pp. 191–122. (Original work published 1896).

28. Hull CL: Hypnosis and Suggestibility: An Experimental Approach. New York: Appleton-Century-Crofts, 1933.

29. Orne MT, Whitehouse WG, Dinges DF, Orne EC: Reconstructing memory through hypnosis: forensic and clinical implications. In HM Pettinati (Ed.), Hypnosis and Memory. New York: Guilford Press, 1988.

30. Dywan J, Bowers K: The use of hypnosis to enhance recall. Science 1983; 222:184–185.

31. Rosenthal BG: Hypnotic recall of material learned under anxiety and non-anxiety-producing conditions. J Exp Psychol 1944; 34:369–389.

32. Erdelyi MH: Hypnotic hypermnesia: the empty set of hypermnesia. Int J Clin Exp Hypn 1994; 42:379–390.

33. Wagstaff GF, Maguire C: An experimental study of hypnosis, guided memory and witness memory. J Forensic Sci Soc 1983; 23:73–78.

34. Sanders GS, Simmons WI: Use of hypnosis to enhance eyewitness accuracy: does it work? J Appl Psychol 1983; 68:70–77.

35. Laurence JR, Perry C: Hypnotically created memory among highly hypnotizable subjects. Science 1983; 222:523–524.

36. Labelle L, Laurence JR, Nadon R, Perry C: Hypnotizability, preference for an imagic cognitive style, and memory creation in hypnosis. J Abnorm Psychol 1990; 99:222–228.
37. Lynn SJ, Weekes JR, Milano MJ: Reality versus suggestion: pseudomemory in hypnotizable and simulating subjects. J. Abnorm Psychol 1989; 98:137–144.
38. Mercer B, Wapner W, Gardner H, Benson FD: A study of confabulation. Arch Neurol 1977; 34:429–433.
39. Sheehan PW, Statham D, Jamieson GA: Pseudomemory effects over time in the hypnotic setting. J Abnorm Psychol 1991; 100:39–44.
40. Kihlstrom JF: Context and cognition in posthypnotic amnesia. Int J Clin Exp Hypn 1978; 26:246–267.
41. Kihlstrom JF: Instructed forgetting: hypnotic and nonhypnotic. J Exp Psychol Gen 1983 112:73–79.
42. Coe WC, Sluis AS: Increasing contextual pressures to breach posthypnotic amnesia. J Pers Soc Psychol 1989; 57:885–894.
43. Silva CE, Kirsch I: Breaching hypnotic amnesia by manipulating expectancy. J Abnorm Psychol 1987; 96:325–359.
44. Kihlstrom JF, Brenneman HA, Pistole DD, Shor RE: Hypnosis as a retrieval cue in posthypnotic amnesia. J Abnorm Psychol 1985; 94:264–271.
45. Holden C: Forensic use of hypnosis on the increase. Science 1980; 208:1443–1444.
46. Wagstaff GF: Hypnosis and witness recall: discussion paper. J R Soc Med 1982; 75:793–798.
47. Wagstaff GF: The problem of compliance in hypnosis: a social psychological viewpoint. Bull Br Soc Exp Clin Hypn 1979; 2:3–5.
48. Orne MT, Soskis DA, Dinges DF, Orne EC, Tonry MH: Hypnotically Refreshed Testimony: Enhanced Memory or Tampering with Evidence? Issues and Practices in Criminal Justice. Washington DC: National Institute of Justice, 1985.
49. Wagstaff GF, Vella M, Perfect T: The effect of hypnotically elicited testimony on jurors' judgments of guilt and innocence. J Soc Psychol 1992; 132:591–595.
50. Orne MT: The use and misuse of hypnosis in court. Int J Clin Exp Hypn 1979; 27:31–341.
51. Timm HW: Suggested guidelines for the use of forensic hypnosis techniques in police investigations. J Forensic Sci 1984; 29:865–873.
52. State v. Mack, 292 N.W. 2d 764 (Minn. 1980).
53. Diamond B: Inherent problems in the use of pretrial hypnosis on a prospective witness. California Law Rev 1980; 68:313–349.
54. Scheflin AW: Forensic hypnosis: unanswered questions. Aust J Clin Exp Hypn 1994; 22:23–34.
55. Spiegel D: Dissociating damage. Am J Clin Hypn 1986; 29:123–131.
56. Phillips M: Turning symptoms into allies: utilization approaches with posttraumatic symptoms. Am J Clin Hypn 1992; 35:129–137.
57. Brown D: Pseudomemories: the standard of science and the standard of care in trauma treatment. Am J Clin Hypn 1995; 37:1–24.
58. Yapko MD: Suggestibility and repressed memories of abuse: a survey of psychotherapists' beliefs. Am J Clin Hypn 1994; 36:163–187.
59. Janet P: Psychological Healing: A Historical and Clinical Study, Vol. 1. New York: MacMillan, 1925.
60. American Medical Association: Scientific status of refreshing recollection by the use of hypnosis. JAMA 1985; 253:1918–1923.

15

Cognitive Therapy of Dissociative Identity Disorder

Cognitive therapy was first developed by Aaron Beck and colleagues[1] for the treatment of depression. Since then it has been applied to a wide variety of different mental health problems, including anxiety disorders,[2] personality disorders,[3,4] and dissociative disorders.[5] It is also used in marital therapy[6] and as an adjunctive modality throughout the mental health field. The cognitive therapy of depression is one of the few psychotherapies that has been subjected to systematic treatment outcome studies, and it has proven to be as effective for the treatment of unipolar nonpsychotic depression as antidepressant medication.[7] In some of its modifications, cognitive therapy involves techniques and strategies not described by Beck: this is true of the cognitive therapy of dissociative identity disorder (DID).

The cognitive therapy of DID, formerly called multiple personality disorder, has been described by Ross and Gahan,[8] Ross,[5,9,10] and Fine,[11,12] but no treatment outcome data are available. My model of cognitive therapy of DID involves a blend of systems, and cognitive and psychodynamic principles, as described in a collection of case histories[9] and a book on treatment of DID patients with Satanic ritual abuse memories.[10] The purpose of this chapter is to describe the cognitive therapy of DID in the context of the controversy about the accuracy of recovered memories of childhood trauma. From a strict cognitive therapy perspective, the therapy to be described is not cognitive: I refer to it as cognitive therapy to emphasize that component of the treatment method.

I have restricted my discussion to DID because that is my area of expertise, however, most of what I will say in this chapter can also be applied to borderline personality disorder, posttraumatic stress disorder, acute stress disorder, and dissociative disorder not otherwise specified. The target of the cognitive interventions in the treatment of

DID is sometimes diagnostically specific cognitive errors, such as the belief that different parts of the self are different people, but more often is cognitive errors arising from trauma, such as a victim's belief that childhood sexual abuse occurred because of the badness of the victim.

The plan of this chapter is to review some general principles of cognitive therapy; discuss the benefits and limitations of the cognitive model in the 1990s; explain how the cognitive therapy of DID is exempt from the usual criticism of trauma psychotherapy; and then discuss several core principles of the cognitive therapy of DID. These include behavioral principles, the problem of attachment to the perpetrator, the locus of control shift, and orientation of the alter personalities to being in the same body in the present.

Although I have not coined a name for the method of therapy described here, one might call it cognitive-systems trauma therapy.

General Principles of Cognitive Therapy

The basic idea behind cognitive therapy is that thoughts influence feelings and behavior. Clinical correction of disturbed thinking can improve pathological mood and behavior, resulting in the remission of Axis I and II disorders. I view the cognitive, mood, sensory, and motor functions as elements of a unified field; intervention at any point in the field can affect other elements. It is not necessary to postulate linear causality with thoughts causing feelings in a simple unidirectional manner in order to do cognitive therapy; I assume the existence of numerous feedback loops and causal arrows in the psyche.

Thoughts can occur at one of two levels, which roughly correspond to implicit and explicit memory. They can be within conscious awareness, or function largely outside the sphere of the executive ego as automatic thoughts, schemas, or basic assumptions about the world. Although the word *dissociation* is not used in the cognitive therapy literature, the basic model implicit in cognitive therapy is one of dissociated cognition and modularity of mental function. It is the thoughts one isn't aware of thinking, the dissociated thoughts, which cause the clinical problems. The cognitive model lends itself naturally to a therapy focused on the thoughts of alter personalities; alter personalities are abnormally personified containers of schemas and cognitive errors.

A number of basic types of cognitive errors have been catalogued in the literature, and all occur frequently in patients with DID. These include *overgeneralization,* in which an accurate observation about one event or experience is overgeneralized and applied to life in general. The patient with DID who reports a male perpetrator of childhood sexual abuse often overgeneralizes her negative feelings about the perpetrator to all men. For instance, since Uncle Jim wore a blue baseball cap when he abused his niece, all men in blue baseball caps trigger abreactions in the adult survivor. More broadly, all men get perceived as rapists and liars.

Overgeneralization is closely linked to *dichotomized thinking,* also referred to as *black-and-white thinking* or *all-or-nothing thinking.* In psychodynamic vocabulary, the patient with DID often has a pervasive negative transference to most or all men, including her male psychiatrist. In cognitive terms, people are thought of as all good or all bad due to dichotomization of cognition, with the entire class of men being bad. This is a dissociation of cognition, but would be called *splitting* in psychodynamic theory.

Another common cognitive error in DID is *personalization,* which I will discuss in more detail below in terms of what I call the *locus of control shift.* In personalization, one attributes causality for events to oneself or takes them too personally, which is a form of attributional error. DID patients universally blame themselves for their childhood trauma.

Castastrophization is a cognitive error more characteristic of panic disorder than depression, and it involves activation of an alarm response in reaction to relatively minor environmental stimuli. When this happens to DID patients it is often called *triggering* or *spontaneous abreaction.*

I am illustrating the relationship between cognitive and other models of psychopathology in a cursory and simplistic manner to make the point that cognitive therapy principles are in many ways not much different from those of psychodynamic psychotherapy. The differences are often more a matter of vocabulary and accompanying theory than of the basic ideas involved. Very similar therapeutic interventions can be cast in the language of cognitive therapy or in more psychoanalytic terms.

Advantages of Cognitive Therapy Vocabulary in the 1990s

In the current managed-care environment, the vocabulary of cognitive therapy is much more palatable to reviewers than that of psychoanalysis. Insurers are less likely to certify treatment for the analysis of traumatic transference, and more likely to approve billings for the correction of trauma-related cognitive errors, although the treatments might be more similar than different. For this reason, it is better strategically to talk the language of cognitive-behavioral therapy, and to explicitly include the behavioral component, than to talk in psychoanalytic terms.

There are advantages to cognitive therapy vocabulary which are grounded in science. For instance, if one speaks of attributional errors rather than cathexis of negative introjects, one's clinical model is grounded in a large experimental social psychological literature. The existence of attributional errors and their effects on perception and behavior are well demonstrated, but there is no laboratory evidence of any kind for the existence of introjects or any other postulates of object relations theory.

Similarly, if one speaks of the inner world of the DID patient in psychoanalytic terms, one appears to hostile critics to be unscientific. The charge has been made that there is no scientific evidence for the reality of repression, and this then leads skeptics to the conclusion that the foundation of the psychotherapy of DID is unscientific and based on belief only. In fact, DID can be treated to stable integration in the language of cognitive therapy, and the theory of repression is an unnecessary postulate.

There is abundant scientific evidence for modularity of mental function, dissociated processing of sensory input, parallel processing of information, state-dependent learning, and related phenomena.[13,14] The entire edifice of psychoanalytic theory could disappear, and DID could still be a valid diagnosis treatable to stable integration. Therefore, in the current political climate, it is strategically advisable to ground one's clinical vocabulary in a broad base of social psychology, cognitive science, and developmental psychology.

Limitations of the Cognitive Model for Treatment of Trauma

The major trauma-related disgnoses in DSM-IV are DID, dissociative disorder not otherwise specified, posttraumatic stress disorder, acute stress disorder, and borderline personality disorder. All of these contain dissociative symptoms in their diagnostic criteria, and in fact, acute stress disorder and posttraumatic stress disorder can be diagnosed on the basis of a preponderance of dissociative symptoms by DSM-IV rules. Any treatment model for these disorders needs to take dissociation into account. Classical cognitive therapy does not do this explicitly.

DID is the extreme example of trauma-driven dissociation, therefore it best illustrates the limitations of the cognitive model for treating trauma victims. In the cognitive therapy of depression, an implicit assumption is made that the patient is inherently normal, except for her depressogenic cognitive errors and core beliefs. Once these are corrected, the depression remits, and treatment is over, except for perhaps some brief relapse prevention work. There is no need to consider any possible vacuum left by the dissappearance of the cognitive errors.

In patients with DID however, the cognitive errors serve defensive and systemic–strategic purposes. They are there for a reason. The errors cannot be removed, with nothing to take their place, because they are serving intrapsychic and interpersonal functions: they need to be transformed into healthier cognitions. Dissociative defenses and cognitive errors are over relied on in the DID patient, and there is a deficit in normal, adaptive defenses. The patient must unlearn excessive reliance on dissociation and learn a wide repertoire of new, more flexible coping strategies.

The strict cognitive models don't take the function of the cognitive errors into account. In discussing the cognitive therapy principles of my work, then, I am deliberately restricting my focus to what is one component of the treatment. This component is contained within the broader cognitive-systems trauma therapy.

Cognitive Therapy, Dissociative Identity Disorder, and the Theory of Repression

A current attack on the validity of the psychotherapy of DID is the argument that there is no scientific evidence for the reality of repression. Hostile skeptics state that since repression theory is wrong, recovered memories of childhood trauma must always be false: the mind cannot store traumatic memories in the way psotulated by repression theory, according to these skeptics.[15]

The first problem with this skeptical argument is that it is backwards. Freud originally proposed a trauma-dissociation theory[16] in which reasonably accurate dissociated memories of real childhood trauma were driving symptoms. He then repudiated the seduction theory and hypothesized that most of the remembered childhood sexual abuse never actually happened. In the next step in his intellectual development, Freud then developed a theory to explain why so many women were presenting to him with false memories of childhood sexual abuse. This was repression theory. Repression theory is designed to explain why the memories are false: it is when the memories are false that repression theory is true.

A second problem with the attack on repression theory as a way of proving that recovered memories are false is based on another failure in Freudian scholarship on the part of the skeptics. Repression is a mental mechanism postulated by Freud to explain how the mind deals with inner drives and wishes which cause conflict between the id and the ego. The assumption of repression theory is that repression is an intrapsychic mechanism focused on material emerging from deep in the inner world. It is not a mechanism for dealing with information coming into the mind from the environment. Repression is a fundamentally different psychological mechanism from trauma-driven dissociation, although the two words are widely used as synonyms.

A third problem with the skeptical attack on repression theory is that it assumes Freudian postulates about the nature of the unconscious. In psychonanalytical theory, the id works by *primary process* using magical thinking, symbolism, and other "irrational" processes. In contrast, the adult ego uses *secondary process* which involves rational cognition and adult mental functions. According to the skeptics, recovered memories are either always false, or they are more likely to be false because they have been *repressed*. According to psychoanalytical theory, this means that the memories are actually symbolic expressions of wishes and by definition, never happened. The skeptics, however, simultaneously talk about the *distortion* and *elaboration* of memories that occur during the period of repression, which then results in their being recovered in an inaccurate form. This could only occur if real memories had been repressed into the id and subjected to primary process there. The skeptical critcism is self-contradictory—it assumes both that the memories were never real, and that they are real but distorted.

The debate about repression and the accuracy of recovered memories is irrelevant to DID, because repression is not involved in its formation and no memories are recovered from the unconscious during its treatment. Herein lies the key difference between the trauma-dissociation theory of DID, and its cognitive therapy, and repression theory.

What one sees clinically in DID patients is dissociated modules of mental function which are abnormally personified, which take turns being in executive control, and which are capable of secondary process mental function. From the point of view of the alter personality that holds the memory, at a clinical phenomenological level, the traumatic memories have never been repressed and subjected to primary process in the id. They have been held in the ego of an alter personality, who never forgot them. The memories of the alter personalities, therefore, are not subject to the contaminating primary process of the id anymore than the incest memories of non-DID individuals which have never been "repressed."

The memories are dissociated packets of information about traumatic stimuli brought into the mind through the senses, not repressed drives expressed in symbolic form. A person with DID cannot be treated with "recovered memory therapy" because his or her traumatic memories have never been lost: they have been held in dissociated windows. The purpose of the therapy is not to "recover" the memories, but to erode the abnormal amnesia barriers between modules and to correct the cognitive errors arising from the trauma. In DID there are many sub-egos, all of whom hold memories in secondary process, and they are separated by varying amnesia barriers. The machinery that maintains these modules, identities, or personality states in abnormal dissociation from one another is an interlocking network of cognitive errors.

The scientific research bearing on the accuracy of traumatic memories held by alter personalities, the nature of alter personalities, and the mind's ability to maintain separation of modules and restrict information flow between them has nothing to do with psychoanalytical theories of repression. Even if one accepted that there is not scientific evidence for the reality of repression, this would be irrelevant to the question of whether DID is a valid diagnosis, or whether the memories processed during the cognitive therapy of DID are accurate.

The relevant literatures are those on hypnotic amnesia, traumatic amnesia, parallel processing, modularity of mental function, state-dependent learning, artificial intelligence, and the organization of complex systems. Anyone who has used a WINDOWS-based word processing program has experienced an analogue of DID, with dissociated subsystems holding discrete packets of information in a secondary process mode. If word processing programs can do this, why not the human brain?

It is an unanswered question whether the neuropsychological mechanisms of post-traumatic stress disorder, acute stress disorder, and borderline personality are akin to those of DID. My view is that DID is the extreme case and that these disorders are all closely interrelated. In trauma-related diagnoses other than DID, the dissociated information is held in windows that are less personified, and the cognitive error that these windows are separate people is absent.

DID and its treatment can be protected from the ideological hostility of extreme skeptics if proponents ground their vocabulary and theories in cognitive science and social psychology.

Behavioral Management of Dissociative Identity Disorder

Designing effective behavioral management strategies for DID inpatients is a subtle, challenging, and creative art, one grounded in scientific principles. The principles are less necessary on an outpatient basis, but still are used frequently. The behavioral component of cognitive-behavioral therapy is a key element of any specialty unit with reasonable lengths of stay and acute treatment outcomes. On our Dissociative Disorders Unit at Charter Behavioral Health System of Dallas, 56% of 103 patients with DID met structured interview criteria for borderline personality disorder. Many of our behavioral management strategies are the same as those used for borderlines without DID.[4]

The foundation of successful behavioral management of DID is a positive counter-transference, and this is the major element missing in most clinical settings where these patients are misdiagnosed. Inversely, there must be a relative absence of hostile countertransference. In object relations terms, the main source of staff burnout is the effort required to deal with the massive doses of hostile projective identification inflicted by the patients.

The major behavioral management strategy we have in place at Charter Behavioral Health of Dallas is transferring patients to another floor if their behavior falls below tolerable levels in terms of acting out and disruptiveness. Institution of this measure on our unit resulted in a two-thirds reduction in nursing incidents for 9 months of observation compared with a baseline of 4 months of observation, and this difference was highly statistically significant using a t test. The threat of transfer off the Dissociative Disorders Unit only works because the Unit is highly valued by the patients.

On an outpatient basis, one must be prepared to terminate a session, terminate therapy, or set whatever other limits are necessary to maintain a healthy treatment frame. It is essential not to be bribed and manipulated by self-mutilation.

An example will illustrate the required flexibility in behavioral strategies. A patient who had abused her children through complex Munchausen's-by-proxy behaviors was also highly sadistic towards her own skin in the form of cutting and burning herself with cigarettes. She stated that she had physically harmed her children, some of whom had died, in order to make them undesirable for a Satanic cult, and was superficially cutting herself. The patient believed that she had grown up in a multigenerational orthodox Satanic cult, and that she was still being harassed by cult members who had a detailed knowledge of her personality system. I assumed that the Satanic ritual abuse was not real because of its inherent implausibility, the lack of evidence that organized Satanic human sacrifice has ever occurred anywhere in North America, the apparent defensive function of the belief, and the extreme nature of many of the details she reported.

According to medical records, the children were treated for seizures, fevers of unknown origin, frequent infections of lungs, bowels, and bladder, unexplained somnolence, and unexplained toxic blood levels of medication. No definitive biomedical explanation for these symptoms was ever obtained. It was not possible to tell for sure whether the children had died from Munchausen's-by-proxy overdoses, as some of the patient's alters claimed, or complications of actual neurological illnesses. Although there were definite brain abnormalities on post-mortem examination, these could have been long-term complications of the Munchausen's-by-proxy or independent disorders.

It was not possible to challenge the woman's belief about the Satanic cult directly because the risk of completed suicide was too high should the belief be dismantled precipitously. The belief that she had abused her children to protect them from a cult was a defense against accepting responsibility for her Munchausen's-by-proxy behavior, and against dealing with her guilt and remorse. According to her distorted cognitions, she was abusing the children in order to protect them from the cult, and therefore the Munchausen's-by-proxy was proof that she was a good mother.

While the host personality was working on accepting the reality of the Munchausen's-by-proxy abuse that she had perpetrated, which was supported by the medical records I obtained and reviewed with her, she was also self-mutilating as a key Satanic holiday approached. Her behavior included scratching her arms hard enough to draw blood and leave large scabs, and burning them with cigarettes. The persecutor alter personalities in her system believed that the host should be punished for not returning to the cult. The function of the persecutors, who were actually disguised protectors, was to protect the host personality by reinforcing her belief in the reality of the cult.

The question was how to intervene behaviorally, given the patient's conflicted desire to avoid responsibility for the Munchausen's-by-proxy and simultaneously punish herself for abusing her children. The self-mutilation was functioning both as punishment for the Munchausen's-by-proxy and as a defense against it. Sending her to the other floor would be perceived as a reward by the aspects of herself that wanted to avoid the guilt for the Munchausen's-by-proxy, and also by the parts that wanted to punish her for it. On the other floor the host personality would be able to avoid any real therapeutic work, but could feel guilty for being bad enough to be banished from the Dissociative Disorders Unit. The cognitive error that the reason for transfer was the recent bad behavior of the host gave her an explanation for her guilty feelings: in psychoanalytical terms, the cognitive error permitted a displacement of guilt from the Munchausen's-by-proxy to recent behavior by the host personality.

I held the strategy of transfer to another program in abeyance and attempted to ride out the remaining days till the Satanic holiday was past, using increased doses of benzodiazepine, which I tapered back down immediately after the holdiay. My behavioral strategy was to use *extinction* as the primary behavioral intervention. Focusing on the self-mutilation, I decided to try to ignore the convoluted psychodynamics and cognitive errors.

When the patient showed me or the nurses her wounds, we did not particularly react to them. This strategy became intolerable because the amount and degree of self-injury was too great. I therefore transferred the patient to another floor. While a nurse was explaining the transfer order I had given by telephone, the patient seriously assaulted the nurse. The next day I discharged her. The discharge could be understood as *negative reinforcement*. What I did was reward the patient with removal of the noxious stimulus of intolerable therapy when she displayed the desired behavior of asking to be discharged. My prediction was that the undesired behavior, the self-mutilation, would quickly extinguish once the noxious stimulus was removed. The treatment for the self-mutilation was to stop treatment.

It might appear incomprehensible from a conventional point of view to discharge a patient because she was self-mutilating. From a behavioral point of view, this measure made perfect sense, even though self-mutilation was also the reason for admission. At the time of admission, the reinforcers were different because the alters who wanted the host personality to deal with the Munchausen's-by-proxy abuse of her children wanted the host to meet inpatient criteria so she would be compelled to listen to them, which they achieved through cutting. The persecutors were punishing the host for not listening, but also believed that the Satanic cult was real, therefore they were being destabilized by the approaching cult holiday. As the host personality began to glimpse the reality of having abused her children through Munchausen's-by-proxy, the balance in the system shifted towards host denial, with discharge and avoidance of therapy functioning as rewards.

A complicating factor in the case was a body-image distortion in which the patient showed me fresh cigarette burns which she claimed she had inflicted the night before, but which were clearly many days old. This meant that the behavioral analysis had to take into account both actual and delusional self-mutilation. The body image distortion was probably being deliberately inflicted by the persecutors to increase the degree of intimidation of the host personality. The patient's effort was to defend against what appeared to be real Munchausen's-by-proxy with a delusion of Satanic ritual abuse, self-mutilation to force discharge, and delusional amplification of the self-mutilation. The woman was not psychotic and a trial of antipsychotic medications was not warranted.

The subtlety of behavioral analysis required in treating DID is driven by the ambivalence of the patients. Too often, setting limits and instituting behavioral management involves staff identifying with and reinforcing one side of the patient's ambivalence, which leads to temporary stabilization but inevitable relapse when the staff reinforcement disappears post-discharge.

In other situations, identification with one side of the patient's ambivalence can be countertherapeutic even in the short term. Telling this patient that her alters and their claims of Satanism were not real, through staff identification with one side of her ambivalence, could have been rationalized as not feeding into Satanic ritual abuse hysteria. The problem was that the Munchausen's-by-proxy appeared to be real, as did the highly convoluted pathological grief experienced by the host personality during the many years since her children had died. Telling her that the cult was not real might have overwhelmed her defenses and escalated the self-mutilation.

The view that DID can be treated solely by benign neglect, on the grounds that it is an iatrogenic artifact that will remit through the behavioral strategy of extinction alone, is wrong because it is simple-minded. It was possible that the DID of the woman who abused her children through Munchausen's-by-proxy was a mixture of factitious and iatrogenic elements, and that it had not existed prior to contact with a previous therapist. Even if that was the case, however, simple extinction as the primary or sole treatment plan could never have worked at this stage of her illness.

Although it is true that extinction is a useful behavioral strategy in the treatment of DID, no adequate behavioral analysis could ever result in a treatment plan relying exclusively on one set of reinforcers or one behavioral principle. The idea that extinction alone represents an adequate treatment plan for DID is proven in the minds of skeptics by tautology, based on the initial assumption that the disorder is always an iatrogenic artifact. This tautology is not supported by any systematic treatment outcome data, and therefore is an untested hypothesis. Clinically, it does not make sense from psychoanalytic, cognitive, or behavioral perspectives.

The Problem of Attachment to the Perpetrator

DID can be understood as fundamentally a disorder of attachment driven by the problem of attachment to the perpetrator. This perspective is rooted in a vast literature on mammalian attachment, learned helplessness, disturbed attachments of traumatized young monkeys, and other related literatures.[17,18] As Jennifer Freyd[19] has pointed out, the main driver of traumatic amnesia in children who are victims of incest might not be a need to defend against traumatic affect. Rather, it might be the attachment to the perpetrator.

In cognitive therapy group, which I do three times a week on our Dissociative Disorders Unit, I often explain this problem to the patients in the following way.

Case Study

What you've just said is an example of the problem of attachment to the perpetrator. Let me explain what I mean by that. When you were 4 or 5 or 6 years old, there were two things you had no control over, and no choice about. One was that you were being abused. You couldn't make the abuse stop, and you couldn't get married and move out of the house, run away to live on the street, or go away to college because you were just a little girl. You were stuck in the home. In reality you were a small, defenseless girl who did not have the power to control her abuser.

There was another reality you had no choice about or control over. This was the fact that you were attached to your perpetrator, your father, for three reasons. First, you were attached to him biologically, just like all mammals attach to their parents, including little foxes, rabbits, lions, and human beings. This attachment was built into your body by evolution. The second kind of attachment was caused by the fact that you depended on your father for food, clothing, a roof over your head, and all the everyday things you needed to survive. You could not survive on your own, and if you tried to separate from your perpetrator at this age you would have faced a huge, overwhelming, frightening world as a very lonely, scared little girl. This was impossible to do.

The third thing that kept you attached to your perpetrator was the emotional reality of your family, and the fact that you are a human being. You didn't have any choice about this either. As a human being you had to want love, attention, and approval from your parents very deeply, whether you got it or not. And since you were starved for normal love, you made do with whatever you could get, which some of the time was the incest. Therefore, you became attached to the incest and the perpetrator. The attention and affection you received during the sexual abuse, including any sexual pleasure your body may have experienced, reinforced this attachment.

If you did get any pleasure from the abuse, this doesn't prove that you wanted to be abused. What you wanted was what every child wants, simply to be loved and to grow up in a healthy family. If your body reacted the way normal bodies do to sexual stimulation, this doesn't prove that what you wanted in life was to be a victim of incest. No child is born into the world wanting to be an incest victim.

The problem you are describing today is based on this attachment to the perpetrator. You are looking at present-day reality from the emotional perspective of an abused child who is trapped in her reality, and you are afraid to separate from your current abuser based on the actual reality of the past. The problem is that this is not the reality of the present. In fact, in the present your body is 30 years old, you have a master's degree, you have many skills and abilities that you didn't have at age 6, you have social supports and a therapist at home, and you can now detach from your perpetrator and survive.

You need to take care of the little ones inside who don't realize it is 1995. They are reacting with an emergency response to the reality of the present as if it were the reality of the past: the past really was an emotional emergency from which there was no escape.

If your child alters could realize that they are in a 30-year-old body in 1995, and the abuse happened in another state over 20 years ago, they would feel much safer and you would have far fewer symptoms. You can teach them this, and provide them the TLC you missed out on as a child. That's the kind of work we do here, and many people get an amazing amount of work done while they are in our program.

The problem of attachment to the perpetrator manifests itself in numerous ways in the transference triad of childhood relationships, therapeutic transference, and current relationships outside therapy. It can be analyzed and treated in terms of dichotimized thinking and other cognitive errors: the only options are to be attached and abused or intolerably lonely and separate, in the patient's mind. The treatment can be framed in terms of separation/individuation conflicts which are part of the normal life work of all of us. It is clear to everyone that a basic mammalian developmental task is separation from parents. DID patients are often either rigidly separated in an unhealthy way that in psychoanalytical terms would be called *reaction formation,* or are obviously pathologically enmeshed.

The primary purpose of the traumatic amnesia, from this perspective, is not to reduce conflict about affect, but to help the organism maintain its biologically encoded and developmentally protective attachment to a parent who is also an abuse perpetrator. The brain modules responsible for attachment must not be contaminated by experiential input that would threaten to deactivate them, because this would lead to failure to thrive. The solution to this conflict, from the brain's point of view, is to interrupt the flow of information from the modules processing the traumatic events to those responsible for attachment behavior. It is as if, at an emotional level, the child has to be amnesic for intermittent food poisoning in order not to starve herself to death.

The unique feature of DID is that these different modules are abnormally personified and can take turns being in executive control, while maintaining the necessary amnesia barriers. This property of DID is also what makes it treatable, and its treatment rational and highly structured: the different modules and their cognitive errors can be accessed directly, and all are capable of secondary process cognition. The child alters can learn that it is 1995 and they are in an adult body more quickly than someone would who had been in a coma for 20 years. This is because they are housed in a brain which has undergone adult psychological development and can tap into more mature developmental skills quite readily.

The Locus of Control Shift

The second key element I practice in the cognitive therapy of DID is what I call the *locus of control shift.* It is directly related to the problem of attachment to the perpetrator, and it is imbedded in large literatures on internal versus external locus of control, attribution theory, and other social psychological concepts with empirical validation.

In cognitive therapy group I explain the locus of control shift as follows.

Case Study

In your childhood you had a problem which couldn't be dealt with by using dissociation. You could use dissociation effectively to block out the memory of part of a particular day when something bad happened. But there was a more pervasive problem you had that was with you all the time, and that couldn't be solved by blocking out any one event. This was the fact that you were trapped in the situation. You couldn't get the abuse to stop, and if you told anyone about it, you wouldn't be believed and would be abused more. Therefore the only escape was in your mind.

A problem you had to face every day in your childhood, but couldn't do anything about, was the fact that you were overwhelmed, helpless, and powerless to do anything about the abuse. You lived in an unpredictable world of arbitrary violence. You were a frightened, lonely, abused little girl who couldn't change her world.

What you did to solve this problem is what I call the *locus of control shift*. You took the qualities that were in fact in the perpetrator, and shifted them inside yourself. This was a smart and strategic thing to do, and it helped you survive. You took the badness, control, power, and mastery that were in the perpetrator and shifted them inside yourself. Now, instead of being small and overwhelmed, you were in control and calling the shots. You were big and strong like the perpetrator.

The locus of control shift created an illusion in your mind that you were causing the abuse and in control of it. This wasn't actually true, but it worked for you emotionally nevertheless. Now you weren't so overwhelmed and frightened because you were big and bad too. This is also called *identification with the aggressor*. Interrogators around the world work on their victims systematically to try to get them to identify with the aggressor. When this happens, the political prisoner feels like the interrogator is his friend, and his friends are his enemies. He then provides the interrogator with information about the members of his underground political group.

The locus of control shift involves magical thinking that is developmentally normal for a young child. Young children tend to see themselves as being at the center of things and causing things to happen when really the cause lies outside them. An example is the child who thinks her parents divorced because she didn't keep her room tidy enough. Also, children have a magical sense of causality. So it was normal for you to think that you were causing the abuse and controlling the perpetrator. Sometimes the perpetrator says things to reinforce this belief in the child victim.

Why was it smart to blame yourself for the abuse? Because this actually worked to protect you emotionally from the overwhelming feeling of helplessness, betrayal, and powerlessness. Although the locus of control shift is an illusion, and not actually true, it actually works to protect you emotionally. Because abuse causes children to have bad feelings, the bad feelings reinforced and proved your belief that you were bad. It was good to be bad, because then you could be powerful, strong, and in control. The cost of this strategy was that you had to believe and feel that you were bad, and you carry that belief with you today. Those feelings of badness were a heavy price to pay for an illusion of power, but what else could you do? You were only a little girl.

What you need to understand is that the parts inside who are telling you that you are bad are actually protectors, not enemies. The voices you hear saying bad things about you are working hard to keep the locus of control shift in place, which is good. The problem is that outside reality has changed. Although it was an excellent strategy to believe you were bad and causing the abuse as a child, now as an adult, that belief is interfering with your function. It isn't necessary to be bad to be strong anymore, and it was never actually true that you were bad; that was just the magical thinking of a child's mind trying to protect itself. The belief that you are bad and to blame isn't working for you anymore, and your skin is paying a heavy price for it, in the form of cutting and burning. Really, your skin has already had far more abuse then it ever deserved, and in fact, it never deserved any abuse at all.

In family systems terms this would be described as a *paradoxical intervention* because the patient is being defined as strong and smart for believing that she is weak, bad, and stupid, which most DID patients do. The cognitive therapy of DID resembles dialectical behavior therapy of borderline personality disorder[4] in its use of this range of interventions.

The most frequent response of DID patients to my explanation of the locus of control shift in cognitive therapy group is amazement that it is so simple and makes so much sense. The format of the group is rotating individual cognitive therapy with group feedback, and the patient to whom I am directly explaining the shift in terms of her own life content may cry deeply during the session. Discussion of attachment to the perpetrator and the locus of control shift results in therapy moving off of Satanic ritual abuse themes, as I describe in more detail in my book *Satanic Ritual Abuse. Principles of Treatment.*[10]

The locus of control shift underlies the formation of *paternal introject alters,* a common form of persecutor personality with whom it is essential to form a treatment alliance.[5,20] These alters are understood by themselves and the host personality as literal psychic intrusions of the father's identity into the inner world of the patient. The formation of a treatment alliance with these parts involves correction of the pathognomonic DID cognitive error that different aspects of the self are different selves.

Orientation of Alters to the Present and the Body

Almost without exception, alter personalities directly involved in the presenting symptoms that justify inpatient admission do not realize it is 1996 or that they live in the same body as the host personality. Since writing my 1989 text,[5] I have shifted further away from abreactive work and more into cognitive-behavioral interventions. Since arriving in Texas in 1991, I have treated patients to integration without a single full abreaction occurring in my office. I am referring to abreactions in which the patient is lost in the past, fully reliving a trauma, and mistaking me for a figure from the past. Such abreaction does not appear to be necessary for full recovery, and it is usually destabilizing and regressive.

Before, I would have been more inclined to seek out and abreact a specific traumatic event driving the current symptom, and I did observe remission of specific symptoms with this method, which I never used more than sparingly. Now, however, I go straight to orienting the alters to present reality, and regard the symptoms as an artifact of the alters' cognitive errors. These changes in practice are all a matter of degree and emphasis, and do not represent dichotomized shifts from bad to good techniques.

If a triggering event in the present was in fact evidence of impending paternal rape, then an alarm response would be realistic and accurate. In present reality, however, a man wearing a blue baseball cap is not necessarily a rapist, despite the fact that the incestuous uncle wore such a cap. This is an example of overgeneralization and it can be treated with a cognitive and psychoeducational approach. One element of the intervention is to have the triggered child alter assume executive control, following which I explain that it is 1996, and uncle Jim is far away in both space and time.

A second element is to assign protector alters the job of soothing, orienting, and protecting the children internally on an ongoing basis. Elaborate guided imagery exercises for building safe places are not necessary to achieve this goal. The third element is to foster co-consciousness and interpersonality communication and cooperation. This helps the child alters learn from ongoing experience and maintain their grounding in the present.

Sometimes, from the viewpoint of the child alter personality, there is no overgeneralization taking place. This is because the child alter holds only a narrow range of experience involving interaction with perpetrators and has no experiential evidence available that there are nonabusive men in the world. I work with these alters in a mode of *collaborative empiricism,* and test their contention that it is 1965 by having them look at their adult body, look out the window, read the newspaper, and watch TV. All of those things can be done in session and between sessions through co-consciousness with the adult alters. The child alter can access a broad store of disconfirmatory experience by becoming aware of the experience base of the adult alters.

I have found that when the alters that are doing the cutting and burning really grasp the fact that they are in the same body, it is not long before the cutting stops. The best way to do this is to have them examine their arms while in executive control and try to explain how they got into the room, why they have the host's clothes on, and where the host is currently. This is particularly effective with adolescent male alters who are disturbed to find that they are in a female body with long hair, breasts, earrings, and a dress. Ordinarily, the belief that one is a male with male genitalia would be a delusion and a symptom of psychosis if stated by a biological female, but in DID it is a cognitive error that responds well to psychotherapy.

There are a number of reasons why the cognitive therapy of DID takes much longer than the cognitive therapy of depression and averages 3–5 years instead of 10–20 sessions. One reason is the complexity and quantity of psychopathology involved in DID, along with its extensive comorbidity. Another is the large amount of learning of new skills and unlearning of maladaptive defenses required in the cognitive therapy of DID, compared with the cognitive therapy of depression. Additionally, the network of cognitive errors in DID is much more intricate than that in major depressive disorder. The cognitive errors of a major depressive episode are a subset of those in DID.

To oversimplify, one can say that when the depressogenic cognitive errors are corrected in a classical Beckian therapy, the patient walks away cured and armed with relapse prevention strategies. In DID, this does not occur because of the massive amount of new skills that have to be acquired to replace the cognitive errors. The generic depressed patient treated successfully with classical Beckian cognitive therapy is assumed to be an intact competent adult, but this is not true for patients with DID, who are impaired across a wide range of functions. Put another way, there is much more wrong with DID patients than just their DID.

In DID, the cognitive errors have systemic and intrapsychic functions which must be taken into account in planning the therapy.

Conclusion

The purpose of this chapter has been to provide an overview of the cognitive principles and techniques of the therapy of DID, and to illustrate some of the key principles. The content of the traumatic memories is not a primary target in this method of treatment, and the same interventions are used whether the memories appear to be accurate or confabulated. This is because the targets of therapy are the problem of attachment to the perpetrator, the locus of control shift, the cognitive errors, and the lack of communication, cooperation, and free information flow in the system—not the content of the memories.

The clinical problem requiring solution is the blockage in information flow, not the content of the information as such. Within the model I have outlined, the purpose of the amnesia barriers and abnormal personification of parts of the self in DID is not primarily to protect the self against affect or the information component of memory. The amnesia is designed more to serve strategic social psychological purposes and to keep modules responsible for attachment uncontaminated by traumatic information.

The basic problem being managed by DID amnesia is attachment to and separation/individuation from the perpetrator, a task we all accomplish with some degree of denial and dissociation, even when our parents were never abusive. The problem of attachment to the perpetrator exists in a muted form in all of us, since we all have ambivalent feelings about imperfect parents. Most of us do not have full DID because our minds did not develop in an emergency alert mode during traumatic childhoods. If they had, we, too, might have DID and might require amnesia barriers to maintain our attachments.

Current concerns abour repression theory and recovered memory therapy are not relevant to the cognitive therapy of DID, nor are the criticisms directed at psychotherapies in which abreaction, guided imagery, hypnosis, and memory recovery predominate. The information content of traumatic memories is not the target of DID cognitive therapy, just as the specific content of a simple phobia does not determine the structure of its systematic desensitization. Much of the cognitive therapy of DID can be understood as a systematic desensitization, with the phobic stimuli being dissociated and internal.

In terms of the larger debate about the accuracy of recovered memory, the purpose of this chapter has been to argue that DID and its treatment do not require an adherence to repression theory. Neither the diagnosis nor its treatment depend on any psychoanalytical postulates, and both can be grounded in extensive literatures about traumatic mammalian attachment, information processing in the brain, hypnotic amnesia, developmental psychology, and social psychology. There are psychoanalytical theories of depression, psychosis, DID, panic disorder, and fetishism: all of these can be valid and reliable diagnoses with specific effective treatments, even if psychoanalytical theory is rejected.

DID cannot be treated with pure cognitive therapy alone because it is too complex; its treatment requires a blend of cognitive, systems, and psychodynamic principles. If a given memory of paternal incest is judged to be confabulated, then the memory is a symbol of ambivalent attachment to that parent, and the target of therapy remains the ambivalent attachment. In many cases, no definitive proof of the reality of the childhood trauma is available, even with reasonable efforts at collateral history taking, nor is there definitive proof that the incest did not take place. Denial by the alleged perpetrator is not decisive one way or the other, since both falsely and justifiably accused perpetrators can be expected to deny the accusations. The solution to this uncertainty is to design one's treatment model and interventions such that they are the same no matter what the accuracy of the memories. In cases in which definitive proof is available one way or the other, the target of therapy is still the ambivalent attachment.

References

1. Beck AT, Rush AJ, Shaw BF, Emery G: Cognitive Therapy of Depression. New York: Guilford Press, 1979.
2. Beck AT, Emery G: Anxiety Disorders and Phobias: A Cognitive Perspective. New York: Basic Books, 1985.
3. Beck AT, Freeman A: Cognitive Therapy of Personality Disorders. New York: Guilford Press, 1990.
4. Linehan MM: Cognitive-Behavioral Treatment of Borderline Personality Disorder. New York: Guilford Press, 1993.
5. Ross CA: Multiple Personality Disorder: Disorder: Diagnosis, Clinical Features, and Treatment. New York: John Wiley & Sons, 1989.
6. Freeman A: Cognitive Therapy With Couples and Groups. New York: Plenum Press, 1983.
7. Rush AJ, Altshuler K: Depression. Basic Mechanisms, Diagnosis, and Treatment. New York: Guilford Press, 1986.
8. Ross CA, Gahan P: Cognitive analysis of multiple personality disorder. Am J Psychother, 1988; 42:229–239.

9. Ross CA: The Osiris Complex: Case Studies Studies in Multiple Personality Disorder. Toronto: University of Toronto Press, 1994.

10. Ross CA: Satanic Ritual Abuse: Principles of Treatment. Toronto: University of Toronto Press, 1995.

11. Fine CG: Thoughts on the cognitive perceptual substrates of multiple personality disorder. Dissociation 1988; 1:5–10.

12. Fine C: The cognitive sequelae of incest. *In* R Kluft (Ed.) Incest-Related Syndromes of Adult Psychopathology. Washington, DC: American Psychiatric Press, 1990, pp. 161–182.

13. Hilgard ER: Divided Consciousness: Multiple Controls in Human Thought and Action. New York: John Wiley & Sons, 1977.

14. Ornstein R: Multimind. Boston: Houghton Mifflin, 1986.

15. Ofshe R, Watters E. Making Monsters: False Memories, Psychotherapy, and Sexual Hysteria. New York: Scribner's, 1994.

16. Breuer J, Freud S: Studies on Hysteria. New York: Pelican Books, 1986. (Original work published in 1895).

17. van der Kolk BA: Psychological Trauma. Washington, DC: American Psychiatric Press, 1987.

18. Barach P: Multiple personality disorder as an attachment disorder. Dissociation 1991; 4:117–123.

19. Freyd J: Theoretical and personal perspectives on the delayed memory debate. Paper presented at Controversies Around Recovered Memories of Incest and Sexual Abuse, A Continuing Education Conference for Mental Health Professionals, Ann Arbor, MI, August 1993.

20. Putnam FW: Diagnosis and Treatment of Multiple Personality Disorder. New York: Guilford Press, 1989.

16

Memories of Trauma in the Treatment of Children

MARIA C. SAUZIER

Trauma, our capacity to forget and our ability to remember, has long been a leitmotif in psychiatry, as well as being of interest to anyone attempting to understand human nature. Childhood trauma, and particularly sexual abuse, has been the focus of controversy for well over 100 years. In 1860, Ambroise Tardieu, a forensic pathologist, described the effects of sexual abuse, torture, and murder on the child bodies he had studied in the Paris morgue. His textbook became a medical sensation, was reprinted three times—and then disappeared.[1] In 1896, Sigmund Freud told his Viennese colleagues that he had discovered sexual abuse to be the root of hysteria.[2] He was met with cold rebuke and the threat of losing all credibility and academic standing. When fact became fantasy, in the Oedipus conflict, Viennese society sighed with relief—except for Sandor Ferenczi. In 1933, Ferenczi's paper about incest, "Confusion of Tongues Between Adults and the Child," was met with more than just stony silence. It was literally destroyed: not only the paper but the printing plate disappeared. An English translation escaped, which allowed a reprinting in 1949.[3] In the early 1950s, Kinsey and his colleagues found that 24% of white, middle-class married women reported childhood sexual abuse and were still upset by it. This finding was downplayed, as it ran counter to Kinsey's agenda of liberating contemporary Americans from the shackles of Victorian prudery and hypocrisy.[4]

In the 1960s and 1970s, health professionals and child advocates mobilized around physical child abuse, beginning the Child Protection Movement.[5] Starting in the late 1970s, a new coalition of child advocates and feminists focused on the sexual abuse of children. The issue drew media attention, mobilized public support, and at first, remained relatively uncontested. Controversy erupted in the late 1980s, when the child abuse issue was shifted into the legal arena. Mandated reporting of serious abuse and particularly of incest to district attorneys led to an increased threat of potential prosecution. VOCAL (Victims of Child Abuse Laws) accused Child Protective Services and district attorneys of interfering in family life. Other legislative changes, particularly the extension of the statute of limitations, which allow prosecution that is based on newly remembered data, gave victims the possibility to sue in adulthood. This potential shift in the balance of legal power between victim and alleged victimizer was reacted to by the formation of the False Memory Syndrome Foundation.[6]

Seen from a historical perspective, our society seems to have come to a point where the occurrence of child sexual abuse has been accepted. Yet there is still a discrepancy between the theoretical "yes it happens" and the practical "but not in this case."

Currently, the issue of "repressed memory" vs. "false memory" has led to considerable controversy in the psychiatric literature on adults. The impact of this controversy on individual patients, families, and therapists whose lives have become public case illustrations, examined in the courts and the media, has been disturbing. The impact on scientific inquiry and on psychiatric practice parameters has the potential for being most useful by promoting the integration of new findings in biology,[7-9] memory,[10-13] early development,[14,15] and trauma.[16-18]

In child psychiatry, trauma theory has not been well integrated. In the literature, there is still a dichotomy between general child psychiatry and the writings of sexual abuse and trauma experts who describe specialized evaluation and intervention techniques.[19-22] This separation is also found in most training programs where learning about trauma is relegated to a rotation on a specialized trauma unit and is not well integrated into the main training setting.

Furthermore, in practice, children seem to be triaged a priori into those referred to specialized trauma clinics, and those sent to generalists, child clinicians who have neither a focus on, nor any particular training in the detection of abuse and trauma. In specialized clinics, children are evaluated by clinicians trained in utilizing a methodology which is constantly evolving in response to new data and scrutiny. This requires focused attention to the alleged events, as well as a broad look at all aspects of the child's life, and leads to the generation of several hypotheses that need to be considered in order to best understand the child's presentation.

For the generalist, however, there is no equivalent body of literature to help her identify what, in the course of an evaluation or therapy with a child, should raise the index of suspicion sufficiently to warrant a different approach, a switch from play therapy to a more focused inquiry, or even a consultation with or referral to a trauma expert. More specifically, there is no literature that this author is aware of that addresses the issue of unsuspected abuse or trauma memories emerging in the course of therapy with a child or young adolescent.

This chapter will focus on children whose presentation in the course of ongoing treatment led to the questioning of whether unsuspected early trauma had to be considered and explored. These situations raise issues on many levels. The encoding and retrieval of memory, nontraumatic or traumatic, is the focus of Chapters 4, 6, and 11 in this volume. Here, only clinically relevant observations and questions will be addressed as they pertain to the presentation of the 6-, 10- and 16-year-old patients described below. These kinds of cases also raise questions of technique, such as how to handle the sense of emergency in the therapist; how and when to involve the parents; when to involve Child Protective Services; whether and how to change the therapist–patient interaction to a more directive, evaluative one; or when and whether to request a consultation or make a referral to a trauma expert. The goal of this chapter is to offer a point of view integrating dynamic child psychiatry and trauma-focused approaches.

The cases described here have been significantly altered and do not correspond to any one identifiable case.

Case 1

Andy is a 6-year-old boy who is referred because he is "hyperactive" in his kindergarten class. He is repeating this grade because of his social and academic immaturity. His parents are appropriately concerned and come to the evaluation with the request for treatment, as a trial of psychostimulant medication had not been effective. Andy's 3-and-a-half-year-old sister Ally is seen as developing normally.

Pertinent history to this case includes the maternal stepgrandfather, who had joined the family late in life and was an important father figure and babysitter. He died suddenly when the patient was 20 months old. Andy's mother was subsequently sad, preoccupied, and at times physically absent while settling her ill mother into a nursing home.

During his sessions with me, Andy is a very active boy who likes to move around, throwing dart balls and playing loud games. He also plays with puppets and animals, but not long enough to develop a story line. Only the make-your-own-puppet kit engages his repeated and somewhat prolonged interest, and soon becomes part of a weekly ritual: on a Velcro head, he attaches various pieces, creating a great variety of noses surrounded by furry parts.

After several weeks of meetings, Andy's mother reports an incident that upset everyone. As they were talking about grandfather, she brought out a family photo album. Ally pointed to a picture of the grandfather, commenting that he is "all bald and smooth." Andy disagreed vehemently, saying grandfather was *not* bald, and started crying, then screaming, which turned into a temper tantrum. He was put in his room and soon fell asleep. His mother also reports that he has become inseparable from his favorite teddy, now brought to therapy. Andy says that Joe, the bear, used to have stiff hair, but that he has always loved the soft velvety paws best. In the next hour, he is distressed about having forgotten Joe at home. He makes a puppet and buries his face in its fuzzy cheeks. He seems distraught. The therapist mentions separation and loss (from the bear, but implying grandfather's death and mother's absences). Andy cries, quietly sucking his thumb before wildly dashing about the room. At home, his parents wonder whether he is masturbating more openly. They see him as battling against his sad feelings which he has called "babyish."

A new play activity with clay emerges in treatment. The sequence seems quite stereotyped: a ball of clay, digging holes into it with his fingers, and rolling it into a cigar or snake shape. A later variation of the clay play involves sticking the tops of magic markers into the clay, smoothing clay over them, and tricking the therapist into believing it is soft instead of hard. Sometimes Andy adds fuzzy balls or feathers and tickles his own cheek. Once, when he accidentally pokes himself, he seems surprised, gets very excited and cries "grandfather did have hair and he had a beard too." He seems to be rubbing himself against the back of the small chair and looks dazed before dashing about the room, making incoherent grunting noises. As it is time to go, his mother needs to come in to help him leave. She says that she has heard the grunting noises before, when Andy gets overexcited.

An update on Andy's history, with his parents, focuses on his normal to precocious development until his grandfather died, after which he spent more time with adequate, but in his parents' eyes, less stimulating babysitters. Andy always seemed very excited to see his grandfather. He was usually asleep when his parents came back, even if it was not his nap time. They remember laughing about how he wore himself out with excitement. They cannot understand why Andy insists that his grandfather had hair and a beard, and refuses to look at pictures confirming the opposite. Andy seems to be getting increasingly distressed, waking up with amorphous bad dreams, acting more clinging as well as restless and angry, especially at bedtime.

This presentation raises a variety of complex questions of a theoretical nature as well as a practical one. Why does Andy appear agitated when remembering his step-grandfather? What is Andy saying, in words and in play? Is it something based on fact, or fantasy, or impulse? Is it a combination of fantasy, metaphor and actual experience? How important is it to know the difference? How can one ever gain access to what has shaped his memory so early in his life? How should parents and the therapist react in the face of such uncertainty? Whose need to know drives the exploration: the child's (as measured by his distress), the parents' (because of their distress, or their own histories), or the therapist's (because he is eager to help, or because he has a particular bias)?

Andy seems to be grappling with something unsettling, triggered by reminiscing about his stepgrandfather's physical appearance. His vehement contradiction of his sister's description of the man in the picture shattered what had been a cozy family time, with him sitting on his father's lap, and Ally on his mother's. State-dependent retrieval of memories is particularly important in young children. Sexual abuse disclosures often surface accidentally, in the context of being bathed, or diapered, or having a seemingly unrelated conversation.[23,24] The young child may be unaware of the importance of the information shared, and become confused and upset by the emotions elicited in his caregivers. In other cases, the child's accidental disclosure may run counter to his wish to hide the abusive experience—because he has been bribed to do so, or told to expect punishment. In both situations, the child's momentary disclosure may be followed by normal or distressed behavior, without further verbal divulging, or the child may even insist on retracting the statements made.

In Andy's case, his intense statement was met with incomprehension. There was no empathic connection, no affective support for his contradicting what the image showed, or for his intense emotions. Everyone was taken by surprise. His reaction became a behavior problem (temper tantrum) leading to isolation (time-out). Falling asleep followed, preventing the short discussion with which his parents usually ended his time-out.

The typical memory talk that families with young children engage in often follows the meanderings of the child's associations, with older siblings and adults making additions and corrections.[25] What evolves is a family narrative that gets rehearsed every time the story is told, and is more likely to remain retrievable as a declarative (verbal) memory as the child grows older. The child's own nonverbal implicit memories may remain disconnected from this co-constructed narrative, which can never capture the complexity of the real experience of each individual participant. The child's own implicit, emotional, somatic, and behavioral memories may not fit (even if the child gives clues, they may be overlooked), or they may be unavailable (the child gives no clues). In these cases, the child may be left with a discrepancy between his verbally retrievable recollections of his early years and the implicit memories which will guide some of his deepest views and feelings throughout life, including transference. While minor discrepancies are unavoidable, major disjunctions between verbal and nonverbal memories affect the child's growing sense of self, and may lead to psychopathology.

In childhood, implicit memory colors the child's play. If the play is repetitive or disruptive, and thus gets special attention, it may be possible to help the child translate the meaning of his play into more conscious information that can be shared verbally.[26] This is most likely to happen in play therapy, where the goal is to help the child make sense of his inner life, his impulses, his fantasies, conflicts, as well as his relationships. In that context, words outside of the play are mostly an adjunct, stage directions, or reality intrusions. Therapeutic interventions, when indicated, are meant to facilitate the play or to add relatively minor twists that help the child develop new coping skills. The therapist stays in the zone of proximal development of the child. The goal is to help the child make sense of who he is, as shaped by his life experiences and attachments, and make the best of it.

When children are seen because of preexisting suspicion of abuse, the therapist has a specific task to fulfill: is this child safe in his or her environment now, and has this child been abused? The verbal therapist–patient interchanges are of critical importance and follow a protocol prescribed in the literature.[19–21] The clinician is aware of operating at the medicolegal interface, where the difference between focused and leading questions is highly significant. In this context, the evaluator is more likely to respond to an attempt at disclosure because he or she notices it, however momentary or well hidden in displacement it may be. This is particularly important with young children, who may be in an active phase of disclosure one week, and deny it all the next.

Can a threshold be defined, indicating when the index of suspicion is high enough to warrant a switch from play therapy to abuse-focused intervention? Andy's therapy provides an opportunity to examine this issue as faced by a therapist trained in dynamically oriented child therapy as well as in trauma and abuse reactive interventions.

In Andy's case, the therapist began constructing several alternative hypothetical pathways leading to the current presentation. They were on a continuum rather than either/or, and went from loss of an important attachment figure to overstimulation to sexual abuse. Andy's play was observed more carefully for clues, and he was invited, somewhat more insistently, to settle down and play. He was offered a variety of toys that could portray family configurations (puppets, small animals, dolls). He chose elephants, and included a grandfather when the therapist suggested that relatives might be coming to visit. The grandfather often stood over the little elephant, or poked him with his tusks until he rolled over, all in good fun. His physical boundaries were different from those of other elephants. Overstimulation emerged as an issue in the play, but had Andy been traumatized?

Parallel to the work with the child, Andy's parents were introduced to these hypotheses, which had already crossed their minds. They contacted the stepgrandfather's biological family, who had often seemed angry and cold towards him. They were told of several incidents of inappropriate sexual behavior.

With Andy, the parents' instinctive reaction was to avoid all mention of his grandfather. On the advice of the therapist, they brought the grandfather back into the realm of what could be talked about. They asked nonspecific questions, remaining affectively open but neutral. They wondered about Andy's special times with him, asking what he remembered. Andy remembered lollipops. His parents commented that he hates them. He sometimes made gagging and grunting sounds. His parents, containing their intense affective reaction, asked if he ever felt hurt. Andy seemed surprised, but said he didn't remember.

At this point, parents and therapist together decided that the issue should be pursued more actively in the therapy, rather than waiting for things to unfold. This was due mostly to the parents' difficulty tolerating their intense anxiety, which they saw as starting to interfere with their relationships with both children. Andy was more ''hyper'' than ever, in school and at home, and sleeping poorly. In the next session, the therapist explained that there were some real-life questions she needed to ask, that were different from the play and pretend that had ruled so far. She ascertained that Andy did, indeed, understand the difference between real and pretend. Andy was suddenly very attentive, as if he had been waiting for this moment. Asked a general question about his grandfather, he said he had a ''secret dream'' he couldn't tell his parents, especially his mother who loved her (step)father so much. He described himself as being in a ''forest of sort of white hair'' in which he searches for something and then sucks on it. The dream ''comes back'' to him when he tries to fall asleep. He had wanted to tell me before, but it was "too gross." He looked very sad. Asked whether this dream could mean something real, he said "I did it, I sucked it."

The practical considerations raised by this case are comparatively simple: the parents are supportive, there is no threat of family disruption or feud following the disclosure, there is no question of whether to contact Child Protection Services, or to press charges. Yet the technical and theoretical issues raised are of paramount importance. Without the family interchange about the grandfather's appearance, would the experiences troubling Andy have surfaced during his childhood? Although it is impossible to answer that question, it can be said that this new understanding of Andy's history had important consequences. Diagnostically, Andy's "hyperactivity" is now more likely a post-traumatic stress disorder (PTSD)-related reaction. Cognitively, he is now free to use his brain to remember, in all areas. In the family, the dynamics have changed. His parents' ability to reach out affectively and effectively, to listen and to understand, to help him make sense of his life history, his impulses and conflicts, has been put back on the right track. He is now truly back in the lap of his family, as opposed to having a secret, unspeakable past that was on the verge of becoming encapsulated as a verbally unretrievable piece of himself.

This family outcome may not be attainable when multigenerational abuse forces parents to cope with their own memories of abuse as they are trying to respond to their child's disclosure. Unravelling what really happened when can be a near impossible task, leading to hypotheses that are difficult to validate. In addition, many parents find it impossible to remain calm or listen empathically to what their child is trying to say or show without jumping to conclusions, which can be false positive or false negative.

Andy's therapy continued. He talked about his grandfather, and played out elephant stories that became more aggressive, as the little elephant started to fight back. At home and at school, after an initial period of intense affective lability, Andy seemed much calmer and focused. He stopped being the class clown, made two friends, and started to catch up academically. Periodic follow-up into his ninth year indicated normal adjustment.

Case 2

Beth is a 10-year-old fifth grader evaluated for recent onset of school failure and depression: failing grades, seemingly half asleep in class, reduced contact with friends. A school-based evaluation had found high-average functioning, but only when given constant encouragement. Beth was seen as unable to take any risk, which sapped her scholastic motivation and her self-esteem.

Beth's parents are very concerned. Her mother has recently been diagnosed with chronic fatigue syndrome, after being incapacitated for over a year. Her father is away on business more than ever, attempting to compensate for the loss of his wife's income. Her brother Colin, who is 8 years old, spends most of his time out of the house playing sports. Her half brother David, 19, is the product of her mother's first marriage to her high school boyfriend, who left when David was 3. David is said to have been "wild" since age 13, exhibiting seriously rebellious behavior, including alcohol and drug use. He has been off all substances for a year now, and he is in therapy. He has taken a semester off and plans to transfer to a more challenging college. He drives the children to their various appointments and events.

During the evaluation, Beth expresses a variety of emotions about her family: concern for her mother, as well as resentment about her unavailability (mother sleeps or rests a lot); mixed feelings for the absences of her short-tempered father; contempt and some envy for her "eager beaver" competitive brother. About David, she complains that she doesn't know how to talk to him. She remembers admiring him a lot, before his partying became too much.

Beth wants to talk. However, once weekly psychotherapy is agreed upon, she becomes more reticent. She wants to play board games, but seems to pay little attention to what she is doing. At times, Beth seems to be barely there, at others she reminds the therapist of a bat—seemingly blind, but artfully avoiding contact.

One day, about 6 weeks into the therapy, David is not in the waiting room at the end of Beth's session. While the therapist calls home, Beth looks out the open window. When a door slams loudly, she screams "No", seemingly scared. The therapist comforts her verbally, then acknowledges that she too found the noise loud and startling. Beth talks about feeling so alone in her house. But it had not always been so, she says. David used to be such fun to follow around, and he often told her secrets. When Beth is silent again, the therapist asks her for an example, but she doesn't remember any. At this point, her eyes become evasive again, and the therapist realized that for a brief moment there had been a light, and life, in them.

What had brought life into Beth's eyes? The empty waiting room, the slamming door startling her into screaming "No", the affective connection with her therapist? A physiologic event seemed to have occurred as much as a psychologic one.

Following this session, Beth's parents report what they call mood swings: one moment she is alert and talkative but anxious, the next, dreaming and withdrawn. In therapy, Beth also vacillates, seeming either hypervigilant or avoidant. She describes two nightmares about suffocating. She is afraid of being afraid. She is talking again, mostly about feeling alone, bereft, abandoned: she feels "alone down to my bones." The therapist wonders whether, in addition to depression, Beth is beginning to show signs of an anxiety disorder, specifically, PTSD.

In contrast, the family situation is improving, with her mother starting to feel better and stronger, and David actively pursuing his college reentry.

Sexual or physical abuse or trauma had been asked about during the evaluation. The issue is now revisited. Beth's parents state that she had been very independent as a baby, which was somewhat disappointing to her mother who expected a girl baby to be more cuddly. As soon as Beth could move by herself, she sought out her half brother. Nothing specifically related to trauma emerges in the meeting with the parents. They then talk to David who acknowledges that Beth had been his "little accomplice" until she was about 5, but denies ever having involved her, or taken advantage of her. After discussing the range of possible consequences in therapy, Beth decides to tell David of her startle reactions to loud noises, her fear of suffocating (in her dreams) and her fear of being afraid and alone. He requests to join her next session. He states that he remembers something he feels guilty about. When he was 13 or 14 and alone in the house, he invited a few friends. Together they experimented with a variety of substances including glue, spray cans, and alcohol, leading to a moment of crisis when one of the boys had an asthma-like attack, and was gasping for air. When his friends noticed Beth standing by his room, David just slammed the door in her face and forgot about her. At some later point he told her she had to keep this secret or he would be kicked out. He remembers the incident as the boy with asthma was later hospitalized. Beth has no memory of the incident that she can translate into words, but she feels that her brother is describing something real.

What is the importance of this revelation? It implies loss, but was the experience traumatic? Was it a real but minor incident among more abusive ones?

Current research on childhood trauma points to its profound and lasting effects on the developing central nervous system (see chapter 3) and underscores the importance of adopting a developmental perspective.

In contrast to the current delineation of its consequences, the definition of trauma itself is still broad, vague, and changeable. Classically, trauma was seen as an extraordinary event that overwhelms the organism's capacity to survive with physical and/or psychological integrity. DSM-I related war experiences to "gross stress reactions."[27] DSM-III and DSM-IIIR described an event "outside the range of usual human experience."[28,29] DSM-IV has omitted the notion of extraordinariness and describes the event by its consequences only (loss of or threat to physical integrity or death).[30] Recent research on vicarious traumatization, as experienced by adolescents who "heard about" a trauma they were not personally involved in, has further broadened the concept.[17]

There seems to be a contradiction between trauma, which is seen as exceptional, and its consequences, posttraumatic stress symptomatology, which are seen as widespread. This paradox can be better understood if one takes a developmental approach and defines trauma by including more clearly the perspective of the traumatized person. A better definition of trauma thus needs to consider the relationship between the power of the experience and the strength of the available protective factors. Conversely, the definition of resilience must include both the protective factors and the psychological or actual events challenging them. This definition implies a shift from trauma as a static event to trauma as a dynamic interplay. Similarly, resilience has to be seen not as a static achievement but as a constantly changing equilibrium. These definitions require a knowledge of child development, family dynamics, and a close look at the protective factors within and outside the child. An additional advantage of this view is that it protects against biases based on the cultural viewpoint of the clinician that may define certain events as traumatic, while overlooking others.

In childhood, a major protective factor related to resilience in the face of trauma is the availability of an adult who can listen, empathize, and reality test.[31] One striking feature of children and adults whose experiences of trauma require psychiatric intervention is the sense of aloneness they experienced during and after the event. When trauma is secret, like sexual abuse, for example, the abuse and its emotional consequences occur in psychologic isolation. There, the only affective connection possible is to the abuser, and often becomes a component of the deep and tenacious bond that binds victim to victimizer. When the event is a collective one, like a natural disaster or family violence, the child may be emotionally connected or alone.

The benefits of telling about a confusing, frightening, or traumatizing experience are multiple.[32,33] On an affective level, the child can reexperience some of the traumatizing emotions in the context of a safe relationship. A child attacked by a dog, for example, may need to tell and retell the experience many times. The aim is to undo the state of helplessness and aloneness experienced at the time of the trauma, and prevent it from permanently shaping the child's development. A caregiver who is empathically attuned to the child has to be able to tolerate the profound emotions elicited each time he or she listens to the child, until the intensity fades for both of them and the child has regained some measure of control over her inner and outer reality. On a cognitive level, a child who talks about a trauma has the opportunity to air her developmentally appropriate but possibly false views, for example, attributing causality egocentrically. In addition, the child has the opportunity to cope with the memory of the traumatic experience by utilizing new cognitive and affective capabilities as they develop and mature.

Trauma that is never talked about is more likely to remain inaccessible to affective and cognitive review and reprocessing and to stay encapsulated and difficult to access verbally. The adult who remembers such early trauma in therapy can be helped to see the discrepancy between his or her usual cognitive functioning and the arrested understanding of the trauma. In children and adolescents, the discrepancy is more subtle, and can be more difficult to perceive.

In order to understand how an event has affected a child, it is therefore important to evaluate the child's developmental level when it took place. Equally important is a review of the child's connection to others before, during, and after the potentially traumatizing event.

This viewpoint was first anticipated in an early large-scale, longitudinal study of sexually abused children, which reported that the severity of symptomatology was not only related to abuse factors (primarily the identity of the perpetrator and the degree of violence), but also to the mother's reaction to the abuse and the need for out-of-home placement.[34,35] These last two factors, pertaining to the characteristics of the mother–child relationship and the quality of the family milieu, are of critical importance and point to contemporary notions on the complex effects of infant–caregiver attachment.

It is important to consider that the child's ability to seek and find a caring other to share a secret with has a long history predating the impact of the trauma, and originating in the earliest mother–infant interactions. Attachment theory has not only delineated various types of early interactions but also pointed to their later consequences and provided a framework for the intergenerational transmission of such patterns.[14,15]

The child's ability to connect, therefore, has a developmental component, based on the child's past experiences and quality of attachment. In addition, there are critical reality–based components. Children who hold a secret that they know can hurt someone, or that can destroy the fabric of their family, carry a special burden—one far more complex than the good secret/bad secret taught in prevention programs. They face the most complex of moral dilemmas—dilemmas that are sometimes parralleled in our struggle about whether to involve Child Protective authorities.

Beth's case underscores the importance of looking at potentially traumatizing experiences from a developmental point of view. She was referred for depression, which was obscuring her pervasive avoidance and numbing symptoms. The startle reaction to the slammed door was the first such experience she was aware of, as she could not remember whether other things had startled her before. After that, she had nightmares, generalized anxiety, and was described by her parents as "moody," which was their description of her alternating states of avoidance and vigilance. The therapist suspected a traumatic etiology, but had, at first, no indication whether it was past or present, sexual or physical in nature. Fear of suffocating can be associated to many experiences, ranging from medical mishaps (e.g., anesthesia before adequate sedation), to accidents, to rough play, to attempted suffocation or to fellatio—or, as in this case, to a complex but vicarious experience. Constructing various hypotheses to guide one's attempt to understand a patient's traumatic memories should always leave room for the unexpected. The goal is to let the child tell her story in words or play by helping her focus on that task but not leading her.

When Beth's half brother provided an explanation for her distressing symptoms, the therapist was skeptical, and thought that more abusive behavior might yet surface. But for Beth, David's confession was the beginning of a renewed connection with him. They could talk again and she felt more understood by him than by her conservative parents. There was no fear or anxiety around him, and she showed general improvement. Beth's grades improved because she was able to listen in class and concentrate on her work. Her fears became more philosophical in nature: she was passionate about pollution and saving the rain forest. She related better to her peers, although she still lacked a best friend.

In therapy, Beth focused on her distant relationship with her mother and her conflicts with her father, both issues predating her mother's illness. Without David, she had felt very alone. Affectively, he had been her primary object and caretaker. Reviewing Beth's relationship with her mother, it became clearer that there had never been a close, easy, and flexible connection between them. Beth's mother had felt confused and rejected when her infant girl did not seem to need the physical and emotional contact she had hoped to have with her baby. She had felt hurt by her daughter's seeming indifference to her good-byes and hellos. The therapist questioned whether there was a history of insecure attachment of an avoidant type.

This case illustrates how a developmental perspective, focusing on the interplay between the traumatic experience and the available protective factors, allows a broader range of experiences to be considered as potentially traumatizing.

Case 3

Cathy is a 16-year-old living in a stable foster home. She ran away from her biologic family at age 8. She is pregnant but does not really believe it. She is frequently involved in fights. She often gets hurt, as she seems to provoke other adolescents who do not usually get along to rally together against her. After being accidentally struck by a bicycle and hitting her head on the edge of a parked car, she has a miscarriage, becomes depressed, and is briefly suicidal. Her school counselor, who has a long-standing relationship with her, is very concerned and requests a psychiatric consultation.

Cathy wants to forget about her family of origin, and is only willing to say that she ran away because of the constant fighting. When describing the bike accident, she denies any loss of consciousness. As she describes the scene, it becomes clear that she is depicting it from a bird's eye view. Cathy is not aware of her perspective until it is mentioned to her. She is surprised, noting that "it's as if I was out of my body," and then adds, "I think I spent a lot of my childhood like that." She puts finger puppets on as many fingers as she can and hits one fist against the other. Somehow they stay on one hand, whereas only one puppet is left on the other. The evaluator asks her to describe what she can see from that bird's eye perspective. She refuses.

When Cathy sees her counselor again, she tells about this strange perspective. Over time, she shares memories which she tells in words and in action—using pencils, action figures, or anything available. It seems that in order to remember, she needs to get the position of the bodies correctly, and has to make the hitting and colliding movements real. The essence of her life story is that her mother tried to kill her many times, often hitting her head against furniture, walls, or most dangerously, the metal radiator. Most of the worst physical abuse occurred before she was 5. The other children were neglected and abused, mostly verbally. No one ever helped her, and she remembers not helping her siblings. Her father would sometimes get violent, but mostly seemed in a daze. She adored him, and thought he knew nothing of the abuse. She never thought of telling him. To the outside world, the family presented a normal middle-class facade.

Did Cathy really forget and then remember? What is the boundary between being forced to keep an event secret and forgetting it?

This case points to the importance of being alert to signs of dissociation in the presentation or history. When Cathy was asked whether her eyes were open as she lay on the ground after the accident, she said "I can't see my eyes." Without challenging this response, the evaluator asked her to describe the scene as best she could, with all the activity around her. It became clear that she saw everything from above—for example, the rounded backs of the people bending over her. The differences were subtle, as Cathy seemed quite adept at translating her viewpoint into the more normal and acceptable perspective, but they were heightened by a sense of unreality.

Once Cathy started sharing some of her history with her school counselor, she acknowledged that she just wanted to forget it and that therapy made it harder for her to "have a life." Her counselor had the difficult task of coordinating three distinct approaches: Cathy's need for help in the here and now, and her wish to be as distant as possible from her past; the counselor's own feeling that helping Cathy must include working through the abuse trauma; and the consultant's view that Cathy's current developmental needs may well preclude any in-depth investigation of her abuse history. Balancing available ego strengths, developmental tasks, and the potential regression inherent in exploring an abuse history is an essential task for the therapist. With adolescents, who experience normative fluctuations in functioning and face constantly changing developmental challenges, an ongoing review of the patient's coping skills is especially important.

This case highlights how knowledge of the abuse, however incomplete, is useful to help the patient mature. Therapeutic work can be done on a cognitive level, leading to more intellectual insight and control, even without fully exploring the history and connecting specific traumatic moments with affect. But without knowledge of the abuse history, the patient's current state would be much more difficult to understand and empathize with.

Conclusion

To summarize a vast, complex, and growing field of inquiry, recent research has postulated a variety of mechanisms for the "forgetting" of early childhood experiences. From neuropsychiatric research comes a new look at childhood amnesia and a beginning delineation of posttraumatic memory pathways; from infant research a beginning connection between early attachment and later development; from memory research a new sense of the vagaries of memory.

Childhood amnesia, once understood as the psychological rite of passage distancing us from our primitive infantile selves, is now seen as biologically programmed. Early memories, good or bad, influence subsequent development. They affect lifelong core attitudes and feelings, but they are not easily accessible to verbal recall.

Traumatic memory most likely follows a different biologic pathway, which facilitates implicit behavioral memory and hinders verbal retrieval. Furthermore, events and emotions experienced in a dissociated state may only be retrievable in a similar state of mind. They may thus be unavailable when conscious and focused attempts at remembering are made.

Insecure avoidant attachment, which is seen as a normal variant in the early mother–infant relationship, has been correlated with reduced autobiographical memory in later childhood and in adulthood. There is a paucity of memories, good or bad. A bland sense that ''it was just a regular, typical, fine childhood'' makes retrieval of any meaningful memories very difficult, thus impeding therapeutic inquiry.

All these findings seem to indicate that, from a biologic perspective, lack of verbal access to memories of early childhood trauma is the favored outcome. From a psychologic perspective, one must add multiple complicating factors enforcing silence and forgetting: children are bribed and manipulated; children are threatened; children are made to feel responsible; children feel responsible due to their developmental self-attribution of blame; children are told they are guilty; children identify with the guilt projected on to them by their abuser; children are told abuse is love; children need to be loved and to love, and cannot afford to see the price.

Why do children ever remember traumas in the face of these powerful hindrances? Perhaps it is because, since birth, they are trying to make sense of their world and to find meaning. One of our roles as therapists is to help them gain access to their history, revisit their helpless aloneness in the company of an empathic witness, and then return to their current developmental tasks and challenges.

References

1. Tardieu A: Etude medico-legale sur les sevices et mauvais traitements exercés sur les enfants. Annales d'hygiene publique et de medecine legale 1860; 13:361–398.
2. Freud S: The Etiology of Hysteria. *In* E Jones (Ed.), Collected Papers, Vol I. New York: Basic Books, 1959, pp. 183–219. (Original work published 1896).
3. Ferenczi S: Confusion of tongues between adults and the child. *In* The Problems and Methods of Psychoanalysis. New York: Basic Books, 1955. (Original work published 1933).
4. Kinsey AC, Pomeroy WB, Martin CE, Gebhard PH: Sexual Behavior in the Human Female. Philadelphia: WB Saunders, 1953.
5. Kempe CH, Silverman FN, Steele BF, Droegmueller W, Silver HK: The battered child syndrome. JAMA 1962; 181:17–24.
6. Finkelhor D: The ''backlash'' and the future of child protection advocacy: insights from the study of social issues. *In* JEB Myers (Ed.), The Backlash: Child Protection Under Fire. Thousand Oaks, CA: Sage, 1994, pp. 1–16.
7. Perry BD, Pate JE: Neurodevelopment and the psychobiological roots of PTSD. *In* LF Koziol, CE Stout (Eds.), The Neuropsychology of Mental Disorders: A Practical Guide. Springfield, IL: Charles C. Thomas, 1994, pp. 81–98.
8. van der Kolk BA: The body keeps score: memory and the evolving psychobiology of posttraumatic stress. Harvard Rev. Psychiatry 1994; 1:253–265.
9. Johnson MK, Hirst W: Processing subsystems of memory. *In* RG Lister, HJ Weingartner

(Eds.), Perspectives in Cognitive Neuroscience. New York: Oxford University Press, 1992, pp. 197–217.

10. Lewis M: Memory and psychoanalysis: a new look at infantile amnesia and transference. J Am Acad Child Adolesc Psychiatry 1955; 34:405–417.

11. Ceci S, Bruck M: Suggestibility in the child witness: a historical review and synthesis. Psychol Bull 1993; 133:403–409.

12. Loftus EF: The reality of repressed memories. AM Psychol 1993; 48:518–537.

13. Saywitz K, Goodman GS, Nicholas E: Children's memories of physical examinations involving genital touch: implications for reports of child sexual abuse. J Consult Clin Psychol 1991; 59:682–691.

14. Biringen Z: Attachment theory and research: application to clinical practice. Am J Orthopsychiatry 1994; 64:404–420.

15. Alexander PC: Applicaton of attachment theory to the study of sexual abuse. J Consult Clin Psychol 1992; 60:185–195.

16. Erickson MT: Rethinking Oedipus: an evolutionary perspective of incest avoidance. Am J Psychiatry 1993; 150:411–416.

17. Horowitz K, Weine S, Jekel J: Post-traumatic stress symptoms in urban adolescent girls: compounded community trauma. J Am Acad Child Adolesc Psychiatry 1995; 34:1353–1361.

18. Gaensbauer T, Chatoor I, Drell M, Siegel D, Zeanah CH: Traumatic loss in a one-year-old girl. J Am Acad Child Adolesc Psychiatry 1995; 34:520–528.

19. Jones DPH, McQuiston MG: Interviewing the Sexually Abused Child. London: Gaskell, 1988 (distributed by APA Press).

20. American Academy of Child and Adolescent Psychiatry: Guidelines for the Clinical Evaluation of Child and Adolescent Sexual Abuse. Washington, DC: American Academy of Child and Adolescent Psychiatry, 1990.

21. American Professional Society on the Abuse of Children: Guidelines for Psychosocial Evaluation of Suspected Sexual Abuse in Young Children. Chicago: American Professional Society on the Abuse of Children, 1990.

22. Finkelhor D, Berliner L: Research on the treatment of sexually abused children: a review and recommendations. J Am Acad Child Adolesc Psychiatry 1991; 34:1408–1423.

23. Sorensen T, Snow B: How children tell: the process of disclosure in child sexual abuse. Child Welfare 1991; 70:3–15.

24. Sauzier M: Disclosure of child sexual abuse: for better or for worse. Psychiatr Clin North Am 1989; 12:455–469.

25. Nelson K: The psychological and social origins of autobiographical memory. Psychol Sci 1993; 2:1–8.

26. Terr L: What happens to early memories of trauma? A study of twenty children under age 5 at the time of documented traumatic events. J Am Acad Child Adolesc Psychiatry 1988; 27:96–105.

27. American Psychiatric Association: Diagnostic and Statistical Manual of Mental Disorders. (1st ed.) Washington, DC: American Psychiatric Association, 1952.

28. American Psychiatric Association: Diagnostic and Statistical Manual of Mental Disorders (3rd ed.). Washington, DC: American Psychiatric Association, 1980.

29. American Psychiatric Association: Diagnostic and Statistical Manual of Mental Disorders, (3rd ed, rev.). Washington, DC: American Psychiatric Association, 1987.

30. American Psychiatric Association: Diagnostic and Statistical Manual of Mental Disorders (4th ed.). Washington, DC: American Psychiatric Association, 1994.

31. Rutter M: Protective factors in children's responses to stress and disadvantage. *In* MW Kent, TW Rolf (Eds.), Social Competence in Children. Hanover NH: University Press New England, 1979, pp. 49–74.

32. Pynoos RS, Eth S: Witness to violence: the child interview. J Am Acad Child Adolesc Psychiatry 1986; 25:306–319.

33. Pynoos RS, Eth S: Special intervention programs for child witnesses of violence. *In* M. Lystad (Ed.), Violence in the Home. New York: Brunner/Mazel, 1986, pp. 193–216.

34. Gomes-Schwartz B, Horowitz JM, Sauzier M: Severity of emotional disorders among sexually abused preschool, school age and adolescent children. Hosp Community Psychiatry 1985; 36: 503–508.

35. Gomes-Schwartz B, Horowitz JM, Cardarelli AP, Sauzier M: The aftermath of child sexual abuse: 18 months later. *In* B Gomes-Schwartz, JM Horowitz, AP Cardarelli (Eds.), Child Sexual Abuse: The Initial Effects. Newbury Park, CA: Sage, 1990, pp. 132–152.

17

Diagnosis, Pathogenesis, and Memories of Childhood Abuse

LISA A. UYEHARA

The debate about memories of childhood abuse can be conceptualized as a diagnostic argument: on the one hand, that psychopathology resulting from childhood sexual abuse can be diagnosed with reasonable accuracy; and on the other, that clinicians erroneously diagnose a traumatic syndrome when no such events occurred. In the midst of this furor, we are forced to reconsider our theories of diagnosis and pathogenesis and our procedures for evaluating patients and reconstructing their histories.

Several issues related to diagnosis and pathogenesis recur in these discussions. The relationship of childhood trauma to diagnosis or symptom, and vice versa, confronts the clinician considering childhood abuse as an explanation for a patient's difficulties. There is also controversy over what constitutes clinical data, and how one obtains them. And we face the question of whether an accurate picture of a patient's history is critical to the patient's therapy and mental health. These questions are considered below. I have bypassed the easier target of radical techniques in order to examine the dilemmas encountered in ''diagnosing'' trauma through using general therapeutic practices. The chapter draws most heavily from the analytic literature, both because it is the literature with which I am most familiar, and because it remains unparalleled in the detail provided about the therapeutic process.

The following case illustrates the kinds of diagnostic difficulties that may be encountered when the question of childhood sexual abuse emerges during the course of an ''ordinary'' psychotherapy. The case is not representative of cases in which sexual abuse is explored—indeed, its conclusion is atypical in my experience—but it demonstrates evolving diagnostic formulations, both psychodynamic and biological, in the course of a therapy.*

Case Study

Mrs. A, a married mother of two, entered therapy in her early thirties to resolve recurrent concerns about her sexual orientation. Though heterosexual in her relationships, she had worried intermittently since adolescence that she might be a lesbian. Her anxiety generally took the form of thinking ''there is something wrong with you—you're probably gay.'' Although she had crushes on boys from early adolescence, she had heen fearful of physical contact, and did not have sexual intercourse until she was 25. She remained sexually inhibited in fantasy and behavior, was often anorgasmic, and felt she lacked a sense of femaleness.

She came from an intact working-class family with an alcoholic, though affectionate father, and brothers 1 year and 3 years older who often bullied her physically. Her mother, who usually worked second shift, was described as a classic ''enabler'' who denied her husband's alcoholism, did not curb her sons' bullying, and told the patient that she was lucky to have such a loving father and brothers. The patient denied any history of sexual abuse.

She was an intelligent, insightful, and very anxious patient, who repeatedly asked for reassurance that she was heterosexual, as well as for direct advice on what to do. Ten months into the therapy, after beginning to talk more explicity about her sexual thoughts, Mrs A came into therapy sobbing. With many fits and starts, she told me of a stream of associations that had led to her thinking the phrase ''I want to lick your cunt.'' She then thought that perhaps something sexual had happened with her year-and-a-half older brother, and calmed down. I said it was possible that she had heard these words in childhood, but also noted that sexual exploration may occur in siblings close in age. She felt reassured, in part by the thought that something other than her being a lesbian was giving rise to her sexual anxieties, and also that the obscene thoughts might not be coming from her.

As she attempted to piece together her history, thoughts arose as disjointed visual images and verbal phrases, detailed and sexually explicit, and often told with intense distressing affect. Most of these thoughts focused on her next older brother, but others concerned her oldest brother, father, and a friend of her father's. For example, she had fragmented images of her brother's penis, and of the attic wall; a thought of her brother putting his finger in her vagina; she heard phrases, sometimes in the voices of family members, such as ''take it off,'' ''spread your legs,'' ''I have been raped,'' and ''tell–tell.'' Some of her thoughts had a highly dissociative quality, such as her thought

*I am grateful to Mrs. A for granting permission to me to describe her case without distorting the biographical data.

"just look at the wall," and her talking about her childhood self as "the little girl."

There were times when she and I were fairly convinced that there had been incestuous trauma and times when we were doubtful, our views not necessarily coinciding. Once she said she felt we were playing a bizarre game in which I was getting her to say weirder and weirder things. When she pleaded with me to tell her whether she had been abused, I responded that I didn't know, though sometimes adding that it seemed plausible or possible. She approached her mother, who listened to her concerns, but said she had no knowledge of anything having happened. Throughout this work I interpreted various aspects of a maternal transference, including her wish to please, her anger when she thought I was withholding or blaming, and her fear that I wished to replace her with a more satisfying patient.

Her fragmented thoughts continued, at times becoming more violent. However, after a year of twice weekly therapy, nothing had pulled together into a more coherent memory. This work stood in contrast to other work we did on her childhood, particularly about her mother. We reconstructed a coherent narrative of her sense that her mother preferred her brothers, did not encourage her femininity, and had actively discouraged her sexual development. She felt she had not satisfied her mother, as she often feared she had not satisfied me.

The patient gained a more positive sense of her femininity, was more convinced that she was heterosexual, and more comfortable with her sexuality. However, I began to wonder if the persistent homosexual thoughts were a symptom of obsessive-compulsive disorder, and asked the patient about other symptoms. She indeed had a few other symptoms, including a few checking behaviors. After treatment with an SSRI (selective serotonin reuptake inhibitor antidepressant), her intrusive sexual thoughts gradually diminished, and a low-level chronic dysphoria also improved. The patient still had occasional memory fragments about her childhood, but increasingly felt it was unproductive to explore them further. She terminated, convinced that there had been no childhood abuse. Her relationships with her husband and children and female friends were warmer and freer, and she was deeply gratified about resuming the artistic interests that she had abandoned in adolescence. Her improvement remains in the 3 years since terminating.

I began this case with the formulation that the patient had neurotic-level conflicts about her sexual orientation and femininity. In the mid-phase of treatment, this formulation vacillated with the idea that the patient had been incestuously abused by her brother or father, and I wondered about a dissociative disorder. In the final work, I saw her homosexual thoughts as a symptom of OCD, with both a biological basis and a psychological determinant from her developmental conflicts about her femininity.

Was she abused in childhood? Her fragmented thoughts could have been dissociated memories, which she abandoned pursuing because of a resistance to remembering. However, neither the transference nor the patient's other relationships were typical of someone brutally abused; her brother's close age made him an unlikely violent perpetrator in childhood, and her vivid visual imagination might explain her "memories." I was aware, of course, that the biological explanation was more palatable to the patient.

Trauma, Pathogenesis, and Diagnosis

Childhood sexual abuse is not a diagnosis, yet the notion of diagnosis arises frequently in these discussions. Before addressing the controversies of diagnostic process and procedure, I would like to touch upon some of the differing views of the role of trauma in diagnosis.

As described by Levine[1] and Galatzer-Levy,[2] Freud replaced the seduction theory, which was essentially a trauma theory of neurosis, with the theory of infantile sexuality. While he continued to recognize that actual sexual abuse was a pathogenic factor in neurosis, Freud proposed that universal childhood conflicts over sexuality and aggression were sufficient factors to produce neurosis in adult life. The basic postulate that adult character and psychological symptomatology are rooted in childhood experience, the genetic principle, remains a central tenet in contemporary analytic theory. However, the outcome of childhood experiences is regarded as highly variable bacause of the mediating influence of the individual's unique psychic functioning. Shengold, the psychoanalyst probably best known on the subject of trauma, applies this principle to the trauma patient as well when he declares that patients cannot be reduced to a diagnostic category, nor can they be defined by what happened to them.[3] He borrowed the poetic term of "soul murder," taken from the writings of Freud's paranoid patient, Dr. Schreber, to describe "a certain category of traumatic experience: instances of repetitive and chronic overstimulation, alternating with emotional deprivation, that are deliberately brought about by another individual"[4] (p. 2). He acknowledges that "the term does not define a clinical entity; it applies more to pathogenic circumstances than to specific effects"[4] (p. 16).

This focus on unique individual meaning is reflected in a general lack of interest among analysts in diagnosis. In 1963, Karl Menninger urged psychiatrists, at that time predominantly psychoanalysts, to abandon psychiatric diagnoses entirely, and instead use individual dynamic formulations broadly grouped by level of dysfunction in a continuous spectrum.[5]

In contrast, the descriptive-empiric tradition, which was utilized in the formulation of DSM-III and its successors, emphasizes discrete categories of illness which are defined by strictly operationalized criteria. The genetic principal, along with the rest of psychoanalytic theory, was dropped from DSM, and theories of psychological etiology were included only when "clearly known." In contrast to the psychodynamic formulation, the multiaxial diagnoses were independent of one another.[6–8]

Herman has criticized both the traditional psychodynamic approach to the role of trauma, as well as the trauma-related diagnoses in DSM categories. She argues that the current diagnoses of borderline personality disorder, multiple personality disorder, multiple personality and somatizing disorder, as well as the older diagnoses such as hysteria and masochistic character, have blamed the patient by omitting the etiologic significance of trauma.[9]

Neither the survivor of chronic child abuse nor the Holocaust survivor described by Niederland[10] appear in the DSM-IV. Pointing out that the diagnosis of posttraumatic stress disorder (PTSD) is more appropriate to the victim of single trauma, Herman proposes a new diagnosis of complex posttraumatic stress disorder, with disturbances of affect, consciousness, self-perception, perception of perpetrator, relationships, and belief systems resulting from "a history of subjugation to totalitarian control over a prolonged period"[9] (p. 121). This diagnostic approach includes descriptive, psychodynamic, existential, and social concepts—the latter three are unrecognized in DSM diagnostic principles.

Protesting that investigations into the personal characteristics of the trauma victim typical of an analytic formulation have often blamed the victim, Herman instead emphasizes the external event. This social and political agenda propelled the assumption that PTSD was a normative response to an extreme stressor. However, as described by Yehuda and MacFarlane, these original presumptions have been contradicted by subsequent research findings, which show a heterogeneous response to traumatic events.[11] Not only is PTSD not the inevitable outcome of trauma, it is not even the majority response. While the incidence of PTSD rises with the severity and duration of the trauma, it is clear that there are individual variations in the level of trauma required to induce PTSD. Moreover, the study of predisposing factors, including previous trauma, intelligence, and personality, is once again acceptable and shows promise.[12–14]

A traumatic stressor, defined in DSM-III as an event "outside the range of usual human experience," was modified in DSM-IV to reflect the fact that trauma is common. The criterion is now "actual or threatened death or serious injury, or a threat to the physical integrity of oneself or others." With reports of PTSD symptoms in pathological grief[15] or in the close friends of adolescents who committed suicide,[16] the strength of the connection between experience and syndrome is further brought into question.

The diagnosis of PTSD highlights other controversies engendered by the diagnostic philosophy underlying DSM-III and its successors. While many felt that the empirical basis of the DSM-III brought psychiatric diagnosis in line with the standards of the medical model, others argued that the criteria for making a diagnosis were now stricter than in other areas of medicine. Pointing out that symptoms that were not diseases or syndromes (e.g., diarrhea or headache) were acceptable throughout other areas of medicine, Pinsker argued that the heavy research orientation disconnected DSM-III from clinical realities.[17] This difficulty applies to many trauma patients as well, who would not meet the criteria either of PTSD or of the complex posttraumatic stress disorder proposed by Herman.

Some of these patients meet criteria for other DSM diagnoses, such as major depression, dysthymia, panic disorder, or dissociative disorders. However, converging factors, including the declining influence of psychodynamics, a diagnostic system emphasizing superficial symptoms, and insurance pressures toward brief, standardized, symptom-focused treatments, have contributed to a fractured approach to diagnosis and a lack of interest in individual formulation. Reiser designates this lack of diagnostic synthesis the "loss of the mind."[18] For example, a patient with a history of childhood sexual abuse who develops a major depression and alcohol abuse following a rape will have these two diagnoses listed on Axis I, the rape acknowledged in an Axis IV footnote, and possibly little or no formulation integrating the diagnoses with her childhood history.

The uncomplicated and unintegrated checklist format of DSM III has been imitated by various authors and self-help books in guidelines for the diagnosis of sexual abuse. As personal history which is not an integral part of diagnosis is pushed further to the margins, therapists may diagnose PTSD when the patient has a significant history of childhood trauma, even if criteria for the diagnosis are not met, if only to insert some psychological meaning into the assessment of a patient.

What Constitues Evidence?

Different diagnostic systems require different diagnostic procedures. MacKinnon and Michels,[19] writing on psychiatric interviewing at a time when psychoanalysts dominated the field of psychiatry, characterized these different approaches to diagnostic evaluation:

> Interviews in the non-psychiatric branches of medicine generally emphasize medical history taking, the purpose of which is to obtain facts that will facilitate the establishment of a correct diagnosis and the institution of appropriate treatment. The interview is organized around the present illness, the past history, the family history, and the review of systems. Data concerning the personal life of the patient are considered important if they have possible bearing on the present illness. . . . [The medical patient] is usually willing to tell the doctor anything that he thinks may be related to his illness. . . . [A]lthough the psychiatric patient is motivated to reveal himself in order to gain relief from his suffering, he is also motivated to conceal his innermost feelings and the fundamental causes of his psychological disturbance.[19] (p. 5–6)

It is illustrative of the massive shift in American psychiatry away from psychoanalysis that the interview here characterized as nonpsychiatric is closer to what is widely accepted as a standard psychiatric interview today.

McHugh's arguments about the overdiagnosis of sexual abuse represent a traditional medical model. For example, he maintains that a psychiatric diagnostic evaluation includes not only a history and mental status examination, but also "searching with family doctors, teachers, schools, and other records for evidence."[20] In the case of accusations of incest, he asserts that the clinician should interview the patient's parents. McHugh feels that a proper diagnosis is necessary to instituting appropriate treatment and sees his approach to evaluating allegations of incest as consistent with general medical practice. He contends that conducting an evaluation without seeking external proof is malpractice.[21] The presentation of these principles of psychiatric diagnosis by a highly regarded academic psychiatrist, widely quoted by members and attorneys from the False Memory Syndrome Foundation, deserves careful consideration.

McHugh's recommendations on outside verification holds memories of childhood sexual abuse, whether always remembered or recalled after a period of forgetting, to a higher standard than is generally applied to a patient's history—in psychiatry or other branches of medicine. When adult patients in individual therapy attribute their problems in part to other childhood events, the clinician is not expected to seek outside corroboration. Some events, such as a death in the family, one might expect to be provided from the outset. However, within the course of therapy, other "facts" of a patient's childhood may be deduced or uncovered, including a parent's alcoholism, physical or mental illness, marital infidelity, or inadequate caretaking. Patients often enter therapy without having identified some major problem in the family, especially when the issue has been denied, avoided, or minimized by the parents, consciously or unconsciously.[22]

Obviously, when an allegation of sexual abuse enters the legal system, the issue of outside evidence must be confronted. McHugh feels that seeking outside corroboration even when there is no question of legal proceedings is indicated to avoid "wreaking havoc on the family."[20] Frankel likewise contends that a therapist's "acceptance" of a claim of childhood sexual abuse without verification is legally and *ethically* dubious.[23] However, disruption of family relationships is accepted as an outcome of therapy in other circumstances. Patients in individual therapy may proceed to divorce without the therapist having interviewed the spouse; adult patients may minimize contact with family members as a healthy outcome to therapy. With the unfortunate exception of the *Ramona* judgment and a handful of similar cases, the therapist's traditional clinical responsibility has been to his patient, not his patient's family.[24] The therapist's role is to help the patient understand his relationship with his family, not to advise the patient what to do.

Even if the clinician wants to obtain outside information, his contact with others and access to previous records is contingent upon the patient's granting such permission. There are circumstances in which we decide to abide by the patient's restrictions, even when outside contact might be useful.

Gathering data from outside sources is of limited usefulness. Witnesses to child molestation and confession by perpetrators are rare. If the child never reported the abuse to an adult, if the allegation was never evaluated by a professional who was both receptive to the possibility and knowledgeable about what to look for, documentation of the event is unlikely to exist. Signs and symptoms of abuse, which are difficult enough to determine even when abuse is the focus of an evaluation, are easily overlooked in routine pediatric exams. Paradise, for example, cautions against the "inappropriate reliance on physical findings" because of problems of both false negatives and false positives, and concludes that "clinician comfort aside, the diagnosis of sexual abuse inevitably rests not on a genital measurement but on descriptive statements made by the child."[25] If the events occurred two or three decades ago, when the incidence of child sexual abuse, especially incest, was believed by most mental health professionals to be a rare phenomena, it is conceivable that even contemporaneous psychological evaluation could have overlooked the possibility of abuse.

A more pointed objection to the clinician's demand for outside corroboration is that the level of skepticism implied about the patient's reliability is inimical to establishing a therapeutic relationship. Decades before the emergence of the false memory controversy, MacKinnon and Michels wrote: "The interview that is oriented only toward establishing a diagnosis gives the patient the feeling that he is a specimen of pathology being examined, and therefore actually inhibits him from revealing his problems"[19] (p. 7). McHugh's diagnostic stance is closer to Gutheil's characterization[26] of a forensic expert witness than to a therapist. In order to testify to "reasonable medical certainty" in an adversarial judicial proceeding, a forensic expert witness must evaluate all of the available information from both sides. Gutheil contrasts this function with the therapist's need to establish an alliance with a patient, in part by seeing the patient's experience through his eyes. While a therapeutic alliance does not imply an unquestioning acceptance of the historical accuracy of all the patient presents, it differs from the skeptical position of the forensic examiner. On the other hand, Gutheil states equally strongly that the therapist cannot properly bring this subjective therapeutic view of the patient's experience into the courtroom in the form of expert testimony.[26]

Among child psychiatrists, including child analysts, there is less variation in the scope of diagnostic evaluation. Because of the child's cognitive immaturity and legal incompetence, a child diagnostic assessment routinely includes interviewing the parents. The assessment may also involve obtaining medical and school records and observing the child outside of the therapist's office.

In cases of suspected incest, the child therapist, charged with legal responsibilities in most jurisdictions to report cases of suspected abuse, must come to some tentative conclusion about the reality of such an issue, even if not seeing the child in a defined forensic context. Unlike most therapists who primarily treat adult trauma patients, Lenore Terr insists that the psychiatrist *must* function as a detective. At a clinical case conference at the 1994 American Psychiatric Association Annual Meeting, Terr took issue with the psychiatrist presenting a case of a patient with an extraordinary history of abuse for failing to seek corroboration in birth and death certificates and hospital records.

The importance of a diagnosis in determining appropriate psychiatric treatment is arguable. Initial treatment interventions are often related more to levels of impairment or dangerousness than to diagnosis. Even in psychopharmacology, where one would expect the highest correlation between diagnosis and treatment, medications are frequently prescribed by symptom across diagnostic categories. Diagnostic accuracy often emerges from the treatment process—e.g., the diagnosis of a psychotic patient will be affected by a positive response to lithium. Therapeutic approaches for a given diagnosis vary both by the clinician's preferred treatment modalities and by a number of features in the patient which may be independent of the diagnosis, including available supports, level of functioning, reliability, ability to tolerate affects and contain impulses, current stressors, and motivation for treatment. In the specific issue of childhood sexual abuse, one may initiate psychotherapy without knowing the accuracy, significance, or even the existence of a history of abuse.

In psychoanalysis with adults, the analyst eschews obtaining information from sources other than the patient. Few analysts seek previous treatment records. To the analyst, the relevant information for an analytic formulation is found not in external sources, but in what is revealed in the patient's actions and productions when engaged in an analytic dialogue. Wallace argued that the elimination of psychodynamic data from DSM-III conceptualization did not reflect greater objectivity: "longitudinal history, the pattern of interpersonal relations, including those with the physician, the individual's experience of self-in-world phenomenology, motivation, and the inner life of fantasies, attitudes, meanings, expectations, conflicts, avoidances, and so forth: this reflects theory-driven decisions about what constitutes relevant information and reliable methodology."[27]

Far from accepting the patient's presentation at face value, the analyst assumes that the patient's defenses and conflicts produce distortions in the way the patient perceives, remembers, and relates his experiences. From these observations, the analyst constructs a tentative formulation of the patient's overall development and functioning as well as identifies specific areas of conflict which might make an analysis useful. Simultaneously, the analyst attempts to ascertain whether the patient is analyzable—that is, capable of tolerating the intense, regressive, and depriving conditions of an analysis.

In psychoanalytic therapies, the process of formulation is intertwined with the process of therapy. The analyst begins an analytic treatment with an assessment of the patient's analyzability, a formulation of the patient's developmental history, character, and current neurotic symptoms, and the expectation that the formulation will evolve through the course of the treatment. Greenson's observation that "sometimes one can arrive at a reliable diagnosis only at the end of a long analysis" is not atypical.[28] Moreover, many an analysis concludes with unresolved questions about the patient's history.

Trauma therapists point out that both the standard psychiatric interview and the open-ended psychodynamic interview failed to include explicit questions about childhood trauma, thereby frequently missing this possibility. Now attuned to the many conscious and unconscious barriers to a patient's disclosure of a history of abuse, therapists struggle with how to phrase these inquiries to allow for the fact that patients who remember childhood molestations may not label them as "trauma" or "incest" or even "unwanted touching." The more medically oriented interviewer expects straightforward answers to specific questions, and is suspicious that techniques pursuing "hidden" data suggest responses that the patient would not otherwise have.

When patients pursue their own searches for external validation during the course of therapy, many of the problems engendered by the therapist's search for evidence are obviated.[29,30] It may be appropriate for the therapist to explore why a patient has not sought corroboration for certain memories. Good, for example, in his analysis of a middle-aged woman with a memory of having had a clitoridectomy at age 5, expressed surprise that she had never sought confirmation of her memory from any of her gynecologists. Six months later, when the patient finally raised the question with her gynecologist, she was informed unequivocally that her genitals were intact.[31]

Considering Uncorroborated Memories

Although the preponderance of skepticism has been directed at the accuracy of recovered or reconstructed memories, the "always-held" memory is not above suspicion, and has not been exempted from demands for corroboration. The prototypic always-known false memory is Piaget's memory of a kidnapping attempt in early childhood—a story which turned out to have been fabricated by his nanny, but remembered as an experience by Piaget. Good's patient's false memory of having undergone a clitoridectomy was "always known."[31] However, generally clinicians do not question the gist of always-held memories. It seems as unreasonable to seek outside verification of a patient's initially presented, plausible memories of abuse as it would to request a death certificate from a patient who presented himself as a bereaved widower. Good was unable to find any case in the analytic literature—admittedly not a representative sample of a general psychiatric population—of a patient whose *memory* of sexual abuse was disproven.

On the other hand, it is equally illogical to exempt a story of a traumatic experience from the same considerations of differential diagnosis that would be applied to any piece of a patient's presentation. Malingering, Munchausen's syndrome, psychotic delusion (in delusional disorder, schizophrenia, mania, or depression), condensation of different experiences, and confabulation have all been mentioned as possibilities. Intrusive sexual thoughts may also be a symptom of OCD, as in the case of Mrs. A. A colleague described a more flagrant case of a child with severe OCD who began to complain to his parents that people were breaking into the house and forcing him to have sex—during times when the parents were at home with the child.

Of course, a psychotic patient may also have an accurate memory of abuse. Like children, the mentally ill and the mentally retarded are more vulnerable to experiences of abuse, but their stories are less likely to be regarded as credible.

As described by Levine,[1] the analytic view of memories of childhood has a long and convoluted history. The classic analytic position maintains that memory of an event is distorted by internal meanings both at the time of the occurrence of the event and with persistence of the memory through time. Arlow defined psychic reality in this way: "It is not a fantasy that is taken for real truth, for an actual event, but the 'real' recollection of a psychic event with its mixture of fact and fantasy. This becomes the dynamic reality for the patient under the influence of the traumatic events which live on in his inner fantasy. Subsequent events and perceptions of reality are selectively organized into memory schema consonant with inner fantasy thinking."[32]

For many decades analysts regarded both reconstructions and memories of incest as primarily fantasy driven, because of the belief in the powerful and universal influence of the Oedipus complex.[33] Simon found a remarkable dearth in the analytic literature of writing on the impact of actual incest until the last decade.[34] His title, "Incest—see under Oedipus complex," drawn from the index of an analytic text, exemplifies the degree to which external reality was subordinated to psychic reality. Greenacre, decrying the loss of interest among analysts in the effects of actual trauma, postulated that the coincidence of internal fantasy and external reality had a uniquely powerful pathogenic effect: "If the reinforcement [by reactions of others] has been much influenced by a single disturbing experience, verifying the infantile fantasy and making it powerfully real, the organizing effect of such an event is very great and the fantasy behind it gains much force"[35] (p. 440).

"Delayed" memories of trauma have elicited the greatest skepticism. Part of the current controversy reflects a lack of agreement about basic concepts such as forgetting, suppression, repression, dissociation, or amnesia. Some critics make no distinctions among reasons for the delay, casting blanket suspicion on any memories of trauma which emerge during the course of therapy. Memories of trauma are often omitted during an initial evaluation for conscious reasons. In a study by Della Femina and others, subjects with documented histories of significant abuse in adolescence were interviewed about their histories 9 years later. Of those with documented severe abuse who denied it in the follow up interview, the subjects explained the discrepancy by not wanting to talk about something upsetting, not liking or trusting the interviewer, or wishing to protect their parents.[36]

Similarly, in Williams's prospective study of women with documented childhood sexual abuse, some of the 38% of subjects who "forgot" their trauma consciously avoided discussing the incident.[37] In a follow-up analysis of her original study, Williams further demonstrated that some patients who eventually described the index incident of abuse did not initially respond positively to broad questions about childhood physical or sexual abuse. Some patients, for example, needed to be prompted by specific questions of sexual experiences in childhood with someone 5 years or more older—because the subjects otherwise did not label the incident as sexual abuse.[38] In initial evaluations, some patients who do not volunteer a history of abuse make no connection between their histories and their current difficulties.

Analysts regard the recall of childhood events during treatment as frequently the result of a lifting of repression, i.e., that unconscious defenses which interfere with remembering are weakened, allowing a return of a memory to consciousness.[39] The emergence of new memories in response to an interpretation is considered one aspect of confirmation of the interpretation, and no less accurate than other memories, with their mix of fact and fantasy. Conversely, the lack of actual memories to substantiate an interpretation of dreams, associations, or symptoms is taken as an indication that the interpretation may be incorrect. On the other hand, some analysts may conclude that the preponderance of clinical evidence supports a formulation of childhood abuse, even when no memories emerge.

Although clinicians generally agree that memory is complex and may be inaccurate, the nature of traumatic memories remains controversial. As analysts have turned their attention more to traumatized patients, differing opinions have emerged about the fate of memories of severe trauma. Galatzer-Levy's view in this volume[2] that traumatic memory is dissociated rather than repressed does not represent a consensus among psychoanalysts. For example, Burland and Raskin, summarizing several years of a discussion group of the American Psychoanalytic Association on the psychoanalysis of adults who were sexually abused as children, found that repression of memories occurred in most instances, with recovery of memories in the course of analysis.[40] This general psychodynamic view that repressed memories of childhood can be accurately recovered has been supported by cases in which some external corroboration was eventually obtained by the patient.[39,41] Still, at least some analysts maintain that massive trauma is never repressed. Adler, for example, recently wrote: "Severe traumas, unlike so-called normal traumas, can never be forgotten, nor can they be integrated by means of screen memories with their anxiety binding functions."[42]

Psychotherapy cases in which some external validation of recovered memories of childhood trauma was obtained have also been cited.[43,44] Nash described a case in which a memory of childhood trauma recovered during a therapy that included hypnosis was confirmed by a witness;[45] Nagy described a patient undergoing hypnosis for panic symptoms, not memory retrieval, whose recovered memory of childhood sexual abuse was supported by photographs and family members.[30] The widely cited Herman and Schatzow study, though describing both examples of amnesia and corroboration, is difficult to evaluate because the cases were composites and because the incidence of complete amnesia with subsequent corroboration of recovered memories is not spelled out.[29]

The proliferation of studies of trauma victims has renewed interest in dissociation rather than repression as the defense most commonly associated with trauma.[46–49] Dissociative phenomena include depersonalization and derealization as well as amnestic states. However, considerable disagreement about the characteristics of a dissociated memory remains.

Some view a dissociated memory as a "flashbulb" retaining a highly accurate picture of the original event—one more accurate than normal memory. Terr, for example, whose research of children's memory of trauma showed misperceptions, although the "gist" might be correct,[50,51] nevertheless characterized James Ellroy's memories of being informed of his mother's murder as "burned in visual memories . . . horror registered clearer than clear. A photo by Ansel Adams. A Vermeer painting."[52] Ross argues that the dissociated memory is not unconscious and is therefore not susceptible to contamination by unconscious elements of fantasy or drive.[53] Galatzer-Levy[2] similarly states that although a repressed memory cannot be accurately recalled later, a dissociated memory is conscious but inaccessible, and therefore reliable when it is recalled. Neither Ross nor Galatzer-Levy clearly explain how dissociated and repressed memories are clinically distinguishable, and their arguments for the accuracy of dissociated memory are tautologies. van der Kolk argues that traumas are remembered differently from normal memories, but places his emphasis on nonverbal, sensory components of memory rather than altered states of consciousness.[49]

Spiegel, who also regards dissociation as a trauma-related defense, expects a dissociated memory to be *more* fragmented and less coherent than other memories because of the distorting influence of dissociation at the time of the traumatic event. He differentiates dissociation, as an ongoing defensive response at the time of trauma, from repression, as a post-event phenomenon. Spiegel's testimony for the defense in the Franklin trial was partially based on his belief that the trauma described by Eileen Franklin (witnessing her father's murder of her best friend at the age of 8) would have produced a dissociated memory that would have been far less coherent than her testimony.[54] Spiegel's view that dissociated memories are subject to later influence and alterations contradicts Terr, Ross, and Galatzer-Levy.

Others dispute the connection between dissociation and trauma. The core of these arguments is that dissociative phenomena are insufficiently distinguished from hypnotizability or "fantasy proneness," which are distributed throughout the population. Ganaway, for example, considers memories of a patient with a dissociative disorder *more* suspect in their historical accuracy than other memories.[55] He proposes that patients with dissociative disorders, like the Grade V highly hypnotizables described by H. Spiegel, are subject to spontaneous trance states in which they are vulnerable to confusing fantasy with memory, especially if suggestive influences are present.

Clinicians' judgments about the validity of memories reflect their beliefs of what is possible and what is likely. Clinical and experimental data demonstrate that detailed verbal memories, including traumatic memories, of events before the age of two and a half rarely arise from the patient's own recall.[50] Alien abduction and past lives are readily placed in the category of the impossible. Satanic ritual abuse, although possible, is dismissed by most on the basis of a lack of corroboration by law enforcement. Others hold a more jaundiced view of the reliability of law enforcement or other official reports. Personal or professional experiences with sexual abuse may bias the clinician to greater or lesser degrees of suspecting the possibility of abuse. The therapist with a personal history of abuse may see abuse everywhere—or need to remain blind to its existence.

McHugh and others argue for a high degree of skepticism of the likelihood of incestuous abuse by the stably married, pillar-of-the-community, biological father.

Spence found Greenacre's reconstruction of a primal scene experience implausible because the father in the case was a Calvinist minister whom he thought would be highly private in his sexual practices. The essence of Freud's legacy is a vision that beneath the niceties of civilization lurk the dark, the violent, the irrational, and the infantile; beneath the veneer of middle-class, church-going respectability may lie spousal abuse, alcoholism, drug addiction, sexual perversion, and venomous relationships. It wasn't long ago that sexual abuse by a Boy Scout leader, a parish priest, a teacher at a prestigious prep school, or a respected psychiatrist (including some presumably well-analyzed analysts) seemed unlikely—all occurrences which have been substantiated in recent years.

Given the difficulties in ascertaining the truth of memories, some therapists opt to abandon this seemingly impossible task. Arguing against this epistemological despair, Shevrin reminds us that *all* human interaction contains the possibility that a communication is true, fantasied, or a lie: ". . . we all remember, misremember, and fail to remember many times during the day. We act as if we know when we are *really* remembering and when we are fantasizing. Moreover, we apply the same judgment to what others tell us, deciding if they are 'telling the truth,' selectively recalling, lying, or simply making things up. Life with others (and with ourselves) would be impossible if we failed to make such judgments and, *most important, if we were not right a good deal of the time*"[56] (second italics mine).

Suspecting Abuse When No Memories Are Present

In 1983, Gelinas described the disguised presentation typical of a history of incest as "a characterological depression with complications and with atypical impulsive and dissociative elements."[57] In the years since, the list of signs, symptoms, and diagnoses which could be correlated to a history of childhood abuse has steadily grown. In addition to PTSD, dissociative disorders, self-mutilating behavior, sexual dysfunction, borderline personality disorder, and eating disorders have been suggested as outcomes of childhood abuse.[9,58–62]

It is widely agreed that there are no pathognomonic signs and symptoms of a history of childhood sexual trauma.[1,43,47] However, pathognomonic symptoms are rare in psychiatric diagnoses, and many pathogenic factors have multiple possible outcomes. It may well be that childhood sexual abuse is a nonspecific risk factor for a wide range of adult psychiatric disorders.

The attempt to ascribe specific outcomes to childhood sexual trauma is complicated by the wide variety of experiences which might be included by the term. Weil documented a range of events, from observation of adult sexual activity to overt sexual abuse, with marked pathological impact because of their overstimulation of sexual and aggressive instincts in the child, particularly at specific developmental phases.[63] Elements of violence, repetition, the identity of the abuser, and responses to disclosure at the time are significant variables.[64] Other bodily traumas, such as medical problems or procedures, may be experienced as intrusive, overwhelming, frightening, or damaging. When Sherkow proposed guidelines for the psychoanalytic evaluation for sexual abuse in little girls,[65] Good argued that the clinical presentations described could also have resulted from a child's viewing pornographic material.[66] Moreover, in cases of incest, the actual sexual abuse is not the only trauma to which the child is subjected. A general lack of parental empathy and nurturance provides a potent backdrop to the impact of aggressive and sexual traumas, and the clinical picture will include a mix of depriving and overstimulating environmental influences with the individual's temperamental endowment through different phases of development.[1–4]

Guidelines have been proposed which might lead an analytically oriented therapist to suspect a history of sexual abuse. Dissociative symptoms, promiscuity, somatization, sexual dysfunction, castration fears, repetitive traumatic dreams, depressive affect, pathological doubting, sadomasochistic relationships, gaps in reality testing, poor capacity to symbolize, and learning problems have been cited.[43,47,64,67–69] Levine, with many caveats, proposes that the best, though by no means foolproof, indicator, is the nature of the transference that develops. This transference, characterized by an intensity more typical of psychotic transferences, at times loses its "as if" quality for the patient. The content of the transference typically includes profound fears of being abused or exploited by the therapist.

Currently, the diagnostic syndromes considered to be most specifically associated with extensive childhood trauma are the dissociative disorders. Certainly, some dissociative symptoms occur in patients without a history of major trauma. Brenner described an analysand who responded to intense painful affects by going into a dreamlike state.[70] Ludwig regarded the walling off of catastrophic experiences as only one of several functions of dissociation, which also included automatization of behaviors, such as driving on the highway; resolution of irreconcilable conflicts; economy and efficiency of effort, allowing single-minded focus on a task; escape from reality, as in many religious trance states; and cathartic discharge of feelings, as well as social cohesion in group trance rituals or behaviors.[71] I consulted on a young male patient who had debilitating depersonalized, out-of-body responses to severe social anxiety. He had been a sensitive child who had felt overwhelmed by his parents' arguing and his older brother's bullying, and had dissociated in response to interpersonal anxiety since adolescence.

Many clinicians agree with Matthews and Chu that severe dissociative pathology is rare in the absence of significant trauma. Bitter controversy has erupted over the diagnosis of multiple personality disorder (MPD), renamed dissociative identity disorder (DID) in DSM-IV. Mersky,[72] McHugh,[73] and Weissberg[74] maintain that the sharp rise in the diagnosis of what was previously believed to be a very rare disorder is iatrogenically produced by suggestive therapeutic techniques. Proponents of the diagnosis such as Kluft[75] and Ross[76] explain that the increase in diagnosis results from years of underdiagnosing the syndrome by clinicians who did not know what to look for. For example, they feel that many patients previously diagnosed as schizophrenic were really suffering from DID.

The highest rates of histories of childhood abuse have been found in adults with DID—up to 97% in a study by Putnam et al.[77] The bulk of these patients report incest, and the reports of satanic ritual abuse have largely come from patients with DID. Many clinicians therefore consider a diagnosis of DID as a posttraumatic one.[46,53,78] Frankel has questioned this association, since many of the studies reporting the correlation of sexual abuse with MPD lacked outside verification.[79] In fact, arguments about most studies correlating a clinical diagnosis with rates of childhood abuse hinge upon the reliability of patient reports.[80] A different contradiction arises from studies such as the case reports of DID in India, in which none of the three patients described had a history of trauma, despite the researchers' openness to such a possibility. In two of the three cases the precipitating factor appeared to be a love interest that was strongly disapproved by the family—an etiology closer to a neurotic conflict.[81]

Some clinicians assert that a diagnosis of DID may be missed unless special diagnostic procedures are followed. Recommendations such as the use of hypnosis or extraordinarily long interviews to bring out alter personality states are exceptional to both traditional medical and psychodynamic evaluative procedures. Other special techniques are applications of the symptom-focused interviews typified by DSM-III. Lowenstein advocates incorporating questions regarding symptoms such as amnesia and autohypnotic states into the mental status exam,[82] while Ross promotes structured clinical interviews such as the Dissociative Disorders Interview Schedule (DDIS) he developed.[83] Critics charge that either special procedures or focused diagnostic questions may create rather than uncover the condition,[72,73] although proponents of the diagnosis retort that hypnosis produces only a partial version of symptom picture of MPD.[84]

Should the therapist communicate to a patient her suspicions of a forgotten history of abuse? Sauzier has characterized the disclosure process in psychotherapy as a series of three dialogues: one within the patient, one within the therapist, and one between therapist and patient.[85] On the basis of the patient's overall picture, the therapist may ask more specifically about childhood trauma, even if these questions were initially denied. These inquiries may trigger questioning in the patient.

A further step is an interpretation that raises the possibility that abuse occurred. Herman[9] and Matthews and Chu[43] warn that a premature confrontation of the patient could be retraumatizing. Psychoanalysts, concerned with the suggestive and contaminating impact of such an intervention, would not present such a formulation until well into a treatment, when there was an accumulation of a great deal of relevant material. Ross, however, routinely informs patients at the time they are diagnosed with MPD that the disorder is ''a survival strategy for the abused child.''[86]

There is a wide spectrum of concern about the therapist's inadvertent influence on the patient's reconstructions. Ever since Freud repudiated hypnosis, psychoanalysts have fretted over the degree to which suggestion might contaminate the analytic process. Many contemporary analysts now renounce the classic analytic view of the ''pure gold'' of interpretation, instead conceptualizing transference and interpretation as unavoidably affected by the analyst's subjectivity. Raphling, for example, asserts that all analytic interpretation has an interactional component of suggestion that cannot be avoided at the time of interpretation, but only mitigated by post hoc exploration by patient and analyst. He writes: ''It is difficult for the patient not to experience an interpretation as advocating something, and difficult for the analyst to frame an interpretation that is not, in fact, advocating something''[87] (p. 105). For example, a patient with a plausible history of paternal incest described a series of obscene phone calls she had received. Although the calls continued after she changed her number to a new, unlisted one, they stopped immediately after she told her father that a trace was being put on her line. I pointed out that she was not saying what she obviously suspected— that her father was making the calls. While not stating that her father was the caller, my comment nevertheless implied this.

The increasingly common phenomenon of the patient who comes to therapy with suspicions of childhood abuse, requesting help in memory retrieval, has been explored in several cases in the analytic literature. Raphling discussed a patient who began analysis believing she had been incestuously abused, but having no memories. He observed that the patient's thoughts of abuse intensified at points in the analysis when she was struggling with Oedipal conflicts. The patient repeatedly pushed him to confirm her sense of having been abused. Eventually, Raphling interpreted the patient's belief of having been abused as a defense against Oedipal disappointment, and the analysis ended with both patient and analyst concluding that no incest had occurred. His conclusion was based not only on the pattern of when her concerns about incest arose but also on the lack of transference enactments and other signs and symptoms which analysts now associate with histories of abuse.[88] Shengold described three patients who sought treatment with him because of his reputation for working with traumatized patients. These patients' initial beliefs of having been sexually abused were not borne out in their analyses, which instead generated pictures of a type of narcissism.[89]

In contrast, Herman and Schatzow accepted into their groups for incest survivors some patients who had no memories of abuse prior to beginning the group therapy. Several of these patients indicated that their goals for participating in the group were to recover memories of abuse. For example, ''Doris'' was referred by her couple therapist who suspected abuse, presumably on the basis of the patient's presentation of increasing panic attacks during intercourse. Placing a patient who is suspected of having an abuse history in a group identified for incest survivors is clearly suggestive, though Herman and Harvey are critical of therapists who make ''unwarranted inferences about their patient's histories without waiting for their stories to unfold.''[90]

Special techniques such as hypnosis or sodium amytol interviews have been advocated to retrieve forgotten memories. Freud abandoned hypnosis for memory retrieval for the same reason that has put it again under attack: the problem of suggestion inherent in the technique. In Yapko's recent survey, clinicians with various levels of training and experience revealed a disturbingly high level of confidence in the validity of memories generated under hypnosis, including memories of past life experiences.[91] Frankel's partial review of the MPD literature in 1993 cited frequent use of hypnosis and sodium amytal interviewing in the large case series reported by Putnam et al. and Ross on the incidence of childhood abuse in MPD patients.[79]

Hypnotherapists are increasingly divided on the use of hypnosis to enhance memory of childhood events. Although Frankel in 1978 described "the other traditional role of hypnosis in therapy, namely, that of aiding in the exploring and recovering aspects,"[92] he now cautions that "there does not seem to be substantial evidence to support the claim that hypnosis can be a dependable instrument in the recovery of memory."[93] Herman[9] and Matthews and Chu[43] opine that hypnosis for the recall of traumatic childhood memories is rarely necessary, but neither delineate when the procedure is indicated nor its possible drawbacks. Guidelines to minimize the introduction of suggestion during hypnosis have been proposed.[94] However, Frankel maintains that even when direct suggestion is scrupulously avoided, memories are often confabulated as a result of the suggestive context of hypnosis. Such memories hold greater credibility for the patient because of the beliefs most people hold about hypnosis (Frankel, personal communication). Erdelyi concluded from experimental data that "no hypnosis-specific effect on memory enhancement had been demonstrated," thereby disputing the basic rationale for using hypnosis for memory retrieval[95] (p. 386). Although continuing to regard hypnosis as "inevitably a part of these (DID) patients' treatments," Kluft now acknowledges that "the cautions of those who fear iatrogenic . . . generation of confabulations and pseudomemories are not without substance"[84] (p. 370).

The Question of the Therapist's Validation of the Patient's Memories

The principle of analytic neutrality is frequently invoked in the discussion of the therapist's role in validating the patient's memories. The trauma patient may sorely test the psychotherapist's adherence to neutrality by demanding that the therapist declare whether what she remembers is true. Levine conceptualizes this entreaty as an enactment of the universal childhood wish for an omniscient parent, and describes the optimal analytic role as helping the patient work through the pathological doubting which is often a residue of incest. He views pronouncements by the analyst of "what really happened" as an abandonment of neutrality, although he recognizes that not all patients can tolerate the uncertainty required by a sustained analytic inquiry. Levine regards the reconstruction of trauma as a *possible* historical reconstruction.[67] Although many analysts[4,96] take the position that the analyst must leave it to the patient to struggle with the question of certainty, some advocate the analyst's verifying the experience. Kramer[68] supports this stance from her experience that she has never seen a fabricated case of incest—an argument also advanced by Herman and Harvey.[90]

Matthews and Chu argue for neutrality in the psychotherapy of trauma patients. They suggest that the therapist acknowledge to the patient the general reality of child abuse—and therefore the plausibility of the patient's reconstruction—while explaining the limits of the therapist's knowledge of what happened to the patient. They also emphasize the important supportive function of the therapist's empathic attempts to help the patient bear the painful uncertainties of sorting out what happened.[43]

Psychodynamic therapists such as Matthews and Chu also recommend minimizing suggestive influences on their patients. Psychoanalysis, with its greater focus on all aspects of the transference, provides more opportunity than psychotherapy for monitoring positive transferences and the compliant interactions which may ensue.

Herman seems ambivalent about the power of the transference to affect the patient. In describing the patient's vulnerability to abuse by a therapist, she writes: "[the patient] submits herself to an unequal relationship in which the therapist has superior status and power. Feelings related to the universal childhood experience of dependence on a parent are inevitably aroused. These feelings, known as transference, further exaggerate the power imbalance in the therapeutic relationship and render all patients vulnerable to exploitation" [9] (p. 134). Yet, in her response to the accusation that therapists plant false memories in their patients' minds, Herman minimizes these determinants: "patients will respond only when those suggestions [of the therapist] resonate with their own feelings and experiences. If the therapist is on the wrong track most patients simply say so."[90]

Ross implies that so long as he does not explicitly validate a specific unsubstantiated memory of abuse, there is little reason to be concerned with suggestion. His interventions assume abuse as a fact of the patient's history—e.g., "[y]ou are looking at present day reality from the emotional perspective of an abused child who is trapped in her reality, and you are afraid to separate from your abuser based on the actual reality of the past,"[53] (p. 370) as does his informing of the newly diagnosed DID patient that the syndrome is a response to trauma.[86]

Other therapists, noting that the patient's initial experience of abuse was often compounded by being disbelieved when she reported the abuse to an adult, advocate validating a patient's traumatic memory by explicitly stating a belief that what the patient says is true. For example, Olio and Cornell write: "[B]ecause of the years of silence, the family denial, and the victim's own disconnection from personal history, in the therapeutic effort to resolve abuse, the question 'Did it really happen?' is of critical importance. Therapeutic validation requires an acknowledgment of the abuse as an external reality"[97] (p. 520). The wording here is critical. It is one thing to convey to the patient that the therapist believes her story, and another for the therapist to say "I *know* what happened to you."

Although there are patients who cannot tolerate a therapy in which a therapist is unwilling to take this stand, the therapist's early validation may complicate the therapy. Ganaway[55] warns that the therapist's confirmation may force the patient into further doubt by occupying one side of the patient's ambivalence. Furthermore, by claiming a more knowing position than the patient, the therapist encourages the patient to experience herself as dependent and less competent.

Matthews and Chu, while adhering to a neutral stance, acknowledge that there comes a point in the therapy when certain aspects of history are accepted as true by both patient and therapist. The most neutral therapist may eventually drop such qualifiers as ''from what you've told me . . . .'' or ''you felt that . . . .'' Once the patient has substantially resolved her ambivalence about the reality of certain experiences, and the therapist feels that sufficient work has been done to minimize distortions and to explore defensive functions of such memories, the therapist's persistence in interjecting doubt about the memories would be unnecessarily undermining to the patient.[43,98]

A neutral position regarding the reality of what happened differs from the medical model. McHugh regards the clinician faced with a question of sexual abuse as having both the ability and the responsibility to make a reasonable determination of what happened—a position also held by some trauma therapists. For example, Butterfield, arguing against McHugh on the reality of memories of childhood sexual abuse, also implied the clinician *could* and *should* arrive at an accurate conclusion about what had happened, though she concluded that the memories were invariably true.[99] In a case on which I was consulted, a psychiatrist had evinced the obverse bias when he informed a bipolar patient that the memories of sexual abuse by her stepfather that she had recovered in therapy were false, despite the fact that the patient's mother and father believed that their daughter's story explained concerns they had about her childhood. The psychiatrist asserted that because severe trauma is never forgotten, the patient's memories must be false.

Does History Matter?

One of the more remarkable arguments against the reconstruction or exploration of a traumatic history is that it doesn't matter anyway. This proposition emerges from several different sources.

The genetic principle, no longer relevant to DSM categories, has been further eroded by advances in biological psychiatry. Schizophrenia seems to have little to do with schizophrenogenic mothers; obsessive-compulsive disorders appear to be determined more by serotonin levels than toilet-training experiences. Many psychiatrists see little reason for needing to know much about a patient's childhood history.

Ross advances a pragmatic argument for the irrelevance of a traumatic history.[53] Having abandoned reconstructive and abreactive techniques which he found unnecessarily regressive and destabilizing, he now uses an amalgam of psychodynamic and cognitive behavioral techniques for traumatized patients. (The techniques Ross discontinued are not derived from current psychodynamic practices, but from a model of psychoanalytic technique which predated the development of ego psychology.) Because cognitive behavioral techniques focus more on the here-and-now than do psycho-dynamic therapies, he argues that the techniques work (i.e., produce symptom relief) even if the associated childhood memories are not accurate. Levine agrees that the false reconstruction of trauma may nevertheless produce symptom relief in a patient, by providing a simplified, sanctioned, and less conflicted identity as a trauma victim.[1]

However, Ross' case examples raise thorny questions. He describes a patient who justified having abused her children with the delusion that she was actually protecting the children by making them undesirable to a Satanic cult. Although in the vignette he explains his decision not to confront the patient with the inaccuracy of this belief, it is not difficult to argue that at some point, if the patient is to be well, she must recognize this belief as a delusion used to absolve her from guilt. Therapy generally includes helping a patient with reality testing.

In his influential book *Narrative Truth and Historical Truth*,[100] Spence took the more radical position that the proper role of the psychoanalyst is in working with his patient only to establish a narrative or psychic truth. He urged analysts to relinquish their attempts to make historical inferences and instead measure their interpretations by the narrative coherence and "pragmatic power" that they imparted to the patient.

Shengold, while sharing Spence's appreciation of the poetic and creative aspects of psychoanalysis, denounced the view that the historical truth is irrelevant to the analytic enterprise. He compared Spence's statement that "we can create truth by statement" to the totalitarian control of history described in Orwell's *1984:* "For when it [the past] has been recreated in whatever shape is needed at the moment, then this new version *is* the past, and no different past can ever have existed"[4] (p.30). Shengold holds that actual trauma is a decidedly different experience that the fantasy of trauma. He writes: "Being able to define the limits of 'did it really happen?' almost always helps the patient; this has been true even in those sad instances where the patient has had to conclude, and therefore know, only that he or she can simply never know"[4] (p.40).

Two types of errors regarding a patient's history are cited: the positive error of assuming a history of trauma when none existed, and a negative error of failing to establish the existence of a significant trauma history. However, other errors might occur: erroneously attributing pathogenic influence to a childhood experience that had occurred but had not been traumatic, or conversely, failing to recognize such an influence of a remembered event, and vast possibilities for partially true memories of childhood trauma. For example, a patient might correctly recall having been molested, but be mistaken about who the molester was, or at what age it occurred, etc. What harm, if any, develops from which errors?

A 1967 paper by Sachs[101] was unusual in the analytic literature for the author's conclusion that his failure to distinguish between real and fantasied elements led to a patient's need for further analysis—a negative error. In this case, the reality consisted of certain events that confirmed to the then six-and-a-half-year-old child that her mother was having an affair. What the analyst felt had been repressed was the mother's injunction to the patient not to tell. As in cases of incestuous abuse, the analytic formulation here is that the event was particularly pathogenic because of its resonance with deeply conflicted Oedipal wishes.[101]

Williams described her reconstruction of a sexual molestation of her male patient at about the age of 2 by a beloved male servant. She was startled to hear for the first time from the patient that his previous analyst had made a similar interpretation. However, while the first analyst had not attributed a great deal of significance to this reconstruction, Williams saw it as one of several critical developmental experiences for the patient. She felt that the patient's much greater improvement in the second analysis resulted from working through the meanings of the trauma. Though the patient had some confirmatory sense of the location in which the repeated molestations occurred, he never recovered any actual memories, which Williams thought was explained by his young age and the intensity of the trauma.[102]

In Good's case of the patient who falsely believed she had been subjected to a clitoridectomy in childhood to end her recurrent masturbation, he concluded that "uncovering the distorted fantasy [of the clitoridectomy] appeared to make more extensive analytic treatment unnecessary." He compared this outcome to some analytic interventions with children that were also more in the nature of "reconstructing the child's misinterpretation of events rather than the events themselves"[31] (p.96). In this case, the patient's fantasy had a profound pathogenic effect.

Even when there is a believable history of trauma, analysts struggle with the question of the relative importance of trauma and internal wishes as pathogenic factors. Person and Klar[47] refer to Joseph's argument that overemphasizing the former may "reinforce a defensive view of oneself as a passive victim of events which denies the patient's creative role in his adaptation," while focusing entirely on the role of wishes may "suggest that patients are omnipotent in determining their intrapsychic reality and thereby denying human helplessness and limitation in the face of external reality"[103] (p.175).

Raphling, while noting the pathogenic impact of childhood sexual abuse, also provides a psychodynamic explanation for a patient's false belief of having been sexually abused. He writes that "the concept of sexual abuse trauma offers one ready explanation for the misery endured in life, for it allows one to assign blame, to feel entitled to compensation, and to enjoy vengeful wishes" and moreover "explains a neurosis that is otherwise complicated and difficult to understand."[88] In my case of Mrs. A, the possibility that she had been sexually abused was preferable to her believing she was a lesbian. On the other hand, many patients who have been profoundly neglected and abused by their parents cling to the fantasy of having been loved—a phenomena that Shengold labeled a "quasi-delusion."[4]

While emphasizing the importance of truth telling in the therapeutic process, Herman is the least troubled of the authors disscussed here by the difficulties in establishing what is historically true. After creating a safe therapeutic relationship, she recommends that "the next step is to reconstruct the traumatic event as a *recitation of fact*"[9] (my italics; p. 177). In *Trauma and Memory,* there is virtually no discussion of the problem of distorted or confabulated memories. Her discussion of the therapist's, as well as the patient's, need to tolerate uncertainty refers to the gaps of memory which may persist— not to possible inaccuracies.

Most psychodynamic therapists consider the remembrance and abreaction of childhood trauma as a necessary but not sufficient curative factor.[42] Analysts emphasize the "working through" of sequelae of childhood events, including their influence on character formation and interpersonal relationships, as in Williams's case above.[1,47,102] Bernstein writes that "repair of ego deficits seemed more dependent on the analysis of the consequences and conflicts related to maternal deprivation than on uncovering the details of the incest experience itself"[69] (p.89). Contemporary psychoanalysts now share with their cognitive behavioral colleagues the perspective that their greatest interest in their patients' childhood histories is in the light it sheds on what the patient has carried forth from the experience.[104]

Herman adds moral, social, and existential arguments to the importance of establishing a history of trauma: "Remembering and retelling the truth about terrible events are prerequisites both for the restoration of the social order and for the healing of individual victims"[9] (p.1). Herman and other trauma therapists clearly feel that the greatest moral failing is the therapist's failure to align with the traumatized victim. However, any psychotherapy based upon an entirely inaccurate view of the patient's experiences must damage the patient's sense of reality and authenticity, including the false positive as well as the false negative mistakes. The patient with pseudomemories of a happy childhood may be alienated from his perceptions, feelings, thoughts, and behaviors, which have been stripped of any meaningful context. Shengold writes: "To feel that we have an identity, we must know (or at least feel that we know) what is and was 'real'; we must trust that at least some of our memories, if not most of them, are true, and be able to set them apart from our conscious fantasies"[4] (p.16). Even if the patient shows symptomatic improvement with fallacious memories of childhood, whether happy or tragic, it is morally objectionable for the therapist to knowingly—or even non-chalantly—participate in sustaining these beliefs.

Conclusions

Authors often conclude reviews of the complexities of trauma and memory with calls for further research. The research needs to be done and will help to deepen and refine our understanding of these patients, and to untangle some of these disputed issues. However, the notion that research can completely resolve these dilemmas is an illusion. If current trends in research continue, we will accumulate more data that the response to trauma is heterogeneous: some people remember and some, by whatever mechanism, don't. We may learn more about predisposing factors to one response or another, or prevailing rates of remembering fully, partially, not at all, always, sometimes, or never. Nevertheless, faced with an *individual* in one's office, uncertainty will remain about the accuracy of specific memories.

In uncertain circumstances, is the best course that advised by Hyman and Loftus,[105] or Frankel,[23] the Hippocratic principle "to do no harm?" Hyman and Loftus compare withholding therapy from a patient with an unsubstantiated abuse history to not giving chemotherapy to a patient without a definitive diagnosis of cancer. However, active treatment in the face of an uncertain diagnosis abounds in medicine. We offer potent medication to a migraine patient on the basis of history alone; the surgeon must proceed to operate on the acute abdomen on the *suspicion* of appendicitis, fully knowing that sometimes the surgery, with all of its risks, may prove to have been unnecessary. The psychiatrist evaluating a suicidal patient may employ clinical guidelines drawn from the vast research literature on suicide, but must then decide whether an involuntary hospitalization in the long run is more or less likely to help this individual.

Clinicians may err more in one direction or the other but cannot avoid acting in the face of ambiguity. Whether using a diagnosis or a dynamic formulation, the clinician must constantly reconsider his hypothesis. The medical model advocated by McHugh, with its challenging stance toward the patient, narrow diagnostic criteria, and heavy reliance on external proof, is likely to result in significant rates of false-negative diagnoses and to discourage a traumatized patient from seeking treatment; trauma therapists who diagnose early without external corroboration risk making false-positive diagnoses.

The therapist needs to take a humble position regarding knowledge of a patient's history. When relying upon internal, psychodynamically derived observations, the clinician must be able to apply criteria which might refute, as well as substantiate, suspected histories of abuse. The clinician who seeks external verification must also be aware of the limitations of such an approach. In any case, often the best that the clinician can do is to seek to construct the most plausible explanation for the totality of the patient's experience. The psychotherapist should be as free to raise the possibility that the patient was sexually abused as he is to question such a hypothesis.

It may remain impossible to escape the problem so clearly delineated by Brenneis: that the therapeutic conditions necessary to allow a patient to disclose and work through experiences of abuse may be the very conditions which also give rise to inaccurate suggestions of such a history.[106] However, we cannot be so paralyzed by this conundrum that we abandon the practice of psychotherapy, which is still the best that we can offer to many of our patients. As argued by J. M. Ross:[107]

> These past occurrences matter. History matters . . . lies and even half truths can be dangerous. While the vicissitudes of psychic reality make the search for actualities a difficult one . . . nonetheless they still matter. . . . Remembering and reconstructing the past, or simply trying to remember and reconstruct it, are vital if only to provide hope. If we can't do them right, not just yet, we should keep on trying. We should keep on trying . . . for the sake of truth, whatever the consequences, and however imperfectly. (p. 570)

References

1. Levine HB: Psychoanalysis, reconstruction, and the recovery of memory. *In* PA Appelbaum, LA Uyehara, MS Elin (Eds.), Trauma and Memory: Clinical and Legal Controversies. New York: Oxford University Press, 1997, pp. 293–315.
2. Galatzer-Levy R: Psychoanalysis, memory, and trauma. *In* PA Appelbaum, LA Uyehara, MS Elin, (Eds.), Trauma and Memory: Clinical and Legal Controversies. New York: Oxford University Press, 1997, pp. 138–157.
3. Shengold L: Child Abuse: "Did it really happen?" paper delivered at the Sixth Susan J. Wise Memorial Lecture, Boston Psychoanalytic Society and Institute, Cambridge Mass., April 29, 1995.
4. Shengold L: Soul Murder. New York: Fawcett Columbine, 1989.
5. Menninger K, Mayman M, Pruyser P: The Vital Balance. New York: Viking Press, 1963.
6. Frances A, Cooper A: Descriptive and dynamic psychiatry: a perspective on DSM-III. Am J Psychiatry 1981; 138:1198–1202.
7. Klerman GL, Vaillant GE, Spitzer RL, Michels R: A debate on DSM-III. Am J Psychiatry 1984; 141:539–553.
8. Wilson M: DSM-III and the transformation of American psychiatry: a history. Am J Psychiatry 1993; 150:399–410.
9. Herman J: Trauma and Recovery. New York: Basic Books, 1992.
10. Neiderland WG: Clinical observations on the "survivor syndrome." Int J Psychoanal 1968; 49:313–315.
11. Yehuda R, MacFarlane AC: Conflict between current knowledge about post traumatic stress disorder and its original conceptual basis. Am J Psychiatry 1995; 152:1705–1713.
12. Bremner JD, Southwick SM, Johnson DR, Yehuda R, Charney DS: Childhood abuse and combat-related posttraumatic stress disorder in Vietnam veterans. Am J Psychiatry 1993; 150:235–239.
13. Pitman RK, Orr SP, Lowenhagen MJ, Macklin ML, Altman B: Pre-Vietnam contents of PTSD veterans' service medical and personnel records. Compr Psychiatry 1991; 32:1–7.
14. Schnurr PP, Friedman MJ, Rosenberg SD: Premilitary MMPI scores as predictors of combat-related PTSD symptoms. Am J Pschiatry 1993; 150:479–483.
15. Horowitz MJ, Bonanno GA, Holen A: Pathological grief: diagnosis and explanation. Psychosom Med 1993; 55:260–273.
16. Brent DA, Perper JA, Morritz G, Liotus L, Richardson D, Canobbio R, Schweers J, Roth C: Posttraumatic stress disorder in peers of adolescent suicide victims: predisposing factors and phenomenology. J Am Acad Child Adolesc Psychiatry 1995; 209–215.
17. Pinsker H: Memorandum to the Task Force on Nomenclature and Statistics, Jan 1, 1975. *In* Robert L Spitzer Papers. New York: New York State Psychiatric Institute.
18. Reiser MF: Are psychiatric educators losing the mind? Am J Psychiatry 1988; 145:148–153.
19. MacKinnon RA, Michels R: The Psychiatric Interview in Clinical Practice. Philadelphia: WB Saunders, 1971.
20. McHugh P: Viewpoints—Do patients memories of sexual abuse constitute a "false memory syndrome?" Psychiatr News Dec. 19, 1993, p. 18.
21. McHugh P: The do's and don'ts for the clinician managing memories of abuse. Paper delivered at Memory and Reconciliation Conference, Baltimore MD, December 1994.
22. Kestenberg J: What children remember and parents forget. Int J Psychoanal Psychother 1972; 1:103–123.
23. Frankel F: Discovering new memories in psychotherapy—childhood revisited, fantasy, or both? Sounding board. Engl J Med 1995; 333:591–594.

24. Appelbaum PS, Zoltek-Jick R: Psychotherapists' duties to third parties: *Ramona* and beyond. Am J Psychiatry 1996; 153:457–465.
25. Paradise JE: Predictive accuracy and the diagnosis of sexual abuse: a big issue about a little tissue. Child Abuse Negl 1989; 13:169–176.
26. Gutheil T: True or false memories of sexual abuse? A forensic psychiatric view. Psychiatric Ann 1993; 23:527–531.
27. Wallace ER: What is truth? some philosophical contributions to psychiatric issues. Am J Psychiatry 1988; 145:137–147.
28. Greenson R: The Technique and Practice of Psychoanalysis. Madison, CT: International Universities Press, 1967, p. 53.
29. Herman J, Schatzow E: Recovery and verification of memories of childhood trauma. Psychoanal Psychol 1987; 4:1–14.
30. Nagy TF: Incest memories recalled in hypnosis—a case study: a brief communication. Int J Clin Exp Hypn 1995; 43:118–126.
31. Good M: Reconstruction of early childhood trauma. J Am Psychoanal Assoc 1994; 42:79–101.
32. Arlow J: Fantasy, memory, and reality testing. Psychoanal Q 1969; 38:28–51.
33. Dewald PA: Effects on an adult of incest in childhood: a case report. J Am Psychoanal Assoc 1989; 37:997–1014.
34. Simon B: "Incest—see under Oedipus complex":the history of an error in psychoanalysis. J Am Psychoanal Assoc 1992; 40:955–988.
35. Greenacre P: Re-evaluation of the process of working through. Int J Psychoanal 1956; 37:439–444.
36. Della Femina D, Yeager CA, Lewis DO: Child abuse: adolescent records vs. adult recall. Child Abuse Negl 1990; 14:227–231.
37. Williams LM: Recall of childhood trauma: a prospective study of women's memories of child sex abuse. J Consult Clin Psychol 1994; 62:1167–1176.
38. Williams LM: Adult reports of documented child abuse. Paper delivered at American Psychiatric Association Annual Meeting, New York, May 1996.
39. Viederman M: Repressed sexual molestation. J Am Psychoanal Assoc 1995; 43:1169–1195.
40. Burland JA, Raskin R: The psychoanalysis of adults who were sexually abused in childhood: a preliminary report from the discussion group of the American Psychoanalytic Association. *In* HB Levine, (Ed.), Adult Analysis and Childhood Sexual Abuse. Hillsdale, NJ: The Analytic Press, 1990, pp. 35–41.
41. Lisman-Pieczanski N: Countertransference in the analysis of an adult who was sexually abused as a child. *In* HB Levine, (Ed.), Adult Analysis and Childhood Sexual Abuse. Hillsdale, NJ: The Analytic Press, 1990, pp. 137–148.
42. Alder H: Recall and repetition of a severe childhood trauma. Int J Psychoanal 1995; 76:927–943.
43. Matthews JA, Chu JA: Psychodynamic therapy for patients with early childhood trauma. *In* PA Appelbaum, LA Uyehara, MS Elin (Eds.), Trauma and Memory: Clinical and Legal Controversies. New York: Oxford University Press, 1997, pp. 316–343.
44. Kluft RP: The argument for the reality of the delayed recall of trauma. *In* PA Appelbaum, LA Uyehara, MS Elin, (Eds.) Trauma and Memory: Clinical and Legal Controversies. New York: Oxford University Press, 1997, pp. 25–57.
45. Nash MR: Memory distortion and sexual trauma: the problem of false positives and false negatives. Int J Clin Exp Hypn 1994; 42:346–362.
46. Spiegel D: Dissociating damage. Am J Clin Hypn 1986; 29:123–131.

47. Person E, Klar H: Establishing trauma: the difficulty distinguishing between memories and fantasies. J Am Psychoanal Assoc 1994; 42:1055–1082.

48. Brenner I: The dissociative character. J Am Psychoanal Assoc 1994; 42:819–846.

49. van der Kolk BA: Traumatic memories. *In* PA Appelbaum, LA Uyehara, MS Elin (Eds.), Trauma and Memory: Clinical and Legal Controversies. New York: Oxford University Press, 1997, pp. 243–260.

50. Terr L: What happens to early memories of trauma? A study of twenty children under age five at the time of documented traumatic events. J Am Acad Child Adolesc Psychiatry 1988; 27:96–104.

51. Terr L: Chowchilla revisited; the effects of psychic trauma four years after a schoolbus kidnapping. Am J Psychiatry 1983; 140:1543–1550.

52. Terr L: Unchained Memories. New York: Basic Books, 1994.

53. Ross CA: Cognitive therapy of dissociative identity disorder. *In* PA Appelbaum, LA Uyehara, MS Elin (Eds.), Trauma and Memory: Clinical and Legal Controversies. New York: Oxford University Press, 1997, pp. 360–393.

54. Spiegel D: Dissociated or fabricated? Psychiatric aspects of repressed memory in criminal and civil cases. Int J Clin Exp Hypn 1994; 42:411–432.

55. Ganaway G: Historical vs. narrative truth: clarifying the role of exogenous trauma in the etiology of MPD and its variants. Dissociation 1989; 2:205–219.

56. Shevrin H: The uses and abuses of memory. [editorial] J Am Psychoanal Assoc 1994; 42:991–996.

57. Gelinas D: The persisting negative effects of incest. Psychiatry 1983; 46:312–332.

58. Romans SE, Martin JL, Anderson JC, Herbison GP, Mullen PE: Sexual abuse in childhood and deliberate self harm. Am J Psychiatry 1995; 152:1336–1342.

59. Brodsky BS, Cloitre M, Dulit RA: Relationship of dissociation to self mutilation and childhood abuse in borderline personality disorder. Am J Psychiatry 1995; 152: 1788–1792.

60. Herman J, Perry C, van der Kolk B: Childhood trauma in borderline personality disorder. Am J Psychiatry 1989; 146:490–495.

61. Rorty M, Yager J, Rossotto E: Childhood sexual, physical, and psychological abuse in bulimia nervosa. Am J Psychiatry 1994; 151:1122–1126.

62. Kinzl JF, Trawager C, Guenther V, Biebl W: Family background and sexual abuse associated with eating disorders. Am J Psychiatry 1994; 151:1127–1133.

63. Weil JL: Instinctual Stimulation of Children: From Common Practice to Child Abuse, Vols. 1, 2. Madison, CT: International Universities Press, 1989.

64. Steele B: Some sequelae of the maltreatment of children. *In* HB Levine (Ed.), Adult Analysis and Childhood Sexual Abuse. Hillsdale, NJ: The Analytic Press, 1990, pp. 21–34.

65. Sherkow S: Evaluation and diagnosis of sexual abuse in little girls. J Am Psychoanal Assoc 1990; 38:347–369.

66. Good M: Letter to the editor. J Am Psychoanal Assoc 1991; 39:630–632.

67. Levine H: Clinical issues in the analysis of adults who were sexually abused as children. *In* HB Levine (Ed.), Adult Analysis and Childhood Sexual Abuse. Hillsdale, NJ: The Analytic Press, 1990, pp. 197–218.

68. Kramer S: Residues of incest. *In* HB Levine (Ed.), Adult Analysis and Childhood Sexual Abuse. Hillsdale, NJ: The Analytic Press, 1990, pp. 197–218.

69. Bernstein AE: The impact of incest trauma on ego development. *In* HB Levine (Ed.), Adult Analysis and Childhood Sexual Abuse. Hillsdale, NJ: The Analytic Press, 1990, pp. 65–92.

70. Brenner I: The dissociative character: a reconsideration of "multiple personality". J Am Psychoanal Assoc 1994; 42:819–846.

71. Ludwig AM: The psychobiological functions of dissociation. Am J Clin Hypn 1983; 26:93–99.
72. Merskey H: Manufacture of multiple personality disorder. Br J Psychiatry 1992; 160:327–340.
73. McHugh P: Multiple personality disorder. Harvard Ment Health Lett 1993; 10:4–6.
74. Weissberg M: Multiple personality disorder and iatrogenesis: the cautionary tale of Anna O. Int J Clin Exp Hypn 1993; 41:15–34.
75. Kluft RP: Unsuspected multiple personality disorder: a common source of protracted resistances, interruption, and failure in psychotherapy. Hillside J Clin Psychol 1987; 9:100–115.
76. Ross CA: Epidemiology of mutiple personality disorder and dissociation. *In* Lowenstein R. (Ed.), Psychiatric Clinics of North America, Vol. 14. Philadelphia: WB Saunders, 1991, pp. 503–517.
77. Putnam FW, Guroff JJ, Silberman EK, Barban I, Post RM: The clinical phenomenology of multiple personality disorder: review of 100 recent cases. J Clin Psychiatry 1986; 47:285–293.
78. Ross CA: Current treatment of dissociative identity disorder. *In* ML Cohen, JN Berzoff, MR Elin (Eds.), Dissociative Identity Disorder: Theoretical and Treatment Controversies. Northvale NJ: Jason Aronson, 1995, pp. 413–434.
79. Frankel F: Adult reconstruction of childhood events in the multiple personality literature. Am J Psychiatry 1993; 150:954–958.
80. Bursten B: Validity of childhood abuse memories [letter to the editor]. Am J Psychiatry 1995; 152:1533.
81. Adityanjee MD, Raju GSP, Khandelwal SK: Current status of multiple personality disorder in India. Am J Psychiatry 1989; 146:1607–1610.
82. Lowenstein RL: An office mental status examination for complex chronic dissociative symptoms and multiple personality disorder. *In* RJ Lowenstein (Ed.), Psychiatric Clinics of North America; Multiple Personality Disorder, Vol. 14. Philadelphia: WB Saunders, 1991, pp. 567–604.
83. Ross C: The Dissociative Disorders Interview Schedule: a structured interview. Dissociation 1989; 2:169–189.
84. Kluft R: Current controversies surrounding dissociative identity disorder. *In* LM Cohen, JN Berzoff, MR Elin (Eds.), Dissociative Identity Disorder: Theoretical and Treatment Controversies. Northvale NJ: Jason Aronson, 1995, p. 370.
85. Sauzier MC: The role of the therapist in the emerging disclosure process. Paper delivered at the Sixth Susan J. Wise Memorial Lecture, Boston Psychoanalytic Society and Institute, Cambridge, Mass., April 29, 1995.
86. Ross C, Gahan P: Techniques in the treatment of multiple personality disorder. Am J Psychother 1988; 42:40–52.
87. Raphling D: Interpretation and expectation: the anxiety of influence. J Am Psychoanal Assoc 1995; 43:95–112.
88. Raphling D: A patient who was not sexually abused. J Am Psychoanal Assoc 1994; 42:65–78.
89. Shengold L: A variety of narcissistic pathology stemming from parental weakness. Psychoanal Q 1991; 55:86–92.
90. Herman J, Harvey M: The false memory debate: social science or social backlash? Harvard Ment Health Lett 1993; 9:4–6.
91. Yapko M: Suggestibility and repressed memories of abuse: a survey of psychotherapists' beliefs. Am J Clin Hypn 1994; 36:163–171.

92. Frankel F: Hypnosis and altered states of consciousness in the treatment of patients with medical disorders. *In* TB Karasu, RI Steinmuller (Eds.), Psychotherapeutic Approaches in Medicine. New York: Grune and Stratton, 1978, pp. 181–201.

93. Frankel FH, Covino NA: Hypnosis and hypnotherapy. *In* PA Appelbaum, LA Uyehara, MS Elin (Eds.), Trauma and Memory: Clinical and Legal Controversies. New York: Oxford University Press, 1997, pp. 344–359.

94. Bloom P: Clinical guidelines in using hypnosis in uncovering memories of sexual abuse: a master class commentary. Int J Clin Exp Hypn 1994; 42:173–178.

95. Erdelyi MH: Hypnotic hypermnesia: the empty set of hypermnesia. Int J Clin Exp Hypn 1994; 42:379–390.

96. Davies JM, Frawley MG: Treating the Adult Survivor of Sexual Abuse: a Psychoanalytic Perspective. New York: Basic Books, 1994.

97. Olio KA, Cornell WF: The therapeutic relationship as the foundation for treatment with adult survivors of sexual abuse. Psychotherapy 1993; 30:512–523.

98. Chu J: Ten traps for therapists in the treatment of trauma survivors. Dissociation 1988; 1:24–31.

99. Butterfield M: Viewpoints—Do patients memories of sexual abuse consititute a "false memory syndrome?—No" Psychiatr News Dec 19, 1993, p. 18.

100. Spence D: Narrative Truth and Historical Truth. New York: W W Norton, 1982.

101. Sachs O: Distinctions between fantasy and reality elements in memory and reconstruction. Int J Psychoanal 1967; 48:416–423.

102. Williams M: Reconstruction of an early seduction and its aftereffects. J Am Psychoanal Assoc 1987; 35:145–163.

103. Josephs L: The paradoxical relationship between fantasy and reality in Freudian theory. Psychoanal Rev 1987; 74:161–177.

104. Beck AT, Rush AJ, Shaw BF, Emery G: Cognitive Therapy of Depression. New York: Guilford Press, 1979.

105. Hyman IE, Loftus E: Some people recover memories of childhood trauma that never really happened. *In* PA Appelbaum, LA Uyehara, MS Elin (Eds.), Trauma and Memory: Clinical and Legal Controversies. New York: Oxford University Press, 1997, pp. 3–24.

106. Brenneis CB: Belief and suggestion in the recovery of memories of childhood sexual abuse. J Am Psychoanal Assoc 1994; 42:1027–1053.

107. Ross JM: King Oedipus and the postmodernist psychoanalyst. J Am Psychoanal Assoc 1995; 43:553–571.

V

THE TRAUMA DEBATE AND
THE LEGAL SYSTEM

18

Legal Rights of Trauma Victims

WENDY J. MURPHY

Victims of sexual trauma can seek justice through civil or criminal proceedings or both. This chapter will discuss the similarities and significant differences between these proceedings as well as recent developments in the law regarding victims' privacy rights and the admissibility of ''repressed'' memory testimony.

The first section will provide a comparative overview of criminal and civil sexual trauma litigation.

The second section will discuss victims' privacy rights and counseling privileges in sexual trauma litigation, the constitutional rights of the accused, and limitations on confidentiality.

The third section will discuss recent court decisions involving the admissibility of ''repressed'' memory testimony in sexual trauma litigation.

Criminal vs. Civil Litigation—an Overview

As a preliminary matter, whether a victim can pursue a criminal or civil case requires an initial determination that the statutory limitation period, within which a legal action must be filed, has not expired. In most states, such limitation periods do not begin to run until the victim reaches a certain age. In many states, civil time limits are extended to compensate for factors that impaired the victim's ability to initiate a claim within the strict time limits. This is known as the ''discovery rule,'' and is discussed in the next chapter.

Criminal Litigation

One major purpose of criminal sexual trauma litigation is to punish persons who commit acts of sexual violence in violation of criminal laws or penal codes. The attorneys in such cases are limited to the prosecutor and defense counsel who represent the government and the accused, respectively.

Sexual trauma charges in criminal litigation typically involve various degrees of rape and/or indecent assault and battery. Different, but similar, charges apply when the victim is a child, but a significant distinction is that with children, the prosecution is not required to establish lack of consent on the part of the victim. Related claims may include civil rights violations, indecent exposure, lewd and lascivious conduct, child pornography, incest, assault and battery, threats, kidnapping, and charges under the recently enacted federal Violence Against Women Act.

As a witness to her own violence, a sexual trauma victim has a civic, if not legal, obligation to report the crime, to cooperate with prosecuting authorities, and to testify before the grand jury and/or at a probable cause hearing—all before the case even formally begins. Thereafter, the victim awaits resolution of the case during an extensive pretrial period involving discovery requests, hearings, and other legal proceedings. The victim is not a party to the criminal proceedings and is not represented by an attorney but is merely a witness for the government. Not being a party to the criminal case, the victim has no control over the proceedings, which can be difficult to endure in the aftermath of a crime characterized by a loss of power, dignity, and control.

During the criminal proceedings, many victims require the advocacy, insight and support of an attorney, but the system does not provide such representation. While many believe the prosecuting attorney represents and advocates for the victim, in reality, the prosecutor's job is to defend the interests of justice, which can sometimes conflict with the needs and desires of victims.

Many victims fear retribution during the pendency of criminal proceedings and feel they cannot move forward and begin the healing process until the case is over. As a result, delays in criminal proceedings can be very difficult for victims to endure. Ironically, although the accused has a Constitutional right to a speedy trial, it is a common defense strategy to delay the trial for as long as possible. This is because witnesses die or move away, memories fade, and the emotional impact of the crime diminishes. This delay strategy is described in an oft-cited adage of the defense bar: "a good defense, like a good wine, gets better with age."

The trial process itself can also be very painful for victims of sexual trauma, as the typical defense tactic in such cases involves accusing the victim of being mentally ill or otherwise assailing the victim's character and blaming her for the crime. In the end, even if the perpetrator is convicted or pleads guilty, the punishment in a criminal sexual trauma case is not likely to be severe.[1]

Congress and most states have passed laws giving victims various "rights" during the processing of a criminal case. For example, in Massachusetts, a victim has the following rights: to be informed by the prosecutor about the victim's rights in the criminal process; to be heard at sentencing and at any other time deemed appropriate by the court; to confer with the prosecutor prior to any hearing on motions by the defense to obtain psychiatric or other confidential records; to request confidentiality of personal information such as an address, telephone, place of employment, or school; to be notified by the prosecutor when a court proceeding to which they have been summoned will not go on as scheduled; to be informed of procedures for receiving any witness fee to which they are entitled; to be informed of the right to decline an interview by defense counsel; to request that restitution be an element of the final disposition of the case and if ordered, to receive a copy of the schedule of restitution payments and the name and telephone number of the probation officer responsible for supervising the defendant's payments; to be informed that they may have a right to pursue a civil action for damages relating to the crime against the defendant or others, regardless of whether there has been an order for restitution; to be provided with reasonable safeguards to minimize contacts with defendants, including the right to a safe and secure waiting area in the courthouse during court proceedings; to an explanation of the criminal process at the outset and any subsequent significant event; to be present at all court proceedings; to receive protection from law enforcement from harm and threats of harm arising out of the victim's cooperation with the criminal justice process; to be informed of and to receive assistance in applying for financial assistance and other social services, such as victim compensation; to confer with the prosecutor before the start of a trial, prior to the dismissal of charges against the defendant and prior to proposing the Commonwealth's sentence recommendation and to have the court informed of the victim's position on the prosecutor's recommendation; to a prompt resolution of the case; to be informed of procedures for applying for any witness fees to which they may be entitled; to receive employer and creditor intervention services, including protection from discharge from employment or penalty as a result of the victim's participation in the criminal justice process; to confer with the probation officer prior to the filing of a full presentence report; to submit a victim impact statement to the parole board for inclusion in the prepetrator's records; to be informed by the prosecutor of the final disposition of the case, including an explanation of the type of sentence imposed by the court and to receive a copy of the court order setting forth the conditions of probation within 30 days of the order; to have all seized property returned within ten days or as soon as possible once it is no longer needed for law enforcement purposes; to be provided by the parole board with information regarding a convicted offender's parole eligibility and status in the criminal justice system; to be notified in advance by custodial authorities whenever the defendant received a temporary, provisional, or final release from custody or escapes and whenever a defendant is moved from a secure facility to a less-secure facility.[2]

It should be noted, however, that such "rights" are often toothless tigers, as most legislation in this area expressly provides that victims' rights are not enforceable via the initiation of a cause of action.[3]

In most states, a victim may file a claim for financial assistance from the government. These funds are partly comprised of fees levied against convicted felons, which are then deposited in a crime victim compensation fund. This money is then distributed to victims and their families by another government agency.[4] In Massachusetts, claims for such funds are filed under the Victims of Violent Crime Act[5] and processed pursuant to regulations promulgated by the Attorney General.[6]

Such funds may be given to victims and their families to cover uninsured medical treatment, unreimbursed lost wages, and other benefits. To be eligible for benefits in Massachusetts, the claimant must report the crime to law enforcement authorities within five days of its occurrence and cooperate with law enforcement, unless there is good cause not to do so. Regulations also require that the victim file her claim within three years of the date of the crime.

For adult survivors of child sexual abuse, the three-year time limit is extended such that a claim need only be filed within five days of remembering the abuse. Seemingly generous at first blush, this requirement effectively bars claims of most victims who have always remembered the abuse but did not appreciate until adulthood that the abuse was wrongful, let alone criminal.

Regulations in Massachusetts also provide that the crime must have resulted in a criminal complaint or an administrative determination that a crime occurred. Again, this presents a significant hurdle for many adult survivors of child sexual abuse, given that prosecutors, in their discretion, will generally be unwilling to proceed with a criminal case involving an extended passage of time and a lack of fresh corroborative evidence.

While the criminal justice system is designed to punish and rehabilitate criminals, protect society and deter crime, a victim's individual needs are not entirely satisfied by the processing of a criminal case or by the imposition of penal sanctions. To that end, a victim should also consider filing a civil lawsuit to recover financial compensation and to economically punish those legally responsible for causing the sexual trauma.

Civil Litigation

Civil lawsuits are explicitly designed to benefit victims by compensating them in the form of money damages for losses suffered as a result of sexual trauma. Claims in civil cases may include assault and battery, negligence, emotional distress, civil rights violations, sexual harassment and/or discrimination, and claims under the federal Violence Against Women Act.

Unlike a criminal case, a civil lawsuit is initiated by a victim who, as the Plaintiff, is a formal party to the litigation and has significant control over the proceedings. In addition, civil lawsuits are easier to win than criminal cases because the standard of proof is lower; "more probable than not" in the former, "beyond a reasonable doubt" in the latter.

Whether criminal proceedings are pending or not, a victim may engage her own attorney and initiate a civil action. It should be noted, however, that the pendency of a civil lawsuit can be used during the criminal trial to undermine the victim's credibility on the grounds that she is fabricating the allegations due to the possibility of future financial gain. In addition, the defendant can use the civil proceeding to perpetuate discovery, such as taking the victim's deposition, for use in the criminal case. In many states, such discovery is not allowed in criminal cases.

A civil action is sometimes the only option for a victim where, for example, there has been a significant passage of time between the sexual abuse and a report to the authorities. In such cases, the criminal statute of limitations will likely have expired or the prosecutor will exercise his discretion not to initiate a criminal case due to the passage of time and a lack of sufficient "fresh" evidence.

Most attorneys who represent victims of sexual trauma in civil lawsuits do so on a "contingency fee" basis. This means the victim is not required to pay the attorney for his or her legal fees unless there is a recovery of money in the case. In the event of recovery, the attorney receives a fixed percentage of the gross award, usually 33 1/3%. While many victims might choose to sue a perpetrator for the moral victory alone, it is unlikely that a civil attorney will represent a victim without a clear possibility that assets are available to be recovered in the event the victim prevails.

A civil lawsuit against the perpetrator directly is not a feasible option for most victims because the perpetrator often has no assets. Nonetheless, there may be a viable cause of action against a third-party with substantial liability insurance to cover the victim's losses. For example, if a child is sexually traumatized at home, a parent, grandparent, or caretaker of the child might be liable for the child's injuries if they knew or should have known of the assault and failed to protect the child from harm. In such cases, despite standard exclusionary clauses in homeowner's insurance policies for intentional misconduct, coverage for losses incurred as a result of deliberate sexual trauma is often available under the theory that it was the negligence of the caretaker, and not only the intentional sexual misconduct, that led to the child's harm.[7]

In another situation, an employer, school, church, or childcare/employment placement agency might be liable for negligently failing to protect the victim and/or negligently hiring or retaining the perpetrator and/or for negligently failing to adopt or enforce adequate policies and procedures to prevent the assault.

In some states, the doctrine of charitable immunity prohibits lawsuits or significantly limits recovery against religious and other charitable entities. In many states, however, this doctrine can be avoided where, as is the case with sexual abuse, the conduct at issue is outside the scope of the charitable purpose. Another exception to this immunity/limitation rule involves naming an individual employee of the institution as the defendant because only the institution, but not the individual employee, is usually protected by charitable laws that preclude or limit recovery.

While both criminal and civil proceedings deter sexual violence through the imposition of sanctions, many advocates for victims believe that as an engine of social change in a capitalist country, civil economic sanctions are more effective than penal sanctions in reducing the incidence of sexual violence. This is particularly true when institutions and insurance companies are made to pay for the victim's losses, because broad-based policy changes generally follow major financial losses to reduce the risk of such liability exposure in the future.

Privacy Rights of Sexual Trauma Victims

In the aftermath of sexual truma, many victims seek counseling services. In most states, such services are available free of charge from rape crisis centers and most legislatures have enacted strict privilege statutes protecting the confidential communications between a sexual trauma victim and her crisis counselor.[8] Such privilege statutes, by their very nature, are designed to restrict access to information which would otherwise be disclosed in judicial proceedings and elsewhere.[9] Protecting privileged communications reflects society's compelling interest in fostering certain relationships.

Confidentiality is the cornerstone of effective sexual trauma counseling, as it enables victims to speak freely about a degrading, debilitating, and deeply personal act of violence.[10] A recent national study found that despite misconceptions to the contrary, the stigma of rape is still a very real concern in victims' eyes, and rape victims want and need meaningful confidentiality.[11] This same study found that victims continue to be extremely concerned about people learning about the rape and finding reasons to blame them for the crime.[11]

The process of speaking freely in a safe environment not only allows the victim to begin recovery but also empowers her to report the crime to law enforcement officials and to stay involved in the criminal justice process. Courts uniformly recognize the importance of providing victims with confidential counseling as a means of encouraging victims to heal in the aftermath of sexual trauma. As one court has written:

> Once it becomes known that confidentialities are violated, other people may be reluctant to use [confidential] services and may be unable to use them to maximum benefit. The purpose of enacting a . . . privilege is to prevent the chilling effect which routine disclosure may have in preventing those in need from seeking that help.[12]

Without strict confidentiality, fewer rape cases will be reported and prosecuted, thereby diminishing the societal value of the criminal justice system. For similar policy reasons, states have enacted so-called rape-shield laws, which protect sexual trauma victims from undue harassment and humiliation during trial by prohibiting the admission of evidence of a victim's prior sexual conduct.[13] Such statutes are often circumvented, however, if the accused can make a plausible showing that such evidence will materially affect the credibility of the victim's testimony. For example, in one case, a victim's prior sexual experience as a prostitute was admissible because when the victim was discovered by the police engaged in sexual activity with the defendant, she told the police she was being raped. At trial, the defense claimed that the victim falsely accused the defendant of rape to avoid being arrested for prostitution. To legitimize this claim, the defense was allowed to avoid the rape-shield statute and introduce evidence of the victim's previous sexual experience as a prostitute.[14]

In several states, access to victims' counseling records is absolutely prohibited by both statute and court decision. In Pennsylvania, for example, the state supreme court recently upheld the constitutionality of legislation providing that rape crisis counseling records are protected by an absolute privilege, impenetrable under any circumstances, reasoning that the rape crisis counseling privilege statute is a reflection of the ''compelling interest in protecting the confidentiality of the rape victim's records.''[15] This court observed that as a direct result of a decision ten years earlier,[16] where defendants were granted ready access to victims' counseling records, data showed that the effectiveness of rape crisis counseling had suffered.[17] In a remarkable example of self-criticism, the court effectively reversed itself, overruled that earlier decision, and held that access to victims' rape counseling records would be denied in all circumstances.[18]

It is noteworthy that the defense in the Pennsylvania case petitioned the United States Supreme Court for review, arguing that an absolute bar to victims' counseling records violates the United States Constitution. The nation's highest court declined the opportunity to entertain the defendant's petition, which may indicate that the Court does not believe absolute protection for victims' counseling records is unconstitutional. The United States Supreme Court has not directly addressed the issue of when privileged material must give way to the Constitutional rights of the accused since 1987,[19] when the Court ruled that the rights of the accused could override the privacy interests at stake in confidential records maintained by a child welfare agency if there was a legitimate need for such records, but only after the court conducted a private judicial screening to determine the materiality of such information to the case on trial. The Court noted, however, that the records at issue there were in the government's file and were protected by only a qualified privilege statute. The Court indicated that its decision was not a reflection of how it might rule if the information requested by the defense was in the hands of a third-party or was protected by an absolute privilege, such as rape crisis counseling records.

In a few states, despite the existence of clear legislative language mandating strict confidentiality for victims' counseling privileges, courts have held that the constitutional rights of the accused can outweigh victims' privacy rights. The rights of the accused in this regard are derived from both state[20] and federal[21] constitutional principles, which guarantee criminal defendants a fair trial, due process,[22] as well as the right to confront and cross-examine witnesses.[23] In states where appellate courts have overridden strict legislative mandates precluding access to counseling records, courts are likely to reason that an absolute legislative bar to such records violates the state, not the federal, constitution. This is because the rights of the accused as protected by the federal Constitution appear not to override victims' counseling privileges, but courts are free to give the accused greater rights under their individual state constitutions.

Defendants typically assert that access to a victim's counseling records is important because they may contain evidence of the victim's capacity to perceive, remember, and articulate the alleged events,[24] or of the victim's bias or motive to lie, misidentification, or inability to identify or describe her assailant.[25] Defendants also argue that a victim's privilege should readily give way to a request for counseling records because the victim's interest is a mere statutory right, whereas the defendant's interest is constitutional. This is an unfair characterization of the balance of interests, as the victim's right to privacy in counseling communications is plainly derived from the Constitution, which has long provided protection for personal matters.[26]

It is particularly important to note here that virtually every federal court that has addressed the issue has found a constitutional right of privacy in therapeutic counseling.[27] While no court has yet recognized such a right on behalf of a victim in a criminal case, there is no legitimate legal basis upon which a constitutional right may be characterized as existing in a civil, but not a criminal, case. While victims may have a constitutional privacy interest at stake, this does not mean their records will receive absolute protection, but status as a fundamental right will help victims' counseling records to be more resistant to disclosure in all legal proceedings.[28] Likewise, constitutional value will help to ensure that due process and proper legal standards are satisfied before any counseling records are forcibly divulged, even to the judge for an "in camera" review.

It should also be emphasized that counseling records are not part of the prosecution's case but are, instead, highly private material belonging to a non-party to the criminal proceeding. Hence, it is not a situation where one party to the litigation has access to the information and the other does not. Counseling records are not investigative or evidentiary in nature; they are designed only to help the blameless victim heal. Thus, while there is always a speculative possibility that a victim's counseling records might contain information relevant to a criminal prosecution, there should be a strong presumption against disclosure of such records unless the accused can demonstrate that unusual circumstances exist such that disclosure is constitutionally warranted.

Circumstances under which criminal defendants may gain access to a victim's privileged counseling records vary from state to state, but generally states provide that disclosure should be ordered, if at all, only in limited circumstances where the defense has submitted an adequate proffer to the court establishing that disclosure is necessary under applicable standards.[29] In many states, even if disclosure is appropriate in a particular case, the victim's records are not turned over directly to the defense, they are, instead, produced only to the court for a private or "in camera" inspection. During this state of review, the judge may determine that despite the adequacy of the defendant's initial proffer, further disclosure to the defense is not warranted. Defense advocates argue that in camera review is harmless and that judges should routinely, without cause, search through victims' counseling records to look for evidence that may prove helpful to the defense. At first blush, this may seem reasonable because the judge is only one person. But he is, after all, the government. Moreover, the Massachusetts Supreme Judicial Court recently rejected a "harmlessness" argument and held that even private judicial screening is a "substantial invasion of privacy."[30] It should also be recognized that routine disclosure of records to the judge enhances the likelihood of further disclosures while placing therapists and counselors in the uncomfortable role of evidence-gatherers.

Whether a defendant's initial proffer constitutes an adequate showing can only be determined on a case by case basis. However, it is clear that mere speculation that the victim's records "may" contain relevant information is inadequate even to justify an in camera inspection by the judge.[31]

In those states which have in camera inspection procedures, an adequate and fact-specific defense proffer is essential, as it enables the judge to conduct an intelligent and focused review with an eye toward matters properly claimed by the defendant. Determining whether evidence bears on a particular issue in the case with the assistance of a fact-specific proffer from the defendant is a far clearer task than asking a judge to determine whether ambiguous information might possibly be helpful to the defense.

Proffers that fall short of establishing an adequate showing reflect no more than "a desire to embark on 'an unrestrained foray into confidential records in the hope that the unearthing of some unspecified information would enable [the defendant] to impeach the witness.'"[32] Such fishing expeditions are usually prohibited.

Some courts recognize a hierarchy of privileges and confidentiality rules such that a stricter access standard is applied if the confidential information at stake is protected by a high-level "absolute" privilege, such as sexual assault victim/counselor or priest/penitent, rather than a conditional or "qualified" privilege or rule of confidentiality, such as social worker/client.[33]

In civil lawsuits, because the defendant's liberty is not at stake, the Constitutional rights of the accused that apply in a criminal setting are not brought to bear on confidential information. Yet, the civil defendant often gains access to privileged records on the theory that the victim has waived her privilege by initiating the action and placing her psychological health at issue by seeking money damages as compensation for her suffering. Courts generally hold that when a plaintiff seeks such compensation, it is fair to allow the defendant access to the plaintiff's counseling records so that the true extent of the victim's damages can be litigated. This is known as the patient/litigant exception.

Oftentimes, even when records are ordered disclosed, courts will impose strict limitations to protect the privileged material. For example, the court might allow access only to certain specified post-incident counseling records, or the court might simply order the therapist to write a summary report of the victim's treatment. In addition, judges will typically issue protective orders for such material, if requested, to avoid needless disclosure of privileged information beyond those individuals necessary to a proper resolution of the case.

The United States Supreme Court recently adopted an absolute federal common law privilege in the social worker/client context, opining that "the mental health of our citizenry, no less than its physical health, is of transcendent importance."[34] The Court expressly declined to view the social worker privilege as less worthy of absolute confidentiality than the doctor/patient privileges, noting that confidentiality is vital in therapeutic counseling, irrespective of the education of the caregiver. The ruling sends an important message but has mandatory application only in federal law cases and makes no mention of the patient–litigant exception. Also, the Court did not indicate how, if at all, the privilege might give way to the rights of the accused in a criminal case. Finally, it remains to be seen whether courts will interpret this decision as applying to non-professional crisis counselors, but sound public policy, and at least one federal district court supports such a view.

Given the risk that counseling records may be disclosed in litigation, victims should be so informed at the outset of treatment. However, caregivers should offset the chilling effect of such a warning by promising to release records only after the victim and/or caregiver has had an opportunity to formally object and only if proper legal standards are met. The surest way to maximize protection for confidentiality is for victims and caregivers to insist on a voice in the legal proceedings, at the trial, and appellate levels. In the absence of aggressive advocacy, courts will wrongly assume that the social value of confidentiality in therapy is insignificant. Such advocacy also helps to prevent attorneys from sending subpoenas for counseling records simply to gain strategic leverage in the litigation. It would also help if victims were advised at the outset of treatment not to reveal to anyone in a criminal case that they have ever received counseling, in the absence of a legitimate court order to do so.

It should also be noted that in matters of sexual violence, unlike gender-neutral crime, there is a knee-jerk willingness on the part of litigants and judges alike to inquire about the mental health of the victim. This gender-bias means that women are more likely than men to be forced to choose between healing and justice. For those who choose healing, the perpetrators enjoys an undeserved ''victory by intimidation.''

Courts have a responsibility to be open-minded in this area and to realize that if the law protects the attorney/client and priest/penitent privileges in order to preserve the integrity of those relationships, there is no legitimate reason to deny similar respect to the relationship between a victim and her therapist. Some judges reject this comparison on the grounds that the attorney and priest privileges are rooted in ancient history— while therapeutic relationships evolved more recently. But this argument is irrational as it ignores the indispensable value of confidentiality in therapy.

While access to counseling records in some cases may be justified, it should be the rare exception to the rule. The current trend appears to be moving toward greater protection for victims' privacy rights, but more than half the states have yet to address the issue, either in the legislature or in the appellate courts.

Memory Evidence

In litigation where it is alleged the victim experienced delayed recovery of memories of sexual trauma, memory evidence will likely be the central focus of the case. This is largely because the so-called false memory syndrome movement has received such significant media attention that it is now part of routine defense strategy.

Public controversy surrounding recovery of traumatic memories is perplexing, given that scientists and clinicians agree with virtual uniformity that the human mind is capable of avoiding conscious recall of traumatic experiences. Cogent proof exists in the very fact that the DSM IV recognizes such a phenomenon. Thus, many victim advocates believe that the false memory syndrome movement is not a legitimate scientific development, but rather a backlash response to increasingly successful civil litigation initiated by victims against their attackers and responsible third-parties.

By far the most disturbing effect of the false memory syndrome movement is that defense attorneys often initiate strategic retaliatory lawsuits against the victim, and her therapist separately, to use as leverage against the victim's filing of a civil lawsuit against the perpetrator or a responsible third-party. Claims against the victim include allegations of libel, slander, malicious prosecution, and abuse of process. Therapists are usually sued for malpractice, including allegations that the therapist "implanted false memories" of abuse in the victim's mind. These strategic lawsuits are not generally designed to recoup money for an injured person but rather to intimidate and pressure the victim into recanting, withdrawing her lawsuit, or accepting a paltry settlement. Of course, when the therapist is sued, there is added pressure because a rift is then created between the victim and her care provider. These strategic lawsuits are often dismissed, by agreement but only after the victim's lawsuit is resolved to the satisfaction of the perpetrator. Such strategic litigation is also being used to force victims to refuse to testify in criminal cases, or to passively accept probation or other insignificant punishment for the perpetrator during the plea-bargain process.

Victims and therapists are increasingly learning to utilize little-known proceedings called "anti-SLAPP-suit" motions to dispose of retaliatory lawsuits immediately after they are filed. "SLAPP suit" (Strategic Litigation Against Public Participation) is the term used to describe any litigation that is not honest in substance but is designed merely to intimidate someone from taking advantage of their fundamental right to petition and seek redress from the government, including the right to file a lawsuit against a perpetrator for sexual abuse. Anti-SLAPP-suit motions are now covered by statute in many states, although they may also be filed as a matter of constitutional right. The benefit of this proceeding is that it puts a burden on the SLAPP-ing party to prove the validity of his litigation within weeks of the date the SLAPP-suit is filed.

Another disturbing effect of the false memory syndrome movement is that defense attorneys routinely file pretrial motions to dismiss cases and/or to completely exclude the testimony of victims. At the heart of these defense motions is the broad-sweeping claim that victims' recovered memories are not reliable enough to be admitted as evidence in a court of law. Such motions effectively seek to deny victims access to justice.

In four recent cases, the defense successfully argued that victims with recovered memories lacked a certain foundational credibility and should be precluded from testifying because the phenomenon of repressed memories is not generally accepted by the relevant scientific community.[35,36] Two of the cases arose in criminal prosecutions and were decided jointly by a single New Hampshire judge. In those cases, the victims' testimony was excluded. The other two cases were civil in nature and were also decided jointly by a single judge. In those cases, out of the District of Columbia, the lawsuits were dismissed.

It is noteworthy, however, that another judge in New Hampshire recently considered the admissibility of recovered memory testimony in a criminal matter and, relying on the same expert testimony elicited in the above-referenced cases, held it admissible.[33] Though the decision is somewhat esoteric, the court ruled that because objective truth cannot be scientifically measured, testimony cannot be barred on the basis that there has been no scientific proof of its reliability. The court went further to say that if testimony were barred on such grounds, all memory-based testimony would be excluded from judicial proceedings. Likewise, the court excluded expert testimony to the effect that recovered memories are reliable or unreliable on the grounds that there was no evidence that such memories are either more or less reliable than ordinary memories. Expert testimony was thus limited to "that body of scientific knowledge that may assist the fact-finder in assessing the plausibility of the traumatic amnesia phenomenon."[37] Although the judge allowed expert testimony on traumatic amnesia, it was precluded on the issue of how traumatic memories are recovered because, according to the court, the victim's memories were "spontaneously" recovered and thus not related to "scientific" knowledge.

Very few state court decisions squarely address the admissibility of recovered memory testimony and those that do have little value as legal precedent, as they are conflicting and have not been adopted by an appellate court. A federal appellate court, however, recently commented favorably on the admissibility of recovered memory testimony of an adult victim who had been sexually abused between the ages of 4 and 16 and then repressed the memories until she began therapy at age 24.[38] The court noted in that decision that even the authority cited by the defense as support for the claim that traumatic amnesia is not generally accepted by the scientific community[39] recognizes that the mind is capable of consciously avoiding traumatic information and reliably recalling it years later. Unlike the state trial court decisions, the federal appellate court decision has significant value as legal precedent.

In two additional recent federal decisions, judges ruled that while repressed memories, like ordinary memories, may not always be accurate, the theory of recovered memories has been established as valid through various studies and has gained general acceptance in the relevant scientific community.[40] In one of these cases, the plaintiff alleged she had been abused during the time period 1940–1945, more than 47 years before she filed her complaint, when she was between the ages of 12 and 17. The plaintiff alleged she had no memories of the abuse until 1990, when, during psychotherapy, she recalled the abuse. The court ruled that the credibility of the allegations was not for the court to decide but only whether the theory of repressed memories was scientifically valid. On this point, the court said that "to reject a diagnostic category generally accepted by those who practice the art and science of psychiatry would be folly. Rules of law are not petrified in the past but flow with the current of expanding knowledge."[41]

Memory Evidence

Most attorneys are accustomed to dealing with the memory of a witness only in terms of passage of time. For example, a typical "memory" question posed to a witness would be, "and your memory was better a year ago than it is today, isn't that true?". Recently, however, memory experts have been testifying in courtrooms all over the country about ways in which the human mind perceives, stores, and retrieves information.

Sometimes, memory is described as being no more complicated than the sensory devices of which it is comprised, such as vision and hearing. In matters of such common sense evidence, expert testimony is not generally allowed because the jury is presumed capable of judging the evidence as the product of ordinary human experience and expert testimony is believed only to distract the jury from a fair resolution of the issues. While this may be true of memory in general, such a simplistic characterization is probably inappropriate where there has been traumatic amnesia and/or a substantial delay between the abuse and the recovery of traumatic information. In such cases, expert testimony is necessary to assist the fact-finder in understanding how the mind copes with trauma.

Experts testifying on behalf of the victim will likely attest to the general reliability of memory. They will also cite extensive clinical evidence demonstrating the strikingly similar accounts of trauma victims who report the experience of traumatic amnesia and delayed recovery of memories. In addition, such experts will cite numerous controlled studies to support their opinion that many victims of sexual trauma do not recall the abuse until long after the trauma has ended.[42]

In delayed recovery cases, corroboration of the long-since ceased abuse can be very helpful in demonstrating the reliability of the victim's memory in particular and traumatic memory in general. The victim's expert will likely testify about the significance of corroboration in support of his or her opinion on reliability.

Corroboration can be found in medical and school records, as well as diaries and old pictures, which may document signs of the abuse, such as symptoms of stress and other unusual behavior. It is also valuable to interview family, friends, and teachers about their observations of the victim's behavior around the time of the abuse. In addition, it is significant if the victim is aware of unusual genital markings or knows of other personal information about the abuser or if the victim has atypical sexual knowledge for her age. In addition, newspaper files, court records, and media attention may prove to be corroborative if they reveal other victims.

Finally, the victim's expert will likely attest to the lack of scientific support for false memory syndrome and why such a defense theory in a particular case is implausible.

Experts for the defense are likely to focus generally on the imperfection and malleability of memory and specifically on suggestibility factors that they contend influenced a particular victim's memory. Defense experts may also testify that there is no "scientific proof" of repression or traumatic amnesia and delayed recovery of memories.

It is also possible for a defense expert to testify that memories which are stored during a dissociative experience are particularly unreliable when recovered. This is curious testimony, however, given that no valid studies support such a claim.

Defense attorneys often try to argue that the process of recovering traumatic memories is akin to hypnosis because hypnotically aided testimony is considered unreliable in many states and therefore inadmissible in civil and criminal cases. This comparison is easily rebutted, however, by distinguishing hypnosis as a deliberate, active process of intervention that places the subject in a state of limited consciousness during the information-gathering process. In addition, hypnosis is largely irrelevant because, for most sexual trauma victims, memories are recovered without hypnosis.

Finally, a defense expert may attempt to testify that the victim is suffering from "false memory syndrome." This testimony generally should be disallowed, as there is no clinically recognized phenomenon known as "false memory syndrome," though some have described it as the process by which a person adopts a memory of a traumatic experience which is in fact not true but which the person believes to be real. The phrase was coined by the False Memory Syndrome Foundation, a support group whose membership comprises largely adults accused of sexual abuse. The group's advisory board members often represent their interests in court.

Although expert testimony is often needed to explain traumatic amnesia in sexual trauma cases, the recovery of memory is only one factor that may bear on the victim's credibility. Hence, memory should not generally become such a cumbersome scientific issue at trial that attention is diverted from the abuse.

Admissibility of Expert Scientific Testimony

Admissibility of expert scientific testimony is typically raised prior to trial when one or both sides of a controversy seek to admit or preclude it. The leading federal case in this area is *Daubert* v. *Merrell Dow Pharmaceuticals, Inc.*[43] In *Daubert*, the Supreme Court discussed the admissibility of "expert" scientific testimony under Federal Rule of Evidence 702 which provides:

> if scientific, technical, or other specialized knowledge will assist the trier of fact to understand the evidence or to determine a fact in issue, a witness qualified as an expert by knowledge, skill, experience, training or education, may testify thereto in the form of an opinion or otherwise.

The *Daubert* Court construed Rule 702 to require "some degree of regulation of the subjects and theories about which an expert may testify."[37] The Court stated further that the "subject of an expert's testimony must be 'scientific . . . knowledge'" and that such evidence must be relevant and reliable.

While some have tried to argue that *Daubert* precludes expert testimony unless the expert's opinions and conclusions are generally accepted by the relevant scientific community, it is important to note that the *Daubert* Court plainly rejected this position and stated that "science" is not "an encyclopedic body of knowledge about the universe" but rather "a process for proposing and refining theoretical explanations about the world."[43] The *Daubert* Court further explained that "[i]n a case involving scientific evidence, evidentiary reliability will be based upon scientific evidence," not universal acceptance, and "[p]ertinent evidence based on scientifically valid principles will satisfy." On this point the court specified that "[t]he focus . . . must be solely on *principles and methodology, not on the conclusions they generate.*"[43]

Daubert's focus on valid methodology is supported by sound legal doctrine, as it has long been held that courts should not determine which expert's conclusions are more in line with the scientific community, but only whether the expert's opinion, even if controversial or unique, is supported by well-founded principles.[44] Clearly then, under *Daubert*, "scientific" refers to methods and procedures—not results and conclusions. Nearly all the federal circuit courts addressing the admissibility of scientific evidence after *Daubert* agree.

It should be noted that because *Daubert* was decided under federal law, it is not binding on state courts. However, many states already have adopted *Daubert's* standards. Some states still apply the standards set forth in an earlier notable decision, *Frye* v. *United States*,[45] or their own case law. Under *Frye,* an expert opinion based on a scientific technique is inadmissible unless the technique is "generally accepted" in the relevant scientific community. The *Frye* standard was later superseded by Federal Rule of Evidence 702 which was, in turn, adopted in its essential form by many states and then interpreted and construed in *Daubert.*

The most significant distinction between *Frye* and *Daubert* is that *Frye* requires the scientific technique at issue to be "generally accepted" before it may be admitted in a judicial proceeding, whereas *Daubert* requires "reliability" as a prerequisite to admissibility.

In applying either *Daubert* or *Frye* to traumatic amnesia cases, courts should be sympathetic to the admission of such evidence, and expert testimony in support thereof, in view of a long history of methodologically valid science,[42] overwhelming clinical data demonstrating the validity of traumatic amnesia, and the very existence of the phenomenon in the DSM-IV. Thus, in most cases, defense criticism of recovered memory testimony should bear on the weight, not admissibility, of such evidence.

At the same time, expert testimony about "false memory syndrome" should not be as readily admitted under *Frye* or *Daubert,* as it is difficult to identify any reliable scientific support for such a syndrome. In fact, no controlled studies support the theory that false memories of sexual trauma can be created by suggestive questioning or therapy. Even if evidence of "false memory syndrome" were admissible under *Frye* or *Daubert,* a judge could still exclude such testimony on the grounds that it would be misleading, confusing, and/or not helpful to the fact-finder.[46]

Types of Experts

Generally, an expert witness in a sexual trauma case in which delayed recovery of memory is an issue will be one of the following: (*1*) a professional therapist who treated the victim, or (*2*) a forensic expert hired for the specific purpose of testifying about the way memory works in general and how it likely worked in the case at issue. Such experts are apt to be either scientists/researchers, clinicians with experience treating victims of sexual abuse, or a combination of both.

Treating experts are usually called to testify about their observations relative to symptomatology and damages, whereas the forensic expert is called to testify about the science of memory and its application to the facts in a particular case. In many instances, the information gleaned from these two types of experts will overlap, as treating experts will be questioned about their knowledge of the science and forensic experts will be asked about their knowledge of particular facts in the case.

Experts for both sides will likely address delayed memory separately from suggestibility, though the issues are related, as each deals with the evidentiary concept of reliability. Thus, many delayed recovery cases involve defense claims not only that recovered memories are per se unreliable but that the particular memories at issue are unreliable because they were the product of undue suggestibility during the investigation and/or therapeutic process.

Finally, even in cases where there is no evidence of traumatic amnesia and delayed recovery of memories, the defense may nonetheless try to claim that the victim's ordinary memories were distorted by undue suggestibility during investigative questioning or therapy. This is particularly true when the victim is a child. In such cases, if allowed by the court, experts will likely testify about the respective cognitive abilities and limitations of adults and children in the context of perception, memory, and suggestibility in general.

Conclusion

Child sexual abuse is a disturbing topic, which makes some people reluctant to believe in its existence. Some people even liken sexual abuse prosecutions to witch hunts from the seventeenth century. But there is a significant difference in that we all know there are no witches.

Historical and political forces encourage society to acquiesce in "explanations" for sexual abuse allegations that typically involve claims that denigrate the character of victims. These stigmatizing claims, in turn, feed biases against victims and perpetuate more sexual abuse by discouraging victims from speaking out. Obviously, unless the abuse is revealed, the deterrent value of civil and criminal litigation is lost.

While there have been a handful of troubling cases involving delayed recovery of memories, recantations, and controversial therapies, the magnitude of negative media attention and intimidation of victims are unjustified. To be sure, each category of crime has its share of disturbing examples of injustice, which is difficult to tolerate in a society that prefers to let 100 guilty people go free rather than convict one innocent person. Yet, the development of an organized effort to showcase and exploit a small number of sexual abuse cases in an apparent effort to undermine the integrity of the mental health profession and the credibility of women and children in general is far more disturbing because it threatens to deny all victims access to justice.

So few sexual abuse cases ever make it to the criminal or civil justice system that it hardly seems appropriate to intimidate a small population of potential cases with such overreaching tactics. On this point, the gender bias implications should not be overlooked. Females are more likely than males to be victims of sexual trauma and are more likely to seek the services of mental-health care providers. Thus, females are more likely than males to be discouraged from participating in criminal and civil justice proceedings.

Sexual abuse is not a ''family'' problem or a sickness best resolved in confidential ''healing'' sessions designed to retain the dignity of the family unit. It is a serious and insidious crime that targets society's vulnerable.

Litigation is an important tool in the continued struggle to eradicate sexual abuse through social accountability, but it is only effective if victims speak out and participate in the process. If privacy rights are protected and courts give due respect to recovered memory testimony, more victims will speak out and the law will work better to deter sexual violence.

Victim advocates and mental health professionals alike should welcome and encourage litigation as a legitimate forum for resolving controversies involving sexual trauma. Through the imposition of criminal and civil sanctions, we not only reduce the risk of victimization, but also give victims a meaningful voice in the development of social policy.

References

1. The Response to Rape: Detours on the Road to Equal Justice, Senator Joseph R. Biden, Jr., May, 1993.
2. Massachusetts General Laws, c.258B, sec.3(a) et. seq; Massachusetts General Laws, c.279, sec.4B.
3. See e.g., Massachusetts General Laws, c.258, sec.10.
4. See e.g., Massachusetts General Laws, c.258B, secs.8, 9.
5. Massachusetts General Laws, c.258C.
6. 940 Code of Massachusetts Regulations 14.00 et. seq.
7. *Worcester Insurance Co., Inc.* v. *Fells Acre,* 408 Mass. 393, 404 (1990).
8. Largen MA: State-by-State Comparison of Sexual Assault/Victim Counselor Privileged Communications, Statutes and Case Law, June, 1989. Distributed by National Network for

Victims of Sexual Assault; The Confidentiality of Communications Between Sexual Assault or Domestic Violence Victims and Their Counselors, Findings and Model Legislation, U.S. Dept. of Justice, Report to Congress, December 1995.

9. 1 *McCormick on Evidence*, sec.72, at 269 (Strong ed., 4th ed., 1992).

10. The Privilege of Confidentiality and Rape Crisis Counselors, 8 Women's Law Reporter, No. 3, Summer, 1985, pp. 186, 195; Existing Confidentiality Privileges Applied to Rape Victims, 5 Journal of Law and Health, No. 1 (1990–1991) pp. 104–196.

11. Rape in America, A Report to the Nation. National Victim Center and Crime Victims Research and Treatment Center, pp. 4, 10 (April, 1992).

12. *Commonwealth* v. *Collett*, 387 Mass. 424, 427–428 (1982); Accord *Commonwealth* v. *Bishop*, 416 Mass. at 176 ("victims of rape or sexual abuse would likely shy away from forthright therapeutic sessions with their counselors if their words were later lent to the perpetrator in aid of his or her defense.").

13. See e.g., Massachusetts General Laws, c.233, sec.21B; *Commonwealth* v. *Widrick*, 392 Mass. 884, 891 (1984); *Commonwealth* v. *Licata*, 412 Mass. 654 (1992).

14. *Commonwealth* v. *Joyce*, 382 Mass. 222, 228 (1981).

15. *Commonwealth* v. *Wilson*, (and a companion case) 529 Pa. 268, 281 (1992).

16. *In the Matter of Pittsburgh Action Against Rape*, 494 Pa. 15 (1981) ("PAAR").

17. *Wilson*, supra, at 276, n.6.

18. For examples of decisions in other states where courts have reached the same result see *People* v. *Foggy*, 521 N.E.2d 86 (Ill. 1988) and *People* v. *District Court of Denver*, 719 p.2d 722 (Colo. 1986).

19. *Pennsylvania* v. *Ritchie*, 480 U.S. 39 (1987).

20. *Commonwealth* v. *Joyce*, 382 Mass. 222, 225–229 (1981).

21. *Davis* v. *Alaska*, 415 U.S. 308, 319 (1974).

22. *Pennsylvania* v. *Ritchie*, 480 U.S. 39, 51 (1987).

23. *Chambers* v. *Mississippi*, 410 U.S. 284, 302 (1973).

24. *Commonwealth* v. *Figueroa*, 413 Mass. 193, 203 (1992).

25. *Commonwealth* v. *Two Juveniles*, 397 Mass. 261, 269 n.7 (1986).

26. See e.g., *Whalen* v. *Roe*, 429 U.S. 589, 599 (1977); *Roe* v. *Wade*, 410 U.S. 113, 153 (1973); *Eisenstadt* v. *Baird*, 405 U.S. 438, 483 (1972); *Griswold* v. *Connecticut*, 381 U.S. 479, 483 (1965); *Borucki* v. *Ryan*, 827 F.2d 836 (1st Cir. 1987); *Nixon* v. *Administrator of General Services*, 433 U.S. 425 (1977).

27. *Whalen* v. *Roe*, 429 U.S. 589 (1977); *Nixon* v. *Administrator of General Services*, 433 U.S. 425 (1977); *Daury* v. *Smith*, 842 F.2d 9 (1st Cir. 1988); *Caesar* v. *Mountanos*, 542 F.2d 1064 (9th Cir. 1976); *In re August 1933 Regular Grand Jury (Clinic Subpoena)*, 854 F.Supp. 1375 (S.D. Ind. 1993); *N.T.S.B.* v. *Hollywood Memorial Hospital*, 735 F.Supp. 423 (S.D. Fla. 1990); *Hawaii* v. *Ariyoshi*, 481 F.Supp. 1028 (D.Hawaii 1979); *McKenna* v. *Fargo*, 451 F.Supp. 1355 (D.N.J. 1978); *Merriken* v. *Cressman*, 364 F.Supp. 913 (E.D.Pa. 1973); *United States* v. *Layton*, 90 F.R.D. 520 (N.D. Cal. 1981); *Lora* v. *Board of Education*, 74 F.R.D. 565 (E.D.N.Y. 1977).

28. Smith, Steven R. Psychotherapy and the Right of Privacy, 49 George Wash Law Rev 1, 56 (1980).

29. For examples of cases setting forth rules and standards that strive to balance the interests of victims and defendants see *Commonwealth* v. *Fuller*, 423 Mass. 216 (1996). *Commonwealth* v. *Bishop*, 617 N.E. 2d 995, 997 (1993) (as a threshold burden, "a defendant must show at a minimum a likelihood that the records contain relevant evidence to justify initial review [by the judge]" . . . "defense counsel shall submit to the judge, in writing, the

theory or theories under which the particular records sought are likely to be relevant to an issue in the case''); *Goldsmith* v. *Maryland*, 651 A.2d 866 (Md. 1995) (defendant must establish a likelihood that the records sought would provide exculpatory information); *State* v. *Howard*, 604 A.2d 1294, 1300 (Conn. 1992) (defendant must establish ''reasonable ground to believe failure to produce records would likely impair defendant's right to impeach witness''); *State* v. *Hummel*, 483 N.W.2d 68, 72 (Minn. 1992) (defendant must make a ''plausible showing'' that information sought is material and favorable to defense); *State* v. *Gagne*, 612 A.2d 899, 901 (N.H. 1992) (defendant must demonstrate a ''reasonable probability'' that the records contain information that is material and relevant); *State* v. *Shiffra*, 499 N.W.2d 719, 721 (Wis. 1993) (defendant must make a ''preliminary showing that the sought after evidence is material to his or her defense'').

30. *Commonwealth* v. *Fuller*, 423 Mass. 216 (1996).
31. For a more detailed look at the application of the rules and standards in practice see *Goldsmith* v. *Maryland*, 337 Md. 112 (1995) (the defendant's proffer was inadequate because he asserted only that (*1*) there was a long delay between the date of the assault and the victim's report to the authorities and (*2*) the victim was in counseling. The court held the defendant's proffer was, at best, only a ''speculative assertion'' that such records ''may'' contain evidence useful for impeachment, which plainly fell short of establishing a ''likelihood'' that the victim's counseling records would provide helpful information); *Commonwealth* v. *Reed*, 417 Mass. 558, 561–562 (1994) (the defendant's proffer was adequate because it was a detailed affidavit which stated specific facts upon which the defendant based his opinion that confidential records of a witness would likely contain certain evidence bearing on a reward the witness had been promised related to her testimony); *Commonwealth* v. *Bishop*, supra, note 25 (school records not discoverable because defendant failed to assert specific theory under which undisclosed school records were relevant); *Commonwealth* v. *Baxter*, 36 Mass. App. Ct. 45, 48 (1994) (psychiatric records disclosed only after defendant submitted a ''detailed offer of proof'' and a specific theory of defense).
32. *People* v. *Gissendanner*, 48 N.Y.2d 543, 549 (1979).
33. For examples of cases where the court acknowledged such a hierarchy see *Commonwealth* v. *Fuller*, 423 Mass. 216 (1996) and *State* v. *Goldsmith*, 337 Md. 112 (1995) (where a defendant seeks disclosure of material protected by an absolute privilege, defendant must show a ''likelihood that records will contain exculpatory evidence.'' Requests for merely confidential information require the defendant to show only a ''reasonable possibility that review of the records would result in discovery of usable evidence''); *Commonwealth* v. *Two Juveniles*, 389 Mass. 261 (1986) (the rape crisis counseling privilege statute, ''like few other testimonial privilege statutes, is a statement of absolute privilege,'' thus, disclosure shall be prohibited unless the defendant can establish a ''legitimate need'' for access); *Commonwealth* v. *Gauthier*, 32 Mass. App. Ct. 130, 135 (1992) (stating without explanation that the priest/penitent privilege is ''absolute,'' the sexual assault counseling privilege is ''semi-absolute'' and the psychotherapist/patient privilege is ''qualified''); *Pennsylvania* v. *Ritchie*, 480 U.S. 39, 57–58 and n. 14–15 (1987) (the court adopted a strict need-based access standard for merely confidential social service agency records but noted that it had not determined the circumstances under which access would be granted, if at all, to material protected by an absolute privilege, such as rape crisis counseling records); *Commonwealth* v. *Wilson*, (and a companion case) 529 Pa. 268 (1992) (citing the ''compelling interest in protecting the confidentiality of the rape victim's records'' the court refused to allow Pennsylvania's rape crisis counseling privilege to be abrogated under any circumstances because the privilege is of a higher status than the lower-level privilege afforded other information

such as psychotherapy records which are available to the defense for inspection.); *State* v. *J.G.* 261 N.J. Super. 409, 619 A.2d 232 (N.J. Super. Ct. App. Div. 1993); *In the Matter of T.M., J.R.*, No. J4367–91 (D.C. Super. Oct 21, 1992).

34. *Jaffee* v. *Redmond*, 116 S. Ct. 1923 (1996).
35. *State* v. *Hungerford*, 94-S-045 (New Hampshire Superior Court); *State* v. *Morahan*, 93-S-1734 (New Hampshire Superior Court).
36. *Doe* v. *Maskell*, 94236030/CL185155 (Dist. of Columbia); *Roe* v. *Maskell*, 94236031/CL185156 (Dist. of Columbia).
37. *State* v. *Walters*, 93-S-211, 2112. (New Hampshire Superior Court).
38. *Hoult* v. *Hoult*, F.2d (1st Cir. 1995).
39. Loftus E: The reality of repressed memories. 48 Am Psychol 1993; 48:518–537.
40. *Shazade* v. *Gregory*, United States District Court, District of Massachusetts, 92-12139-EFH (May 8, 1996); *Isley* v. *Capuchin Province*, 877 F.Supp. 1055 (E.D. Mich 1995).
41. *Shazade* v. *Gregory*, United States District Court, District of Massachusetts, 92-12139-EFH (May 8, 1996).
42. For a recent and comprehensive review of the research in this area see van der Kolk B and Fisler R: Dissociation and the fragmentary nature of traumatic memories: overview and exploratory study. J Traumatic Stress 1995; 8:505–526.
43. *Daubert* v. *Merrell Dow Pharmaceuticals, Inc.*, 113 S.Ct. 2786 (1993).
44. *Cella* v. *United States*, 998 F.2d 418, 426 (7th Cir. 1993); *Christopherson* v. *Allied-Signal Corp.*, 939 F.2d 1106, 1111 & n.9 (5th Cir. 1991) (en banc), cert. denied, 112 S. Ct. 1280 (1992); *Hines* v. *Consolidated Rail Corp.*, 926 F.2d 262, 274 (3d Cir. 1991); *Osburn* v. *Anchor Laboratories, Inc.*, 825 F.2d 908, 915 (5th Cir. 1987).
45. *Frye* v. *United States*, 293 F. 1013 (D.C. App. 1923).
46. See *Robinson* v. *McCloskey*, 676 F.Supp. 351 (D.D.C. 1988) (expert testimony regarding memory excluded because testimony was not supported by valid science, jury would be confused and misled and jury could understand the way memory works without expert guidance).

19

For Whom Does the Bell Toll?
Repressed Memory and Challenges for the Law—
Getting Beyond the Statute of Limitations

Law and psychiatry are fields that share a common goal of trying to resolve issues of the past in the present. The impetus either to seek therapy or pursue a lawsuit is often based on the same need to integrate the past: by bearing witness to the past, to tame rather than bury it, a person is expressing the desire to incorporate one's history into present reality. The meaning of memory is therefore the inescapable foundational element for both disciplines.

While both disciplines are linked in their aim of resolving issues of the past in the present, the meaning that each assigns to the past is very different. For talk-based therapy, historical accuracy has not been, and many argue should not be, the orientation of its focus. What is important is rather the "narrative truth" of memory—how an individual has understood a past event and the role that memory plays in determining the inner life and external choices of the individual.[1] For law, the concern is not with how an individual struggles to construct personal meaning out of the past; it cares about defining in a fair and accurate manner what *is* the past. The very legitimacy of law's power of judgment depends upon civil and criminal verdicts being seen and accepted as accurate statements about the factual reality of, and a resolution of responsibility for, a past event.[2]

Since 1986, with the emergence of the first legal cases raising claims of repressed memory, the law's systemic reliance on both the fragility and the power of memory has been exposed as never before. Legal cases based on repressed memory are founded on an inextricable linkage between the explanation for the delay in the onset of memory and the historical accuracy of the event itself. As such, these cases force the law to recognize its overall dependence on the accuracy of memory and, to the extent that the historical accuracy of these cases is attacked, the concomitant potential of this type of litigation to undermine the legitimacy of all legal verdicts.

The central premise of this chapter is that the ground of defendants' legal arguments is in the process of shifting. For the past decade, the legal doctrine that has borne the brunt of finding a principled way to decide whether and when cases based on repressed memory should enter the judicial system has been the statute of limitations. In order to ensure the fair resolution of legal disputes, all lawsuits must be filed within a legislatively prescribed "limitations period" dating from the occurrence of the act that caused the harm. Standing like Cerberus as a gatekeeper at the courthouse door, the statute of limitations is the traditional legal doctrine by which every defendant can bar any plaintiff's claim at the initial stage of a lawsuit on the basis of the mere fact that the complaint was filed too late. The defendant can ordinarily even admit responsibility for the harm and successfully use the statute of limitations as a defense. The rules governing when to file a lawsuit have been violated and the defendant is entitled to be left in peace.

If a plaintiff claims that she or he could not file a lawsuit within the filing period, not because of inadvertence or a lack of diligence, but because she or he did not even know that an act of sexual abuse had occurred during his or her childhood due to repression of the memories of this abuse, how should the legal system react? Should plaintiffs be afforded access to the legal system through a "discovery" rule which would suspend or "toll" the limitations period until the date when the plaintiff claims to have recovered memories of the abuse, or should defendants be protected through a strict reading of the statute of limitations? On whose side should the legal system err?

In the past two years, we have seen the emergence of new defense strategies that have moved away from the issue of the "discovery" exception to the statute of limitations to strategies that mount a much more sophisticated and multipronged frontal attack on the reliability of recovered memory itself. This chapter is divided into three sections that trace this development. In Part One, I first explain the role that a traditional statute of limitations defense plays in all lawsuits, as an attempt to illustrate the conflicting policies that have shaped the application of this defense over several hundred years of litigation. I then explore the way in which these policy considerations have been understood and applied to cases involving plaintiff claims of recovered memory of childhood sexual abuse. In Part Two, I use the 1986 case of *Tyson* v. *Tyson,* the first reported appellate decision in this area of law, to set out an analytic framework that traces a decade of case law and legislative reform surrounding the statute of limitations in cases involving childhood sexual abuse. In Part Three, I outline new defense legal strategies that have moved beyond the statute of limitations as the primary challenge to a plaintiff's complaint.

The motivation behind this shift in defense strategies is clear. Defendants are no longer content to argue on the basis of the statute of limitations that these lawsuits are indefensible due to the passage of time; the premise of these new defense strategies is that these complaints may be the result of a false (or at least a misguided) accusation. The dismissal of a plaintiff's claim on the grounds of the statute of limitations may end a lawsuit, but it does not necessarily imply that the defendant did not do the acts; it is rather only a statement that the plaintiff waited too long to sue. These new defense strategies more overtly attack the assumption that the plaintiff's claims can be relied on as truth, thereby turning the initial procedural challenges into a mini-trial on the validity of the accusation. If the complaint is then dismissed, defendants can seemingly characterize the decision, at least to themselves, their family and community, as having established their probable innocence of the accusation.

These new defense strategies attempt to shift the factual determination of the accuracy of an allegation of abuse from the trial to a variety of pretrial hearings. By dismissing a lawsuit at a preliminary stage of the proceedings or precluding a witness' testimony in a pretrial evidentiary ruling, defendants are trying to end the lawsuit before a plaintiff even has the chance to develop the case through the normal investigative stages of the legal process. These new defense strategies which are designed to cut the lawsuit off at the very beginning of the process, are problematic insofar as we may never know whether or not the claim *was* valid, unless it can proceed onwards in the legal system. To the degree that defendants are successful, these new strategies have the potential to foreclose the legal system to plaintiffs as an avenue to hear and redress *valid* claims of childhood sexual abuse.

Part One: The Countervailing Policies and Meanings of a Statute of Limitations Challenge

The statute of limitations is the legal doctrine responsible for equitably balancing an inescapable tension. A plaintiff who, although seemingly late in filing, still wants his or her day in court to present a claim is juxtaposed against a defendant who, due to the passage of time, is concerned that the allegations in the complaint can neither be heard in a way that comports with fairness nor the process be trusted to produce a reliable verdict. For hundreds of years before the controversy over "false" memory ever arose and in all types of civil and criminal litigation far removed from the highly charged area concerning childhood sexual abuse, the law has always been concerned with balancing access to legal remedies for deserving plaintiffs against the potential of indefensible or "unfair" lawsuits against defendants. To manage these conflicting purposes, the law has, over time, developed two competing sets of arguments. The first favors strict construction of statutes of limitation so that defendants are protected, and the second (not surprisingly) favors equitable exceptions to strict construction for a deserving plaintiff. In this section of the chapter, I will outline both sets of arguments as they have been expressed in the law generally and then present how they have been construed in the context of litigation over the past ten years in cases of childhood sexual abuse.

Traditionally, courts have given three policy reasons in support of the strict construction of statutes of limitations. The first rationale is to "protect defendants and the courts from having to deal with cases in which the search for truth may be seriously impaired by the loss of evidence, whether by death or disappearance of witnesses, fading memories, disappearance of documents, or otherwise."[3] The desire is to assist courts in their pursuit of the truth through accurate fact-finding by expediting cases to trial before physical evidence is mislaid or destroyed, while witnesses are still available and memories can be relied upon. Both civil and criminal courts here use the terminology of barring "stale" claims and the need to act while the evidence is "fresh."

The second rationale is to protect defendants from the protracted fear of litigation. Here the desire is for finality, letting sleeping dogs lie and allowing people to move on with their lives—to let the documents be discarded and memories fade—without fear that they will be needed in the future. This rationale, though related to issues of proof, is more about efficiency, closure, certainty, and the fears of vulnerability that the potential exposure to financial liability or criminal responsibility entails.[4]

The third rationale is that statutes of limitation, by forcing plaintiffs into action and not allowing them "to sleep on their rights," serve as an initial systemic assurance of the validity of a complaint.[5] If a plaintiff truly has been harmed, the argument goes, then she or he will be ready, willing, and able to file suit as soon as it is possible, and that will be during a period when defendants are able to defend themselves. If a plaintiff files late, there is an increased risk that no harm was done and that the lawsuit or prosecution is motivated by reasons other than remedying the harm. Seen this way, statutes of limitation serve as a procedural device to ensure the substantive validity of a lawsuit.

These three rationales are all powerful arguments for the strict construction of statutes of limitation and have been used by all levels of courts in the Anglo-American tradition to express the importance of this doctrine for the proper functioning of a legal system. For example, in an 1879 case, *Wood* v. *Carpenter,* the United States Supreme Court extolled the virtues of strict construction of statutes of limitations:

> Statutes of limitation are vital to the welfare of society and are favored in the law. They are found and approved in all systems of enlightened jurisprudence. They promote repose by giving security and stability to human affairs. An important public policy lies at their foundation. They stimulate to activity and punish negligence. While time is constantly destroying the evidence of rights, they supply its place by a presumption which renders proof unnecessary. Mere delay, extending to the limit prescribed, is itself a conclusive bar. The bane and antidote go together.[6]

There are, however, equally compelling arguments for plaintiffs. Fairness and equity, access to the legal system, and protecting the integrity of the process are equivalent policy concerns for the judiciary. While the strict construction of a statute of limitation will bar an individual case that is based on a valid complaint, the repeated refusal to allow valid claims to be addressed by the courts could undermine the legitimacy of judicial process as a forum for the redress of individual harm and social wrongs. If similarly placed parties are continually denied access to the legal sytem, they may look elsewhere or to extralegal means to achieve what they see as justice. Since courts can be seen as a way of channeling social unrest, cases in which an entire class of plaintiffs would be affected tend to be more successful, perhaps because their grievances may seem to be more threatening to the social order.

For example, one of the most influential modern U.S. Supreme Court cases to recognize a discovery exception to the statute of limitations, based on arguments of fairness or equity, was the 1948 case of *Urie* v. *Thompson*,[7] a test case for the scope of workers' compensation law. In *Urie,* the plaintiff claimed that he had to leave his job as a fireman on a steam locomotive due to silicosis poisoning and that this amounted to negligence on the part of his employer under the Federal Employers' Liability Act (FELA). The defendant, a trustee of the railroad, made two arguments: first, whatever conditions of employment could or should be attributed to him were not covered by FELA; and second, that in any event, the lawsuit was filed too late. The Supreme Court ruled unanimously for the plaintiff on both issues. Speaking for the Supreme Court, Justice Rutledge said that the negligence statute and its limitation period must be construed together in a "humane" manner so that the legislation does not afford the plaintiff, and those like him, only a "delusive remedy." To do otherwise on the limitations issue, the Court held,

> . . . would mean that at some past moment in time, unknown and inherently unknowable even in retrospect, Urie was charged with knowledge of the slow and tragic disintegration of his lungs; under this view Urie's failure to diagnose within the applicable statute of limitations a disease whose symptoms had not yet obtruded on his consciousness would constitute waiver of his right to compensation at the ultimate day of discovery and disability.[8]

Urie could neither file any earlier than he did nor be expected to, reasoned the court:

> There is no suggestion that Urie should have known he had silicosis at any earlier date. It follows that no specific date of contact with the substance can be charged with being the date of injury, inasmuch as the injurious consequences of the exposure are the product of a period of time rather than a point in time; consequently the afflicted employee can be held to be 'injured' only when the accumulated effects of the deleterious substance manifest themselves. . . .[9]

Similarly, in *Bowen* v. *City of New York,* a 1986 case, the U.S. Supreme Court held that a 60-day period to file a claim with the Social Security Administration should be tolled for equitable reasons when a class of claimants was prevented from knowing its rights by the actions of a governmental agency. Courts must be careful to not be "unduly restrictive" in interpreting the statute of limitations, cautioned the Court, lest they violate the statutory intent to provide victims with access to the court system for a remedy that is consistent with the equities of the situation. Adopting the language of the Second Circuit Court of Appeals' opinion in the case, the Supreme Court held:

> Where the Government's secretive conduct prevents plaintiffs from knowing of a violation of rights, statutes of limitations have been tolled until such a time as plaintiffs had a reasonable opportunity to learn the facts concerning the cause of action. Since in this case the full extent of the Government's clandestine policy was uncovered only in the course of this litigation, all class members may pursue this action notwithstanding the sixty-day requirement.[10]

The Supreme Court has even tolled the applicable statute of limitations using arguments of Constitutional equal protection. In the 1982 case of *Mills* v. *Habluetzel*,[11] the Court found that a Texas statute violated the Equal Protection Clause of the Constitution by mandating the institution of a paternity suit to identify the natural father of an illegitimate child for the purposes of obtaining child support before the child's first birthday.

In addition, for hundreds of years, common law courts have held that statutes of limitations may be tolled whenever there are equitable considerations affecting either party to the dispute. Claims that the defendant has engaged in fraud or duress will toll the limitations period, as will the catch-all exception called "equitable estoppel," which prevents parties from taking legal advantage of a situation that they themselves have created. This would cover those unspecified situations in which a defendant's conduct had somehow interfered with the plaintiff's ability to file to the degree that it would be improper for the court to bar the lawsuit.[12] On the other side, a plaintiff's service in the Armed Forces is equally regarded as a legitimate reason to be exempted from normal filing requirements,[13] as is a claim that the plaintiff was suffering from a mental disability that prevented timely filing of a claim.[14] And, for the reason most germane to this chapter, all limitations periods are tolled during the infancy of the victim, the potential plaintiff. While plaintiffs should be forced to act—and foreclosed from legal remedy if they fail to act—it is unjust to hold minors to this standard of personal accountability until they reach the age of majority.

In *any* situation where the court tolls a limitations period, the potential for lost evidence and disruption in the defendant's life exist, but the legal system nevertheless allows these cases to be heard. It is doing so for important reasons related to its own systemic values and purposes. By providing exceptions to the statute of limitations defense, the courts are allowing a limitation period's potential for undue harshness to be circumscribed, either in an individual case or for a class of plaintiffs. Equitable exceptions guard against the possibility that the limitations period is being manipulated by an individual defendant to deny the plaintiff access to a legal remedy. For both individuals and plaintiffs as a class, applying an equitable exception allows the legal system to prevent itself from being seen as a co-perpetrator of a plaintiff's injury. A legal system's claim to legitimacy will not survive if it is seen as a collusive agent in the creation of harm.

Finally, it should be noted that statute of limitation challenges raise somewhat different issues in criminal trials, where the State is the prosecuting authority, the victim is the notifying witness, and the defendant has a Sixth Amendment constitutional right to a speedy trial. The criminal rights of the defendant would be implicated in a situation where, for example, a district attorney wanted to press assault, rape, statutory rape, or incest charges against a defendant on the basis of a victim's repressed memories of harm. The civil/criminal distinction is also the reason why neither the highly publicized *Franklin*[15] case in California nor the *Slutzker*[16] or *Crawford*[17] trials in Pennsylvania is directly relevant to the issue of a civil statute of limitations. For most of this chapter's discussion of the statutes of limitation, I am concerned exclusively with civil cases, although what I say here has obvious implications for the interpretation of statutes of limitation in criminal cases.

Turning to cases involving a civil tort claim of childhood sexual abuse, if one were to date these cases as one does ordinary personal injury cases from the date of the act that causes injury, the limitations period to bring a civil action would expire 1 to 6 years after the last act of abuse. The variation in the range is dependent on the type of tort theory used in the complaint to describe the abuse (which could be framed as assault, battery, or intentional or negligent infliction of emotional distress) and the limitations period set out in the statutes of the jurisdiction for claims based on that tort theory of recovery. For many victims of childhood sexual abuse, their legal rights to sue might well expire before they reach adulthood. As explained above, all jurisdictions toll or delay the running of the limitations period until a plaintiff reaches the statutorily prescribed ages of majority; the statute then begins to run as if their birthday were the date on which the injury occurred.

For an adult plaintiff alleging childhood sexual abuse, passing over the legal hurdle of the statute of limitations is a necessary requirement in order to maintain the lawsuit. If a defendant raises a sufficient argument that the lawsuit was filed on a date outside of the limitations period,[18] a plaintiff must meet one of two standards in order to go forward in the legal process: either that he or she did in fact remember the abuse or discovered the causal connection on a date within the limitations period so that the judge rules in his or her favor as a matter of law, or that the plaintiff can at least raise sufficient facts showing that the date of filing the lawsuit on which she or he is relying is within the allowable limitations period so that the issue as to which date governs—the plaintiff's or the one alleged by the defendant—can then be turned over as a matter of fact to be decided by the jury. A judge at a statute of limitations hearing therefore has three options: dismiss the case (which the plaintiff can appeal), apply discovery rule as a matter of law (which the defendant can appeal), or leave the question to the jury to be determined at trial.

Only if the plaintiff can convince the judge that the date of filing is within the statute of limitations can she or he progress to the next stage in the legal process or to trial where the plaintiff must establish on a balance of probabilities that the abuse did in fact occur. In the next stage of the legal process, ironically called the "discovery phase" of a civil lawsuit, the plaintiff has the legal authority to depose the defendant and other witnesses and gather other evidentiary material that may be crucial to bolstering his or her own testimony about either the application of the discovery exception, or the circumstances of the abuse itself.

Procedurally, it is important to realize that if a judge rules in a statute of limitations motion to leave the question of which date governs to the jury, which may be the most attractive compromise option, the issue is hardly over. There are several further procedural stages in a civil trial in which the defendant has the right to ask for this defense to be applied,[19] and there are motion judges who will re-hear this same issue again even at the same stage in the process. In other words, an initial determination by a single judge to allow a plaintiff to proceed to the next stage of the litigation is not a final order and the issue may be reversed by a later court, precluding an ultimate trial on the merits.

Regardless of when it is raised, the psychological ramifications of a statute of limitations challenge on a plaintiff are troubling. From a plaintiff's perspective, the defendant has turned the tables and has gone on the offense on an issue that seems, at least at first blush, wholly apart from the merits of the case. If *the* question posed by the motion is why the plaintiff is bringing this up so late, then it is no longer a lawsuit about what the defendant did but rather what the plaintiff did not do. For a plaintiff who honestly believes that she or he has been abused as a child, and that coming to terms with either the event itself or the realization of its harmful effects continues to be a protracted struggle, the message of a statute of limitations defense is that she or he is to blame for not having taken the decisive action of filing the lawsuit earlier. When the actions, or more precisely the omissions, of the victim are the sole, contested focus of this preliminary stage of the lawsuit, a statute of limitations challenge has the potential to be an instance of psychological revictimization.[20] Although it may be viewed as self-inflicted (given that the plaintiff controlled the decision about whether to initiate a lawsuit), there are systemic concerns for the law if a statute of limitations challenge, viewed this way, has become a powerful therapeutic disincentive to the seeking of a legal remedy for harm.

Although all jurisdictions ordinarily toll or delay the running of the time period in a civil case until a plaintiff reaches the age of majority, it is still arguably the rare childhood sexual abuse plaintiff, even in a case of documented abuse, who is sufficiently emotionally stable and independent to mount a legal action against a perpetrator by the time the limitations period expires somewhere between the age of 19 to 24. But if a plaintiff, regardless of whether she or he is deserving or deluded, brings a lawsuit beyond the statutory time limit, the court is ordinarily required to dismiss the complaint: hence, the importance of the discovery rule and all equitable exceptions to the limitations period.

Plaintiffs in childhood sexual abuse cases have tried to use the traditional common law exceptions such as mental disability, fraud, duress, and equitable estoppel either as additional or alternative arguments to the discovery rule to toll the limitations period. These efforts have been largely unsuccessful, except for rare instances in which the facts strictly conform to the arguments ordinarily recognized in nonsexual abuse cases.

For example, the mental disability exception to the statute of limitations (styled also as mental incompetency, unsound mind, and insanity) ordinarily demands that a plaintiff be "incapable of caring for his or her personal safety and providing for basic human needs."[21] As a result, plaintiffs who allege a "mere post-traumatic neurosis"[22] or "multiple personality disorder"[23] but who were still able to live in the community have been barred from using the mental disability exception. On the other hand, in cases where there has been a history of hospitalization and facts indicating severe mental impairment, courts have recognized the tolling provision so long as the plaintiff can show that "she repressed the memory of the facts upon which her claim is predicated, such that she could not have been aware of the rights that she was otherwise bound to know."[24]

Similarly, courts have rejected arguments that the fraud exception should be applied even in circumstances when the defendant told the child that the sexual act was not wrong or where the defendant told the child that she had been the one at fault for the sexual encounter. Only if the victim is deceived as to the *sexual* nature of the act, will fraud toll the limitations period. Fraud has been successfully used to toll the statute in a case where, for example, the defendant who was the plaintiff's father medicated her, acting as her doctor.[25]

Courts have uniformly rejected duress as grounds to toll the statute of limitations past the date when the plaintiff moved away from the situation in which the defendant was in physical control of the plaintiff's person.[26] Courts have rejected arguments that the power differential between an adult and a child constituted duress, even when there are facts in the complaint that describe threats to the child or others if they were to *ever* reveal the abuse.[27]

Lastly, although legal commentators favor this exception,[28] courts have also rejected arguments based on equitable estoppel as a means to overcome the statute of limitations.[29] Here, a plaintiff argues that because it was the *defendant's* acts which created the inability to sue within the ordinary running of the limitations period, the defendant ought to be precluded from using the statute of limitations as a defense. Perhaps because this argument could potentially result in any childhood sexual abuse plaintiff's open-ended ability to bring suit, no court has accepted equitable estoppel as the sole reason for tolling the limitations period.

For adult plaintiffs in childhood sexual abuse cases, the discovery exception has been the only legal argument by which they have, as individuals and as a class of plaintiffs, succeeded in tolling the statute of limitations. The "discovery" exception to the statute of limitations, unlike other common law equitable exceptions, has been part of the American legal system for only over forty years. Used originally for late diagnosis of physical injuries or progressive diseases, as in *Urie* v. *Thompson* discussed earlier, it now has a complicated legal life of its own that is not often understood by those lay advocates for childhood sexual abuse victims who seek to use the discovery rule in civil cases. Several jurisdictions, for example New York, take a highly restrictive view of the discovery exception generally and limit its use in medical malpractice to cases where a foreign object is left in the body of the patient.[30] Not surprisingly, therefore,

New York is a jurisdiction that consistently has refused to recognize the validity of the discovery exception as applied to the facts of childhood sexual abuse cases absent explicit legislative authorization.[31]

The argument to apply the general discovery exception to cases involving childhood sexual abuse and repressed memory seems simple in terms of equity. It would be unjust to consider that the action has accrued until the plaintiff knew, or at least reasonably should have known, the facts that would form the basis of the legal claim to be pursued. Even if this delay causes problems for a defendant in terms of proof or inconvenience, how can a plaintiff be held responsible for failure to bring a lawsuit if he or she did not know that there was a lawsuit to bring? If a plaintiff's cause of action is not known until a certain point, then that moment of "discovery" ought to mark the commencement of the running of the statute of limitations and not a moment sooner. For a decade, the entire goal of the legal reform efforts on behalf of plaintiffs in this area of law has therefore been to achieve the legal recognition that the discovery exception ought to be applied to the issue of childhood sexual abuse. This legal strategy first manifested itself in the 1986 case of *Tyson* v. *Tyson,* to which I now turn.

Part Two: The Patterns of Litigation Strategies: 1986 to Present

In this section of the chapter, I trace the litigation strategies that have characterized the hodgepodge of case law and legislative amendments in this fast-breaking area of law. The first case raising the intersection of recovered memory and sexual abuse was *Tyson* v. *Tyson*[32] in 1986. Any discussion of litigation in this area over the past decade must begin with a detailed examination of this case which has set the landscape in terms of the political agenda, legal strategies, and rhetorical tone for activity on all sides of this dispute.

Nancy Tyson alleged that she had totally repressed the memory of abuse from the age of 3 to 11 at the hands of her father, Robert, until she entered therapy. She then began to recall the abuse and understand its causal role in her emotional problems as a young adult. She filed suit in 1983, one year after starting therapy, at the age of 26.

The defendant moved to dismiss the complaint as time-barred by the statute of limitations. The defendant noted the 3-year statutory limitations period on the tort claim brought by the plaintiff, arguing that the last possible date for his daughter to have filed suit was 1978, 3 years past her eighteenth birthday and the date of majority. In reply, the plaintiff argued that the traditional discovery exception to the statute of limitations should be applied to her complaint, stating that the limitations period ought not to begin to run until she had discovered through therapy that she had a legal cause of action against the defendant. How could she sue, she argued, when she did not even "discover" that she had been abused until she recovered her memories and understood the psychological harm that the childhood sexual abuse had caused?

The Washington Supreme Court rejected Nancy Tyson's argument. Over two separate dissenting opinions, Justice Barbara Durham for the majority of the court held that it would not apply the discovery rule because Tyson's claim was based solely on repressed memory rather than objective, verifiable evidence of the wrongful act. Had the plaintiff discovered "hard" evidence, like a sponge inside her abdomen as in a case of surgical malpractice, then the discovery rule could be used to permit late claims for a new fact situation like childhood sexual abuse. With a sponge or other physical evidence, the court reasoned, "the objective nature of the evidence makes it substantially certain that the facts can be fairly determined"[33] despite the passage of time. However, the risk to the defendant of an inaccurate verdict was too great where the only evidence that is discovered is *memory* of the abuse, and the only further proof would come from experts drawn from the therapeutic community or lay witnesses contemporaneous to those long-ago events. In addition, in reasoning that was prescient in its ability to forecast litigation strategies that would emerge only a decade later, Justice Durham noted the imprecision of psychiatry and psychology as disciplines as contrasted with the biological sciences and questioned whether therapists have any special ability to ascertain historical rather than narrative truth of an event, raising the possibility that memory may be distorted through therapeutic suggestibility.

The Washington state court held that when there is no means of "independently verifying" in whole or in part the allegations in a complaint, the discovery rule is inapplicable as a matter of law and dismissed Nancy Tyson's complaint as time barred by strictly constructing the statute of limitations. Two years following the dismissal of the case in 1988, after public hearings, the Washington legislature amended its code of civil procedure to permit the state courts to use the discovery rule in cases of childhood sexual abuse for cases in which a plaintiff "discovered or reasonably should have discovered the injury or condition was caused by the act or discovered the act, whichever period expires later,"[34] thereby undoing by legislation what the *Tyson* court had done.

We are now 10 years removed from the *Tyson* case, in which time we have seen a complicated mix of case law, legislative reform efforts, changes in statutory requirements to sue, and legal commentaries on the application of the discovery exception to this type of litigation. These legal moves have transpired in the larger social context of the furious pace and high-pitched tone of mass media coverage of sexual abuse generally,[35] the emergence of the false memory movement,[36] and rising concern about overreaching therapeutic practices in this area.[37] The larger legal landscape against which these issues also must be measured includes other complicated phenomena such as concern in the criminal law about the rise of the "abuse excuse"[38] and attempts to cut back in tort liability in the law more generally.[39] When variations across states as to the existence, definition, or interpretation of the discovery rule are added to the mix, it is very hard to predict how any individual case will be decided.

It is now clear that the litigative patterns for the past decade were definitively established by the *Tyson* case in three different ways. First, *Tyson* set up a typology for legal reform, reproduced in many states, in which the highest appellate court in a state case decision upheld the dismissal of a lawsuit on statute of limitations grounds and then was overturned by legislative action enacting some version of a discovery exception for childhood sexual abuse. The second effect was to set in motion a litigative framework around which both plaintiffs and defendants had to formulate their legal strategies. For plaintiffs, their goal was to distinguish the *Tyson* precedent as inapplicable in order to succeed with their own claims that the discovery rule should indeed be applied or recognized in their case by the courts. Conversely, defendants tried to use the arguments in *Tyson* to maintain a time bar on this type of lawsuit. The third effect of the decision was to set up a particular rhetorical paradigm for the traditional balancing of the equities as between plaintiffs and defendants in statute of limitations arguments.

The first effect of the *Tyson* decision was to set a pattern of how discovery rules have come into existence in many jurisdictions. A court in another state hearing a childhood sexual abuse case based on repressed memory for the first time had to justify what result it reached in light of the *Tyson* precedent. A defendant in that new jurisdiction would argue on the basis of *Tyson* and its subsequent history that it is a *legislative* function to amend the statute of limitations to include this type of case as an instance for the application of the discovery rule. A plaintiff would have to urge the court to act on its own in the face of what the Washington court had done. The *Tyson* court, by treating the question of whether Washington's existing discovery rule should be applied to claims of childhood sexual abuse as if it would have been an issue of judicial "legislation" rather than ordinary interpretation, set up a persuasive precedent for other state courts not to act on their own initiative—even if they wanted to as a matter of social policy.

In jurisdictions that followed this pattern of dismissal of an initial case seeking to use the discovery rule, several legislatures have indeed responded by enacting some sort of amendment to their code of civil procedure. Although legislation in those states may differ in the definition given "discovery," *Tyson* set the historical pattern as to how many of the states that do have the discovery rule for these cases arrived at this legal result: a case law dismissal, public hearings, followed by legislative reform designed to reverse the holding of the court.[40] Viewed this way, *Tyson* can be understood as an example of how legal reform is and is not accomplished.

The second way to understand the effect of the *Tyson* decision is to see the case as a frame for the litigative strategies used by plaintiff and defense lawyers to argue about the applicability of the case to a different set of case facts in a different jurisdiction. As the first case emerging in this field, *Tyson* set the stage for how both sides thought about the success of the claims that they wanted to bring and how the legal issues surrounding the application of the statute of limitations should be raised. Since *Tyson* itself resulted in the dismissal of the claim, plaintiffs' lawyers had the burden of persuasion to convince the court that *Tyson* should not be followed, either because it was wrongly decided as a matter of law or because their case was different enough as a factual matter to be distinguishable.

Regardless of which tack plaintiff lawyers used to distinguish *Tyson,* the first task for any plaintiff's counsel was to grapple with the scope of the Court's power to interpret legal rules. Since *Tyson* was a case where the court dismissed the complaint due to the absence of an existing explicit legislative mandate, a plaintiff had to address the structural issue of which branch of government has the authority to act to craft the new legal rules, or at least to apply old rules (i.e., the already existing discovery exception) to a new situation.

Using the same arguments as Justice Utter, one of the two dissenting judges in *Tyson,* many plaintiffs have succeeded in arguing that courts could and should take the lead in applying the discovery rule to situations involving childhood sexual abuse. Plaintiffs have succeeded first by framing the issue before the court as narrowly as possible (i.e., this is traditional interpretation, not legislation), convincing the court that judicial action to apply the discovery rule is an entirely appropriate action. Then, using Justice Pearson's separate dissenting opinion in *Tyson,* these plaintiffs have detailed the reality of the phenomenon of sexual abuse and highlighted the inequities of denying a blameless plaintiff access to the legal system, particularly when it was the defendant's actions that prevented timely filing. If a plaintiff succeeded in convincing a court hearing this kind of case for the first time to proceed, it was because of the conjunction of two forces: that the court was in favor of judicial activism in the larger national debate over strict construction of statutory language and legislative supremacy, and that when the court balanced the equities, the plaintiff's argument for access to the legal system prevailed.

Conversely, during the period in which plaintiffs were trying to establish some version of the discovery rule in each jurisdiction, defendants used the majority opinion in *Tyson* to dismiss cases in one of two ways: either by convincing a sympathetic court not to act in the absence of legislation or by using the lack of "objective evidence" to block cases where memory serves as the sole or primary means of proof of the abuse.

The requirement of objective evidence of the abuse and its repression in order to toll the statute of limitations, seemingly the crux of the *Tyson* majority's reasoning in the dismissal of the case, has been adopted in a few jurisdictions as part of a judicially crafted discovery rule[14] and as a prerequisite to the application of the insanity tolling provision.[24] In these jurisdictions, courts will allow the lawsuit to proceed only in the presence of some reliable evidence independent of the plaintiff that "corroborates" the facts in the complaint. However, some courts[41] and commentators[42] have opposed requiring corroborative proof at the preliminary stages in order to file a case or toll the limitations period. Corroboration, they argue, is an evidentiary matter unrelated to the applicability of the statute of limitations and should be left to the trier of fact as a matter going to the ultimate proof of the lawsuit.

The concerns expressed by the majority opinion in *Tyson* in 1986 as to the reliability of a complaint in the absence of independent proof of the abuse also have resurfaced in recent statutory amendments. Fearing that discovery provisions to toll the statute of limitations may have gone too far in sexual abuse cases, several jurisdictions have begun to impose new procedural obstacles to the filing of childhood sexual abuse claims. Seemingly designed to ensure that the discovery provisions are not perceived as allowing meritless claims to be filed, these procedures uniformly offer protections to defendants that normally do not exist in other tortious actions but that are consistent with the concerns about protecting defendants against meritless claims expressed in the *Tyson* opinion.

The most severe procedural limitation enacted so far has been the amendments to the discovery provisions in California which require the filing of a ''certificate of merit'' with every civil claim for the recovery of damages suffered as a result of childhood sexual abuse before a complaint is served on the defendant.[43] The certificate is to be executed by the plaintiff's attorney and by a licensed mental health practitioner selected by the plaintiff. The attorney has to attest, after reviewing the facts of the case and consulting with a licensed mental health practitioner, that there is ''reasonable and meritorious cause'' for the filing of the lawsuit. The mental health practitioner has to conclude that, in his or her professional opinion, there is a reasonable basis to believe that the plaintiff had been subject to childhood sexual abuse. A single judge in camera (alone in judicial chambers) reviews the certificate of merit and, if there is found to be reasonable and meritorious cause for the lawsuit, then and only then may the defendant be served with the complaint. Failure to file a certificate results in dismissal of the case.

Since the ordinary civil rules demand that every case be reviewed by the plaintiff's attorney to establish that there is a substantial basis in law and fact before it is filed,[44] this certificate of merit represents an unprecedented upping of the ante for lawyers who take this kind of case. The statute specifies that failure to file a certificate of merit may constitute unprofessional conduct and be grounds for discipline personally against the attorney. Since the demands of the ordinary civil rules have their own sanctioning provisions and failure to consult with a mental health professional in this kind of a case may violate those rules, it is hard not to regard the certificate of merit as a measure designed to erect a higher threshold of reliability for such claims, thereby providing a further financial and systemic disincentive to plaintiffs to bring these cases and a caution to lawyers about the risks involved in taking these cases.

Furthermore, requiring the involvement of a licensed, practicing mental health practitioner imposes a level of verification from an outside party not normally associated with civil claims outside of the medical malpractice area. The 1994 amendment to the California statute that clarified that the licensed mental health practitioner who must sign off on the certificate of merit can not be the plaintiff's current or past treating therapist is a provision purportedly designed solely to increase the probative value of the attestation, but which also serves as a financial and emotional disincentive to the plaintiff and counsel at the earliest stages of the litigation.[45]

In addition, at least two jurisdictions have amended their discovery provisions to protect a defendant's privacy. In 1994, in California's latest amendments to its discovery provisions for repressed memory cases, the state now requires those cases to be filed using the name ''Doe'' in the title of the lawsuit until a plaintiff makes a ''showing of corroborative fact.'' In order to name the defendant personally, a plaintiff over the age of 26 who brings a claim for childhood sexual abuse (and whose claim is therefore based on the discovery provisions to toll the statute of limitations) must file with the court a ''certificate of corroborative fact'' executed by the plaintiff's attorney, declaring that the attorney has discovered at least one fact corroborating the abuse alleged in the complaint. If the corroborating fact is a witness, the identity of the corroborating witness must be revealed; if it is a document or a record, its location must be specified. This corroborative fact may not be the opinion of a mental health practitioner, but rather must be a ''fact'' that confirms or supports the allegation of abuse. This showing of corroborative proof is also reviewed in camera by a judge and must satisfy the judge before the defendant can be named or served or the complaint made public.[46]

In Vermont, a different methodology is used to keep the defendant's identity secret at the preliminary stages of a lawsuit. If a plaintiff is using the discovery provisions in order to bring a lawsuit based on sexual abuse that took place more than six years prior to the filing of the action, then the complaint is sealed by the court clerk and remains sealed until the answer is served. This allows the defendant to move to dismiss the case before his identity is made public. The provisions further mandate that any motion to dismiss be held in camera so as further to protect the identity of the defendant.[47]

All of these legislative amendments strengthen some of the protections that statutes of limitations are themselves designed to achieve. If one of the purposes of statutes of limitation is to protect defendants against the filing of claims that ultimately cannot be proven due to the passage of time, these legislative changes require that a plaintiff show some nonmemory, nonplaintiff-based ''objective'' fact that can serve as corroborative evidence of the abuse at trial. If another of the traditional purposes of statutes of limitation is to protect defendants from harassment, then the requirements that the records be sealed gives defendants some procedural protections before they are served with the complaint and have their identity revealed. And lastly, if statutes of limitation are designed as an initial check on the validity of a complaint, then the initial opportunity for judicial review of the case serves that purpose.

From a legal policy perspective, it may be tempting to see these amendments as achieving the same results as a statute of limitation but doing so explicitly, by addressing each concern embodied in a statute of limitation with a specifically tailored procedure that meets the concern without totally barring a deserving plaintiff on the basis of the arbitrary criterion of the passage of time. As such, these legislative changes might be seen as carefully crafted, policy-specific provisions designed for the protection of an individual defendant *if* they operated *instead* of, rather than as a supplement to, already existing statutes of limitation.

However, by targeting only this kind of case for additional corroborative proof and privacy protections, these defendant-oriented legislative changes are not merely an attempt to restore a balance that was presumably tipped in favor of plaintiffs in the original adoption of the discovery rule. Nor can these amendments be explained simply as measures designed to provide the public some assurance that there are controls on cases involving repressed memory. Their reach extends to those cases where the plaintiff did not repress the memory of abuse but rather failed to make a causal connection between the abuse and the harm suffered.

For plaintiffs and their advocates, these recent amendments represent the first tangible evidence of a backlash against the public airing of the issue of childhood sexual abuse. They signal a return to an era when an accusation of sexual abuse was greeted with skepticism. Requiring additional proof in only this kind of case reminds us that the impulse to disbelieve the existence of sexual abuse is still with us. Wigmore's caution first enunciated almost a century ago, that the testimony of women and children is not to be accorded the same degree of credibility as those of other witnesses,[48] finds its modern expression. As it stands today, childhood sexual abuse cases are the only place in law where testimony of a witness is not allowed to stand or fall based on its own inherent credibility.

The third aspect of the *Tyson* case is at the same time its most intangible and its most important effect: by deciding the case on the issue of the lack of "objective evidence" to support Nancy Tyson's claim of remembered abuse, Justice Durham established the rhetorical paradigm that has shaped this decade's characterization of the dangers with which defendants are faced. These lawsuits are not indefensible due to the mere passage of time; rather, their indefensibility stems from the fact they could not be proven, or perhaps more importantly, be disproven, due to the lack of objective evidence. As such, the issue of time and proof became blended in the analysis of the statute of limitations in a manner that inextricably linked indefensibility to the specter of falsity.

Tyson's linkage of indefensibility to falsity was the central orientation of defense strategies for a decade. With memory (and repressed memory at that) as the only evidence against a defendant, these cases have been deemed to carry too great a risk for the legal system to allow these complaints to proceed. Statutes of limitation need to be strictly construed so that unsubstantiated lawsuits do not undermine the legitimacy of the legal system and defendants need additional procedural protections so that, in the event that these cases do proceed, we have a heightened sense of assurance as to their reliability and merit.

In the decade since *Tyson*, defendants' central strategy in challenging these lawsuits has been to frame the debate as if it were about the reliability of repression in the absence of corroborative proof. But if lack of proof is the perceived danger, then corroboration can also be its adequate remedy. It is for this reason, I argue, that new defense strategies have emerged that are designed to change the terms of the debate away from the possibility that a charge of abuse is unsubstantiated toward establishing the image that every public accusation of abuse is unreliable. The rhetoric is shifting from indefensibility to inaccuracy. It is to these new defense strategies and their implications that I now turn.

Part Three: The Emerging Assault on Repressed Memory and Its Implications for the Law

In the previous section, I argued that the importance of the 1986 *Tyson* case was its focus on the lack of objective, nonplaintiff-based proof in its analysis of the application of the discovery rule. Although the lack of corroborative proof resulted in the dismissal of the lawsuit on statute of limitations grounds, as a defense strategy it represents only a side-swipe at the accuracy of repressed memories. Lack of proof is at most a statement that we cannot trust the victim–plaintiff's memory when it stands alone; taken strictly, it says nothing directly about the truth of the accusation.

As we enter the second decade of litigation in this area, we are now seeing the emergence of three new, interdependent legal strategies that directly attack the accusation as false so that a dismissal of the case can be portrayed as a finding that the lawsuit was without merit. The first defense strategy is to attack the trustworthiness of the complaint due to therapeutic intervention in the process of recalling the memory or integrating the effects of the abuse into the plaintiff's current sense of self. The second is a related attack on the difference between narrative and historical truth in therapeutic treatment and the inability of the healing community to assess the accuracy of their patients' memories of trauma. The third legal strategy capitalizes on the fact that there is controversy within the academic and scientific communities about the reality and reliability of repression. Here, defendants argue that if the scientific community is itself divided about whether therapeutic intervention irrevocably distorts memory or whether memories once repressed can be relied on as accurate accountings of the events that they purport to describe, then the rules of evidence should render the evidence inadmissible. Without an expert's testimony to explain the nature of repressed memory or the plaintiff's testimony (to the extent that it is held to be based on repressed memory), the case will be substantially weakened, if not futile. As such, this third strategy, incorporating the first two, has to date proved to be the most fertile ground for overtly attacking the reliability of repressed memory cases.

Outlining a pattern that is just emerging is difficult enough, although I will do that shortly; assessing its implications may be even more hazardous. It seems clear, however, that the general attack on the validity of repressed memory, orchestrated in some measure by the False Memory Syndrome Foundation,[36] is now being picked up by individual defense counsel as litigative fodder for their legal challenges to the validity of plaintiff complaints. Defense strategies seem no longer to be bound by the statute of limitations, as we see the emergence of challenges in the form of motions to dismiss and pretrial evidentiary motions to exclude the expert or the plaintiff's testimony. Defendants are no longer content with having the dismissal of the plaintiff's complaint be seen as mere late filing or even lack of proof; they want it to be viewed as a repudiation of the truth of the allegation. The concentrated attack in the popular culture and in the academic community on the "myth of repressed memory"[49] is finally making its way into the legal arena in a discernible manner.

It should be noted that both of the first two "new" defense strategies center around therapeutic intervention in the recovery of memory. Why is this so? If the accusation is false, defendants—particularly those who are parents—need to find a coherent explanation that accounts for why and how they could be accused of such a devastating wrong; that explanation is the therapist. Playing on the suggestibility of the vulnerable patient, it is the therapist alone who has manipulated personal unhappiness or dysfunctional family relations into "memories" of sexual abuse. Perhaps in order to keep alive the possibility of family reconciliation, this new strategy simplistically makes the therapist, instead of the parent, the perpetrator of harm, and the therapist, rather than the child, the instigator of the accusation. For cases involving accusations of incest, this strategy allows for the possibility of two dissonant ideas both to be true at the same time. A plaintiff child can honestly believe that she or he was abused and the defendant-parent can present the accusations as false. In intrafamily abuse, this provides a comprehensive explanation that can, at least in a few cases, be seen as supporting those therapists who urge a "third reality" towards familial reconciliation in these cases.[50]

Although the motivation behind these triangulated attacks on the therapeutic community may seem clear, the first of the three "new" defense strategies is itself a complicated mix of phenomena. Defendants who argue that memory is not to be trusted because it has been distorted by the therapeutic process are capitalizing on a variety of legal, scientific, and popular concerns that center on therapeutic overreaching in "memory" therapy and other techniques, with their potential for unmonitored negligent practice. These issues are beginning to manifest themselves in the legal arena in cases brought by family members of sexual abuse plaintiffs against therapists for negligent practice.[51] As in lawsuits between the victim and the alleged perpetrator, the therapist becomes the causal link between psychological intervention and the falsity of the accusation of sexual abuse.

To the extent that this strategy succeeds, on its own or linked to the arguments of scientific reliability, it will do so by trying to build on the already existing legal framework of rules on hypnosis[52] (which arguably may not be applicable to this category of plaintiffs[53]) and on the dicta in *Tyson,* in which the majority 10 years ago expressed its concern for the distortive potential of the therapeutic process on memory. In that opinion, Justice Durham questioned the testimonial trustworthiness of both the plaintiff–victim and the treating therapist and whether evidence from these sources could be relied upon:

> [T]he psychoanalytic process can even lead to a distortion of the truth of events in the subject's past life. The analyst's reactions and interpretations may influence the subject's memories or statements about them. The analyst's interpretations of the subject's statements may also be altered by the analyst's own predisposition, expectations, and intention to use them to explain the subject's problems.[33]

Quoting from an article by Marianne Wesson, a Professor of Law at the University of Colorado Law School, in which she draws out the distinction between narrative and historical truth,[54] the *Tyson* court continued:

> [T]he distance between historical truth and psychoanalytic 'truth' is quite a gulf. From what 'really happened' to what the subject or patient remembers is one transformation; from what he remembers to what he articulates is another; from what he says to what the analyst hears is another; and from what the analyst hears to what she concludes is still another.[33]

While the *Tyson* court used this argument to draw a distinction between soft evidence like testimony and objective evidence like a surgical sponge, this new, more sophisticated challenge to the veracity of a plaintiff's memory is focused on a slightly different, though related, argument. Here, defendants argue that psychotherapeutic interventions have so distorted the plaintiff's memories that we are no longer able to distinguish the plaintiff's *own* memories from the therapist's interpretations, promptings, or premature interventions. Memory's inherently reconstructive nature has been taken advantage of by the therapist, goes the argument, producing either wholly false memories, or at the very least, plaintiffs who are falsely confident about the veracity of their recollections of the historical event. Regardless of whether the memory is wholly implanted or improperly enhanced, defense counsel argue that it should not be relied upon as the basis for a lawsuit which will represent a binding account of the critical event. Dismissal of a lawsuit is justified even at the earliest stages of a lawsuit because to do otherwise is to sanction judicially the high probability that, given the emotional nature of the case, false accusations will ultimately turn into false verdicts in a jury's hands.

The first case to explore this new strategy in depth has been the 1994 Ohio Supreme Court case of *Ault* v. *Jasko*.[55] The plaintiff, Kathy Ault, initially appealed the dismissal of her lawsuit on statute of limitations grounds to the Court of Appeals of Ohio, the first appellate level in that jurisdiction.[56] She won there; her father, whom she accused of having sexually abused her from the age of 12, appealed. The Ohio Supreme Court dismissed his appeal and recognized the discovery rule in Ohio for the first time, holding that a one-year limitations period for sexual abuse begins to run when a victim recalls or discovers that she or he was abused or when through the exercise of reasonable diligence, she or he should have discovered the abuse.

In dissent, Justice Wright lambasted the Court's decision in an opinion that is ironically and strangely reminiscent of Justice Pearson's powerful dissent on behalf of plaintiffs 9 years earlier in the *Tyson* case. Just as a decade earlier, when Justice Pearson in *Tyson* railed at the majority for having ignored the phenomenon of sexual abuse and relegating its discussion of this issue to a single line in the majority opinion, Justice Wright in *Ault* takes the Ohio Supreme Court to task for summarily adopting the discovery rule regardless of the conditions under which the alleged victim subsequently recovers the repressed memory. Because of the majority's failure to address this issue properly, just as Justice Pearson had done a decade earlier, Justice Wright took it upon himself to discuss at length his concerns as to the potential unreliability of repressed memory. In doing so, he may have created the legal framework for the next decade of litigation in this area.

Relying on two articles by Elizabeth Loftus, and particularly on the law review article she co-authored with Gary Ernsdoff,[57] Justice Wright began his discussion of the issue of reliability of memory by noting that "while all three stages of memory—perception, retention and retrieval—are susceptible to influence and suggestion, the last stage, retrieval, is especially prone to new inputs and suggestive questioning."[58] When memory is retrieved with the aid of a professional, as opposed to being recovered naturally or spontaneously (which he notes may be on a different footing legally), Wright expressed his concern about the "growing body of evidence" that many "repressed memories" may have been implanted in patients' minds, unwittingly or otherwise, by therapeutic suggestion.[59]

In trying to understand how such implantation could occur, Wright drew a distinction between forensic and clinical therapists. A forensic psychotherapist is trying to elicit evidence admissible at trial and therefore will not try to "prepare" the patient, make suggestions, or ask leading questions during therapy. However, because a clinician's goal is the treatment and rehabilitation of the plaintiff–patient, she or he will ask leading questions, reveal expectations, make suggestions, and encourage plaintiffs to use their imaginations. Drawing a parallel to polygraphy, Wright noted that memory retrieval places unusual responsibility on the examiner and that very reliance may be the source of unreliability.

In light of these concerns, Justice Wright stated that he would have refrained from having the judiciary recognize the discovery rule in Ohio in the absence of a resolution of this issue by the legislature. The Ohio General Assembly, Wright concluded, is the appropriate body to conduct hearings, consider expert testimony and fashion standards. In the absence of an explicit legislative mandate, Wright dissented from the court's adoption of a discovery rule, at least for those plaintiffs whose memory was retrieved with the aid of a therapist.

Only Justice Alice Robie Resnick answered Wright's arguments for the majority. In a separate concurring opinion, she wrote that although she shared Justice Wright's concern about the potential unreliability of recovered memories, this case was not at the stage where dismissal of the action on a defense challenge would be the appropriate solution. Dismissal would "totally slam the door of our courtrooms shut on all plaintiffs claiming repressed memory of sexual abuse who seek redress after their nineteenth birthday."[60]

For Justice Robie Resnick, the determinative factor was the timing of the legal challenge mounted by the defendant. A motion to dismiss, coming at the very beginning of the legal process, is a singularly inappropriate moment to dismiss a case in that it did not "leave the courthouse door ajar for a plaintiff with a valid claim"[61] of abuse who had repressed his or her memory.

To understand this part of the holding, it is necessary to know that in the initial stages of a complaint, when a defendant challenges a lawsuit in a motion to dismiss, the court is procedurally required to treat all of the factual allegations in the complaint as true. The defendant's motion in *Ault* v. *Jasko* was asking the court in effect to hold that a plaintiff could find no set of facts that would ever entitle her to succeed. At this stage, the judge stated, it is too early to know how the case will evolve factually and it must be allowed to proceed to the discovery phase of the legal process.

To counter Wright's argument that courts should do nothing until the Ohio legislature acted, Justice Robie Resnick ended her opinion with a brief but powerful closing paragraph. Using a quotation from the same law review article by Gary Ernsdorff and Elizabeth Loftus used by Justice Wright, she states:

> Doing nothing would penalize the individual who has subconsciously invoked a coping mechanism to survive the effects of cruel abuse. I am impressed by the argument that 'the law should not protect perpetrators who successfully traumatize their victims into repression.'[62]

The second of the new strategies being used by defense counsel is also derived from the *Tyson* case and is equally an attack on the therapeutic community. However, here the focus is on whether psychotherapy is able to uncover the historical accuracy of events—the question of narrative versus historical truth with which we began this chapter. Although there are no legal cases that turn on this point per se, the issue of narrative versus historical truth did figure largely in Justice Wright's concerns about whether a person who has had contact with therapeutic process can be relied on to give a personal or accurate account of a past event. As Justice Wright stated in *Ault* v. *Jasko*:

> The clinician's purpose, however, is completely different. The clinician's goal is rehabilitation. The treatment program is provided solely to benefit the patient. If a patient's rehabilitation can be accomplished by assisting the patient to recall a traumatic memory heretofore repressed, whether the memory is fact or fantasy, the clinician will encourage the patient to recall that memory in whatever form. . . . For it is not necessarily the recalling of an accurate memory with which the clinician is concerned, but with the patient's overall rehabilitation.[63]

This language recalls the words of the majority opinion in *Tyson* a decade earlier when Justice Durham expressed alarm at the prospect of a treating psychiatrist's testimony being regarded as corroboration of the event:

> It is suggested that the subjectivity of plaintiff's claim can be eliminated at trial through the testimony of witnesses such as family, friends, schoolteachers and treating psychologists. . . . [T]he testimony of treating psychologists or psychiatrists would not reduce, much less eliminate, the subjectivity of plaintiff's claim. Psychology and psychiatry are imprecise disciplines. Unlike the biological sciences, their methods of investigation are primarily subjective and most of their findings are not based on physically observable evidence. The fact that plaintiff asserts she discovered the wrongful acts through psychological therapy does not validate their occurrence. Recent studies by certain psychoanalysts have questioned the assumption that the analyst has any special ability to help the subject ascertain the historical truth. . . .
>
> While psychoanalysis is certainly of great assistance in treating an individual's emotional problems, the trier of fact in legal proceedings cannot assume that it will produce an accurate account of events in the individual's past.

The purpose of emotion therapy is not the determination of historical facts, but the contemporary treatment and cure of the patient. We cannot expect these professions to answer questions which they are not intended to address.[33]

Two examples demonstrate how this specific issue of historical versus narrative truth may play itself out in the law. The first is embedded in the history of the recent California cutbacks on the discovery rule discussed above in Part Two. Legislatures, like the courts, seem to be increasingly unwilling to trust the clinical therapeutic community's judgment as to the validity of these complaints. The second example arises from the recent development of parents suing therapists for negligence. Family members who feel themselves to be falsely accused are arguing for the necessity and role of historical accuracy in therapy, especially when dealing with the explosive ramifications that an accusation of sexual abuse will certainly cause in the family. The essential element in negligence claims made in the *Althaus*[64] case, for example, was that the treating psychiatrist neither cared nor tried to verify the accusation, nor did she take into account the consequences of that failure to verify on the (falsely) accused parents and her patient. If a legal duty to third parties in negligence actions becomes more widely recognized,[65–67] the conception of a therapist may include the role of historical detective.

The difference between historical truth and narrative truth has always been a great concern to forensic clinicians, but the psychological literature is still somewhat skeletal with respect to this issue.[68] The literature is even more underwhelming in the area of how treating therapists should behave when called to testify[69] at hearings or trials on issues that may turn on the accuracy of the recollections being examined.

However, the American Medical Association,[70] the American Psychiatric Association[71] and the American Psychological Association[72] have all recently issued position papers or resolutions on this intersection of historical truth, childhood sexual abuse, and repressed memory. Couched in the language of compromise and self-protective risk management concerns, these resolutions are certainly going to be used by defendants to make the point about the inability of the treating professions to authenticate abuse. These resolutions, much like the Diagnostic and Statistical Manual (DSM) and its ''Cautionary Statement'' that accompanies each successive volume, fail to appreciate that regardless of what stand they take, their words are capable of being used by one side or the other to support their position. There is no safe place to hide in this debate: demanding, as the AMA resolution does, ''external validation'' before assuming the ''authenticity'' of a patient's trauma history *is* a position in this sharply drawn area, and it is one most helpful to defendants.

The third new defense strategy is an attack on the existence and reliability of repressed memory as a matter of scientific consensus. This strategy is a totally new phenomenon in two ways. First, it is unrelated to the *Tyson* opinion and the multiple effects this case has had on this area of law, and second, it does not arise as a statute of limitations issue at all, but rather as an evidentiary motion to exclude a witness' testimony due to its unreliability. Using the 1993 U.S. Supreme Court case of *Daubert v. Merrell Dow Pharmaceuticals, Inc.*[73] and its revision of the 60-year-old standard as to admissibility of scientific evidence enunciated in the case of *Frye* v. *United States,* defense lawyers are asking for the exclusion of the testimony either of an expert or of the plaintiff qua witness due to the fact that the accuracy of previously repressed memory has been disputed in the scientific and medical community, and as such, is unreliable as a matter of law. Indeed, the very title of the book in which this chapter is found, *Trauma and Memory: Clinical and Legal Controversies,* may itself become a citation as to the questionable admissibility of the main witness' testimony in a civil or criminal trial to the extent that a witness' testimony is based, in whole or in part, on repression.

However, as different as this new strategy may appear at first, it is important to realize its total dependence on the arguments and assumptions contained in the previous two defense arguments. Only *if* the process of therapy or the particular methodology used in any individual case can be attacked as unreliable can the *Daubert* standard for testing scientific reliability be used to exclude the witness' testimony. A defendant here must argue that the process of therapy, as a discipline or in terms of the particular methodology used, leaves us unable to rely on a witness' testimony, because it eradicates the ability to give either a personal or an historical account of the events and as such, is inadmissible as a matter of law.

At this point in time, there are just a handful of cases in the legal reporters and available through on-line services that reflect this strategy. By the time this chapter is published, there may be many more, and the cases that I briefly discuss here may themselves have been appealed or reversed. However, it is clear that this approach has enormous potential as a defense strategy, for it allows a defendant the best of all possible worlds. This strategy accomplishes everything that a statute of limitations hearing could do by allowing a case to be dismissed at an early pretrial motion and it does something that the limitations period challenges have never been able to address fully—allowing the plaintiff's claim to be dismissed in the forum of public *and* private opinion as meritless and suspect. Dismissal on grounds of scientific controversy allows defendents to argue much more convincingly that the accusation was found to be false, their argument substantiated by their expert witness' explanation as to how the false accusation came into existence.

The first case to raise the possibility of this line of defense attack was (perhaps now not surprisingly) the same dissenting opinion in *Ault* v. *Jasko* discussed earlier, in which Justice Wright argued that a discovery rule should not be judicially enacted in Ohio without reference to the methodologies by which the memory was recovered. In discussing the intersection of the methodologies of therapeutic intervention and the standard of scientific reliability, Wright noted that there is sharp disagreement in the academic psychology community as to whether a repressed memory actually can be retrieved and, if it can, whether the memory is accurate.

Again, relying exclusively on the two articles by Elizabeth Loftus referred to above,

Justice Wright noted that it is undisputed that memory may be repressed. Repression can be caused by extreme physical injury (such as that experienced by the "Central Park Jogger" who was brutally beaten and repeatedly raped and yet retained no memory of the incident), or by sheer mental shock as for a war veteran who represses memories of battle even though he or she personally was not injured. Wright noted, citing the two articles, that repression is more likely to occur in children than in adults and that a child who is sexually abused at an early age has a greater likelihood of repressing the memory than a child who is abused at an older age. Likewise, children who experience a particularly violent or intrusive type of abuse and those who experience it over a prolonged period of time are more likely to repress memories of these experiences. Wright noted that scientists generally agree that memories can be repressed, although admittedly, there are few empirical data demonstrating exactly what occurs during the three stages of memory regarding repression. He stressed that, according to Loftus, there is little agreement among scientists about whether a repressed memory can be retrieved and, if it can, whether the memory is an accurate product.

Justice Wright's particular concern was of course the case in front of the court and as that was a case in which the memory of the abuse was recovered with the aid of a therapist, he was careful to confine his opinion to those cases in which memory was recovered with therapeutic intervention. He left for another day the situation of an adult who naturally and without the aid of a therapist recovers a repressed memory, because that situation is factually, and therefore perhaps legally, different from the one faced by the court in *Ault* v. *Jasko*.

To Justice Wright, cases in which there was therapeutic intervention are unmistakably parallel to the practice of testing memory through the "science" of polygraphy. This parallel carries particular resonance in the law since courts consistently have been reluctant to accord credibility to the results of a polygraph test. This reticence can be traced back to the landmark 1923 case of *Frye* v. *United States*,[74] in which the federal district court for the District of Columbia decreed that, in order to be admissible, a scientific technique from which a deduction is made must be sufficiently established to have gained general acceptance in the particular field to which it belongs. This axiom has since been adopted by most courts as *the* standard in determining the admissibility of evidence based on a particular scientific technique. This 60-year-old standard changed in 1993 with the case of *Daubert* v. *Merrell Dow Pharmaceuticals, Inc.* to a standard that uses a different, more flexible legal test for the determination of the admissibility of the evidence into court. In *Daubert,* the Supreme Court held that

> [w]idespread acceptance can be an important factor in ruling particular evidence admissible, and 'a known technique that has been able to attract only minimal support within the community' . . . may properly be viewed with skepticism.[75]

For Justice Wright, polygraphy was still relevant after *Daubert* as an *example* of how the new standard of reliability should be applied to a particular claim of scientific authenticity. For him, polygraphy is parallel to the issue of memory retrieval due to the unusual responsibility placed on the examiner. For Justice Wright, therefore, if techniques of memory recovery are fraught with the same transformative nature as polygraphy, then the judicial system should receive it with the same skepticism and deny its admission into evidence.

With under a dozen cases decided so far on the issue of scientific reliability, it is very dangerous to even suggest trends or prematurely draw the lines of argument. In the past decade of litigation, we have seen the early entrenchment of the legal typology of Type One (nonrepressed memory) and Type Two (repressed memory) plaintiffs that emerged from the *Johnson* case[76] and we should be aware of the distortive, punitive results that may emerge from any legal categorization that fails to capture the meaning or breadth of individual experience.[77] Nevertheless, I offer several tentative observations about this emerging trend in the litigation.

First, the issue as to admissibility of a witness' testimony cuts across civil–criminal and victim–witness distinctions. For example, one of the unreported cases that uses this new strategy is a criminal decision in New Hampshire, *State* v. *Hungerford* and *State* v. *Morahan*.[78] This case was, in fact, two separate cases joined together by the court because they both seemingly presented the same legal issue to be addressed: whether two sexual abuse victims who claimed to have repressed memories of the assaults against them could testify against their alleged assailants at their criminal rape trials. Judge Groff of the New Hampshire Superior Court trial division treated the two victims in the same manner and held that in both cases, the victims' evidence was not admissible because the phenomenon of memory repression and the process of therapy used in these cases to recover the memories have not gained the general acceptance in the field of psychology necessary to allow admissibility in a criminal proceeding. Without the victims' evidence, neither case was able to proceed to trial and the ruling is currently under appeal.

Raising the issue of scientific reliability is the way in which most criminal cases will arrive at an examination of the issue of repressed memory. Through pretrial "motions in limine" to exclude evidence, the defendant will ask the court for a *Daubert* or a *Frye* hearing (depending on whether the state court uses the new federal standard or sticks with its own *Frye*-based formulation) to present arguments that the issues associated with repression are so controversial that the witness' testimony should be excluded from trial. This is certainly one of the ways in which the defense in the *Franklin* case could have asked the court to deal with the issue of the admissibility of Eileen Franklin-Lipsker's testimony had the prosecution re-tried the case.

Second, the Courts will have to address the threshold question as to whether the *Frye* or the *Daubert* standard is even appropriate for evaluating the admissibility of a lay as opposed to an expert witness. Ordinarily, the scientific reliability standard is reserved exclusively for the admission of expert witnesses whose testimony would be helpful to the jury in explicating concepts beyond their ordinary experience or knowledge. A recent case from the federal district court in Massachusetts, *Shahzade* v. *Gregory*,[79] used the *Daubert* standard to decide that repressed memory is a valid clinical and scientific theory. This type of decision would allow either side to bring in an expert to testify as to the phenomena associated with repression—to explain, for example, why the witness may have repressed the memories in the first place or why the methodologies used to retrieve the memory undermine the reliability of the memory or why the witness' own belief as to the accuracy of the memory may not reflect its trustworthiness. These insights would be a contribution to the jury's understanding of the issues. However, to go the extra step and argue that the standard for general acceptance in the scientific community controls the admission of the testimony of an *ordinary* witness for which the only criterion traditionally has been only personal knowledge[80] of the relevant information is somewhat unprecedented and subject to debate. Judge Groff's opinion in the *Hungerford* case, currently under appeal, is that of trial judge and as such is not a binding determination in New Hampshire or elsewhere on this issue. It may be accurate that there is a "raging, robust debate" on these issues but its effect should not be the exclusion of the testimony of the lay witness with the memories.

Third, it is entirely possible that what will emerge in the area of the admissibility of repressed memory are a series of distinctions between categories of memory cases: between those witnesses who "repressed" totally and those with some memory disturbances who appear more like ordinary witnesses who forget; between witnesses who recalled their memories with therapeutic intervention and those who recalled on their own or spontaneously, like the chief witness in the *Slutzker* case; between those witnesses whose therapist used questionable methodologies and those who were nonjudgmental or more "forensic" in their approach. We may also see distinctions being drawn that parallel the law relating to hypnosis, with pre-therapeutic recollections having a different legal status that post-therapeutic memories.

This raises a fourth issue that will certainly be part of the continuing legal debate surrounding the admissibility of this evidence. Should the determination of the reliability of the evidence and the credibility of the witness be a question for the judge or the jury? Should the judge under the *Daubert* and *Frye* test rule as a matter of law and exclude the evidence, thereby crippling if not ending the legal case, or should the judge let the jury decide issues of reliability and credibility? In *Hungerford,* the Court held that the issue of repressed memory was too volatile, uncertain, and problematic to leave it to a jury. However, in the 1995 case of *Isely* v. *Capuchin Province et al.,*[81] a federal district court judge ruled in a pretrial motion *in limine* that the credibility of a witness and the reliability of repressed memory are questions for the jury. The Court deferred ruling on this issue at trial when the defendant made a motion to dismiss at the end of the plaintiff's case, but reiterated his ruling after the defendants had concluded their presentation of the evidence. The judge in *Isely* held that although the Court does have a "gatekeeper" or "screener" function in evidentiary determinations to ensure that there is the necessary foundation for the evidence, questions as to reliability and credibility are ultimately to be left to the jury.

Another way of framing the judge–jury question is whether the subject of an admissibility ruling is the issue of repression per se or is confined to the general acceptance of the methodologies used in a particular case to retrieve memory. For *Ault,* the point that concerned Justice Wright was that of questionable methodologies; he affirmed the existence of repressed memory as a phenomenon. Two other courts have agreed with this approach. Judge Harrington in *Shahzade* v. *Gregory* stressed that the role of the court in a *Daubert* hearing was not to "rule on the credibility of this individual plaintiff's memories, but rather on the validity of the theory itself."[82] Similarly, in *Isely,* the district court accepted the evidence of an expert witness who had in her testimony distinguished between the controversy that exists over the "elicitation of memories, not with the concept itself."[83] The *Isely* court ruled that an expert may testify on direct examination only as to whether the witness' behavior is consistent with someone who is suffering from repressed memory or posttraumatic stress disorder and that then the defendant is free to cross-examine on a range of issues relating to how the memories came into existence, including

> whether the symptomology is also consistent with somebody who fantasizes about such event and believes them himself, or is susceptible to having 'memories' implanted in his subconscious, or any other range of issues that may go to the basis of [the expert's] opinion as to whether or not Mr. Isely's symptomology is consistent or inconsistent [with repression].[84]

In *Hungerford,* where the specific methodologies used in the cases (visualization and guided imagery) seemed to the Court to be highly suspect, the result was the exclusion of the witness' entire testimony, rather than leaving the issue of reliability to be explored on cross-examination. This may be in part because *Hungerford* is a criminal case, with its potential of imprisonment.

Fifth, the shift in the rhetoric from Stage One litigation is now taking shape. For the first decade, the issues in this area of litigation were largely framed as the need for procedural protections, including the strict construction of the statutes of limitation, so as to prevent the courts from possibly letting an unsubstantiated accusation be heard. Plaintiffs juxtaposed the truth of their pain and the reality of sexual abuse and the effects it causes (including repressed memory) as the counterpoint to defendants raising the specter of falsity.

In Stage Two, the paradigm is not one of truth versus falsity but rather an image that holds truth and falsity together at the same time—a deluded plaintiff honestly deceived and a loving, unjustly accused parent. The new defense strategies ask the law to "save" the family through its recognition of the lack of consensus in this area and to therefore step back from the dispute, allowing another forum be the site for arriving at justice in this case. However, with therapists' doors potentially closing in a self-protective panic due to the lawsuits against them by accused family members, the question of whether there will be any place left for victims' voices to be heard should be of no small moment as a legal and social concern.

Lastly, the issues raised by these cases are problematic precisely because these frontal attacks on reliability of repressed memory could arise in *any* case at *any* stage in the legal process and are applicable far beyond these narrowly drawn, though inflam-matory, cases of sexual abuse. Attacks on a witness' memory after therapy could affect many witnesses who seek psychological counseling for a variety of reasons—to deal with being the victim of crime, or because they witnessed an accident, or because of the impending dissolution of a marriage. Memory and therapy interact in many cases and to the extent that these decisions raise a specter of doubt as to the reliability of the testimony of any witness who has sought professional counseling, the implications of these multipronged attacks on the reliability of memory may prove too much for the legal system to incorporate. The potential exclusionary impact of such an approach would have a far-reaching impact and there does not seem to be an obvious principled means of drawing the exclusionary line around only those victims of sexual abuse who have gone for therapy.

Moreover, these attacks on repressed memory have implications for the status of memory generally in the law. The central enterprise of any litigation is the resolution of conflicting and contested views about past events, with a verdict resolving the historical accuracy of one version of events over another. As all litigation is perforce about the past, and virtually all litigation involves witnesses who are testifying about memories of the past, issues as to the accuracy of memory lie at the very core of the legitimacy of litigation as a means for the resolution of interpersonal and social conflict.

While it is true that all witnesses testify from memory, trial verdicts never merely reflect the testimony of any *one* witness on direct examination reciting his or her version of a remembered event. Every witness is subject to a myriad of procedures honed by the adversary system and designed to test, as best it can, whether the witness' testimony under oath is worthy of belief. Every witness is subject to cross-examination by the party opposed to that witness' interest, so as to uncover the defects in the witness' recollection, whether caused by problems in the witness' original perception of the event, or the process of recollection, or the accuracy of the narration of the event, or a witness' bias or motive to misrepresent.[85] Any witness may be contradicted by another witness or by physical or documentary extrinsic evidence. A witness' testimony, in appropriate circumstances, may be undermined or bolstered by expert opinion.[86] In the end, it is up to the jury collectively to weigh all the evidence and decide which portions of each witness' testimony it accepts and rejects.

Although evaluating the reliability and accuracy of a witness' memory is seen as an ordinary jury function, as just another part of its overall assessment of the evidence, the final jury verdict—guilty, not guilty, liable, not liable—is in its simplicity no more than an opaque reflection of its view of the accuracy of the memory of any *one* witness. Even when there are interrogatives or a special verdict which give us a window into the jury's deliberations, the overall verdict is a statement as to the responsibility of the defendant for the historical event that is the subject of the litigation rather than a focused commen-tary on the reliability of an individual's memory.

The question of what happened is supposed to be resolved at trial, where a full airing of all of the issues can be put to a jury. The biggest implication of these new defense strategies is that, if they succeed, they will foreclose the possibility of a real trial and turn a statute of limitations motion or a pretrial evidentiary motion into something that these procedures were never meant to be: a mini-trial on the merits.

If these new defense challenges to the reliability of memory could guarantee that as a result of the issues they raise, only "worthy" cases would be brought forward, this might be seen as a salutary result. However, if the past decade of litigation is any indication, it is highly unlikely that we will see such a rational result. Moreover, if we could tell from the outset *which* defendants were falsely accused, there would be no need for a trial. Which cases are worthy is something that can only be established at trial, where both plaintiffs and defendants have a chance to present their evidence and leave the determination to the jury.

The ramifications of these legal developments on plaintiffs will be to force them to get ready for "trial" earlier, thereby putting even more pressure on counsel to prepare a case fully before bringing it to the legal system. This, in turn, will create pressure on victims who are considering suits to consult lawyers earlier and earlier. For a victim who is in therapy, that pressure may be counterproductive, as legal pressures to "discover" and sue may influence the course of treatment.

Moreover, if these legal challenges take hold, lawyers are now likely to tell plaintiffs who bring them these cases not only that the result of their case is unpredictable at best, but that the accuracy of their memory will be under fierce scrutiny and attack from the very beginning of the lawsuit. These new challenges, coming either in a statute of limitations hearing or a motion to dismiss on a pretrial evidentiary motion to exclude, represent a defendant's opportunity, under the guise of initial legal procedures, to put the plaintiff's complaint on trial. Plaintiffs will get the message and lawyers, especially those on contingency fee arrangements, will have no incentive to urge them to fight what seems like an ever-increasing uphill battle to get the case heard on the merits before a jury.

If defendants succeed in these new challenges, we may be seeing the beginning of the end of a brief era when courts were open to hearing accusations in the public forum of the courthouse about events that occurred in the most secret of private spaces. Although cases will still be brought for many years to come, fewer and fewer will succeed in making it through the legal process to be heard at trial. Eventually that message too will get out, and although the discovery rule may still exist on the law books in a formal sense, as a reality, childhood sexual abuse will be effectively pushed out of the legal arena, at least for those cases in which repressed or disturbed memory plays a central role.

The politics and emotional grip of this area of law sometimes make it hard to recognize that the legal system's own values and concerns are also involved. These new defense strategies raise tough questions for the legal system about its openness to serve as a forum for the remedy of harms and as a site for decisions in the face of scientific controversy. But perhaps the toughest questions raised for the law by these defense strategies relate to the legal system's reliance on the historical accuracy of memory.

Despite legal academics who, under the influence of postmodernism and literary criticism, may question the existence of a single reality,[87] the traditional legal system has reason to fear that the legitimacy of *all* of its verdicts—not merely those based on repressed memory—may be threatened by this class of complaints. In the words of Judge Lowell Jensen, the federal district court judge who overturned George Franklin's murder conviction on appeal, repressed memory cases are another memory case, just like any other.[88] If that is so, then given the stakes for the legal system with its core reliance on memory, one should not be optimistic about the future prospects in this area of the law for victims of childhood sexual abuse.

In this troubling intersection of law and psychiatry, this area of interrelated legal and clinical doctrines, the legal system must decide how it will meet the central challenge with which it is faced: in the world where deserving plaintiffs and falsely accused defendants may both exist, and when these cases have the potential to threaten the authority of all legal verdicts, on whose side will the law err in fashioning and applying legal rules?

References

1. Spence DP: Narrative Truth and Historical Truth. New York: W.W. Norton, 1982.
2. Nesson C: The evidence or the event: on judicial proof and the acceptability of verdicts. Harvard Law Rev 1985; 98:1357–1392.
3. *United States* v. *Kubrick*, 444 US 111, 117 (1979).
4. *Board of Regents* v. *Tomanio*, 446 US 478, 487 (1980).
5. *Burnett* v. *New York Central Railroad*, 380 US 424, 428 (1964).
6. *Wood* v. *Carpenter*, 101 US 135, 139 (1879).
7. *Urie* v. *Thompson*, 337 US 163 (1948).
8. *Urie* v. *Thompson*, 337 US 163, 169 (1948).
9. *Urie* v. *Thompson*, 337 US 163, 170 (1948).
10. *Bowen* v. *City of New York*, 476 US 467, 481 (1985).
11. *Mills* v. *Habluetzel*, 456 US 91 (1982).
12. Corman CW: Limitation of Actions. Boston: Little, Brown, 1991.
13. *Falk* v. *Levy*, 180 F 2d 562, 564 (2d Cir 1952).
14. *Olsen* v. *Hooley*, 865 P 2d 1345 (Utah 1993).
15. *Franklin* v. *Duncan*, 884 F Supp 1435 (D Cal 1995).
16. Schmitz J: Court upholds murder conviction based on son's old memory. Pittsburgh Post-Gazette, Oct 8, 1993, p. B1.
17. Man recalls '74 scene of murder. Pennsylvanian had repressed memories of scene he witnessed as teen; suspect charged. Rocky Mountain News, May 28, 1994, p. A49; *Commonwealth of Pennsylvania* v. *Crawford*, 682 A 2d 323 (Superior Ct).
18. *Archambault* v. *Archambault*, 846 SW 2d 359 (Texas 1992).
19. Federal Rules of Civil Procedure, Rule 56 (summary judgment); Rule 50 (judgment as a matter of law).
20. Davis L: Foreward to Crnich JE, Crnich KA: Shifting the Burden of Truth. Lake Oswego: Recollex, 1992, pp. vii–viii.
21. *Olsen* v. *Hooley*, 865 P 2d 1345, 1347 (Utah 1993).

22. *Smith* v. *Smith*, 830 F 2d 11, 12 (2d Cir 1987).
23. *Lovelace* v. *Koehane*, 831 P 2d 624 (Okla 1992).
24. *Meiers-Post* v. *Schaefer*, 427 NW 2d 606 (Mich Ct. App 1988).
25. *Hildebrand* v. *Hildebrand*, 736 F Supp 1512 (Ind 1990).
26. *Schmidt* v. *Bishop*, 779 F Supp 321 (NY 1991).
27. *Overall* v. *Klotz*, 52 F 3d 398, 399 (2d Cir 1995).
28. Rosenfeld A: The statute of limitations barrier in childhood sexual abuse cases: the equitable estoppel remedy. Harvard Women's Law J 1989; 12:206–219.
29. *Smith* v. *Smith*, 830 F 2d 11 (2d Cir 1987).
30. N.Y. Civ. Prac. L & R. 214-a (McKinney 1990).
31. *Bassile* v. *Covenant House*, 575 NYS 2d 233 (NY 1991).
32. *Tyson* v. *Tyson*, 727 P 2d 226 (Wash 1986).
33. *Tyson* v. *Tyson*, 727 P 2d 226, 229 (Wash 1986).
34. Revised Code of Washington, Section 4.16.340(1), 1988.
35. Shapiro L: Rush to judgment. Newsweek, Apr 19, 1993, pp. 42–48.
36. Butler K: Marshaling the media. Family Therapy Networker 1995; 19:36–39, 80.
37. Yapko MD: Suggestions of Abuse: True and False. Memories of Childhood Sexual Trauma. New York: Simon & Schuster, 1994.
38. Dershowitz AM: Abuse Excuse and Other Cop-outs, Sob Stories, and Evasions of Responsibility. Boston: Little, Brown, 1994.
39. Labaton S: GOP preparing bill to overhaul negligence law. New York Times, Feb 19, 1995, p. A1.
40. Montana Code Annotated, Section 27-2-216; Minnesota Statutes Annotated, Section 541.073.
41. *Osland* v. *Osland*, 442 NW 2d 907 (N. Dakota 1989); *Lemmerman* v. *Fealk*, 507 NW 2d 227 (Mich. Ct. App 1993).
42. Roegge BJ: Comments: *Lemmerman* v. *Fealk:* A ''reasonableness'' solution allows Michigan's incest victims greater access to the courts. Univ Detroit Mercy Law Rev 1994; 71:943–963.
43. California Code of Civil Procedure, Section 340.1 (e).
44. Federal Rules of Civil Procedure, Rule 11.
45. California Code of Civil Procedure, Section 340.1 (e)(2).
46. California Code of Civil Procedure, Section 340.1 (g)-(m).
47. Vermont Statutes Annotated, Title 12, Section 522 (b).
48. Wigmore JH: Evidence in Trials at Common Law, section 934a. Edited by Chadbourne J. Boston: Little Brown, 1970.
49. Loftus EF, Ketchum K: The Myth of Repressed Memory. New York: St Martin's Press, 1994.
50. Barrett, MJ: The third reality: getting beyond the false memory debate. Paper presented at the 17th Annual Family Therapy Network Symposium (taped address), Washington, D.C., March 1994.
51. *Ramona* v. *Ramona*, No 61898 (Napa Cty Super Ct 1994).
52. Kanovitz J: Hypnotic memories and civil sexual abuse trials. Vanderbilt Law Rev 1992; 45:1185–1262.
53. *McGlauflin* v. *Alaska*, 857 P 2d 366 (Alaska Ct. App 1993).
54. Wesson M: Historical truth, narrative truth, and expert testimony. Wash Law Rev 1985; 60:331–354.
55. *Ault* v. *Jasko*, 637 NE 2d 870 (Ohio 1994).
56. *Ault* v. *Jasko*, WL 46658 (Ohio App 9 Dist 1993).

57. Loftus EF, Ernsdorff GM: Let sleeping memories lie? Words of caution about tolling the statute of limitations in cases of memory repression. J Crim Law Criminol 1993; 84:129–174.
58. *Ault* v. *Jasko,* 637 NE 2d 870, 875 (Ohio 1994).
59. *Ault* v. *Jasko,* 637 NE 2d 870, 876 (Ohio 1994).
60. *Ault* v. *Jasko,* 637 NE 2d 870, 873 (Ohio 1994).
61. *Ault* v. *Jasko,* 637 NE 2d 870, 873 (Ohio 1994).
62. *Ault* v. *Jasko,* 637 NE 2d 870, 874 (Ohio 1994).
63. *Ault* v. *Jasko,* 637 NE 2d 870, 876–877 (Ohio 1994).
64. Weidlich T: 'False' memory, big award. National Law J Jan 9, 1995, p. A6.
65. Appelbaum PS, Zoltek-Jick R: Psychotherapists' duties to third parties: *Ramona* and beyond. Am J Psychiatry 1996; 153:457–465.
66. Bowman CG, Mertz E: A dangerous direction: legal intervention in sexual abuse survivor therapy. Harvard Law Rev 1996; 109:551–639.
67. Rock SF: Note—A claim for third party standing in malpractice cases involving repressed memory syndrome. William & Mary Law Rev 1995; 37:337–379.
68. Appelbaum PS: Memories and murder. Hosp Community Psychiatry 1992; 43:679–680.
69. Gutheil TG: True or false memories of sexual abuse? A forensic psychiatric view. Psychiatr Ann 1993; 23:527–531.
70. American Medical Association: Report of the Council of Scientific Affairs: Memories of Childhood Abuse. Chicago: AMA, 1994.
71. American Psychiatric Association: Statement on memories of sexual abuse. Washington, DC: APA Office of Public Affairs, 1993.
72. American Psychological Association: Questions and Answers about Memories of Childhood Abuse. Washington DC: APA, 1995.
73. *Daubert* v. *Merrell Dow,* 113 S Ct. 2786 (1993).
74. *Frye* v. *United States,* 293 F 1013 (D.C. Cir 1923).
75. *Daubert* v. *Merrell Dow,* 113 S Ct. 2786, 2796 (1993).
76. *Johnson* v. *Johnson,* 701 F Supp 1363 (ND Ill 1988).
77. Lamm JB: Easing access to the courts for incest victims: towards an equitable application of the delayed discovery rule. Yale Law J 1991; 100:2189–2208.
78. *State of New Hampshire* v. *Hungerford* v. *Morahan,* WL 378571 (NH Super Ct 1995).
79. *Shahzade* v. *Gregory,* 923 F Supp 286 (D. Mass 1996).
80. Federal Rules of Evidence, Rule 602.
81. *Isely* v. *Capuchin Province,* 877 F Supp 1055 (ED Mich 1995).
82. *Shahzade* v. *Gregory,* 923 F Supp 286, 290 (D Mass 1996).
83. *Isely* v. *Capuchin Province,* 877 F Supp 1055, 1066–1067 (ED Mich 1995).
84. *Isely* v. *Capuchin Province,* 877 F Supp 1055, 1067 (ED Mich 1995).
85. Federal Rules of Evidence, Rule 611.
86. Federal Rules of Evidence, Rule 702.
87. Sherwin RK: Law frames: historical truth and narrative necessity in a criminal case. Stanford Law Rev 1994; 47:39–83.
88. *Franklin* v. *Duncan,* 884 F Supp 1435, 1438 (ND Cal 1995).

20

Ethical and Clinical Risk Management Principles in Recovered Memory Cases: Maintaining Therapist Neutrality

ROBERT I. SIMON
THOMAS G. GUTHEIL

The current controversy among mental health professionals, their patients, and families over recovered memories of sexual abuse threatens to undermine the credibility of the mental health professions. The debate has generated intense passions that have driven an increasing number of recovered memory cases into the courts. Patients alleging recovered memories of abuse have sued parents and other perpetrators. In a number of instances, the alleged victimizers have sued therapists, who they claim negligently induced false memories of sexual abuse. In other cases, patients have recanted and joined forces with individuals (usually their parents) to sue therapists.

The memory debate has polarized a number of therapists into "believers" and "disbelievers." In fact, most therapists hold personal beliefs about the validity of recovered memories of sexual abuse that are somewhere between the extremes. It is these personal biases that, left unchecked, represent a new occupational hazard for clinicians that can undermine the therapists' duty of neutrality to their patients, creating deviant treatment boundaries and the provision of substandard care.

Litigation in recovered memory cases is expected to soar in the coming years. Multimillion dollar verdicts against mental health practitioners are predicted. In fact, a jury has already awarded $2.7 million to the plaintiffs in a case alleging that the therapist implanted memories of sexual abuse.[1] A fundamental allegation in these cases will be that the therapist abandoned a position of neutrality to suggest, persuade, coerce, and implant false memories of childhood sexual abuse. The guiding principle of

477

clinical risk management in recovered memory cases is the maintenance of therapist neutrality and the establishment of sound treatment boundaries.

Recent highly publicized litigation has been brought in cases of so-called recovered memories, where adult patients, usually in therapy at the time, have unearthed long-buried or repressed memories of sexual abuse during their childhoods. The cases run the gamut from criminal charges against parents for childhood abuse recently recalled to memory by adults, to recanter suits against treaters, to parental suits against treaters for everything from malpractice to slander. This uproar has left many clinicians concerned and bewildered about how to deal with the implied risks and uncertainties.

Further complicating the matter is the empirical evidence about memory mechanisms, which, as is typical of any emerging science, includes contradictory findings about how and what persons in various settings retain in memory and forget (see, for example, references 2–10). Empirical studies often fail to distinguish whether allegedly repressed memories are not retrieved or simply not reported to researchers. Controversy rages over the mechanism of repression—does it really exist or is it a fiction?[11] Moreover, laboratory studies that inflict harm upon individuals in order to study traumatic memory cannot be conducted. Studies that arise from natural or human disasters usually test "single-blow" trauma.[12] In addition, many "recovered memory" therapies have proliferated far from the mainstream, including "past life" therapy and treatment for the traumatic consequences of alien abduction.[13]

Several attempted cures of this problem may be worse than the disease. These include stringent informed consent legislation whereby only the approved forms of psychotherapy may be used that have empirically justified their effects on particular maladies. Yet another well-meant approach, this from the American Psychiatric Association (APA) insurance risk managers, involves highly restrictive instructions on how to practice "careful psychotherapy."[14] Unfortunately, the recommended approach—giving patients cautions about the APA's official professional uncertainties about the validity of recovered memories—constitutes a glaring example of defensive practice, a kind of "misinformed consent." Though it is stated that such informing is not meant "to discourage the patient but rather to educate," it is likely to have a chilling effect on treatment. Would-be reformers also show poor discrimination between ordinary psychotherapy and the alternative, "non-mainstream" therapies such as past life regression. It is unclear at this point what goal, other than the death of psychotherapy as we know it, these efforts at reform will accomplish.

The Context

Before we address what we believe to be valid and clinically based approaches to malpractice prevention in this troubled area, it may be useful to outline the context in which all this activity is taking place. Paradoxically, whereas psychoanalysis, as a dominant theoretical framework and mode of practice, may be in the decline, the notion of the therapeutic effect of recovery of the repressed memory alone has taken hold among a wide spectrum of practitioners. Unfortunately, what has been sacrificed is the notion of therapist neutrality, so that an advocacy for recovered memory, in the name of support of abuse victims, is commonly seen. It is important to distinguish between the ideologic posture of the zealot who *will* find abuse in every case and the legitimate inquiry about abuse that belongs in every psychiatric history.

The advocacy described above has, in some cases, extended to significant interference with and intrusion into the patient's life, often in the form of multiple and extensive boundary violations, which are themselves a possible basis for litigation. These trends have been coupled with growing sensitivity to childhood abuse and the extent to which this event was underreported and unrecognized.[11] The pendulum swing has now reached an extreme where, among certain therapists, almost every symptom of dysphoria is seen as probative of early abuse.[15]

A second dimension is the lack of training and skill that seems to be replaced in some practitioners by advocacy. To the patient's quest for understanding of distress, the therapist supplies a clear answer, a magic bullet: "You were abused as a child," which provides a solution to an "effort after meaning," as well as a mechanism for understanding symptoms (e.g., through the use of "syndrome evidence," where the presence of a particular current symptom is taken inappropriately as solid evidence of a past actual event). This model also may seem to absolve some patients of responsibility for their own lives. The treatment is likewise predetermined in all too many cases, through enrollment in an "incest survivor group" (or, at worst, participation in a "memory mill" or what one author has called the "incest-survivor machine")[16] and validation (or, depending on one's attitude, contamination) by one's alleged peer group.

Confounding all this activity is the fact that *all* psychotherapy, because it encourages self-directed attention, involves voluntary or involuntary recovery of memory. The distinction among repression, suppression, dissociation, avoidance, and simple forgetting or redirection of attention is often hard to establish. Thus, many of the problems, fears, and recommendations about this issue overlap problematically with issues regarding psychotherapy itself. Even when memories are known to be true, there can be significant mistakes in recall, as the study of children's memories following the Challenger spacecraft explosion demonstrates.[17] Hence, any risk-management guidelines for proper conduct should be constructed so as to leave regular psychotherapy intact.

Other Contextual Factors

The True versus the Real

The distinction here has been called by some authors "historical truth" (what actually happened) vs. "narrative truth" (the more-or-less coherent story the patient tells himherself about the past that affords clarity and comprehension of one's "history").[15,18]

What comes up in therapy is the patient's view, which is subjective, selective, erroneous, or accurate—the objective, factual validity of which cannot be determined without data external to the therapy itself. Hence everything a patient tells us is "true" in the sense of coming from the wellspring of the patient's conscious and unconscious database, but it may or may not be "real," in the sense that neutral observers or videotapes on the scene at the time would report the same story. The patient's convincing demeanor and the plausibility of the narrative alone—even coupled with our own deep convictions, as our work with character disorders should tell us—do not in themselves constitute objective proof of the reality of events. Nor does the presence of eating disorders, personality disorders, or multiple personality disorder prove that the patient was sexually abused as a child. All psychiatric conditions have multiple causation.

The Office versus the Courtroom

A second dimension of the issue is that the clinician's office and the courtroom are different worlds with different rules. The role of clinician as empathic, intuition-driven partisan in the patient's world is markedly different from the adversarial, evidence-driven world of litigation. In therapy it is our empathic subjectivity which allows the therapeutic alliance to build. To doubt our patients is to invalidate their personal experience and to doom treatment.

At another level, litigation itself is typically portrayed by unsophisticated therapists as the solution to the problem of healing, empowerment, and closure; you must sue to heal, they suggest.[19] In fact, over and above the reality that any case can be lost, the law is a "blunt instrument." Litigation has many destructive effects as well (we have referred to these as *critogenic harms*),[20] which are often underestimated by such treaters. These include arrest of therapeutic development at the point of suit; prolongation of closure during the pendency of the litigation; entrenchment, at least partly for legal purposes, in the dead-end "victim" posture; revictimization through the stresses of litigation; and in some cases, pathological attachment to the abuser through the "bonds" of litigation. Lenhart and Shrier[21] state that "litigation in cases of sexual harassment is an option that should be resorted to only after careful evaluation of the likely costs and benefits and consideration of a range of nonlegal interventions." Their recommendation holds true for recovered memory cases as well.

Clinically Based Risk-Management Principles

It should be clear from the foregoing that the only valid risk-management principles in this area would be those that rest solidly on a clinical footing and are secondarily informed by awareness of the legal context. Clinical risk management combines the therapist's detailed understanding of the patient with a working knowledge of pertinent legal requirement primarily to provide good clinical care and, only secondarily, to reduce the risk of legal liability. We offer the following as a contribution to this process.

Abstinence and Therapist Neutrality

The *duty of neutrality*, a fundamental clinical and ethical principle, is based upon the *rule of abstinence*, which states that the therapist must refrain from obtaining personal gratification at the expense of the patient.[22] The concept of therapist neutrality also extends to the limitations on clinicians' interference in the personal lives of their patients. This principle allows for the patient's personal agenda to be given primary consideration. The personal views and biases of the therapist concerning, for example, politics, religion, abortion, and divorce should not be inflicted upon the patient.

Similarly, in recovered memory cases, the therapist must guard against reacting from personal biases that may lead to prejudging the cause of the patient's emotional difficulties or the veracity of the patient's report of sexual abuse. For example, a strong belief or disbelief in the validity of patients' reports of recovered memories of sexual abuse will likely interfere with appropriately objective evaluation and treatment. Therapists must not influence or pressure their patients into believing that they were or were not victims of sexual abuse. Suggesting to a patient that he or she was sexually abused as a child, as proven by the fact that he or she now has an eating disorder or some other psychiatric condition, is fallacious, scientifically insupportable, and in today's context, substandard practice. Conversely, a clinician's expression of disbelief in the validity of a recovered memory of abuse may revictimize patients who as children reported sexual abuse to their parents or other trusted significant figures and were not believed. Expression of disbelief by a therapist may further cause the patient to withdraw from treatment and not seek further help.

Some therapists, terrorized by the fear of legal involvement, panic when they hear a patient speak of sexual abuse. A few therapists have gone so far as to squelch such reports or to require patients to sign exculpatory contracts in a vain attempt to preempt litigation. The ultimate expression in destructive defensive practices occurs when therapists are afraid even to inquire about abuse as a routine aspect of their clinical evaluations.

Clinicians should maintain an empathic, nonjudgmental position toward reported memories of sexual abuse. The therapist must be careful that empathy is used in the service of supporting the patient's therapeutic efforts rather than lending weight to the patient's own belief or disbelief in his or her memories. As a rule, it is probably best not to suggest to patients that they read books or newsletters or attend seminars on recovered memories of sexual abuse. Therapists who do decide to make such recommendations should refer the patient to balanced, scientifically based sources of information. Therapists must consider that prematurely referring the patient to abuse recovery or incest survivor groups may be unduly suggestive to the patient, both by the therapist's prescription and the influence of the group.

Using technical terms such as *repression, dissociation,* and *alters* to explain the patient's difficulties adds an air of scientific validity that suggestible patients may seize upon as further evidence of abuse. They may thus resist addressing more pressing current symptoms and problems that often bring patients to treatment. Moreover, extratherapeutic activities such as attending sexual abuse seminars with patients is likely associated with other significant boundary deviations in the therapy.

Clinical experience shows that false beliefs are likely to arise in psychotherapy when four primary risk factors interact.[23] These include (*1*) high hypnotizability; (*2*) uncertainty about past events; (*3*) clear evidence of the influence of suggestive questioning; and (*4*) extratherapeutic social influences by peers and families, but especially self-help group experiences and facilitating sociocultural beliefs. Recovering memories of sexual abuse may represent such a false belief in some treatment situations.

These primarily dynamic psychotherapeutic principles of abstinence and therapeutic neutrality are of particular value here, though their decline in other areas of psychotherapy is lamentable. The necessary "sitting back" that these principles require does not imperil empathy (indeed, they may make undistorted empathy possible), but they successfully avoid advocacy for the *facts,* rather than advocacy for the patient's welfare, which is proper.

Although psychoanalytic neutrality has a more narrow meaning as to the analyst's position in relation to psychic elements (equidistant among ego, id, superego, and reality), we are here referring more broadly to a general clinical—and legal[24]—duty of neutrality, perhaps best defined as the therapist's obligation, absent emergencies, to avoid intruding on the patient's life or imposing his or her beliefs or values on the patient.

A challenge clinicians may face in this context is the patient's query, "Do you believe me?" The clinician's possible answers, "I must," "I should," "I do," though perhaps reassuring to the patient, become irrelevant in the courtroom context, where the clinician's faith is not evidence. Some patients are reassured by a temporizing response: "Let's accept that view now but remain open to deeper or different understanding as we learn more." Most patients do not have complete amnesia for childhood traumas but wish they did. At the same time, these same patients do not have complete recollection and wish they did. Although this may seem illogical, it is consistent with the "trance logic" of how traumatic past events are held, which is both wanting to forget while trying to discern and remember.[25]

There is much to be said for the classic analytic contract whereby the patient agrees to postpone (or at least, bring first into therapy for discussion) major life decisions during the emotional flux of therapy. Going to court should be identified as one of such issues that should be first discussed to see if indeed the expected benefits outweigh the resulting harms. Litigation should be first a treatment issue. The patient who impulsively sues an elderly parent as a resistance to looking inward to dynamic issues is not being aided in the therapeutic growth process. Another such issue would be the patient's completely cutting ties and contact with family, as some overzealous therapists suggest. As a general rule, the therapist should probably abstain from recommending litigation.

The passionate professional and public debate over recovered memories of sexual abuse should not cause clinicians to abandon fundamental clinical and ethical principles expressed in the *Principles of Medical Ethics with Annotations Especially Applicable to Psychiatry* that supports therapist neutrality.[26] The following ethical guideline is particularly relevant in recovered memory cases:

> The psychiatrist should diligently guard against exploiting information furnished by the patient and should not use the unique position of power afforded him/her by the psychotherapeutic situation to influence the patient in any way not directly relevant to the treatment goals. (Section 2, Annotation 1)

It is known that memories can be significantly influenced by the manner of questioning, especially in young children. Memories of childhood abuse can even be implanted by therapists who insistently and undeviatingly suggest abuse as an explanation for mental conditions or disorders, even though the patient initially lacks memory of abuse and resists the suggestion. Furthermore, repeated questioning about childhood sexual abuse may cause some patients to report memories of abuse that may never have occurred. The imperative ethical principle here is, ''first do no harm.''

Maintaining Clinical Focus

Most patients in therapy who report the recovery of memories of childhood sexual abuse have initial diagnoses of mood, personality or adjustment disorders. The clinician should not be distracted from providing adequate evaluation and treatment for the patient's presenting problems and symptoms. In a number of patients, a diagnosis of multiple personality disorder (MPD) is made when previously hidden personalities emerge that harbor memories of childhood sexual abuse. When MPD is diagnosed, the clinician should not automatically assume that sexual abuse occurred in childhood. Other kinds of traumatic experiences may have been etiologic.[27] If the patient's condition has not improved within a few months of beginning treatment, a reexamination of the initial diagnosis and the consideration of a differential diagnosis should be undertaken. Consultation may also be helpful. The therapist's tenacious pursuit of abuse memories, as with any persistent boundary violation, may lead to a deteriorating clinical course in the patient.[28] The multiaxial diagnostic system presented in the *American Psychiatric Association Diagnostic and Statistical Manual (4th ed.)* (DSM-IV)[29] is always a useful format to follow.

The enemies of competent psychiatric diagnosis and treatment of patients reporting recovered memories of sexual abuse are multiple: inexperience, clinical naiveté (poor training), unfettered therapeutic ambition, and zealotry. These problems may be masked by the therapist's wish to seek the easy answer to complex mental disorders. The American Psychiatric Association has issued a "Statement on Memories of Sexual Abuse" that presents helpful clinical guidelines for the clinician.[30]

Documentation and Consultation

These timeless standbys of sound risk management are highly relevant to the present situation since they record the rationale for one's therapeutic approach, as well as bring the therapist in line with standard practice through peer or expert consultation. Careful documentation of memory recovery, therapist questions and comments, and the sequence in which memories returned may aid in avoiding even the appearance of suggesting abuse.

The therapist should document any doubts or uncertainties he or she has about the veracity of memories. Such documentation establishes the therapist's position of neutrality. The progress note is not the place to memorialize the therapist's personal feelings and biases about the patient or the recovered memory debate. The medical record should contain clinical and patient-centered information.[31]

Patient Autonomy and Self-Determination

In addition to the duty of neutrality, other clinical–ethical principles underscore the management of recovered memory cases. *Fostering patient autonomy and self-determination* sustains the patient's separateness in therapy while facilitating the treatment goal of independence. Patient self-determination requires that the therapist's clinical posture toward the patient be expectant; that is, the patient generally determines the content of the session. Particularly in sexual abuse cases, the normal process of separation–individuation has been impaired. The patient's wish for the good parent and a therapist's need to rescue the patient may set the stage for progressive boundary violations. Fostering patient autonomy and self-determination should help negate later allegations that the therapist implanted memories of sexual abuse and manipulated the patient into believing them.

The ethical principle of *compassion and respect for human dignity* underlies all of the treatment boundary guidelines. The clinical correlate of this principle is that the competent therapist strives to maintain the healthy self-esteem of the patient during the course of treatment. Sexual abuse is extremely damaging to a patient's sense of personal goodness and worthiness. Patients who believe they have been sexually abused are more vulnerable to exploitation both by the therapist and others outside the therapy. This is another important reason why therapists must be extremely diligent in not suggesting the specter of childhood sexual abuse to patients beyond inquiring about the absence or presence of abuse as part of a routine psychiatric examination.

Managing Countertransference

Despite the recognized horrors of sexual abuse, clinicians should not become swept away in associated emotional storms. Remaining calm in the "therapeutic chair" permits the greatest degree of help to the patient in working through past trauma. Therapists must be ever vigilant to the emergence of countertransference that may impair therapist neutrality. Recovery of childhood memories of parental sexual abuse in therapy can be particularly evocative of countertransference reactions in therapists. Fears of professional annihilation by litigious patients, feelings of helplessness and uncertainty, as well as reparenting and rescue needs in the therapist are commonly encountered countertransference feelings and fantasies. Some therapists may become personally outraged when they hear reports of abuse, urging the patient to "go public" against the perpetrators. If the therapist begins to cross treatment boundaries, the destabilizing pull of covert countertransference on therapist neutrality must be considered.[32]

Therapists may be vulnerable to loss of perspective because of their own abuse histories, which Pope and Feldman-Summers documented.[33] While such an issue is technically no different from other conflicts in regard to countertransference and over-identification with the patient, our consultative experience suggests that the temptation to work out one's own abuse history through the patient may pose significant counter-transference challenges for the therapist. The attempt to reparent the patient is one of the central countertransference problems that may lead to the loss of therapist neutrality, treatment boundary violations, and inappropriate involvements with patients claiming sexual abuse. The primary therapeutic task of the therapist and the patient is to help the patient grieve painful losses. Trying to be the good, all-loving parent to the patient does not cure; it merely casts a spell that will ultimately disappoint, if not revictimize, the patient.

The following ethical statement found in the *Principles of Medical Ethics with Annotations Especially Applicable to Psychiatry*[26] is central to effectively managing countertransference:

> The psychiatrist shall be ever vigilant about the impact that his/her conduct has on the boundaries of the doctor/patient relationship, and thus upon the well-being of the patient. (Section 1, Annotation 1)

This guideline is especially critical when the therapist treats patients who seek help for mental conditions and disorders that are associated with boundary violations in their childhood. Therapists must be particularly careful in recovered memory cases since, for a variety of reasons, some of these patients may repeatedly test the limits of treatment boundaries.[34]

Understand the Difference Between Historical and Narrative Truth

The therapist and patient strive to understand the "narrative truth" (the patient's version) and the "historical truth" (what actually happened). During the course of treatment, therapist and patient work primarily with the patient's version of historical events without scanting historical truth when it is available. However, confirmatory evidence of childhood sexual abuse is often unavailable for a variety of reasons.

When a patient recovers memories of childhood abuse in the course of psychotherapy, it is important to observe and document the genesis of this recovery to avoid later allegations that the memories of abuse were suggested by the therapist. How did it arise? Why do the memories emerge at this time? What were the precipitating factors? For example, memories of abuse recovered under hypnosis will not likely have the same probative value in court as memories sparked by a current traumatic situation that keys into a reported memory of childhood abuse. Moreover, not all childhood sexual contact leads to a sustained emotional trauma. A brief episode of sexual abuse may or may not prove to be pathogenic of a later psychiatric disorder, depending on the severity of the abuse, the nature and age of the child, the relationship with the perpetrator, as well as numerous other factors.

Pope and Hudson[35] assert that recent studies suggesting that childhood sexual abuse is a cause of adult psychiatric disorders suffer from methodological problems which casts doubt on any presumed causal link. Very little is known about what kinds of factors or circumstances influence positive or negative outcomes following sexual abuse.[36] The therapist should apply clinical judgment to the content of recovered memories as he or she would to all clinical data. Note that credibility of memories alleged to have occurred before 3 years of age is highly suspect.[37] For example, memories of abuse around diapering are likely to be false.

Therapists are not detectives. The therapist's efforts are primarily directed at working with the narrative truth from the patient rather than embarking on a quest for the historical truth. A therapist's intrepid search for the historical truth will likely be experienced by the patient as disbelieving and may result in the patient feeling revictimized. The American Medical Association position on recovered memories does not adequately take into account the negative impact on the therapist–patient relationship when it states that memories of childhood abuse are of "uncertain authenticity" and should be "subject to external verification" before considered to be true.[38]

Professional competence, not the search for external verification, is the relevant issue in assessing the clinical significance of recovered memories. The clinician must assess the type and duration of sexual abuse, the presence or absence of physical trauma, the nature of the victim, the intrapsychic meaning of the abuse experience, and the availability of family or community support. All sexual abuse does not necessarily cause permanent psychic injury. The fact that the therapist is willing to maintain a position of neutrality by being open to all evidence in recovered memory cases should be duly recorded in the patient's chart. It should be remembered, however, that no evidence will be available to establish that abuse did not occur (the impossibility of proving a negative).

Of course, what actually happened is very important to the patient and to the clinical strategy employed. If abuse is corroborated, the patient must both recover from the harmful effects of this trauma and mourn the loss of the ''good'' aspects of the abuser, if a parent or family member is involved. If the abuse did not occur in reality, efforts might be directed to repair or preserve the relevant relationships, at the patient's wish, or to support individuation as desired. If the issue is uncertain, patients might be helped to bear the uncertainty and go on with the work and with their lives. The ambiguity again requires that the clinician tolerate uncertainty in the work without rushing to judgment, since ultimately, unequivocal facts may never come to light. Such toleration counters the patient's tendency to ''split'' and avoid healthy ambivalence.

Treater versus Expert

For a variety of reasons, the role of treater and forensic expert witness are clinically and ethically incompatible.[39,40] The subject is too extensive to address here, but some key points may be illuminating.

First, the clinician's obligation to do no harm may be in conflict with the fact that expert testimony at trial may indeed harm the patient's case, especially in the adversarial context of court.[41] Although forensic examiners should always warn the patient about this possibility, treaters often do not and, arguably, should not do so, since treatment should, if at all possible, follow its own course rather than be tied to litigation. The treater's willingness to accept the patient's view as true is in conflict with the expert's need for external corroboration. The very search for corroboration itself may well be experienced by the patient as disloyalty, disbelief, or abandonment of the alliance posture. On the other hand, an investigative role is perfectly appropriate for the forensic expert to undertake.

The treater's benevolent wish to help with the patient's legal difficulties does not alter these considerations. Should the patient elect to go to court, independent forensic assessment should be sought, while the treater remains clinically available to help the patient cope with the stress of litigation. Indeed, the patient's actual intervention to go to court should be explored as carefully as any other impulses to act that arise during the therapeutic process.

An issue that commonly arises in liability cases is the precise role of the therapist whose patient alleges childhood abuse. Plaintiff's attorneys representing accused family members advance the point that the therapist should have performed some sort of independent investigation of the veracity of the allegations or of the factual situation in which the abuse is claimed to have occurred. Presumably armed with ''the truth'' of the matter, the clinician could then dissuade patients from their erroneous views, sparing parents the stigma and stress of being accused. There are several reasons why this is an inappropriate role for a therapist ever to play.

First, to dispense with the obvious, a clinician who hears of *current* abuse of a minor child is, of course, under clear, mandated reporting obligations in every jurisdiction. For past abuse allegedly recalled by an adult patient, the clinician's task is to do therapy; that is, to explore, understand, and work through with the patient the issues raised by these memories. Attempts to go outside the therapeutic frame of the dyad—in addition to representing commonly a problem of countertransference—are almost always ill advised, in that they shift the focus into the external world where the number of variables confound the therapist's task. Second, the therapist's investigations, as noted, may well represent to the patient a form of disloyalty. The patient may justly claim, "I am here to deal with *my* feelings about my mother, not with the kind of person my mother 'really' is; whose side are you on?"

Finally, investigative involvement outside the office may be seen as a failure of empathy, whereby the therapist lets lapse the duty to see the world through the patient's eyes. Patients who are so treated have experienced the therapist's investigative response as disbelief of their statements, criticism, and lack of faith in the patient's intelligence or understanding. On the other hand, if historical corroboration of childhood sexual abuse becomes available through newly discovered photographs or authentic contemporaneous diaries, the therapist must take this evidence into clinical account.

Supervising or Collaborating with Other Professionals

Psychiatrists who work with other professionals should perform independent assessments of patients without relying blindly on previous formulations and diagnoses made by the referring or collaborating clinician. Caution is also recommended in the supervisory relationship. Supervisees may attempt to influence patients with idiosyncratic theories of abuse and its sequelae. In the supervision of other therapists, the clinician should check the experience, education, licensure, and credentials of the supervised therapist. A discussion should reveal whether a compatible diagnostic and treatment approach is shared. The supervising therapist should be notified immediately if memories of sexual abuse emerge. The supervisor should be certain that the supervisee carries adequate malpractice insurance. The receipt of a certificate of insurance should be required annually.

Psychiatrists who participate in the split treatment of patients alleging recovered memories of sexual abuse are at special risk for malpractice liability. Providing medications only, without undertaking a thorough evaluation and acquiring knowledge of the patient, often leads to the provision of substandard care. Unless there is a close working relationship between the psychiatrist and the psychotherapist when memories of sexual abuse emerge, the psychiatrist should seriously consider taking over full responsibility for the management of the patient or withdraw from the case after proper notification of both the patient and the therapist. At even greater risk are clinicians who specialize in recovering memories of abuse, particularly abuse caused by incest or by multigenerational satanic cults, for they risk being sued by multiple plaintiffs.

Role of Family Members

This issue turns out to be among the most critical, since a number of extant ''recovered memory'' cases brought by families (who are usually considered non-parties to the case) turn upon the family's being granted standing to sue on various theories of litigation.[42] Although the courts' reasoning is often obscure, some cases appear to have been decided on the basis that the therapist's support for the validity of the memories (and, regrettably, for the decision to sue) creates a new duty to the parents, even though they are not the designated patients. The duty appears predicated on the parents being foreseeably harmed participants in the treatment. One legal scholar (Rose Zoltek-Jick, personal communication) quips that the duty arises when the therapist ''reaches out and touches someone'' beyond the patient.

It is also essential to clarify with family members (and so document) that, if they are brought into the treatment, e.g., for a family meeting with the patient present, they are present purely as adjuncts to the treatment of the defined patient, not as patients themselves. If therapy for the parents is indicated, they should be referred elsewhere for treatment.

In *Ramona* v. *Isabella*,[43] California courts permitted a father accused of sexually abusing his daughter to sue his daughter's therapists. Holly Ramona sought treatment for an eating disorder. One of the therapists allegedly suggested to Ms. Ramona that her eating disorder was caused by childhood sexual abuse, the memory of which she had repressed. Ms. Ramona was told that if the memory of abuse was recovered under treatment with sodium amytal, the memory would be accurate.[44] A jury in Orange County, California, awarded $500,000 to her father Gary Ramona, who charged that his daughter's psychotherapists were responsible for ''planting'' her false memories of sexual abuse through the use of sodium amobarbital. Her father had brought an $8 million malpractice suit against the therapists. Ramona attributed the loss of his $400,000-a-year salary as a winery vice president and the failure of his 25-year marriage and estrangement from his three daughters to charges leveled by his daughter in 1991 that he had sexually molested her. The original suit brought by Holly Ramona against her father for sexual abuse was dismissed on the basis of her father prevailing in the malpractice suit. The dismissal was reversed by an appeals court.[45]

In *Ramona*, California courts abandoned the traditional legal approach that granted only patients the right to sue health care providers for negligence. The new rationale by the California courts considered the father to be a ''direct victim'' of the therapists' negligence, thus traditional limitations on therapists' duties toward Mr. Ramona should not apply. Other courts have used similar reasoning.[46] Appelbaum and Zoltek-Jick,[47] after reviewing *Ramona* and other similar cases, concluded that although concern about practices in recovered memory cases may be warranted, abandoning the traditional rules against non-patient suits would be ill advised. These authors suggest steps that the clinician can take to reduce the risk of becoming involved in such litigation.

Special Therapies

Clinical hypnosis and sodium amytal interviewing are time-honored and useful modalities in clinical work. In the treatment situation, memories recovered with or without the aid of special techniques may be true, false, or a combination of both. The clinical knowledge, judgment, and experience of the practitioner is of critical importance in sorting out fact from fancy. In the context of recovered memories, where possible litigation is contemplated, however, the risk–benefit assessment suggests avoiding these techniques, if only to avoid hopelessly confounding the patient's case. Laypersons, including some mental health professionals, hold a common misconception that individuals undergoing such special procedures as hypnosis or sodium amytal interviews will lead to their revealing the truth. Nothing could be more inaccurate. In fact, people who are deeply hypnotized or under treatment with sodium amytal are quite capable of resisting suggestions to be truthful and continue to lie. Memories obtained under these special procedures may be no more or no less reliable than those elicited through normal recall.[37] People in general and patients in particular are especially susceptible to suggestion when hypnotized or during the amytal interview. Under these procedures, patients may translate their own beliefs and those of the therapist into pseudomemories. In hypnosis, it is not necessarily the hypnotic procedure itself but the patient's hypnotizability that is a risk factor for the induction of false memories.[23] Any therapist bias can contaminate memory.[48] Guidelines have been proposed for the conduct of forensic hypnosis to prevent misuse of this modality in litigation.[37]

In *Ramona* v. *Isabella,* one of the allegations of negligence was that Holly Ramona's therapists misrepresented to her that the amytal interview had confirmed her recovered memory of rape. Gary Ramona's attorney successfully argued that the therapists were negligent in believing and portraying to Holly Ramona that an amytal interview could provide reliable evidence in proving the veracity of her claims. Memories that arise from these special procedures are often inappropriately accorded a high measure of veracity. Thus, the Council on Scientific Affairs of the American Medical Association questions the usefulness of hypnosis to enhance memories at civil and criminal trials.[49]

Some authorities recommend the use of hypnosis as an adjunctive treatment approach with selected patients afflicted with MPD.[50] Therapists should give serious consideration to obtaining written informed consent outlining the specific risks and benefits associated with special procedures before using them in recovered memory cases. Informed consent should also be obtained for other so-called memory-enhancing techniques, such as guided imagery, age regression, and body massages (recovering "body memories") which through heightened suggestibility and the therapist's intentional or inadvertent statements may distort the patient's productions.

Maintaining Professional Competence

Psychiatrists and other mental health professionals have an ethical, professional, and legal duty to stay abreast of new developments and remain proficient in their field. The following ethical guidelines stated in the *Principles of Medical Ethics with Annotations Especially Applicable to Psychiatry*[26] apply:

> A psychiatrist who regularly practices outside his/her area of professional competence should be considered unethical. (Section 2, Annotation 3)

Therapists who routinely and mechanistically diagnose an abuse history as a single theory, because they lack the necessary training to properly assess and treat patients with a broad variety of psychiatric disorders, may harm patients by providing substandard care. They also may increase the patient's resistance in obtaining appropriate future treatment. For example, therapists who advise patients with bulimia nervosa that they have probably been victims of childhood sexual abuse are providing a theory that flies in the face of research that has found no such link.[51] Moreover, special knowledge, experience, and expertise are necessary to properly evaluate and treat patients who report recovering memories during the use of specialized interviewing techniques such as hypnosis or treatment with sodium amytal, or to use these techniques in forensic evaluations.

An additional ethical guideline is pertinent here:

> Psychiatrists are responsible for their own continuing education and should be mindful of the fact that theirs must be a lifetime of learning. (Section 5, Annotation 1)

The psychiatrist's ethical duty to stay abreast of new developments is particularly important when attempting to treat patients who have recovered memories of childhood sexual abuse. Therapists can stay current by following new developments within the emerging field of memory science and in the evolving standards in the treatment of patients claiming sexual abuse.

Managed Care

Managed care settings present special problems for the management of recovered memory cases. If a new patient presents difficulties and symptoms that appear to be associated with recovered memories of childhood sexual abuse, more than brief psychotherapy will not be available under most managed care plans. The patient should be informed of plan limitations as early as possible and of the fact that longer-term therapy will likely be needed. An appropriate referral should be made outside the managed care plan.

Patients who recover memories of sexual abuse within managed care settings also must be informed that more treatment sessions may be required than are currently provided under the managed care plan. However, it is crucial not to summarily discharge and abandon these patients. Appropriate referral should be made for continued treatment outside the managed care plan. Some therapists continue to treat patients under a reduced fee schedule when their insurance benefits or managed care visits are exhausted.

Public Statements

Psychiatrists and other mental health professionals who enter into the public debate over recovered memories have to exercise caution and discretion. The most common occasion for psychiatrists to address the public include radio, television, the print media, and seminars and symposia that are open to the public. The following ethical guideline found in the *Principles of Medical Ethics with Annotations Especially Applicable to Psychiatry*[26] speaks to this issue:

> Psychiatrists may interpret and share with the public their expertise in the various psychosocial issues that may affect mental health and illness. Psychiatrists should always be mindful of their separate roles as dedicated citizens and experts in psychological medicine. (Section 7, Annotation 2)

Psychiatrists who partake in the public debate currently surrounding recovered memories of childhood sexual abuse must carefully distinguish, for themselves as well as for the public, personal opinions from scientifically established facts. Since such a distinction can be quite difficult to make at this time, the clinician may decide to remain silent. Much harm can be inflicted on the public when personal opinions proffered by mental health professionals on recovered memories are passed off as scientific verities. This caveat applies to positions taken both for or against the validity of recovered memories of childhood abuse. Psychiatrists also should avoid making public pronouncements about the truthfulness or other aspects of individual reports of sexual abuse.[30]

Encouraging a patient to make public accusations of sexual abuse against alleged perpetrators will significantly increase the risk of a slander suit (and perhaps other claims) being brought against the therapist. In a number of jurisdictions, charges of slander may be brought against a therapist by accused third parties when only patients themselves can sue for malpractice. Therapists should avoid making public pronouncements about the veracity of sexual abuse reported by patients or other individuals. This caveat includes family members of the patient. In just such a case, a Dallas, Texas jury in 1994 found that a psychiatrist committed slander without malice when he repeated accusations of sexual abuse against the patient's parents that were recovered by sodium amytal interviews.[52] The patient's parents sued and were awarded $350,000. If a patient or family determines that memories of abuse recovered in therapy are false, an intense need for vindication may emotionally drive the litigation against the therapist.

When to Stop

If your patient rushes blindly ahead with the intent to sue the parent for long-ago abuse recalled in current therapy, and your own advice militates against this course, do not blindly continue therapy. Take this up as a treatment issue first. The situation here is one in which the patient has violated the therapeutic contract to explore before acting or acting out. Make an appropriate referral if necessary and terminate the work in a clinically supportive manner (after, of course, discussion with the patient so that an opportunity is afforded to weigh the alternatives).

Conclusion

Most therapeutic issues should be worked out in therapy, not in court. Most patients should work through their past experiences, not obtain current revenge for them. We have offered some approaches which may provide clinical, ethical, and risk-management guidance for clinicians concerned about the current chaos regarding recovered memories. Maintaining therapist neutrality is the guiding principle in the treatment of patients reporting recovered memories of childhood sexual abuse. The goal is preservation of sound treatment boundaries.

References

1. Grinfeld MJ: Psychiatrist stung by high damage award in repressed memory case. Psychiatric Times, October 1994, pp. 1, 22.
2. Loftus EF: The reality of repressed memories. Am Psychol 1993; 48:518–537.
3. Ofshe R, Watters E: Making Monsters: False Memories, Psychotherapy and Sexual Hysteria. New York: Scribners, 1994.
4. Gardner RA: True and False Accusations of Child Sex Abuse. Longwood, NJ: Creative Therapeutics, 1992.
5. Briere J, Conte J: Self-reported amnesia for abuse in adults molested as children. J Trauma Stress 1993; 6:21–31.
6. Williams LM: Recall of childhood trauma: a prospective study of women's memories of childhood sexual abuse. J Consult Clin Psychol 1994; 62:1167–1176.
7. Yapko MD: Suggestions of Abuse. New York: Simon and Schuster, 1994.

8. Schouten R: Allegations of sexual abuse: a new area of liability risk. Harvard Rev Psychiatry 1994; 1:350–352.

9. Terr L: Unchained Memories: True Stories of Traumatic Memories, Lost and Found. New York: Basic Books, 1994.

10. Allen JG: The spectrum of accuracy in memories of childhood trauma. Harvard Rev Psychiatry 1995; 3:84–95.

11. Simon RI: Bad Men Do What Good Men Dream: A Forensic Psychiatrist Illuminates the Darker Side of Human Behavior. Washington DC: American Psychiatric Press, 1996.

12. Terr LC: Unchained Memories: True Stores of Traumatic Memories, Lost and Found. New York: Basic Books, 1994; see also, Terr LC: Childhood traumas: an outline and overview. Am J Psychiatry 1991; 148:10–20.

13. Mack JE: Abduction: Human Encounters with Aliens. New York: Scribners, 1994.

14. Managing the risks involved in cases of recovered memories of abuse. RX for Risk. Psychiatrists' Purchasing Group, Inc. Newsletter 1994; 5:1, 4.

15. Gutheil TG: True or false memories of sexual abuse? a forensic psychiatric view. Psychiatr Ann 1993; 23:527–531.

16. Tavris C: Beware the incest survivor machine. New York Times Jan. 3, 1993, p. 1.

17. Terr LC, Bloch DA, Michael BA, et al: Children's memories in the wake of Challenger. Am J Psychiatry 1996; 153:618–625.

18. Spence DP: Narrative truth and putative childhood abuse. Int J Clin Exp Hypn 1994; 42:288–303.

19. Gutheil TG: Risk management and recovered memories. Psychiatr Services 1995; 46:537.

20. Bursztajn H: More law and less protection: ''critogenesis,'' ''legal iatrogenesis'' and medical decision making. J Geriatr Psychiatr 1985; 18:143–153.

21. Lenhart SA, Shrier DK: Potential costs and benefits of sexual harassment litigation. Psychiatr Ann 1996; 26:132–138.

22. Simon, RI: Treatment boundary violations: clinical, ethical and legal considerations. Bull Am Acad Psychiatry Law 1992; 20:269–288.

23. Brown D: Pseudomemories: the standard of science and the standard of care in trauma treatment. Am J Clin Hypn 1995; 37:1–24.

24. Furrrow BR: Malpractice in Psychotherapy. Lexington: DC Heath, 1980, p. 31.

25. Personal communication with Richard A. Chefetz, M.D., April 23, 1996.

26. American Psychiatric Association: Principles of Medical Ethics with Annotations Especially Applicable to Psychiatry. Washington, DC, 1995.

27. Putnam FW: Diagnosis and Treatment of Multiple Personality Disorder. New York, Guilford, 1989.

28. Allen JF: The spectrum of accuracy in memories of childhood trauma. Harvard Rev Psychiatry 1995; 3:84–95.

29. American Psychiatric Association: Diagnostic and Statistical Manual of Mental Disorders (4th ed.). Washington DC: American Psychiatric Association Press, 1994.

30. American Psychiatric Association: Statement on Memories of Sexual Abuse. Washington, DC: December 12, 1993.

31. Berner ME: To write or not to write: tactics of documentation. *In* LE Lifson, RI Simon, (Eds.), Practicing Psychiatry Without Fear: A Clinical Guide to Liability Prevention. Cambridge, MA: Harvard University Press (in press).

32. Gabbard GO, Wilkinson SM: Management of Countertransference with Borderline Patients. Washington, DC: American Psychiatric Press, 1994.

33. Pope KS, Feldman-Summers S: National survey of psychologists' sexual and physical abuse

history and their evaluation of training and competence in these areas. Professional Psychol Res Pract 1992; 23:353–361.

34. Gutheil TG: Borderline personality disorders, boundary violations, and patient-therapist sex: medicolegal pitfalls. Am J Psychiatry 1989; 146:597–602.

35. Pope HG, Hudson JI: Does childhood sexual abuse cause adult psychiatric disorders? essential of methodology. J Psychiatry Law 1995; 23:363–381.

36. Lamb S: The Trouble with Blame: Victims, Perpetrators, and Responsibility. Cambridge, MA: Harvard University Press, 1996, p. 46.

37. Hammond DC, Garuer RB, Mutter CB, et al: Clinical Hypnosis and Memory: Guidelines for Clinicians and Forensic Hypnosis. Des Plains: American Society of Clinical Hypnosis Press, 1994.

38. American Medical Association. Council on Scientific Affairs: Repressed Memories. (CSA Report A-94), 1994.

39. Schouten R: Pitfalls of clinical practice: the treating clinician as expert witness. Harvard Rev Psychiatry 1993; 1:64–65.

40. Strasburger LH, Gutheil TG, Brodsky A: On wearing two hats: role conflict in serving both as psychotherapist and expert witness Am J Psychiatry (in press).

41. Strasburger LH: Crudely, without any finesse: the defendant hears his psychiatric evaluation. Bull Am Acad Psychiatry Law 1987; 15:229–233.

42. Slovenko R: The study of therapists to third parties. J Psychiatry Law 1995; 23:383–410.

43. *Ramona v. Isabella,* Rose and Western Medical Center, No. C61898. (Cal. Super. Ct. May 13, 1994).

44. Gross J: Suit Asks, Does ''Memory Therapy'' Heal or Harm. New York Times, April 8, 1994, p. 1.

45. *Ramona v. Ramona,* No. B091052 (Cal. App. Dep't Super Ct, Oct. 9, 1995).

46. See, for example, *Caryls v. Child & Adolescent Treatment Services, Inc.* 1994, 161 Misc.2d 563, 614 NYS 2d 661; *Althaus v. Cohen* 1994, Case No. G.D. 92-20893, In the Court of Common Pleas, Allegheny County, Pennsylvania.

47. Appelbaum PS, Zoltek-Jick R: Psychotherapists' duties to third parties: *Ramona* and beyond. Am J Psychiatry 1996; 153:457–465.

48. Orne MT: The nature of hypnosis: artifact and essence. J Abnorm Soc Psychol 1959; 58:277–299.

49. Council on Scientific Affairs: Scientific status of refreshing recollection by the use of hypnosis. JAMA 1985; 253:1918–1923.

50. Treatment of Psychiatric Disorders, Vol 3. A Task Force Report of the American Psychiatric Association. Washington, DC, 1989, pp. 2205–2209.

51. Pope HG, Mangweth B, Negrao AB, Hudson JI, Cordas TA: Childhood sexual abuse and bulimia nervosa: a comparison of American, Austrian, and Brazilian women. Am J Psychiatry 1994; 151:723–737.

52. Hausman K: Psychiatrist commits slander in ''recovered'' memories case. Psychiatric News, January 20, 1995, p. 10.

21

Child Victims in the Legal System

DIANE H. SCHETKY

Child abuse is usually a crime without witnesses. Perpetrators may select victims who are compliant, easily intimidated, and not likely to disclose, and secrecy is the norm. In most substantiated cases of child sexual abuse there is no physical evidence.[1] In the absence of physical evidence, corroboration, or witnesses, prosecutors may have no choice other than to have a child testify in court if they wish to get a conviction. This decision is not made lightly and must balance the child's interests with the need to protect her and other potential victims.

Putting a child on the witness stand is risky business. Typically, much time has elapsed by the time a case finally goes to trial and the child will have undergone multiple interrrogations. Memories may change with the passage of time or be altered in the repeated telling of events. Some investigators may employ leading questions or influence the child in other subtle ways. Questions put to the child may be inappropriate to the child's level of development and misunderstood. Family members may pressure a child to alter his or her testimony. The child may feel intimidated by the courtroom, the presence of the perpetrator, spectators, and by the judge and attorneys. Attorneys may argue that the child's testimony has been tainted by any of the above factors. Finally, jurors may perceive children as less credible than adult witnesses.

These issues will be addressed in this chapter, along with a discussion of how to help prepare children to testify in court. Several authors have written excellent guidelines for interviewing children for alleged abuse.[2-4] This chapter will cover some common pitfalls in interviewing children in a forensic context. It will also discuss recent decisions regarding testimony by children, and what can be done to support child witnesses.

496

Investigating Allegations of Abuse

Investigations of allegations of abuse may proceed along many lines, involving child protective workers, police, therapists, and forensic child psychiatrists. If these efforts are not coordinated, there is likely to be a duplication of efforts, a situation that is confusing to the children and their parents and one which may lead to possible contamination by interviewers. One study notes that the average child witness undergoes seven interviews by police before she gets to court.[5] Investigators should strive to minimize the number of interviews needed and maximize recall. Collaborative efforts between departments also minimize the number of interviews a child has to go through.

Investigators vary greatly in their interviewing skills, and not all are adept at communicating at the child's developmental level. For instance, a police officer asked a retarded adolescent male, ''Did you do anything to resist the assault by the defendant?'' The boy stared blankly at him and the officer repeated his question, this time raising his voice several decibels and further intimidating the boy. A good rule of thumb is that the investigator's language should mirror the child's. If a preschool child is speaking in five-word sentences, the investigator should pare his down accordingly. If a child is not speaking in polysyllabic words, then the interviewer should try to avoid using them. The use of many pronouns is confusing to young children and they should be used sparingly.

Investigators need to be aware of their own possible biases. An investigator who is convinced that the perpetrator was the child's father may fail to inquire about other possible perpetrators. She may selectively follow up on the child's desired responses and fail to validate those that do not fit with her prior assumptions. For instance, differentiating hygienic touching from sexual abuse is difficult in preschoolers. There also appears to be a double standard in terms of what sort of touching is permitted between mothers and their children versus fathers and their children.[6] A child's statement that her father touched her pee pee while bathing her is likely to generate more concern and questions than had she said her mother did the same thing. The interviewer with an agenda may overlook the fact that divorced fathers who have overnight visitation with their preschoolers have no choice but to bathe and toilet them. Bias may also be indicated when the investigator uses the terms *perpetrator* and *victim* prior to any documentation of abuse.

Investigators may influence the child's responses by their own behavior, e.g., becoming more interactive when the child begins to speak of abuse and rewarding desired responses with verbal praise or even treats. Teens are also susceptible to such influence. For instance, 15-year-old Nicole Althaus was made to feel like she was part of the police investigatory team and that she was helping other children. She readily bought in to leading questions by police investigators regarding her participation in an alleged sex ring. She later retracted her outlandish allegations and explained that she had felt a need to please the detectives and did not want to let them down.[7]

Leading questions are problematic at all ages but even more so in preschoolers who are highly suggestible. Narrative recall yields the most accurate memories. However, young children have difficulty with encoding and retrieving memories and may not be capable of much free recall. Their verbal skills are limited and their thinking is often not abstract enough to respond to open-ended and vague questions such as "Did anythong happen at Grandpa's?" There may be times when leading questions or prompts are unavoidable, but they should be used sparingly with awareness of the risks. Generally, the risk of leading a child will be greatest when the erroneous suggestion is strongly made by a person in authority and the child's memory for the event is weak. Furthermore, younger children appear to be more eager to please adults in an interview situation than older ones.

Repeated questions may be problematic. It is appropriate to ask a question more than once to check on a child's consistency. Investigators may also wish to reword a question to make sure the child has understood it. However, if the child is repeatedly asked the same questions, he may either feel he is not believed or take it as a demand for more information. The child may begin to confabulate either to please the investigator or to get her off his back. Confabulation undermines the child's credibility and one is often left with half-truths that are difficult to sort out. A useful technique is to warn the child ahead of time that the investigator may repeat a question. The investigator may also use the technique of playing dumb by saying he wants to make sure he heard the child right.

I sometimes tell children at the onset not to answer questions they do not understand. I might also advise that if they don't remember something to say so rather than guess. However, there is risk that avoidant children may use this to get out of discussing abuse. Five-year-old Jessie told the Child Protective Services (CPS) worker a story that was 180 degrees different from what she had told me. Both of us found her credible. I decided to interview Jessie together with the CPS worker and told her it was alright to say she could not remember if she really could not. This savvy child then proceeded to answer every question about alleged abuse by her father with "I don't remember." I was left feeling foolish and with no further enlightenment as to which of her stories was true.

Inexperienced interviewers may bombard children with a laundry list of questions or either-or questions. These are confusing to children and encourage guessing. If asked, "Did it happen in the bedroom or living room?", the child may feel he has to pick one answer even though neither may be correct. Furthermore, these types of questions discourage the child from telling events in his own way and do not get to important idiosyncratic details that the child might spontaneously divulge.

Children should not be exposed to the testimony of other children. In the Kelly Michaels day care case, children were told in detail what other children had disclosed about the alleged abuse by their teacher, Kelly Michaels.[8] The investigation was further contaminated by use of peer pressure, leading questions, suggested answers, and investigators telling the children that their teacher was "bad" and had done "bad things." Michaels, charged with 115 counts of sexual abuse with 19 children, spent 5 years in jail before her conviction was overturned.

It is often productive to inquire as to whether the child has been coached or prompted in any way. Questions such as, "Did anyone tell you what to say today?" may yield responses such as "Just say the truth," or "Mommy said I should tell you about all the bad things Daddy did." Some children may recite a litany of complaints in adult language but be unable to give any details. For instance, Lenny complained that his Dad regularly "sexed" him. When pressed for details, he had no idea what this term meant. Another useful line of inquiry is to ask, "Is there anything you are not supposed to tell me?" Sometimes children who have been threatened not to talk about their abuse are more comfortable showing what happened with dolls or drawings. Older children may also feel inhibited by using sexual terminology or language they consider "nasty." Reassurance may allay some of their fears.

Recording Interviews

Recording interviews serves to preserve their accuracy and may avoid duplication of efforts if shared with other investigators on the case. It also becomes a check on the interviewer to see whether he has in any way led the child or overlooked important parts of the interview. Videotapes are preferable to audiotapes in that they record nonverbal behavior, including affect. They are not without drawbacks. Some children may be inhibited by the camera or overly distracted by it. It is difficult to keep a very active child within the camera's range. Older children may be concerned about confidentiality if a stranger is operating the camera. There are also risks that videotapes may be shown out of context or fall into the wrong hands.

Decision to Prosecute

Factors that need to be considered in weighing whether to prosecute child abuse cases include the strength of the evidence, the child's competency to testify, whether her testimony is likely to help the prosecution get a conviction, and the emotional risk that testifying poses to the child.

The majority of sexual abuse crimes involving children do not go to court. Myers notes that approximately 66% of these cases end in guilty pleas before trial.[9] Many of these defendants plead guilty to a lesser crime in return for a more lenient sentence. Of those cases that go to trial, most of them end in a conviction.[9]

Myers notes that it is possible for allegations of child sexual abuse to be litigated in as many as ten separate legal proceedings.[10] The most visible of these proceedings are criminal ones, yet children may also testify in dependency and neglect or termination of parental rights hearings, and in child custody proceedings in which there are abuse allegations. In these proceedings, in contrast to criminal ones, the child is more likely to be heard in chambers without the alleged perpetrator present. Another context in which children may testify is in tort litigation in which a suit filed on their behalf alleges damages related to abuse. This type of litigation is likely to be drawn out, extending over many years and, unless settled out of court, involves face-to-face confrontation with the alleged perpetrator. Some unfortunate children may find themselves involved in multiple court proceedings simultaneously.

Children as Witnesses

Children as young as 3 and 4 have been permitted to testify in court. In most states it is now the presumption that children are competent to testify. Judges will often make their own determinations as to whether a child has the moral and cognitive capacities to testify. Occasionally, a child psychiatrist or psychologist may be asked to make a competency determination as to whether limited intelligence or presence of a mental disorder might compromise competency. Elements of competency to testify include being capable of observing, remembering, and retelling events. In addition, the child must be able to understand the difference between truth and falsehood and the consequences of lying, and be able to take an oath. A preschooler may comprehend that saying the judge's robe is red would be a lie. In most courts, this limited test suffices. However, this is not the same as grasping the implications of false testimony, and it is dubious that children of this age can appreciate these consequences. The notion of the truth is also a concept that may be too abstract for children of this age to fully understand. Nonetheless, courts continue to permit testimony by very young children and in some states there are no age barriers when it comes to testifying about sexual abuse.

Additional problems with very young child witnesses include short attention spans, anxiety caused by separating them from parents when they testify, and the need to consider their eating and sleeping habits in scheduling testimony. Children may fall asleep while waiting to testify or become irritable and cranky as the day wears on. One 4-year-old, who was somewhat oppositional to begin with, refused to enter the courtroom and made monkeys out of the people in authority who were trying to coax him into the courtroom. The judge ended up seeing him in chambers, but only after the child insisted he remove his robe and put on his ''Mister Rogers sweater.''

Children's Concepts of the Legal System

Children tend to equate going to court with being bad and confuse the roles of the various people in the courtroom. Four- to seven-year-olds have great difficulty differentiating the roles of courtroom personnel.[11] Saywitz found that young children did not understand the concept of ''jury'' and tended to confuse it with ''jewelry.'' Misunderstandings were common among grade-school children who opted for more familiar definitions of legal terms such as ''court is a place to play basketball,'' ''hearing is what you do with your ears,'' and ''minor is someone who digs coal''[11] (p. 136).

Children understand the importance of telling the truth in court, yet they have difficulty with the reasons behind this. They tend to fear punishment if they do not tell the truth, but do not appreciate the fact-finding and truth-seeking processes of the court.[12] By third grade, accurate concepts of court and the roles of courtroom personnel emerge, although understanding of the concept of a jury comes much later.[11,13] Saywitz notes that 8- to 11-year-olds tend to perceive jurors as spectators; it is not until adolescence that minors are able to appreciate the societal role of the legal system and have better awareness of the functions of the jury. She found that young children also have difficulty grasping the nature of the adversarial system and assume they will be believed in court.[11]

Effects of Testifying on Children

Courtrooms are intimidating to adults as well as to children. However, as noted, children do not have the same cognitive skills as adults to help them process what is going on in court. They must deal with confusing and sometimes incomprehensible questions from attorneys. Questions may be phrased in rambling, complex language which is replete with double negatives, embedded clauses, and legal terminology. Often the semantics and syntax are way beyond the child's cognitive level of development. Anxiety may further impair comprehension, as when the child is worried about speaking in public or the presence of the defendant and spectators in the courtroom.

Child accuracy and suggestibility are not just related to cognitive maturity but are also state dependent. For instance, a child may be able to recall certain information, but is unwilling to if it is embarrassing or creates loyalty conflicts. Bottoms et al. noted reverse age trends in children's willingness to disclose information about transgressions by their mothers.[14] Intimidation by the legal system or the presence of the perpetrator may also affect the child's ability to recall information.[15] One study found children performed significantly better when they did not have to face a live defendant.[16] Bussey et al. found that younger children had difficulty relating transgressions in the presence of the accused.[17] Similarly, Hill and Hill found in a laboratory setting that nonvictimized children had greater difficulty with recall in a courtroom setting than when they were interviewed in a less intimidating setting.[18]

Emotions may affect the child's performance in court in a variety of ways. As is well known, trauma may heighten memories or impair them. The child's affective state at the time of retrieval may also affect recall, as will strategies used for dealing with the stress of testifying, e.g., avoidance. Finally, preexisting emotional problems in the child may compromise the child's testimony and be exacerbated by the stress of testifying.

Runyan et al. studied the impact of legal intervention on sexually abused children and concluded that protracted criminal proceedings may have an adverse effect on children, whereas testifying in juvenile court may be beneficial to the child in that it helps the child overcome a sense of powerlessness and may help develop closure.[19] Goodman et al. studied the effect on children of testifying in criminal court and used as matched controls victims who did not testify. They found that 7 months after testifying the testifiers showed more behavioral disturbance than the children who did not testify. This was particularly true for children who had to testify multiple times, e.g., in preliminary hearings, competency hearings, trials, and in some cases, sentencing hearings. Children who received maternal support during the trial were more likely to improve than those who did not. However, they were also less likely to be related to the defendant or to have been involved with dependency and neglect hearings. Curiously, there was an inverse relationship between length of sentence and improvement in the child. They speculate whether prolonged sentences cause the child to feel guilty or whether the severity of abuse accounts for this correlation. On the other hand, plea bargaining did not seem to have any effect on the children's improvement.[16] One possible explanation for the different outcomes in the Runyon and Goodman studies is that juvenile proceedings involve fewer interviews and delays than do criminal proceedings. They are also likely to be more child centered and the child does not have to contend with a jury. It is also possible that the cases that ended up in criminal court involved more serious offenses.

Preparing Child Witnesses for Court

Victim advocate programs provide children and their families with support during their sojourn through the legal system. Advocates help demystify the maze of the legal system and explain courtroom procedures and personnel. Having children visit the courtroom prior to testifying may help desensitize them.

Therapists also have opportunities to support child victims. Role plays with dolls and puppets may be helpful. Six-year-old Everett, who faced testifying against his father, delighted in playing the trial of Little Green Riding Hood, an alligator puppet, accused of eating Grandma. His repetitive play revealed his many fears about court, including his father bribing the judge and bailiff, people drugging him, mayhem erupting in the courtroom, and no one being able to control his father. His therapist was able to counter some of his fantasies and fears and offer reassurance regarding order in the courtroom and his safety. After months of delays, the trial went forward, and Everett's effective testimony resulted in his father's incarceration.

Saywitz and Snyder have developed techniques for improving the accuracy of children's testimony.[20] They emphasize that preparation for court should not be confused with coaching. These techniques include using cue cards with picures to help children organize their memories, training children to resist misleading questions, and employing strategies to improve their comprehension of questions. Among the children trained to resist leading questions there was a 26% decline in erroneous responses to misleading questions when compared with the control group. Children were taught to recognize incomprehensible questions and ask the attorney to rephrase them. The researchers also emphasizd the consequences of trying to answer questions they did not understand. Once again, children in the training group made fewer errors than controls when confronted with questions which were difficult to answer.

I tried these techniques with an 8-year-old girl who had to testify against her father in a criminal proceeding. The child was devastated when her father was acquitted, and tried to blame herself. She explained: "It was my fault, I gave the wrong answer. Dad's lawyer asked me if it was OK to lie sometimes. I knew it was a leading question but I gave him the answer he wanted because I wanted him to like me." This vignette illustrates the fact that cognitive preparation for court, alone, is not enough.

Jurors' Responses to Child Witnesses

Several researchers have studied jurors' responses to child witnesses. Goodman et al. found that jurors perceived young children as significantly less credible eyewitnesses than adults.[21] Jurors were reluctant to judge a person's innocence or guilt solely on a child's statements and looked for corroborating evidence. The authors also noted that a child's delivery style and lack of confidence could undermine the effectiveness of his testimony. Nigro et al. found that speech style could mediate the effects of age on jurors' reactions to a witness.[22] Powerless speech, characterized by hesitation, hedges, intensifiers, and questioning intonations in declarative statements tended to undermine the effectiveness of testimony, whereas powerful speech had the opposite effect. The child's ability to give detail and the presence of anxiety also have a positive correlation with credibility.[16]

Goodman et al. conducted several studies using mock juries and demonstrated that credibility of eyewitnesses increases with age.[21] In contrast, Ross et al. found no such trends.[23] Duggan et al. studied the credibility of children as witnesses in a simulated child sex abuse trial. Jurors viewed allegations of abuse by a 5-year-old as susceptible to influence, whereas testimony by a 9-year-old was perceived as more credible and less susceptible to influence. Interestingly, jurors viewed a 13-year-old victim as more culpable and this appeared to influence their not-guilty verdict.[24] Similar findings were reported by Isquith et al. who noted a robust and replicable finding that jurors viewed children over the age of 12 as partially responsible for their sexual victimization.[25] These findings have disturbing implications for adolescent victims of sexual abuse. Several studies have found that in all age-groups, juries were not likely to convict without corroboration.[21,24]

Modifying Courtroom Procedures

Many child advocates fear that testifying may retraumatize a child and they have proposed alternatives to the child testifying in the presence of the defendant. However, the legal constraints of the Constitution limit the flexibility of the justice system. The 14th Amendment affords the accused due process rights, including the right to obtain witnesses' on his behalf and the right to cross-examination. The confrontation clause of the 6th Amendment provides the accused with the right to be confronted with the witness against him. There is a presumption that face-to-face confrontation affects witnesses' veracity, communication, and recall. It is unlikely that the framers of the Constitution ever considered child witnesses, let alone child sexual abuse, in formulating these amendments.

Closed-circuit TV has been used in some jurisdictions to get around the child having to be present in the same room with the alleged perpetrator. This allows the defendant and witness to see each other on TV screens in their respective rooms. I participated in one such hearing. The 4-year-old witness, who was thoroughly bored with the proceedings, turned to the judge and asked, ''Could we please switch channels and watch cartoons?''

Videotaped testimony is permitted in some jurisdictions, although in some, the defendant retains the right to cross-examine the child. Some states require a showing that testifying will be traumatic or that the witness is unavailable before videotaped testimony may be introduced. In 1990, the U.S. Supreme Court ruled in *Maryland* v. *Craig* that exceptions may be made to the need for face-to-face confrontation if the encounter is likely to cause serious emotional distress in the child and make it difficult for her to communicate. However, the State must first ''make adequate showing of the necessity.''[26] The Court held that

> The Clause's central purpose, to ensure the reliability of the evidence against a defendant by subjecting it to rigorous testing in an adversary proceeding before the trier of fact, is served by the combined effects of the elements of confrontation: physical presence, oath, cross-examination, and observation of demeanor by the trier of fact. Although fact to face confrontation forms the core of the Clause's values, it is not an indispensable element of the confrontation right.[26]

There is a risk that introducing videotaped testimony may prejudice a jury in that it implies the child has been traumatized by the defendant. Videotapes may also lessen the emotional impact of a child witness on the jury. Furthermore, there is no evidence that testimony on videotape is any more reliable than live testimony.

Simpler means exist of shielding the child from the defendant. The prosecutor may stand in such a way so as to block the child's view or the child may be given the option of looking elsewhere in the courtroom.

Another important U.S. Supreme Court decision concerns the use of hearsay statements in court about child sexual abuse. In *White* v. *Illinois,* the Court affirmed the use of hearsay statements of children in sexual abuse cases for the first time.[27] Statements that a 4-year-old had made to her baby-sitter, mother, doctor, and a nurse shortly after being sexually assaulted were permitted in evidence and the child did not have to testify. The Court ruled that the hearsay was admissible regardless of whether the child testified and that her "unavailability" had no bearing on whether the hearsay should be admissible. Even though the child's statements were admitted under "spontaneous declaration" and "medical diagnosis or treatment" exceptions, the decision was not limited to these exceptions. This decision has profound implications for both trial and appellate courts.

The 1st Amendment of the U.S. Constitution also guarantees the defendant a public trial and the public a right to know. This system of checks and balances promotes justice but interferes with the child's interest in privacy. This issue was put to test in *Globe* v. *Superior Court* where Justice Brennan's majority opinion for the U.S. Supreme Court ruled that a "mandatory closure statute could be justified only if it could be shown that closure would improve the quality of testimony of *all* minor victims."[28] Inasmuch as this is impossible to demonstrate, he ruled that there was insufficient justification for mandating a closed courtroom. In contrast to criminal proceedings, most hearings in juvenile and family court are closed to the public.

Additional reforms have been proposed to render the legal system more sensitive to children. These include prioritizing child sexual abuse cases so as to minimize delays, waiving competency requirements, extending the statute of limitations (which is now being done in some states), abolishing corroboration requirements, coordinating criminal and juvenile proceedings, establishing special child abuse prosecution units, closing courtrooms to the public, and permitting support persons to be present when a child is testifying.[29]

Conclusion

Children who must testify in court about their abuse may be retraumatized by the investigatory process and taking the witness stand. There is also risk that these processes may in themselves affect recall. The legal system needs to adopt measures that will support child witnesses through this stressful process and render their testimony more accurate. Efforts to coordinate or consolidate multiple legal proceedings should be encouraged so as to minimize the stress associated with the child having to testify repeatedly.

References

1. Muram D: Child sexual abuse: Relationship between sexual acts and genital findings. Child Abuse Negl 1989; 13:211–216.

2. Raskin D and Yuille J: Problems in evaluating interviews of children in sexual abuse cases. *In* S. Ceci, D. Ross, M Toglia (Eds.), Perspectives on Children's Testimony. New York: Springer-Verlag, 1989, pp. 184–207.

3. Yuille J, Hunter R, Joffe R, Saparniuk J: Interviewing children in sexual abuse cases. *In* G Goodman, B Bottoms (Eds.), Child Victims, Child Witnesses. New York: Guilford, 1993, pp. 95–116.

4. Quinn K, White S: Interviewing children for suspected sexual abuse. *In* D Schetky, E Benedek (Eds.), Clinical Handbook of Child Psychiatry and the Law. Baltimore: Williams and Wilkins, 1992. Vol. 30, pp. 119–144.

5. Van de Kamp J: Report on the Kern County Child Abuse Investigation. Office of the Attorney General, Division of Law Enforcement Bureau of Investigation, Kern County, CA, 1986.

6. Rosenfeld A, Bailey R, Siegel B, Bailey G: Determining incestous contact between parent and child. Frequency of children touching parents' genitals in a nonclinical population. J Am Acad Child Psychiatry 1986; 25:481–484.

7. *Althaus* v. *Cohen* G.D. No 92-20893 Alleghany Cty. Supr. Ct. 1994.

8. *State* v. *Michaels,* 625 A 2d. 489, 1993.

9. Myers J: Commentary: a call for forensically relevant research. Child Abuse Negl 1993; 17:573–579.

10. Myers J: Adjudication of Child Sexual Abuse Cases. Center for Future of Children: The Future of Children. Los Angeles: Packard Foundation, 1994.

11. Saywitz K: Children's conceptions of the legal system. *In* S Ceci, D Ross, M Toglia (Eds.), Perspectives on Children's Testimony. New York: Springer-Verlag, 1989, pp. 113–157.

12. Tapp J, Levine T: Legal socialization. Stanford Law Rev 1974; 27:1–72.

13. Melton G: Children's concepts of their rights. J Clin Child Psychol 1980; 9(3):186–190.

14. Bottoms B, Goodman G, Schwartz-Kenney F, Sachsenmaier T, Thomas S: Keeping secrets: implications for children's testimony. Paper presented at the American Psychology and Law Meetings, Williamsburg, VA, March 1990.

15. Dent H, Stephenson G: An experimental study on the effectiveness of different techniques of questioning child witnesses. Br J Soc Clin Psychol 1979; 18:41–51.

16. Goodman G, Taub E, Jones D, England P, Port L, Rudy, L, Prado L: Testifying in criminal court. Monogr Soc Res Child Dev 1992; 229:57(5).

17. Bussey K, Lee K, Ross C: Factors influencing children's lying and truthfulness. *In* M DeSimone, M Toglia (Eds.), Lying and Truthfulness Among Young Children: Implications for their Participation in Legal Proceedings. Symposium presented at the Society for Research in Child Development, Seattle, WA, 1991.

18. Hill P, Hill S: Videotaping children's testimony: an empirical view. Michigan Law Rev 1987; 85:809–833.

19. Runyon E, Everson M, Edelsohn G, Hunter W, Coulter M: Impact of legal intervention on sexually abused children. J Pediatr 1988; 113(4):647–653.

20. Saywitz K, Snyder L: Improving children's testimony with preparation. *In* G Goodman, B Bottoms (Eds.), Child Victims, Child Witnesses. New York: Guilford, 1993, pp. 117–146.

21. Goodman G, Golding J, Helgeson V, Haith M, Michelli J: When a child takes the stand: jurors' perceptions of children's eyewitness testimony. Law Hum Behav 1987; 11:27–40.

22. Nigro G, Buckley M, Hill D, Nelson J: When juries "hear" children testify: the effects of eyewitness age and speech style on jurors' perceptions of testimony. *In* S Ceci, D Ross, M Toglia (Eds.), Perspectives on Children's Testimony. New York: Springer-Verlag, 1989, pp. 57–70.

23. Ross D, Miller B, Moran P: The child in the eyes of the jury: assessing mock-jurors perceptions of the child witness. *In* S Ceci, M Toglia, D Ross (Eds.), Children's Eyewitness Memory. New York: Springer-Verlag, 1987, pp. 142–154.

24. Duggan M, Aubrey M, Doherty E, Isquith P, Levine M, Scheiner J: The credibility of children as witnesses in a simulated child sex abuse trial. *In* S Ceci, D Ross, M Toglia (Eds.), Perspectives on Children's Testimony. New York: Springer-Verlag, 1989, pp. 71–99.

25. Isquith P, Levine M, Scheiner J: Blaming the child: attributions of responsibility to victims of child sexual abuse. *In* G Goodman, B Bottoms (Eds.), Child Victims Child Witnesses. New York: Guilford, 1993, pp. 203–228.

26. *Maryland* v. *Craig* 497 U.S. 836 (1990).

27. *White* v. *Illinois* 502 U.S. 346 (1992).

28. *Globe Newspaper Co.* v. *Superior Court* 102 S. Ct. 2613 (1982).

29. Bulkley J: The impact of new child witness research on sexual abuse prosecutions. *In* S Ceci, D Ross, J Toglia (Eds.), Perspectives on Children's Testimony. New York: Springer-Verlag, 1989, pp. 208–229.

VI

REFLECTIONS ON TRAUMA
AND MEMORY

22

Reflections on Trauma and Memory

PAUL S. APPELBAUM

Not long ago, I developed an annoying, angry pimple in the middle of my forehead. As I touched the soreness in the area, I noticed a certain familiarity to the sensation. The pain was not a new pain, but one I was sure I had felt before—and precisely in the same location. Moreover, there was a sense of meaningfulness to the recollection. It wasn't merely the memory of some other bygone epidermal eruption that was being jogged. Something more significant was involved. What was I remembering? How could I be so sure about a connection to something in the past? I searched consciously for the answer without success. And then, when I was not even trying, I remembered the story.

It had happened in high school, 30 years before. A classmate, a bully by inclination, had tried to shove in front of me on a line in gym class as we waited to use the water fountain. When he was unresponsive to my more rational entreaties, I grabbed him by the neck and tossed him aside. Needless to say, he was furious; the encounter had occurred in front of a large group of half-naked boys, in whose eyes his reputation was now in question. But this was neither the time nor place for revenge. Too many teachers were nearby. Revenge, however, was his obsession, and whenever he saw me during the next few weeks, he reminded me that it was only a matter of time until satisfaction would be his.

That time came some weeks later, as I stood with friends outside our high school building, waiting for the doors to swing open at the start of the day. I never saw him coming. In one smooth movement, he pushed me from behind, kicking my feet out from under me, and leaped astride my body as I fell to the ground. There he sat, pummeling my forehead with his fist, the middle finger of which protruded from the remainder of his clenched hand, so that the full power of each blow was transmitted through that single knuckle, aimed at the precise center of my forehead.

511

A few eyewitnesses later claimed that I had put up a good fight, but they were my friends and I think they were just being kind. Clearly my assailant—why can I envisage his face, but not remember his name to this day—had his revenge. The center of my forehead felt as though an auger had been taken to it. That it looked as bad as it felt I knew from the puzzled glances of my teachers, and the somewhat less subtle inquiries of my friends. The swelling and soreness in the middle of my forehead must have lasted for a week or two; the bruise was probably there for a good deal longer.

This was the memory that was evoked by the uneasily familiar twinge of an otherwise insignificant pimple. I do not believe that I had consciously recollected these events for many years, perhaps not since shortly after they occurred. Had I not already been thinking about the phenomena associated with the delayed recovery of memory, it is possible that I would have given the entire episode little thought. However, I believe that this encounter with the recovery of a previously neglected memory—a memory so mundane that it might well reflect a near-universal experience—exemplifies many of the controversies and uncertainties discussed by the contributors throughout this book.

That I had not thought consciously about the fight outside my high school for nearly 30 years is clear. Nor is it difficult to find an explanation for why I might very much want to block the episode from my mind. When I envision myself lying pinned to the sidewalk as my assailant drives his knuckle into my forehead, it evokes a sense of helplessness, even impotence, that threatens my self-image as a capable person, a capable man, able to deal with the challenges of the world. The image of oneself as a victim is not a pleasant one. Moreover, the incident underscores the dangers of sudden violence that lurk around us, dangers from which we in the middle class are usually able to insulate ourselves, and thus ordinarily find it possible to ignore. No one could doubt that I had more than sufficient motivation to put the unhappy occurrence out of my thoughts.

How exactly did I accomplish that? Did I consciously will myself not to remember the unpleasant events, just as experimenters sometimes instruct subjects to forget lists of words they have seen or stories they have heard in psychology laboratories?[1] Or was the process more passive: I simply stayed away from the aversive memories, having no reason to recollect them and many to avoid them altogether? Perhaps the process was not conscious at all. There is no evidence that I dissociated the experience, but did I repress the memory, engaging in whatever active unconscious work that requires?[2] And as clinicians and scientists, is there any way for us to tell which of these mechanisms was operative here?

The manner in which the memory returned raises another set of intriguing issues. It began not with a conscious thought, as would be typical of declarative memory, but with a sensation, just as victims of severe trauma often report initially becoming aware of their memories through noncognitive, sensory modalities.[3] Did the return of my declarative memory require a sensory trigger, or would some other mechanism have had the same effect? How dependent was the effectiveness of the sensory trigger (i.e., the pain in my forehead) on other events going on in my life, including my interest in recovered memories per se? Would the same trigger have been effective at any point in the last 30 years, or was some degree of interaction with other affects or cognitions required?

How potent might other triggers have been on their own? Would the memory have returned if I had simply been asked about it? If so, how specific would the stimulus have to be? Would I have responded accurately to a question asking whether I had ever been in any fights as a child or adolescent, or would my questionner have to be more specific (''Did you ever get into any fights at school?'') or even provide some details of the event (''Can you tell me about the fight you had outside your high school?'')? Is it possible to conceive of experimental models that might help us begin to address questions like these?

Even if we could answer all of these questions, it might still not be clear how generalizable my experience is. Do different mechanisms govern the memory—and the forgetting—of traumatic episodes, compared with the other experiences we have in our lives? If so, should my experience with the class bully count as traumatic? Certainly it pales before the traumata that occupy the attention of the majority of clinical memory researchers today: childhood physical and sexual abuse, rape, near-death experiences in combat, natural or man-made disasters resulting in the deaths of dozens or hundreds of people. Does the answer to whether an experience is sufficiently traumatic to invoke the putative alternative mechanisms of memory depend on the nature of the trauma, the response of the victim, or both? If traumatic memories do differ from other recollections in how they are processed, do they vary along a spectrum or is there some sharp step function that describes the line of demarcation between the groups?

Undoubtedly, many other questions can be spun out of my homely tale of memory lost and found, an experience that I suspect is not rare, although that, too, remains to be determined. It would be wrong to leave the reader of this book, however, with the sense that all that has come out of the recent attention to trauma and memory are questions with unknown, and perhaps unknowable, answers. The controversy highlighted in the introductory chapters by Hyman and Loftus[4] and by Kluft,[5] to be sure, has exposed the gaps in our knowledge of how, why, and when we remember the events of our lives. But it has also pushed us toward empirical exploration of these issues and started in motion efforts that have already resulted in some consensus about certain aspects of treating victims of trauma, and it may lead to common understandings of other aspects of the issue as well. In summing up the message of this book, it may be useful to reflect on the ways in which the diverse contributions of these authors point—even if sometimes only tentatively—toward advances in our understanding of trauma and memory.

Mechanisms of Memory

The trauma and memory controversy erupted at a time of profound disjunction between the dominant popular view of memory and scientific advances in understanding the neural and cognitive bases of memory functions. Lay perspectives on memory had, by the late 1980s, probably changed little from the time that Freud began exploring his patients' recollections, nearly 100 years earlier. As Galatzer-Levy notes in his chapter on psychoanalytic views of memory,[6] Freud incorporated into his metapsychology a conception of memory as a repository of a lifetime of sensory perceptions. Although the expression of memories might be modified by defensive mechanisms that altered their content (e.g., condensation, displacement) or blocked their retrieval altogether (e.g., repression, denial), Freud seemed to have little doubt that the original memory traces were retained. Indeed, early psychoanalytic treatment often was aimed at the recovery of actual memories, with techniques such as free association designed to facilitate the process.

This understanding of memory—what has now come to be called the "video camera" theory of the mind—appears to be deeply embedded in popular culture. It has been reinforced by cinematic images of characters recovering (often traumatic) memories under the influence of hypnosis or sodium amytal, and by the widely publicized experiments of Penfield and colleagues in the 1950s, who probed the cerebral cortices of patients undergoing neurosurgery and noted that they reported discrete memories associated with stimulation at different sites.[7] Although the implications of Penfield's findings have now been called into question,[8] for several decades they provided scientific support for the notion that our memories, even if not consciously recalled, were not lost; they were simply buried in the archives of the brain, awaiting retrieval with the proper stimulus.

Well before the trauma and memory debate surfaced in the late 1980s and early 1990s, however, these popular notions of immutable memory were under attack by researchers from a broad array of disciplines. Psychoanalysts themselves, as Levine (citing the work of Kris[9]) demonstrates in his chapter, came to recognize that "memories of formative events are altered in the course of development as they become absorbed into significant patterns of character and defense."[10] Donald Spence's extremely influential book, *Narrative Truth and Historical Truth,* argued that history, that is, memory of actual events, is not even the proper realm of psychoanalytic treatment.[11] Rather, since such knowledge is inherently unattainable, treatment must focus on the patient's understanding of events (their "narrative truth") and the meaning of that narrative to the patient.

Simultaneously, empirical demonstration of the malleability of memory was forthcoming from the laboratories of psychologists such as Loftus and her colleagues.[12] Hyman and Loftus review much of this work in their chapter.[4] Initially, Loftus's efforts were stimulated by concern over the accuracy of eyewitness testimony in criminal trials.[13] Her research showed that memory for events actually witnessed by subjects was susceptible to alteration by exposure to a variety of post-event information and suggestions. Later, a series of experiments motivated by the trauma and memory controversy itself demonstrated, with increasing ecologic validity, that subjects could be induced to endorse memories for entire episodes that had never occurred.

These dramatic demonstrations of the plasticity of human memory have been augmented by a vast body of work, reviewed in the chapter by Koutstaal and Schacter, on factors affecting recall—for better and for worse.[14] Studies of subjects' recovery of previously presented information suggest that memories are laid down as part of associative webs or networks, so that recall of one element in a web increases the likelihood that related elements of memory will be accessed. Cues that enhance entry into an associative network, even when they relate to incidental variables, like the characteristics of the room in which the event in question took place, increase retrieval.

On the other hand, these associative mechanisms are far from foolproof. Unless reinforced by active remembering, cues tend to fade over time,[15] leading subjects to misidentify the sources of information they recall; incorrectly identify distinct memory elements as related; lose recollection for the details of even accurately recalled memories; condense memories of multiple events into one; unconsciously fill in the gaps in incomplete memories on the basis of preexisting knowledge or beliefs; and alter the certainty with which they endorse their memories.

Careful examination of the phenomenology of human memory by cognitive psychologists has been complemented by recent advances in comprehending the neural basis of memory. Bremner and colleagues, in their chapter, review current understanding of the anatomical structures underlying normal memory.[16] Memory is no longer conceived as a unitary category. At a minimum, declarative (or explicit) memory, or memory for events or information that is subject to conscious recall, is distinguished from implicit memory, which includes memory for how to do things, and affective elements of memory as well. The hippocampus, located in the temporal lobe, appears to play a central coordinating function in laying down and retrieving declarative memories.

In contrast to the conclusions suggested by Penfield's work, it seems unlikely that entire memories are stored in any one area of the cerebral cortex. Rather, memories appear to be distributed throughout the cortex, with particular areas specializing in the storage of different types of information. A single memory, perhaps of a July 4th picnic, may be split into visual images of a volleyball game, stored in the occipital lobe; olfactory memories of the smell of grilling hamburgers, retained in the inferior frontal lobe; and recollections of a discussion one had over a beer that day with a favorite uncle (''Son, the future is in plastics''), stored in the parietal area. These widely distributed memory fragments may be linked together by the hippocampus, which facilitates retrieval of the memory web as a whole when any single element is accessed. Imaging studies of the human brain during memory tasks demonstrate diverse areas ''lighting up'' as the components of a memory are pulled together.[17]

Cellular mechanisms underlying the formation of these memory webs remain to be elucidated. It has been suggested for some years that selective reinforcement of connections between neurons, exemplified by the phenomenon of long-term potentiation in the hippocampus, may be the neurophysiological basis for memory.[8] Work is now underway to identify the corresponding changes that take place within individual cells, down to the level of gene expression.[18] Clearly, a major task for neurobiologists in the coming decade will be to link neural and intracellular events to the phenomena of memory elucidated by the cognitive psychologists. At the same time, it will be critical not to lose sight of the whole organism and to recognize, as Elin describes,[19] the humanistic aspects of memory as the repository of the self.

The trauma and memory controversy has impacted recent work on mechanisms of memory at several levels. Although the much-heralded revolution in cognitive science was well underway before the debate over memories of trauma came to a head, it is unquestionable that many scientists have found in the controversy motivation for further work, often in new areas of memory function. The research documented in the chapters by Hyman and Loftus on implantation of memories,[4] by Leichtman and colleagues on memory in children,[20] and by van der Kolk on memories of trauma in adults[3] exemplify this work. Since science often seeks to answer questions made salient by current social concerns, it in no way denigrates the accomplishments of these researchers to point to the controversy as an important part of their motivation.

A second area of the controversy's impact on memory research has been the impetus it has given to the dissemination of the most recent theories and empirical findings to a broad, and now intensely interested, public. The abandonment of the "video camera theory" of memory is trumpeted in the pages of popular newsmagazines. Daily newspapers carry reports on cognitive psychological research that might once have been considered too esoteric for such forums; it is no longer unusual to see articles on errors in source attribution as the basis for distortion of memory—research now meaningful to the lay public as a potential explanation for false reports of childhood sexual abuse.[21] The dramatic stories of parents, grandparents, and day care workers accused of sexual and even satanic ritual abuse, have provided an unparalleled opportunity for public discussion of basic mechanisms of memory, and the introduction of new paradigms to replace the now-discredited models of the early and mid-twentieth century.

Effects of Trauma on Memory

That trauma can affect the way we process memory is indisputable. Golier et al.[22] along with Bremner and his collaborators,[16] provide graphic evidence of how posttraumatic stress disorder (PTSD) may be marked by changes in memory retrieval, ranging from intrusive recollections and nightmares to amnesia. They suggest, in addition, that the hormonal responses associated with stress, through their actions on brain areas involved in memory function, including the hippocampus and the amygdala, may be the means by which trauma exerts its effects. Although the precise mechanisms for the symptoms of PTSD remain to be elucidated, the scientific agenda seems clear. This is not where the debate has centered.

A second area of inquiry, reviewed in the chapter by Pynoos and colleagues,[23] has centered on the impact of trauma on memories in children. Since so many of the traumatic events that later plague adults occur during childhood, some understanding of the ground on which these memories are laid is crucial to appreciating their impact later in life. Typical of researchers and clinicians in this area (see Sauzier's chapter[24] for confirmation from a different perspective), Pynoos et al. stress the many factors, both developmental and environmental, that can affect what and how children remember. Not only is there no single stereotypic response of a child to trauma, but the variables associated with different outcomes are just beginning to be elucidated.

At the heart of the trauma and memory controversy lies the question of whether trauma, especially childhood sexual abuse, can result in a particular alteration in memory function: prolonged amnesia for the traumatic event, followed by recovery of a veridical memory.[12] Several of our contributors have referenced the small number of studies attempting to document loss and recovery of memory, and other reviews from differing perspectives can be found elsewhere.[25–27] Others in this volume, like Kluft,[5] offer evidence based on their extensive clinical experience. Although it is unlikely that all sides to the debate would endorse any single effort to summarize the data, there appears to be an evolving consensus on several important issues that is worth considering.

A substantial number of studies have reported by now that many persons who give histories of childhood sexual abuse also claim to have been unaware of the abuse at some time in their lives. Figures for the percentage of abused populations reporting such amnesia range from 16% to 59%.[28] Interpretation of the early studies was hampered by use of clinical populations of uncertain representativeness—although a general population survey with similar results has now been reported[29]—and by the researchers' inability to verify the alleged sexual abuse.

Perhaps the most important research to date, therefore, has been done by Williams, utilizing a sample of women with documented childhood sexual abuse who were interviewed 17 years after presentation to a hospital emergency room.[30] She found, consistent with other studies, that 38% of subjects did not recall the abusive experiences. Critics have challenged some aspects of these data, arguing, for example, that the findings may merely reflect a reluctance on the part of subjects to talk about shameful childhood events with interviewers.[12,25] Moreover, they note that some of the abusive events occurred at an age when adults rarely recall what happened to them as children, and thus the data do not demonstrate a unique effect of trauma on memory.

Williams's findings, however, suggest that many subjects without a recollection of the sexual abuse in question were willing to talk about profoundly embarrassing issues, and many of the subjects reporting no memory of the event were, at the time, well beyond the age of ordinary childhood amnesia. Given the consistency across studies of identifying such a group, it is difficult to avoid the conclusion that at least some people who suffer childhood sexual abuse fail to remember the event, when they ordinarily would be expected to. Even some of the severest critics of the studies of memories of childhood sexual abuse now appear ready to grant this point, though they continue to dispute the frequency of the phenomenon.[4,25]

But can such memories, once absent, be recovered? To address this question, Williams interviewed those subjects who acknowledged the abuse recorded in the hospital's records. Sixteen percent of those who recalled their abuse reported that there was a period of time in their lives when they had not remembered what had happened to them.[28] Although the accuracy of the retrospective reports of Williams' subjects can be questioned,[25,26] the new data point strongly to the ability of some traumatized persons to forget and later recover memories of their trauma. Again, the critics now focus less on challenging this conclusion than on arguing that the phenomenon is unlikely to be common.[4,25]

What, however, is the phenomenon in question? Early studies focused on repression as the presumed mechanism for failure to remember sexual abuse in childhood,[31] which fit neatly with psychoanalytic theories about defenses to trauma.[6] But the very existence of repression turned out to be a controversial issue in its own right,[2] and served as a additional reason for opponents of psychoanalytic theories to cast doubt on the recovery of memories of sexual abuse.[32] It is of interest, therefore, that Williams' interviews with her subjects lead her to suggest that at least some of them may have engaged in "a conscious attempt to deal with the abuse by blocking it out," even years after the abuse occurred.[28] Though she still maintains that other subjects' memories may have been affected by repression and dissociation, her acknowledgement that some victims of childhood sexual abuse may engage in deliberate efforts to forget their trauma is likely to represent additional common ground on which previously polarized researchers and clinicians may meet.

However welcome the existence of a nidus around which people of different orientations can coalesce, there remain substantial areas of contention and uncertainty. Why do some people forget the trauma they suffered, while others do not? Individual differences in susceptibility to failed recall are just beginning to be studied, with conflicting results.[28] Moreover, there is little agreement regarding how frequently these phenomena occur, as well as concerning the mechanisms of failed recall, in particular whether repression plays any role at all. Why, having put these unpleasant memories out of their conscious awareness, do some people later remember them? Is it simply a matter of jogging their memories (the Williams data suggest not), or does recall depend on a more complex process with both biological and psychological components?

Also at issue is whether memories of trauma, including childhood sexual abuse, are different in quality from other memories. Bremner and colleagues suggest that the physiologic environment within which memories of trauma are laid down may account for such differences.[16] Yet, many persons exposed to trauma, and presumably its hormonal accompaniments, do not develop memory impairments or the symptoms of PTSD. van der Kolk points to differences in the ways in which memories of trauma are recalled, with increased utilization of implicit memory involving noncognitive sensory systems.[3] Researchers and clinicians who are skeptical of claims regarding the uniqueness of memories of trauma, however, argue that insufficient data exist on the characteristics of nontraumatic memory for us to conclude that the phenomena described cannot be accounted for by the usual mechanisms. So far, the work in this area is only suggestive, with definitive conclusions awaiting further research.

The Role of Memory in Treatment

Just as the debate over memories of trauma has highlighted new models of memory and focused attention on the vicissitudes of memory in trauma victims, so has it raised questions about the role that recovery of memory plays in psychotherapeutic treatment. Although these queries have been posed in the context of treatment of trauma and its aftereffects, they are in fact more generally applicable to psychotherapy as a whole. Among the issues pinpointed are the extent to which memory retrieval is essential or even useful in the treatment of persons who may have suffered childhood trauma; how such memories should be handled when they arise; and the degree to which veridical memories can be recovered in psychotherapy.

Readers of Levine's chapter[10] can be left with little question that psychoanalysis has moved beyond reconstruction and abreaction of traumatic events as a model for effective treatment. But as Matthews and Chu make clear in their contribution, attention to patients' recollections of trauma is an inevitable component of mainstream, psychodynamically oriented treatment.[33] Indeed, it is almost inconceivable that one could seriously explore the emotions and behavior patterns of many patients without evoking—and having to deal with—recollections of events as deeply upsetting as sexual abuse and other traumas. Even the cognitive-behavioral techniques outlined by Ross[34] involve specific discussion of presumed traumatizing events.

As Levine suggests and as skeptics of approaches to recovery of memory in therapy maintain,[25] we lack empirical evidence demonstrating that accurate recovery of memory is essential to effective treatment. There is, therefore, little reason to endorse approaches to therapy that are aimed specifically at encouraging recall of traumatic memories. Even when the memories themselves are accurate, patients may react adversely to their recall, with increases in symptoms and subjective distress. Thus, the survey data that suggest large numbers of therapists employ techniques aimed specifically at memory recovery, including the hypnotic techniques cautioned against by Frankel and Covino,[35] are troubling.[36,37] But whether or not they are sought, many patients will offer such memories, either at the inception of treatment or somewhere along the way. The question that must still be addressed is how to deal with these recollections.

Matthews and Chu offer a carefully nuanced approach that is reflective of the best of the evolving literature on this subject.[33] Cautious therapists will listen empathically to patients' recollections, acknowledging the pain that they must evoke. They will, however, refrain from endorsing the truth (or suggesting the falsehood) of any set of memories, recognizing that therapists lack the means to assess the accuracy of patients' recollections. Indeed, it has even been suggested that therapists underscore for their patients the inherent uncertainty of memory, especially when there has been a period during which the episode has been forgotten.[38] This may be a difficult stance to assume—indeed, Simon and Gutheil in their chapter describe the potential adverse consequences of this approach[39]—but it reflects reality: in the absence of outside corroboration, the validity of recovered memories of abuse will always be uncertain.

Much of the concern over the handling of memories of abuse in therapy is based on the belief that psychotherapy itself can induce inaccurate memories. Hyman and Loftus outline how the characteristics of the therapeutic setting, including the power therapists may have to suggest the recollections they want to hear and the use of techniques that are likely to enhance the production of false memories (such as imagining what abuse might have been like had it occurred), may affect patients' presentations.[4] Having proven that false memories for childhood events can be generated in adults, they point to the similarity between the circumstances that enhance false memory creation and those that may be found in some therapists' consulting rooms: demands to remember, invitations to incorporate new information into memories, suggestions to put aside disbelief. (Indeed, these comparisons have served in some cases as the basis for a broader attack on the legitimacy of psychotherapeutic approaches in general.[32]) The courts are now beginning to see cases involving former patients who claim that the suggestive aspects of therapy induced them to believe that, and to act as if, they had been sexually abused, a belief that they later came to repudiate.[40,41]

Here the table is turned on skeptics of recovered memory, who may grudgingly admit that the phenomenon can occur, but demand proof that it is frequent enough to warrant special treatment. Therapists who work with victims of trauma respond to allegations that false memories frequently arise as a result of suggestion with the insistence that critics document just how common the occurrence is.[42] Although rumors circulate of dozens or hundreds of cases in litigation alleging that therapists created false memories of abuse, there is as yet no careful documentation by unbiased researchers. Clinicians can contend with considerable justification that therapeutic techniques of potential benefit to numerous patients ought not to be discarded on the theoretical grounds that false memories may be generated until a clear demonstration of the phenomenon and its prevalence exists.

The debate over the relationship between psychotherapeutic techniques and memories of abuse is far from over. Although it has been the cause of much friction, particularly between cognitive psychologists relying on findings from their research laboratories and clinicians speaking to the reality they see before them in their offices, it has had some salutary effects as well. The potential impact of suggestion in therapy—a concern, as Levine notes,[10] of Freud himself—is now being considered seriously by thoughtful clinicians. Helpful efforts to limit the scope of the problem, while recognizing that it can never be eliminated in any dyadic relationship, may improve therapeutic technique even in areas unrelated to trauma. Moreover, the renewed attention to epistemological issues in therapy, including whether and how one establishes "truth," should encourage therapists' modesty with regard to their reconstructive abilities. The critique of psychotherapy has been, and continues to be, painful for practitioners, but the therapeutic disciplines are likely to be the better for it in the long run.

Societal Responses to Memories of Trauma

The debate over memories of trauma has forced us to consider what mechanisms should exist to assist victims in gaining help for their problems and vindicating their legal rights. By no means has this discussion been limited to victims of childhood sexual abuse, although as with the other areas reviewed here, they have often received the bulk of the attention. The policy questions can be framed simply, though the answers are far from straightforward: Do the peculiar vulnerabilities of victims of trauma require special accommodation from societal institutions, particularly the courts? And to what extent should the rights of other parties be restricted to enhance the rights of victims?

As Schetky's chapter suggests, prosecution of alleged sexual abuse of children was one of the first places where these questions were raised.[43] Children have a difficult time with court proceedings in general; the dynamics associated with sexual abuse, such as the difficulty a young child may have directly confronting his or her abuser, compound the problem. Here, a society that generally has been solicitous of the interests of children has experimented with a variety of means to facilitate their testimony. States have widened the scope of victims' accounts that can be presented in evidence by third parties, and have allowed modification of courtroom design when that is deemed necessary, e.g., the use of screens to block children from having to look directly at defendants. Individual judges may permit young children to testify from their parents' laps, and otherwise modify courtroom procedures to meet their needs. Nonetheless, there are clearly limits to how far this process of accommodation can go. In a country with a strong tradition of protecting defendants' rights, including the constitutional right to confront one's accuser,[44] appellate courts have indicated that there are limits, as yet not clearly defined, to the changes that can be made to meet the needs of child victims.

Similar tensions are at play where adult victims are concerned. Murphy outlines the conflict between facilitating the access of victims of sexual assault to the courts, and allowing defendants to obtain information that may be helpful, or even critical, to their defense.[45] Many victims seek counseling after suffering an assault, something that in itself is socially desirable. But ordinary rules of evidence in many states allow accused rapists to peruse the records of victims' treatment in search of contradictions or other evidence that may impeach victims' credibility. Under such circumstances, victims may have to choose between protecting their privacy in counseling and pursuing legal action against their attacker. Traditional therapist–patient testimonial privileges, which allow patients to keep confidential material out of court proceedings, often carve out exceptions for criminal trials or fail to cover the unlicensed therapists who perform much rape counseling. Some states have responded by creating distinct rape counseling privileges. Again, though, a conflict arises with the accuseds' Sixth Amendment rights to an adequate defense. Courts sometimes split the difference here, allowing access only to certain kinds of information, perhaps after screening by a judge.[46] But a clear legal consensus has yet to evolve in this inherently difficult conflict of rights.

Striking a reasonable balance of interests is no less problematic where civil remedies for sexual abuse are concerned. As in other circumstances, situations in which memories are only recovered at a later date are the most problematic. The law creates limits on the periods during which legal actions can be brought for both civil and (in most instances) criminal cases. These statutes of limitations, as Zoltek-Jick describes,[47] are intended to protect defendants and the integrity of the legal process by encouraging speedy adjudication before witnesses disappear, memories fade, and documents are lost. Out of fairness to victims of negligent and intentional wrongdoing, exceptions have been carved out in cases in which victims did not know about their injuries or who caused them, or were otherwise unable to pursue a remedy.

As the possibility surfaced in the 1980s that memories of abuse might be lost and then regained, many states added repressed memories of sexual abuse to the categories that might extend the period during which suit could be brought or criminal charges filed.[48] The analogy to a sponge left behind in a surgical operation festering unknown for many years—the classic situation in which a statute of limitations is tolled—was too strong to ignore. With the evolution of the debate over trauma and memory, however, the situation has grown more complex. Why should repression, but not forgetting, toll the statute of limitations, and how can we tell the difference between these cases? Indeed, if fairness to victims of trauma is the goal, why omit those persons who were so psychologically crippled in the wake of sexual abuse that they were unable to contemplate the rigors of a lawsuit, though they always retained the memory of the trauma?

The law is usually reluctant to alter doctrine on the basis of new clinical or scientific findings, fearing that today's scientific verity will become tomorrow's discarded theory. Because of social pressures, recovered memories of child abuse were treated as an exception. With understanding of the phenomenon continuing to evolve, one suspects that many courts regret having entered the area before the dust cleared. Signs of a reversal of the pendulum, Zoltek-Jick points out, are already evident. States are beginning to set tighter bounds on the ease with which their statutes of limitations can be extended, and some courts simply have refused to admit testimony based on recovered memories. In any event, with the question now in play, further legal developments are likely to be dependent on advances in understanding the processing of memories of abuse.

A final area to consider in which countervailing interests are being rebalanced as a result of the trauma and memory controversy deals with the duties of therapists who treat victims of trauma. Clinicians are always obligated to conform to reasonable standards of care in treatment. When new problems like recovered memories arise, however, it may not be entirely clear what those standards are. Simon and Gutheil provide an overview of the likely duties of clinicians, while acknowledging that it may be some time before professional standards evolve to the point that a clear consensus exists on many of these issues.[39] The fourteen risk management principles they ennunciate are anchored by a key premise: that therapists will maintain a stance of neutrality with regard to their patients. This implies primary attention to helping patients resolve their own agendas, rather than a focus on demonstrating the validity of therapists' preconceptions about what happened in the past or what should happen in the future.

Simultaneous with rising concern among therapists about their potential liability for the treatment of patients who have or develop memories of trauma are efforts already underway by clinicians[49] and professional organizations to define professional standards of care.[50,51] Progress on many of the unanswered questions regarding memories of trauma (e.g., how essential is recovery of memories to effective treatment?), however, will be necessary before definitive responses are possible. Clinicians may take some comfort in the fact that the law has always recognized that unitary standards of care are rare; diverse approaches are acceptable as long as they are endorsed by a respectable minority of the profession.

As it has in other areas, the debate over traumatic memories is pushing the law across new frontiers. Two such cutting-edge issues can be mentioned briefly. Standards of care in psychotherapy have usually focused on what transpired in the consulting room. Taking patients' presentations as they are, clinicians have been expected to assess and treat them in reasonable ways. As Uyehara notes, however, the question of whether clinicians should be obligated to seek corroboration of patients' accounts of abuse is now unavoidable.[52] If advocates of this duty, such as McHugh,[53] have their way, therapists may be called on to act as detectives (something Sauzier incidentally suggests may not be avoidable in working with children whose histories suggest abuse[24]). Although this may be possible and even desirable in some circumstances, mandating it as part of a standard of care threatens to turn the traditional therapeutic relationship into something quite different, with clinicians feeling obliged to question patients' accounts and seek confirmation of their claims. It is doubtful that traditional psychotherapy can continue in an atmosphere of distrust. A more reasonable alternative would be for clinicians to bear the obligation of indicating to patients the probable limits of certainty with which newly recollected memories can be held, something that, as noted above, many authorities already encourage.

A second barely explored area of law relates to duties that therapists may have in recovered memory cases to persons other than their patients.[54] Traditionally, caregivers have not been held responsible for harm to third parties as a result of what occurred in treatment, even when the treatment was negligent. A small number of exceptions have existed—the most prominent of them being the duty to protect potential victims of patients' violence[55]—but they have always involved a duty to prevent physical injury. Recently, several highly publicized cases have suggested that therapists who assist patients in the recovery of memories of abuse, especially if they suggest or facilitate actions against the alleged abuser, may thereby acquire duties toward the latter that can be vindicated in court.[41,56] The principles underlying these decisions, so far limited to trial courts, could be applied to other kinds of cases, e.g., an aggrieved spouse who is upset that the patient has filed for divorce after a course of therapy. Thus, unless strictly limited, they threaten severe disruption to therapeutic relationships, and a significant expansion of the scope of clinicians' liability.[54]

It seems likely that the ultimate degree of accommodation of the interests of trauma victims will depend in no small part on how accurate we understand their recollections to be. Uncertainty about the veridicality of memories will reinforce attention to the interests of criminal defendants and alleged abusers in civil cases. In addition, to the extent that therapists are seen as promoting belief in and action on unreliable memories, they are likely to face greater risk of liability to patients and to third parties. In the meantime, the trauma and memory controversy has forced the courts to confront basic issues in law itself regarding the rights of defendants, statutes of limitations, the scope of tort liability, and perhaps the extent to which the law's traditional reliance on witnesses' memory as the "gold standard" of evidence may be misplaced.

Conclusion

Why did the debate over memories of trauma arise when it did in the late 1980s and early 1990s? Surely, a large part of the explanation lies in a decade's worth of increasing attention to the reality of childhood sexual abuse, which gave new credibility to the claims of both children and adults to have been victims of such practices. As their revelations reverberated through our society, they focused a spotlight on the underside of the lives of children, and on the people who abuse them. Inevitably, in the wake of highly publicized cases in which these claims were challenged, the controversy over the validity of memories of sexual abuse as we know it today erupted.[53,56,57]

To those in the trenches working with victims of trauma, especially sexual abuse, the debate at times may seem to threaten the legitimacy of their work and thereby to denigrate their efforts. Although that reaction is understandable, it ignores the very real challenges that our evolving comprehension of traumatic memory poses for multiple disciplines, ranging from cognitive psychology to law. The ferment engendered over trauma and memory, as manifested in the contributions to this book, holds the potential to stimulate inquiry and force careful examination of our assumptions about such diverse areas as the nature of autobiographical memory, the basis for therapeutic efficacy in psychotherapy, and fairness towards victims of childhood abuse. By such tumultuous means is progress achieved.

References

1. Johnson HM: Processes of successful intentional forgetting. Psychol Bull 1994; 116:274–292.

2. Singer JL (Ed.): Repression and Dissociation: Implications for Personality Theory, Psycho-pathology, and Health. Chicago: University of Chicago Press, 1990.

3. van der Kolk B: Traumatic memories. *In* PS Appelbaum, LA Uyehara, MR Elin (Eds.), Trauma and Memory: Clinical and Legal Controversies. New York: Oxford University Press, 1997, pp. 243–260.

4. Hyman IE, Loftus EF: Some people recover memories of childhood trauma that never really happened. *In* PS Appelbaum, LA Uyehara, MR Elin (Eds.), Trauma and Memory: Clinical and Legal Controversies. New York: Oxford University Press, 1997, pp. 3–24

5. Kluft RP: The argument for the reality of delayed recall of trauma. *In* PS Appelbaum, LA Uyehara, MR Elin (Eds.), Trauma and Memory: Clinical and Legal Controversies. New York: Oxford University Press, 1997, pp. 25–57.

6. Galatzer-Levy RM: Psychoanalysis, memory, and trauma. *In* PS Appelbaum, LA Uyehara, MR Elin (Eds.), Trauma and Memory: Clinical and Legal Controversies. New York: Oxford University Press, 1997, pp. 138–158.

7. Penfield W, Perot P: The brain's record of auditory and visual experience. Brain 1963; 86:595–696.

8. Squire LR: Memory and Brain. New York: Oxford University Press, 1987.

9. Kris E: The recovery of childhood memories. Psychoanal Study Child 1956; 11:54–88.

10. Levine HB: Psychoanalysis, reconstruction, and the recovery of memory. *In* PS Appelbaum, LA Uyehara, MR Elin (Eds.), Trauma and Memory: Clinical and Legal Controversies. New York: Oxford University Press, 1997, pp. 293–315.

11. Spence D: Narrative Truth and Historical Truth. New York: W. W. Norton, 1982.

12. Loftus EF: The reality of repressed memory. Am Psychol 1993; 48:518–537.

13. Loftus EF: Eyewitness Testimony. Cambridge, MA: Harvard University Press, 1979.

14. Koutstaal W, Schacter DL: Inaccuracy and inaccessibility in memory retrieval: contributions from cognitive psychology and neuropsychology. *In* PS Appelbaum, LA Uyehara, MR Elin (Eds.), Trauma and Memory: Clinical and Legal Controversies. New York: Oxford University Press, 1997, pp. 93–137.

15. Riccio DC, Rabinowitz VC, Axelrod S: Memory: when less is more. Am Psychol 1994; 49:917–926.

16. Bremner JD, Southwick SM, Krystal JH, Charney DS: Neuroanatomical correlates of the effects of stress on memory: relevance to the validity of memories of childhood abuse. *In* PS Appelbaum, LA Uyehara, MR Elin (Eds.), Trauma and Memory: Clinical and Legal Controversies. New York: Oxford University Press, 1997, pp. 61–92.

17. Andreasen NC, O'Leary DS, Cizadlo T, Arndt S, Rezai K, Watkins L, Boles Ponto LL, Hichwa RD: Remembering the past: two facets of episodic memory explored with positron emission tomography. Am J Psychiatry 1995; 152:1576–1585.

18. Rivera DT, Ortiz SP, Derrick BE, Brooks SA, Meilandt MJ, Rosenzweig MR, Diamond M, Martinez JL: Subtraction cloning of a learning-related cDNA encoding a highly conserved site-specific recombinase. Science 1996 (in press).

19. Elin MR: An integrative developmental model for trauma and memory. *In* PS Appelbaum, LA Uyehara, MR Elin (Eds.), Trauma and Memory: Clinical and Legal Controversies. New York: Oxford University Press, 1997, pp. 188–221.

20. Leichtman MD, Ceci SJ, Morse MB: The nature and development of children's event memory. *In* PS Appelbaum, LA Uyehara, MR Elin (Eds.), Trauma and Memory: Clinical and Legal Controversies. New York: Oxford University Press, 1997, pp. 158–187.

21. Goleman D: Miscoding is seen as the root of false memories. New York Times, p. C-1, May 31, 1994.

22. Golier JA, Yehuda R, Southwick S: Memory and posttraumatic stress disorder. *In* PS Appelbaum, LA Uyehara, MR Elin (Eds.), Trauma and Memory: Clinical and Legal Controversies. New York: Oxford University Press, 1997, pp. 225–242.

23. Pynoos RS, Aronson L, Steinberg AM: Traumatic experiences: the early organization of memory in school-age children and adolescents. *In* PS Appelbaum, LA Uyehara, MR Elin (Eds.), Trauma and Memory: Clinical and Legal Controversies. New York: Oxford University Press, 1997, pp. 272–289.

24. Sauzier M: Memories of trauma in the treatment of children. *In* PS Appelbaum, LA Uyehara, MR Elin (Eds.), Trauma and Memory: Clinical and Legal Controversies. New York: Oxford University Press, 1997, pp. 378–393.

25. Lindsay DS, Read JD: "Memory work" and recovered memories of childhood sexual abuse: scientific evidence and public, professional, and personal issues. Psychol Public Policy Law 1995; 1:846–908.

26. Pope HG, Hudson JI: Can memories of childhood sexual abuse be repressed? Psychol Med 1995; 25:121–126.

27. Berliner L, Williams LM: Memories of child sexual abuse: a response to Lindsay and Read. Appl Cogn Psychol 1994; 8:379–387.

28. Williams LM: Recovered memories of abuse in women with documented child sexual victimization histories. J Traumatic Stress 1995; 8:649–673.

29. Elliott DM, Briere J: Posttraumatic stress associated with delayed recall of sexual abuse: a general population study. J Traumatic Stress 1995; 8:629–647.

30. Williams LM: Recall of childhood trauma: a prospective study of women's memories of child sexual abuse. J Consult Clin Psychol 1994; 62:1167–1176.

31. Herman JL, Schatzow E: Recovery and verification of memories of childhood sexual trauma. Psychoanal Psychol 1987; 4:1–14.

32. Crews F: The Memory Wars: Freud's Legacy in Dispute. New York: New York Review, 1995.

33. Matthews JA, Chu JA: Psychodynamic therapy for patients with early childhood trauma. *In* PS Appelbaum, LA Uyehara, MR Elin (Eds.), Trauma and Memory: Clinical and Legal Controversies. New York: Oxford University Press, 1997, pp. 316–343.

34. Ross CA: Cognitive therapy of dissociative identity disorder. *In* PS Appelbaum, LA Uyehara, MR Elin (Eds.), Trauma and Memory: Clinical and Legal Controversies. New York: Oxford University Press, 1997, pp. 360–377.

35. Frankel FH, Covino NA: Hypnosis and hypnotherapy. *In* PS Appelbaum, LA Uyehara, MR Elin (Eds.), Trauma and Memory: Clinical and Legal Controversies. New York: Oxford University Press, 1997, pp. 344–359.

36. Poole DA, Lindsay DS, Memon A, Bull R: Psychotherapy and the recovery of memories of childhood sexual abuse: U.S. and British practitioners' beliefs, practices and experiences. J Consult Clin Psychol 1995; 63:426–437.

37. Yapko M: Suggestions of Abuse: Real and Imagined Memories. New York: Simon and Schuster, 1994.

38. Managing the risks involved in cases of recovered memories of abuse. Rx. for Risk (Psychiatrists' Purchasing Group). 1994; 5:1, 4.

39. Simon ʀɪ, Gutheil TG: Ethical and clinical risk management principles in recovered memory cases: maintaining therapist neutrality. *In* PS Appelbaum, LA Uyehara, MR Elin (Eds.), Trauma and Memory: Clinical and Legal Controversies. New York: Oxford University Press, 1997, pp. 477–495.

40. Marvel B: Past memories, present tense. Dallas Morning News, July 10, 1994, p. 1F.

41. Parents win suit against psychiatrist in sex case. New York Times, Dec. 17, 1994, p. 9.

42. Pezdek K: The illusion of illusory memory. Appl Cogn Psychol 1994; 8:339–350.

43. Schetky DH: Child victims in the legal system. *In* PS Appelbaum, LA Uyehara, MR Elin (Eds.), Trauma and Memory: Clinical and Legal Controversies. New York: Oxford University Press, 1997, pp. 496–507.

44. Appelbaum PS: Protecting child witnesses in sexual abuse cases. Hosp Community Psychiatry 1989; 40:13–14.

45. Murphy WJ: Legal rights of trauma victims. *In* PS Appelbaum, LA Uyehara, MR Elin (Eds.), Trauma and Memory: Clinical and Legal Controversies. New York: Oxford University Press, 1997, pp. 425–444.

46. *Commonwealth* v. *Bishop,* 617 N.E.2d 995 (Mass. 1993).

47. Zoltek-Jick R: For whom does the bell toll? Repressed memory and challenges for the law: getting beyond the statute of limitations. *In* PS Appelbaum, LA Uyehara, MR Elin (Eds.), Trauma and Memory: Clinical and Legal Controversies. New York: Oxford University Press, 1997, pp. 445–476.

48. Ernsdorff GM, Loftus EF: Let sleeping memories lie? Words of caution about tolling the statute of limitations in cases of memory repression. J Criminal Law Criminol 1993; 84:129–174.

49. Brown D: Pseudomemories: the standard of science and the standard of care in trauma treatment. Am J Clin Hypn 1995; 37:1–24.

50. American Psychiatric Association: Fact Sheet: Memories of Sexual Abuse. Washington, DC: APA, April 1994.

51. Psychologists release statement on abuse memories. Psychiatric News Dec. 16, 1994, p. 4.

52. Uyehara LA: Diagnosis, pathogenesis, and memories of childhood abuse. *In* PS Appelbaum, LA Uyehara, MR Elin (Eds.), Trauma and Memory: Clinical and Legal Controversies. New York: Oxford University Press, 1997, pp. 394–422.

53. McHugh PR: Psychiatric misadventures. Am Scholar 1992; Autumn:497–510.

54. Appelbaum PS, Zoltek-Jick R: Psychotherapists' duties to third parties: *Ramona* and beyond. Am J Psychiatry 1996; 153:457–465.

55. *Tarasoff v. Regents of the University of California,* 551 P.2d 334 (Cal. 1976).

56. *Ramona* v. *Ramona,* No. 61898 (Napa Cty. (Cal.) Super. Ct., 1994).

57. Wright L: Remembering Satan: A Case of Recovered Memory and the Shattering of an American Family. New York: Knopf, 1994.

Index

Ablation, 40
Abortions, 15
Abreaction, 45, 294–98
Abuse excuse, 455
Abuse of process, 435
Acceptance of false information into memory, 9
Access nodes, 110
Accuracy of memory
  assessing, 519
  bizarre recovered memories and, 15–16
  in children, 169–77
  posttraumatic stress disorder and, 230–33
Action, as defense, 147
Active perpetrator, formerly passive victim as, 147, 151
Active remembering, 515
Active retrieval attempts, termination of, 105–7
Activities encouraging memory construction, 12
Acute catastrophic stress reaction, 252
Addiction, 27
Additional dimensions to traumatic experiences, 276
Additional traumatic moments after cessation of violence or threat, 276
Adolescents, early organization of memory in, 272–87
Adoption, 28
Adrenal glands, 83
Advocates for victims of abuse, 429–30, 435, 441
Affective elements of memory, 515
Affirmative case, 25
Age estimates, in posttraumatic stress disorder, 232

Age regression, and maintaining therapist neutrality, 491
Alcoholics Anonymous, 27
Alien abductions, 14–18, 33
All-or-nothing thinking, 362
Alters
  arguments supporting delayed recall of trauma and, 28
  dissociative identity disorder and, 373–75
  maintaining therapist neutrality and, 482
Althaus case, 466, 497
"Always-held" memory, 403
"Always known" events, 325
Ambition, unfettered therapeutic, 484
American Medical Association (AMA)
  Council on Scientific Affairs, 490
  position of on recovered memories, 486
American Psychiatric Association (APA)
  insurance risk managers, 478
Amnesia
  arguments supporting delayed recall of trauma, 29, 33, 37, 39, 44–46
  clinical typology and, 262–63, 265–67
  hypnosis and, 351
  integrative developmental model and, 213–14
  memory retrieval and, 111–12
  neuroanatomy of stress and, 62–63, 65, 68, 74, 81–82, 84
  posttraumatic stress disorder and, 225, 228, 234, 248–49
  uncorroborated memories and, 405
Amygdala
  early organization of memory and, 284
  integrative developmental model and, 194, 200

Amygdala (*continued*)
  neuroanatomy of stress and, 64–66, 69–73, 77–78, 80–81, 83
Anchor points, memory, 279, 287
Anecdotal observations, 53
Anger, in posttraumatic stress disorder, 229
Anna O., 138
Anterior cingulate cortex, 64, 67, 79
Anterograde amnesia, and neuroanatomy of stress, 68
Anteromedial prefrontal cortex, 64, 67, 79
Anticipation, in posttraumatic stress disorder, 227
Anti-SLAPP-suit motions, 435
Aphasic stroke patients, 192
Apology, by abusive parent, 32
Arousal
  neuroanatomy of stress and, 73
  physiological, 144–45
  posttraumatic stress disorder and, 226, 230–31
Ash Wednesday fire, 208
Assessment of trauma patients, in psychodynamic therapy, 326–28
Associative clustering, 102
Associative factors, in memory retrieval, 116–18
Associative network, entry into, 515
Association, and reconstruction, 295
Atmosphere of support, 337
Attachment to perpetrator, 369–71, 375
Attention, and integrative developmental model, 192
Attention span impairment, in posttraumatic stress disorder, 225
Attentional resources, 122–24
Attorney General, and victim rights laws, 428
Attributional processes, 112, 114–16
Atypical sexual knowledge for age, 437
Auditory hallucinations, 77
Auditory Verbal Learning Test (AVLT), and neuroanatomy of stress, 75
Ault v. Jasko, 463–65, 467–68, 471
Authority, in increasing probability of accepting suggestions, 12
Autobiographical events, 10

Autobiographical memory, 106, 108, 119, 122
Autohypnotic trance phenomena, 40, 42
Automobile accident, resulting in death of mother, 274–75
Autonomic arousal, in posttraumatic stress disorder, 227
Autonomy, patient, 484–85
Avoidance behavior
  integrative developmental model and, 196
  intimate relationships and, 145
  mechanisms of, 151
  neuroanatomy of stress and, 81
  posttraumatic stress disorder and, 226, 228–29
Awareness of memory
  disturbances in subjective quality of, 121–22
  regulation of, 146

Babysitter, abuse by, 27
Balance of interests, 432
Basal forebrain damage, 124
Beatings, 37
  psychoanalysis and, 145–46
Beckian cognitive therapy, in dissociative identity disorder, 375
Beginning engagement of therapeutic process, 305
Behavioral avoidance, in posttraumatic stress disorder, 228–29
Behavioral management, of dissociative identity disorder, 366–69
"Behind a veil or screen," 204
"Being in a fog," 190–91, 204
Belief paradigm, 310
"Beyond a reasonable doubt," 154, 428
Bias, 48, 170, 432, 520
  cultural, 155
  investigating abuse allegations and, 497
  maintaining therapist neutrality and, 477, 490
  posttraumatic stress disorder and, 237
Birthday party scenario, 7–8
Bizarre practices, 29
Bizarre recovered memories, 14–18
Black-and-white thinking, 362
Blackouts, and neuroanatomy of stress, 74

Blending, 173
Blocking out, 518
Body massages, 491
Body memories, recovering, 491
Boolean cube, incorporation of time into, 203
Borderline personality disorder, 252, 407
Boring stimuli, 166
Boundary violations, and maintaining therapist neutrality, 485
Bowen v. City of New York, 449
Brain archives, 514
Brain memory systems, 69–73
    normal memory function and, 64–68
    stress-related alterations in patients with stress-related psychiatric disorders and, 73–81
Brainstem, and neuroanatomy of stress, 71
Brainstem startle reflex circuit, 66
Breaks, in transference, 153
Breuer, Josef, 138
Broca's area, in posttraumatic stress disorder, 252, 255
Bulimia, 252
Burden of proof, in cases of unusual recovered memories, 17

California, and statute of limitations, 451, 458, 466
California New Learning Test, and neuroanatomy of stress, 75
California Verbal Learning Test, in posttraumatic stress disorder, 239
Calmness, and maintaining therapist neutrality, 485
Capgras syndrome, 124
Car, being left in as false memory scenario, 7–8
Catastrophization, 362
Category clustering, 102
Caudal lateral hypothalamus-subthalamic area, 66
Caudate, 76
Cellular mechanisms underlying memory formation, 515
Censor, internal, 300
"Central Park Jogger," 468
Central tegmental field, 66

Cerebral cortex, and neuroanatomy of stress, 64–71, 77, 82–83
Cerebral glue, 42
Cerebral ventricles, 72
Certainty, 154
Certificate of merit, filing, 458
Cessation of therapy, 493
Challenger space shuttle explosion, 63, 247
Chaos theory, 201
Chaotic negative transferences, 34
Charitable laws, 429
Childhood amnesia, 15
Childhood neighbor of witnessed abuse, 31–32
Childhood sexual abuse. *See* Sexual abuse, childhood
Child Protection Movement, 378
Child Protective Services (CPS), in investigating abuse allegations, 379, 388, 498
Child sexual abuse accomodation syndrome, 48–49
Child victims, in legal system
    children as witnesses, 500
    children's concepts of legal system, 500–1
    decision to prosecute, 499–500
    effects of testifying on children, 501–2
    investigating allegations of abuse, 497–99
    jurors' responses to child witnesses, 503
    modifying courtroom procedures, 504–5
    overview, 496
    preparing child witnesses for court, 502–3
    recording interviews, 499
Chowchilla kidnap victims, 50, 347
Chronic fatigue syndrome, 384
Cingulate, 69
Circumstantial evidence, 152
Civil litigation, 425, 428–30
Clarity of memories, in posttraumatic stress disorder, 227
Cleopatra, past life as, 17
Clinical experiences supporting memory recovery, 26–29
Clinical focus, maintaining, 483–84
Clinical naiveté, and maintaining therapist neutrality, 483

Clinical typology, of traumatic recall, 261–69

Clitoridectomy, 403, 415

Closed-circuit TV, in courtroom, 504

Closed court rooms, 504

Coaching, in investigating abuse allegations, 499

Co-constriction, 286

Cognitive avoidance, in posttraumatic stress disorder, 228

Cognitive memory, and neuroanatomy of stress, 66

Cognitive/personality difference measures, 8

Cognitive processes, 116, 124

Cognitive psychology, and inaccuracy and inaccessibility in memory retrieval, 93–126

Cognitive therapy, of dissociative identity disorder, 360–76

Cohesion, mental, 42

Coincident recovery, 122

Collaboration, and maintaining therapist neutrality, 488–89

Collaborative empiricism, 374

Collective group experience, 50

Color-naming latency memory, in posttraumatic stress disorder, 232, 235–36

Combat veterans, 50
  integrative developmental model and, 212
  neuroanatomy of stress in, 74–75, 78–79, 81
  posttraumatic stress disorder in, 227–29, 234, 236–39, 248–53

Compassion, 37, 484

Competency, of child witness, 500, 505

Competing retrieval cues, presence of, 104–5

Complexes, repressed or dissociated, 296

Complexity of traumatic experiences, 274–87

Complex posttraumatic syndrome, 322, 398

Compromise mechanism, 151

Compulsions, primary repetition, 151

Computed tomography (CT), 37, 75

Concentration camp survivors
  neuroanatomy of stress in, 74–75

posttraumatic stress disorder in, 249

Concentration impairment, in posttraumatic stress disorder, 225, 229, 238

Concretization, 41

Condensation
  across episodes, 119–20
  of memories of multiple events, 515
  posttraumatic stress disorder and, 256

Conditioned stimulus, and neuroanatomy of stress, 64, 72

Confabulation, 26, 33, 47, 49, 124
  clinical typology and, 261–62
  investigating abuse allegations and, 498

Confession of abuse, 31–32, 34, 38

Confidence in memory, in posttraumatic stress disorder, 231

Confidentiality, 28, 430, 432, 434, 441, 521

Confirmation of abuse, 27–32, 34, 36

Conformation to majorities, 12

Confrontation of constructed memory in experimental setting, 10

Confusion
  between dreams, fantasy, and reality, 26, 33
  in investigating abuse allegations, 498

Congress
  victim rights laws passed by, 426

Conjugate reinforcement paradigm, mobile, 166

Consistency of memory, in posttraumatic stress disorder, 233

Consolidation of memory, and neuro-anatomy of stress, 64, 68

Construction of memories in therapy, 12–13, 293

Consultation, and maintaining therapist neutrality, 484

Contamination, 36, 43
  in investigating abuse allegations, 498
  maintaining therapist neutrality and, 479, 490
  posttraumatic stress disorder and, 256

Context-dependency effect, 99

Contextual information, 110

Contingency fee basis, of fee for victim's attorney, 429

Continuous recall, and clinical typology, 264–65

Continuous recognition paradigm, 117
Contributing factors to false memory creation, 5–10
Control nodes, 110
Controversy over delayed recall of traumatic memories, 3–53
Convergence of internal and external dangers, 273–74
Conviction of accused, 499
Corroboration, 34, 38, 320, 405
    child victims in legal system and, 503, 505
    legal rights of trauma victims and, 437
    statute of limitations and, 457, 459–61
Counseling records, 430–34
Countertransference, managing, 485
Court, preparing child witnesses for, 502–3
Court record confirmation of abuse, 31
Courtroom procedures, modifying, 504–5
Courts of Appeals, 489
    Ohio, 463
    Second Circuit, 449
Crawford trial, Pennsylvania, 451
Creation of memories
    processes involved in, 3, 9–10, 19–20
    in response to demands of therapy situation, 3, 19–20
Creative Imagination Scale (CIS), 8
Criminal litigation, 426–28
Crisis counseling, 430, 521
Critogenic harms, 480
Cryptomnesia, 113–14
Cues
    absence of sufficiently informative, 95–97
    distinctiveness of, 96–97
    entry into associative network and, 515
Cumulative trauma, 143
Current abuse of minor child, 488

''Damming up,'' 300
Daubert v. Merrell Dow Pharmaceuticals, Inc., 438–39, 467–71
Day care setting, sexual abuse in, 46
Death threats, 45
Death wish, and arguments supporting delayed recall of trauma, 28
Deathbed confirmation of abuse, 31–32
Decay, 36

Declarative knowledge, 161
Declarative memory, 515
    neuroanatomy of stress and, 64
    posttraumatic stress disorder and, 246
Default values, 120
Defense hysteria, 296
Defense mechanisms
    psychoanalysis and, 145–49
    structural theory and, 301
Defense tactics, in trauma victim trial, 426, 437–38, 440
Deferred action, 141
Deferred imitation, 167
Dehumanization, 145
Déjà vu, 122
Delayed imitation, 167
Delayed memories, uncorroborated, 404
Delay of trial, 426
Delayed recall of trauma, argument for reality of
    additional remarks on recollection and nonrecollection of trauma, 50–51
    clinical experiences supporting recovery of long-unavailable memories, 26–29
    current literature, 45–46
    dilemma of dissociation in repressed memory debate, 42–45
    dissociative identity disorder pilot study, 29–42
    hypnosis and memory recovery, 39–42
    introduction, 25–26
    paradigm of impact of interpersonal influence, 39–42
    perspectives discrediting possible recovery of repressed memory, 46–49
Delayed understanding, 263–66
Delayed-response tasks, and neuroanatomy of stress, 67
Delusions of familiarity, 122
Demanding interviews, of suspected perpetrator, 15–16
Demand to remember in therapy, 12
Demographics, in posttraumatic stress disorder, 238
Denial, 148, 263, 240
Dentate gyrus, 64–65
Depersonalization, 31
    posttraumatic stress disorder and, 250

Depression
  arguments supporting delayed recall of
    trauma and, 29
  children's event memory and, 175
  posttraumatic stress disorder and, 240
  psychoanalysis and, 143, 145
  therapist instigation of false memories of
    child abuse and, 3
  uncorroborated memories and, 403
Derealization, 31
Derepression, of childhood abuse memories, 15
Derivatives, 299
Desert Storm veterans, posttraumatic stress
  disorder in, 234
Desire to please
  children's event memory and, 176
  as factor in investigating abuse allega-
    tions, 497–98
  therapist and, 396
Desire to remember, influenced by therapist, 12
Destructive updating, 173
Detachment, in posttraumatic stress disor-
  der, 229
Detailed recollections, 36
Details of trauma, in posttraumatic stress
  disorder, 233
"Developmental," definition as term, 272–
  73
Developmental approach to early memory,
  160–64
Developmental domains, and encapsulation
  of traumatic memories, 195–200
Developmental factors, effect of on
  memory, 517
Deviant treatment boundaries, 477
Diagnosis, and memories of childhood
  abuse, 394–417
Diapering, memories of abuse around, 486
Diaries, 488
  maternal, 29
  of pleasant and unpleasant experiences,
    47
Dichotic listening task, 117
Dichotomized thinking, 362
Diffuse encephalopathy, 75
Digit Span Test, in posttraumatic stress
  disorder, 239

Digit Symbol Test, in posttraumatic stress
  disorder, 239
Dilution, and children's event memory,
  173
Diminished interest, in posttraumatic stress
  disorder, 229
Diminished recall for stimuli unrelated to
  trauma, in posttraumatic stress disor-
  der, 236–37
Direct victim of therapeutic negligence, ac-
  cused as, 489
Directed forgetting, 109–11
Disaggregation, 346
Disambiguation, rush towards, 52
Disavowal, and psychoanalysis, 148
Disbelief, as indication of authenticity of
  recovered memory, 13
Discovery exception, 453–54
Discovery phase, of civil lawsuit, 451, 452
Discovery provisions, and statute of limita-
  tions, 456–59, 463–64, 466, 473
Discovery rule, 425
Disenriching environment, 215
Disentanglement, 153
Disproval, difficulty of in terms of unusual
  recovered memories, 17
Dissociation
  definition of term, 216
  and early organization of memory in
    school-age children and adolescents,
    277
  as impairment to mentation, 216
  integrative developmental model and,
    190, 195, 200, 214, 216
  maintaining therapist neutrality and, 482
  posttraumatic stress disorder and, 231,
    240, 250–52
  psychoanalysis and, 146, 148
  psychodynamic therapy and, 320–23
  reconstruction and, 296
Dissociative amnesia
  absence of cogent discussions of in
    DSM-IV, 44
  neuroanatomy of stress and, 84
Dissociative disorder not otherwise specified, 39
Dissociative Disorders Interview Schedule
  (DDIS), 409
Dissociative Experiences Scale (DES), 8

in posttraumatic stress disorder, 250,
252
Dissociative flashbacks, in posttraumatic
stress disorder, 225
Dissociative identity disorder (DID), 408–
9, 411–12
arguments supporting delayed recall of
trauma, 26
attachment to perpetrator in, 369–71
behavioral management of, 366–69
causes, 8
cognitive therapy of, 360–76
locus of control shift and, 371–73
orientation of alters to present and body,
373–75
validation of recovered memories in, 29–
45
Dissociative mechanisms, and early organization of memory in school-age children and adolescents, 277
Distinctiveness of cues, 96–97
Distortion, 43–44, 49, 124, 153, 516
cognitive therapy and, 364
hypnotic, 40–41
mechanisms or sources of, 112–16
posttraumatic stress disorder and, 233–
34
psychoanalysis and, 153
Distortion
children's event memory and, 176
integrative developmental model and,
197
Distractor items, 117, 120
Distress, chronic, 145
District of Columbia, federal district court
for, 468
Disuse, in retrieval capacity, 108–9
Divorce, 149
Doctrine of charitable immunity, 429
Documentation, and maintaining therapist
neutrality, 484
Documented abuse, instances of, 30
"Doe," case filed using name of, 458
Dog, attack by, 280–83, 387
"Dora" case, 70, 143
Dominant mass of ideas, 294
Dorsal-medial nucleus, 65
Dorsal thalamus, 70
Dorsolateral prefrontal cortex, 64, 66–67, 71

Double checks, 122
Double cues, 96
Dread, in posttraumatic stress disorder, 227
Dream-like hallucinations, 77
Dreams, 26
integrative developmental model and,
191, 204–7
interpretation of, 4, 13, 141
memories as, 16, 17
posttraumatic stress disorder and, 234
psychoanalysis and, 144, 148
secret, 383
Dr. Z., 192
Due process, 431, 504
Durational time, 203
Duty of neutrality, 481–83
Dynamically unconscious memories, 139

Ear infection memories, 7–8
Early organization of memory, in school-
age children and adolescents
case studies, 274–76, 280–83
complexity of traumatic experiences,
274–87
convergence of internal and external
dangers, 273–74
intervention fantasies, 279–80
memory marker role in episodic memory
of trauma, 277–78
overview, 272–73
selected developmental issues, 283–87
weakened versions of self-protective
mechanisms in remembering and recounting traumatic experiences, 278–
79
Earthquakes, 43, 274
Eating disorders, 3, 407, 489
Ecological validity, 52
Ego, 294, 301
Ego psychology, 301–2, 413
Elaboration, in cognitive therapy, 364
Elderly, memory retrieval in, 125
Electroconvulsive therapy (ECT), and neuroanatomy of stress, 68
Electroencephalogram (EEG), normal, 37
"Else the elsewhere thought known," 43
Embellishment, in posttraumatic stress dis-
order, 256
Emotional charge, 294

Emotional memory
  neuroanatomy of stress and, 66, 80
Emotional numbing, in posttraumatic stress
    disorder, 228–29
Empirical studies, 478
Encapsulation of traumatic memories along
    developmental domains, 195–200
Encoding conditions, 174–75, 177
Encoding of memory, 153
Enematization practices, bizarre, 29
Enjoyment of sexual abuse, 38
Entorhinal cortex, 64–65
Environmental factors, effect of on
    memory, 517
Episodic memory, 116, 277
Equal Protection Clause, Constitutional,
    450
Equitable estoppel, 450
Errors in memory, 5
Eruption, 295
Estrangement, 27, 229
Ethics, 400
  maintaining therapist neutrality and,
    483–84, 492
  lost in the mall experiment and, 47
Evaluation of trauma and memory, 293–
    417
Evaluative processes, 112
Event memory, children's
  developmental approach to early
    memory, 160–64
  individual differences, 177–79
  long-term memory in first years of life,
    165–69
  nature and accuracy of children's memo-
    ries, 169–77
  overview, 158–60
Event-related potential (ERP), 345
"Everett" case, 502
Evidence
  memory, 434–38
  what constitutes, 399–403
Evil, 32
Evolving developmental expectations
    regarding danger, disturbances in,
    276
Excitement, in posttraumatic stress disor-
    der, 227
Expectancy-congruent behaviors, 170

Expectation, and psychodynamic therapy,
    335
Experimental paradigm for creation of false
    childhood memories, 5–10
Expert testimony, admissibility of, 438–39
Experts, types of, 440
Expert witnesses, forensic, 487
Explicit memory
  legal issues and, 515
  neuroanatomy of stress and, 64–68, 74–75
  posttraumatic stress disorder and, 246,
    256
Explicit motor movements, 213
External factors blocking recall, 105
External validation, 466
Extinction, 80
  dissociative identity disorder and, 367
  neuroanatomy of stress and, 83
Extrastriate cortex, 68
Extrinsic physical context, mismatch of, 98
Eye movement desensitization reprocessing
    (EMDR), 35, 43
Eyewitness memory
  posttraumatic stress disorder and, 230–
    35
  studies of, 5, 8

Fabrication, 34
Face-to-face confrontation with alleged per-
    petrator
  by child in court, 500
Factual knowledge, 161
Fading, of cues over time, 515
Fairy tales, 48
Fallibility of human memory, 5
Fallopian tubes, memories from period fol-
    lowing conception in, 17
False childhood memories
  application to therapy, 10–14, 27
  bizarre recovered memories, 14–18
  evidence for, 5–10
  introduction, 3–4
  lost in a mall scenario, 5–6
  memory construction in therapy, 12–13
  memory recovery therapy, 14
  processes involved in memory creation,
    9–10
  punch bowls at weddings scenario, 6–9
  reality monitoring in therapy, 13–14

False expensive expert syndrome (FEES), 52

False expert syndrome, 52

False memories of child abuse, 3–20
  problems with viewing bizarre recovered memories as, 16–17

False memory production, 520

"False memory syndrome," 438–39

False Memory Syndrome Foundation, 438, 461

False memory syndrome movement, 434–35

False suggestions of childhood trauma, 3–17

Falsifiable arguments, 25

Familiarity, 121

Family materials, 29

Family members, and maintaining therapist neutrality, 489–90

Fantasies, 26, 34, 43
  intervention, 279–80
  Oedipal, 140–41
  psychoanalysis and, 147, 149–50, 153

Fantasy/memory complex, 318, 334

Fantasy proneness, 406

Faulty arguments based on unusual recovered memories, 17–18

Faulty generalization to all recovered memories, 17–18

Fear
  chronic, 145, 147
  neuroanatomy of stress and, 66, 73, 79
  posttraumatic stress disorder and, 226–27, 240
  neuroanatomy of stress and, 66, 79

Fear of going crazy, 226

Fear-potentiated startle, 66

Federal district courts
  District of Columbia, 468
  Massachusetts, 469

Federal Employer's Liability Act (FELA), 449

Federal Rule of Evidence, 702, 438–39

Fellow sufferers, 50

Fever memories, 7

Filing on separate channels, 346

Firefighters, posttraumatic stress disorder in, 233–34, 239

Firestorms, 43

First few years of life, memories of, 14, 165–69

Fixation, 144

Flashbacks, 34, 324
  integrative developmental model and, 215
  intrusive recollections and, 153
  neuroanatomy of stress and, 74, 77, 79
  posttraumatic stress disorder and, 225, 227, 254–55
  psychoanalysis and, 147

Flashbulb memories
  neuroanatomy of stress and, 63
  posttraumatic stress disorder and, 247
  uncorroborated, 405

Floods of old memories, 19

Foci of attention or concern, changes in, 276

Foil items, 120

Foot-kicking response, conditioned, 166

Footshock, and neuroanatomy of stress, 70, 72, 80

Forensic applications, of hypnosis, 351–53

Forensic expert witnesses, 440, 487–88

Forensic pathological assessment, 33

Foreshortened future, sense of in posttraumatic stress disorder, 229

Forgetting
  childhood abuse and, 4, 18
  directed (instructed), 109–11
  neural bases of, 111–12
  neuroanatomy of stress and, 63, 68, 81
  posttraumatic stress disorder and, 233

Forgiveness, begging for, 32

Formation of memory, and neuroanatomy of stress, 64

Fornix, 64

Fostering of patient autonomy and self-determination, 484

Fourteenth Amendment, Constitutional, 504

Fragmentation of memories, 36, 231

Franklin case, California, 451, 469, 474

Free association, 4

Free recall, 109–10

"Fresh" evidence, lack of, 429

Friend as witness and interrupter of abuse attempt, 31–33

Frontal cortex, 67, 69

Frontal lobe, 124–25, 246
Frye v. United States, 439, 467–70
"Functional," definition of as term, 272

Gaps in memory, 50
Gatekeeper function, of court, 470
Gender-based violence, deterence of, 434
Gene expression, 516
General Assembly, Ohio, 464
Generalizability of experimentation, 47
Generalization across episodes, 119–20
"Generally accepted," 439
Generations, transmission of abuse across, 147, 151
Generic memories vs. specific memories, 119–20
Gist, and uncorroborated memories, 405
Gist-like traces, 173
Global memory impairment, in posttraumatic stress disorder, 250
Global statements, 52
Globe v. Superior Court, 505
Glucocorticoids, and neuroanatomy of stress, 69–72, 75
"Going away," 267
Goodness of fit, 26
Gratification, undue, 37–38
Gray matter, and neuroanatomy of stress, 70
Grocery shopping scenario, 7–8
Gross stress reactions, 386
Group therapy, for adults recovering from childhood sexual abuse, 3
Guidance of memory retrieval, 95–97
Guided imagery, 4, 13, 491
Guilty plea to child abuse, 499
Gullibility, 49
Gunshot wounds, 217

Habituation paradigms, 166
Hallucinations, 40
  auditory, 77
  dream-like, 77
  integrative developmental model and, 205, 215
  memory-like, 77
  neuroanatomy of stress and, 77, 79
  psychoanalysis and, 143–44
  visual, 77, 79

Head trauma, 37
Hearsay statements, 505
Height estimates, in posttraumatic stress disorder, 232
Helplessness, sense of, 145, 227, 231
Hemiplegia, 192
Heterohypnosis, 39, 42
High attentional load, 123
High-stress event, and children's event memory, 175
Hindering factors to false memory creation, 5–10
Hippocampus
  early organization of memory and, 284
  integrative developmental model and, 194, 200, 212
  neuroanatomy of stress and, 64–78, 80–81, 83
  posttraumatic stress disorder and, 246, 255
Historical reality, and psychic reality, 304–5
Historical truth, 479–480, 486–87
  nature of memory and, 303
  psychodynamic therapy and, 334
Holocaust survivors, 50
  integrative developmental model and, 188, 190, 194, 199–200, 203–4, 208–9, 217
  neuroanatomy of stress and, 74
  posttraumatic stress disorder in, 226, 230, 233–34
Homeowner's insurance policies, standard exclusionary clauses in, 429
Homes, childhood, 4, 12, 19
Homosexual thoughts, 395–96, 415
Honest lying, 124
Hormones
  integrative developmental model and, 194, 200, 212
  stress and, 516
Hospitalization memory scenarios, 7–9
Hugs, innocent by father, 17
Humanistic aspects of memory as repository of self, 516
Hydraulic metaphor, 42
Hyperactivity, 380, 384
Hyperarousal
  hypnosis and, 353

posttraumatic stress disorder and, 229–
30
Hypermnesia, 44, 108
hypnotic, 349
Hypervigilance, in posttraumatic stress disorder, 229
Hypnoid states, 296, 324
Hypnosis, 4, 8, 13, 514
arguments supporting delayed recall of
trauma and, 27–29, 38–42
facilitation of memory retrieval and, 39–
42, 346–48
forensic applications of, 351–53
maintaining therapist neutrality and, 490
implanted memories and, 349–50
legal rights of trauma victims and, 438
overview, 344–46
posthypnotic amnesia and, 351
psychotherapy and, 353–56
recall and, 348–49
recollections acquired through, 519
review of experimental work on, 348–55
Hypnotherapy. *See* Hypnosis
Hypocrisy, familial, 144
Hypothalamic-pituitary-adrenal (HPA) axis
neuroanatomy of stress and, 71
posttraumatic stress disorder and, 240
Hypothalamus
integrative developmental model and,
200
neuroanatomy of stress and, 69–70, 83
Hysteria, 138, 324
psychoanalysis and, 153
Hysterical paralyses, 252

Iatrogenic dissociation, 26
Id, 301
Identification with aggressor, 372
early organization of memory and, 281
in experimental context, 48
Idiosyncratic learning history, 96
Illusion of remembrance, 121
Imagery treatments for memory recovery, 13
Imagery vividness, 8
Imagining what abuse might have been like
had it occured, 520
Immobilization, feeling of in dream, 17
Immune system, and integrative develop-
mental model, 209–10

Implantation of memories, 435, 477, 516
hypnosis and, 349, 350
maintaining therapist neutrality and, 483,
489
Implicit associative responses, 117
Implicit memory, 36, 115, 518
neuroanatomy of stress and, 64, 68, 80
posttraumatic stress disorder and, 246–
47
Inaccuracy and inacessibility in memory
retrieval
absence of sufficiently informative cues
to guide or permit retrieval, 95–97
amnesia and, 111–12
associative factors and, 116–18
attentional resources and, 122–24
competing (inordinately dominant) retrieval cues and, 104–5
condensation or generalization across
episodes and, 119–20
costs of lack of retrieval strengthening
and, 108–9
directed (instructed) forgetting and, 109–
11
disturbances in subjective quality of
memory awareness and, 121–22
disuse and, 108–9
extrinsic physical context and, 98–101
generic memories vs. specific memories,
119–20
interference and, 107–8
internal subjective and physiological environment, 101–2
intrinsic physical context and, 98
intrinsic semantic context and, 97–98
introduction, 93–94
limited retrieval capacity and, 108–9
mechanisms or sources of inaccuracy or
distortion, 112–25
mechanisms or sources of inacessibility,
95–112
medial temporal lobe and, 111–12
memory monitoring and, 122–24
mental reinstatement and, 99–101
meta-memory assumptions and, 122–24
mismatch of encoding and retrieval contexts, 97–106
neural bases of forgetting and, 111–12
pathological distortion and, 124–25

Inaccuracy and inacessibility in memory retrieval (*continued*)
  physical reinstatement and, 98–99
  relatively more complex preexisting patterns of associations, 120–21
  relatively specific effects or restricted effects of preexisting semantic associations, 116–18
  schemas and, 120–21
  statute of limitations and, 460
  subjective organization and retrieval plans, 102–4
  termination of active retrieval attempts and, 105–7
  verbatim v. gist, 118–19
In camera review, 432
Incest survivor groups, 410, 479
"Incest-survivor machine," 479
Incestuous assault misperceived as contemporary reality, 30
"Incidental" encountering of material, 96
Incoherence, 320
Indefensibility to falsity, 460
Independent assessments, psychiatric, 488
Independent encoding, 102
Index of suspicion, 383
Index patient's abuse, 31
Individual differences, in children's event memory, 177–79
Induction ceremony, 39, 42
Ineptitude, 49
Inexperience, and maintaining therapist neutrality, 483
Infantile amnesia phenomenon, 139
Infantile sexuality, 298–301
Infant memories, 354
Inference from symptoms, 36
Inferences, 112
Inferior cingulate cortex, 68
Inferior frontal lobe, 515
Information-processing models, 43
Informed consent, and maintaining therapist neutrality, 490
Ingram family, 15–17
Inhibitory effect on retrieval, 105
Innocent contacts, viewing of as unwanted abuse, 17
Inordinately dominant retrieval cues, 104–5
Instincts, in emotional life, 298, 300

Instructed forgetting, 109–11
Integration of consciousness and personality, 8
Integrative developmental model
  childhood sexual abuse, 212–16
  encapsulation of traumatic memories along developmental domains, 195–200
  language and, 204–8
  linguistic theory, 208–9
  overview, 188–95
  parallel distributed systems for memory, 200–8
  REM sleep and, 204–8
  self-memory system development, 209–12
Intelligence quotient (IQ)
  children's event memory and, 161, 178
  neuroanatomy of stress and, 75
  posttraumatic stress disorder and, 238–39
Interactive encoding, 102
Interference in memory retrieval, 107–8
Internal strategies blocking recall, 105
Interpersonal influence, paradigm of impact of, 39–42
Interpretation, context of, 154
Intervention fantasies, 279, 280
Interviews of child victims, 496–99
Intimidation
  in investigating abuse allegations, 499, 501
  of victims, 441
Intrafamilial abuse, 31
Intrinsic physical context, mismatch of, 98
Intrinsic semantic context, mismatch of, 97–98
Intrusive inquiry, 26
Intrusive thoughts, 151, 153, 516
  invalid, 107
  neuroanatomy of stress and, 74
  posttraumatic stress disorder and, 225
Investigating allegations of childhood abuse, 497–99
Irrational processes, 364
Irregular recollection, 26
Irrelevant verbal stimuli, in posttraumatic stress disorder, 236
Isely v. Capuchin Province et al., 470–71

Islands of amnesia, 50
Isolation, in posttraumatic stress disorder, 229
Israeli trauma survivors, posttraumatic stress disorder in, 251
Item gains and losses, 106

Johnson case, 469
Journaling, 4
Jurors, response of to child witnesses, 503

Keller, Helen, 113–14
Kelly Michaels day care case, 498
Kennedy assassination (JFK), 63, 195, 247
Kisses, innocent by father, 17
"Known and not known" events, 325
"Know" response, 125
Korean veterans, neuroanatomy of stress in, 75
Korsakoff's amnesia, 65

Lacunae, 152
Language, and integrative developmental model, 204–8
Later-life phenomena, 152
Law
    child victims in legal system and, 496–505
    legal rights of trauma victims and, 425–41
    psychoanalysis and, 154
    repressed memory and challenges for, 445–74
    statute of limitations and, 445–74
    trauma debate and, 425–505
Leading experimental context, false memory creation in, 6–7
Leading interviews, of suspected perpetrator, 15
Leading questions, in investigating abuse allegations, 497–98
Left cerebral hemisphere, 255
Legal rights of trauma victims
    admissibility of expert testimony, 438–39
    civil litigation, 425, 428–30
    criminal litigation, 425–28
    memory evidence, 434–38
    privacy rights, 430–34
    types of experts, 440

Legal system, children's concepts of, 500–1
Lenient reality-monitoring strategies, 17
Libel, 435
Libido, 298–300
Life-and-death decision, 28
Lifting repression phenomenon, 148, 301, 348, 404
"Lighting up" of brain areas, 515
Limbic brain, 69
Lineup identification, and children's event memory, 175–76
Linguistic theory, for memory and trauma, 208–9
Liquidation, of unconscious fixed ideas, 251
Litigation, maintaining therapist neutrality and, 480, 482–83
Little Green Riding Hood, 502
"Lived" transference repetitions, 332
Locus coeruleus, 72, 83
Locus of control shift, 362, 371–73
Long-forgotten memories, genuine recall of, 19
Long-term memory
    of childhood abuse, 3–4
    in first years of life, 165–69
Long-term potentiation, 78
Long-unavailable memories, clinical experiences supporting recovery of, 26–29
Loss of perspective, therapeutic, 485
Lost in a mall scenario, 5–6, 47–48
Low-stress event, and children's event memory, 175
Lure words, 117, 119
Lying, 432

"Magic bullet," 479
Magnetic resonance imaging (MRI), and neuroanatomy of stress, 75–78
Making amends, 32
Malicious prosecution, 435
Malignant memories, 202, 272
Malingering, 403
Malpractice liability, 488
Mammillary bodies, 64
Managed care, and maintaining therapist neutrality, 491–92
Mania, 403

Marlowe-Crowne Social Desirability Scale (SDS), 8
Maryland v. Craig, 504
Massachussetts, victim rights in, 426–28, 432–33
Mastery of traumatic experience, 144
Masturbation, 381, 415
Matching of critical features, 95
Material reality, 152–53, 155, 299
Maternal confirmation of abuse, 34, 38, 215
Maternal transference, 396
Meaning, experience of, 153, 303
Mechanisms of memory, 514
Media attention, 437, 440–41
Medial temporal lobe, and amnesia, 111–12
Medial thalamus, 64
"Medical diagnosis or treatment" exception, 505
Medical records, 29, 437
Memory. *See different aspects and types of memory*
Memory fragments, 13
Memory-jogging techniques, 286
Memory-like hallucinations, 77
Memory markers, in episodic memory of trauma, 277–78
"Memory mill," 479
Memory monitoring, 122–24
Memory recovery therapy, 11–12, 14, 17, 19–20
Mental disability exception to statute of limitations, 452–53
Mental energy, lowered supply of, 42
Mental health of female victim, questioned, 434
Mental reinstatement, 99–101
Mental retardation, 497
"Metabolism" of trauma, 197
Metacognition, 163–64, 273, 285
Meta-memory, 122–24, 164
Metamnemonic insight, 164
Methodology, and legal rights of trauma victims, 439
Middle frontal gyrus, 64, 66
Middle temporal gyrus, 68
Military mind control experiments, 33
Mills v. Habluetzel, 450

Minimization, 263
Miscarriage, 389
Misdirection cues, 49
Misidentification, 432
Misinformation, 5
Misleading information, 62–63
Misleading post-event information, 5
Misleading question paradigm, 102
Mismatch of encoding and retrieval contexts, 97–104, 106
Misperception of reality, 34
Missing periods of time, 28
Mississippi Scale, and neuroanatomy of stress, 79
Mitosis-like quality of memories, 197
Mnemonic monitoring, 122
Mnemonic reinstatement, 99–100
Mnemonic strategy, 164
"More probable than not," 428
Mother, adoptive, 28–29
Motivated skepticism, 46–47
Motivation, 432
Mousetrap scenario, 9
Multiaxial diagnostic system, 483
Multigenerational abuse, 384
Multiple determination, 94
Multiple personality disorder (MPD), 252, 408–9, 411
  arguments supporting delayed recall of trauma and, 26, 28–30, 33
  maintaining therapist neutrality and, 483, 490
  statute of limitations and, 453
Multiple sensory cortices, 82
Multiple simultaneous court proceedings, children in, 500
Multiple traumatic moments, 276
Munchausen's-by-proxy behaviors, 366–68
Munchausen's syndrome, and uncorroborated memories, 403
"Myth of repressed memory," 461

Nachträglichkeit, 141–42
Narcissism, 410
Narrative recall, 498
Narrative revision, 330
Narrative truth
  legal issues and, 514

maintaining therapist neutrality and, 479–80, 486–87
nature of memory and, 303
new, 4
statute of limitations and, 445
Narrative value of memory, 150, 152
Narrowing of attention, in posttraumatic stress disorder, 230
National Guard veterans, neuroanatomy of stress in, 75
Naturalistic studies in nonclinical samples, in posttraumatic stress disorder, 231–33
Nature of children's memories, 169–77
Negative case, 25
Negative stereotypes, 170–72
Negligence, 429
Neocortex, 68, 77, 80
Neodissociation theories, 43
Net increase in level of recall, 106
Neural bases of forgetting, in memory retrieval, 111–12, 515
Neuroanatomical correlates, of effects of stress on memory, 61–84
Neurological disease, 37
Neuromodulation of memory traces, 71–73
Neurons, selective reinforcement of connections between, 515
Neuropsychology
inaccuracy and inaccessibility in memory retrieval and, 93–126
posttraumatic stress disorder and, 235–40
Neurotransmitters
integrative developmental model and, 200
neuroanatomy of stress and, 62, 66, 69–74, 80–83
New Hampshire
legal rights of trauma victims in, 435–36
statute of limitations in, 469–70
New synthesis, 198
New York, statute of limitations in, 453–54
Nietzsche, Friedrich, 113
Nightmares
integrative developmental model and, 204
intrusive recollections and, 153

neuroanatomy of stress and, 74
posttraumatic stress disorder and, 225, 227
Noncognitive sensory systems, 518
Nondeclarative memory
neuroanatomy of stress and, 64
posttraumatic stress disorder and, 246
Nonepileptic seizures, 37
Nontraumatic memory, 518
Nontraumatic stimuli, memory for, 237–40
Normal forgetting, and neuroanatomy of stress, 81
Normal memories
brain mechanisms involved in function of, 64–68
stress effects on, 62–64
Northridge earthquake study, 274
Nucleus reticularis pontis caudalis, 66

Obesity, 143
Objective evidence, and statute of limitations, 457, 460
Obsessive-compulsive disorder (OCD), 396, 403, 413
Occipital cortex, 68
Occipital lobe, 200, 515
Oedipus complex, 140–41, 404, 410, 415
Ohio, statute of limitations in, 463–67
Ohio Court of Appeals, 463
Oklahoma City bombing, 195
Olfactory cortex, 82
Opinion stated as fact, 25–26
Orbitofrontal cortex, 67–69, 80, 83
Organization plans, subjective, 102–4
Orienting reflex (OR), and integrative developmental model, 193–94
Out-of-court settlement, 500
Overall level, 106
Overassimilation, 196
Overgeneralization, 361
Overloaded cue, 96
Overnight hospitalization scenario, 7–8
Overstimulation, 143, 383
Overweening pride, 49
Overwriting phenomenon, 62–63

Panic attacks, 252, 326, 410
Paradigms, 49, 52
new, 516

Paradoxical intervention, 373
Parahippocampal cortex, 64–65, 77
Parallel distributed processing, 43–44, 200–8
Paranoid schizophrenia, of adoptive mother, 28–29
Parental confirmation of abuse, 31–35
Parents, adoptive, 29
Parietal association cortex, 64, 67, 71, 515
Parietal lobe, 200
Partial amnesia, and clinical typology, 265–66
Partial reenactments, 332
Part-set cuing, 103–4
Passive avoidance test of memory, 71–72
Passivity, 147, 151
Past-life regression, 14–15, 17, 33, 354, 478
Paternal confirmation of abuse, 34, 38
Paternal introject alters, 373
Pathogenesis, and memories of childhood abuse, 286, 394–417
Pathological distortion in memory retrieval, 124–25
Patient intent to sue, evaluating, 493
Peer pressure in investigating abuse allegations, 498
Pennsylvania
  statute of limitations in, 451
  victim rights laws passed by, 431
Perirhinal cortex, 64–65
Peritraumatic dissociation, in posttraumatic stress disorder, 239–40, 250–51
Peritraumatic Dissociation Experiences Questionnaire (PDEQ), in posttraumatic stress disorder, 250
Permitting of memory retrieval, 95–97
Perpetrator, bias indicated in use of term, 497
Per se exclusion of hypnotically elicited testimony, 353
Personalization, 362
Phone sex, 143
Photo albums, 29
Photographic recall, 26
Photographs, viewing old, 4, 12, 19, 29, 88
Physical reinstatement, 98–99

Physical context
  extrinsic, 98–101
  intrinsic, 98
Physical evidence, lack of, 15
Physiological environment, internal, 101–2
Physioneuroses, 246
Pilot study, exploring validation of recovered memories in dissociative identity disorder patients, 29–39
Pimple scenario, 511–13
Pituitary, 83
Pituitary-adrenocortical response, 69
Place of remembering, 328–30
Planned abusive experiments, 29
Plasticity of memory, 142, 515
Pleasant experiences, 47
Polarization
  maintaining therapist neutrality, 477
Polarization of researchers, 36, 51, 53, 477, 518
Police
  intervention by, 30
  posttraumatic stress disorder in, 239
Police record confirmation of abuse, 31
Polygraphy, 468–69
Poor training, therapeutic, 483–84
Positive transference, 27
Positron emission tomography (PET), and neuroanatomy of stress, 65, 67–68, 80
Possession by devil, 32
Possibility vs. absolute fact, 11
Possible historical reconstruction, 411
Posthypnotic amnesia, 351
Posttraumatic neurosis, and statute of limitations, 453
Posttraumatic stress disorder (PTSD), 398–99, 407, 516, 518
  avoidance and, 228–29
  and early organization of memory in school-age children and adolescents, 273–74
  emotional numbing and, 228–29
  experimental studies and, 230–31
  eyewitness memory and, 230–35
  hyperactivity and, 384
  hyperarousal and, 229–30
  integrative developmental model and, 196, 215

memory for nontraumatic stimuli and, 237–40

memory for traumatic stimuli and, 235–37

naturalistic studies in nonclinical samples and, 231–33

neuroanatomy of stress and, 62, 71, 73, 75–83

neuropsychological findings in, 235–40

overview, 225, 243–56

phenomenology of memory disturbances in, 226–30

posttraumatic factors in, 240

reliving and re-experiencing, 226–28

sibling abuse and, 385

POWs, posttraumatic stress disorder in former, 237–38

Pragmatic power, 414

Precocious expressions of sexual abuse, 213

Preconscious memories, 139

Preexperimental familiarity, 114

Preexisting semantic associations, relatively specific or restricted effects of, 116–18

Prefrontal cortex, 67, 71

Pregnancy, 15, 389

Premature closure, 52

''Preponderance of evidence,'' 154

Preschool children
false memory creation by, 9
interviewing, 497–98

Presently remembered past, 149

Pressure by therapist to remember childhood abuse, 3–20

Presumption against disclosure of counseling records, 432

Primal scenes, 142

Primary auditory cortex, 68

Primary process thinking, 150, 153, 364

Primary repetition compulsion, 151

Primary repression, 147

Priming, and neuroanatomy of stress, 64, 68, 80

Principal sulcus region, 64, 66

Principles, and legal rights of trauma victims, 439

Privacy rights of sexual trauma victims, 430–34, 521

Private inspection, 432

Proactive interference, 107–8

Probability, 154

Procedural memory
neuroanatomy of stress and, 64
posttraumatic stress disorder and, 247

Professional competence, maintaining, 491

Profound amnesia, and clinical typology, 266–67

Projection, and psychoanalysis, 146

Prompting, in investigating abuse allegations, 499

Prosecution, and child victims in legal system, 499–500

Protection, inadequate, 145

Prototypicality, 116

Pseudomemories, 40, 43
hypnosis and, 350, 354
psychodynamic therapy and, 335

Psychiatric disorders, stress-related, 73–81

Psychic blindness, and neuroanatomy of stress, 69

Psychic reality, 299, 302–3, 324
historical reality and, 304–5

Psychoanalysis
case studies and, 143–46, 149–55
defense mechanisms and, 146–49
memory and, 139–42
overview, 138–39
reconstruction and, 293–312
statute of limitations and, 462–65
trauma and, 142–43

Psychodynamic therapy
assessment of trauma patients, 326–28
case study, 320
goals of treatment, 328–30
overview, 316–17
place of remembering, 328–30
psychodynamic understanding of impact of abuse, 317–19
recollection and, 333–37
reconstruction and, 333–37
role of dissociation, 320–23
stages of treatment, 330–33
trauma and memory, 323–25
truth and, 333–37

Psychogenic amnesia
absence of cogent discussions of in DSM-IV, 44

Psychogenic amnesia (*continued*)
    posttraumatic stress disorder and, 225,
    228, 234
Psychological event, 303
Psychotic delusion, 403
Public statements, and maintaining thera-
    pist neutrality, 492–93
Punch bowl at wedding scenario, 6–9

"Query," of memory, 126
Questionnaire about childhood events,
    6–7

Radical shift in attention or concern when
    physical integrity is violated, 276
Rage, 149, 227
Ramona v. Isabella, 400, 489–90
Random ordering, 103
Rape center assessment, 30
Rape crisis centers, 430
Rape-shield laws, 430–31
Rationality, absence of aspects of, 150
Reaction formation, 371
Reactive synaptogenesis, 202
Reading about abuse as source of memory,
    16
Reality monitoring in therapy, 13–14
"Reasonable and meritorious cause" for
    filing lawsuit, 458
Recall, and hypnosis, 348–49
Recantation, 440, 477–78
Receipt of certificate of insurance, annual
    requirement for, 488
Recently observed event, 5
Recitation of fact, 415
Recollection of memory, and psycho-
    dynamic therapy, 333–37
Reconciliation, family, 462
Reconstruction of memory, 139
    abreaction and, 294–98
    ego psychology and, 301–2
    historical reality and, 304–5
    infantile sexuality and, 298–301
    nature of memory and, 303–4
    overview, 293–94
    psychic reality and, 304–5
    psychoanalysis and, 152, 154–55
    psychodynamic therapy and, 333–37
    seduction theory and, 294–98

    structural theory and, 301–2
    suggestion and, 305–11
    topographic theory and, 298–301
    trauma and, 294–98
    validation of trauma and, 305–11
    validation of truth and, 305–11
Recording interviews of child victims, 499
Recovered memory, avoidance of use of
    term, 25
Recovered memory therapy, 152
    dissociative identity disorder and, 365
    neuroanatomy of stress and, 61
Recovery of memories, of childhood
    trauma that did not happen, 3–20
Recreation of event, 144
Reduplicative paramnesia, 122, 124
Reenactment, 36, 147, 151
Reexperiencing, in posttraumatic stress dis-
    order, 225–28
"Refreshing," 357
Registration, 36
Regressive dependency, 37
Reincarnation, 15
Related self-knowledge, 16
Relation between types of information, 97
Relationship difficulties, and therapist in-
    stigation of false memories of child
    abuse, 3
Relative's confirmation of abuse, 31
Relatively more complex preexisting pat-
    terns of associations, effects of, 120–
    21
Relatively specific effects, of preexisting
    semantic associations, 116–18
Relaxation response, 346
Reliability of memory, 437, 439
Reliving
    hypnosis and, 357
    posttraumatic stress disorder and, 226–
    28
Remembering in action, 321–23
"Remember" response, 125
Reminiscence, 44, 106
REM sleep, and integrative developmental
    model, 204–8
Repeated questioning about childhood
    sexual abuse, 483, 498
Repetition
    creation of false memories and, 5–10

posttraumatic stress disorder and, 226–27, 234
psychoanalysis and, 151–52
Repetition compulsion, 144, 321–22
Repetition of traumatic scenario, unwitting, 51
Repetitive trauma, 50
Replay of memories, in posttraumatic stress disorder, 226–27, 234
Repressed memory
  avoidance of use of term, 25
  as defense of psyche, 216
  dissociative identity disorder and, 42–45
  little evidence for, 18–19
  psychoanalysis and, 146–48
  statute of limitations as legal challenge and, 445–74
Repression
  definition of term, 216
  overgeneralization of use of as term, 25
Repressive defenses, 146–48
Reproductive memory, 167
Repudiation, 520
Reshaping of personality, 146
Respect for human dignity, and maintaining therapist neutrality, 484
Restrained coolness, 331
Restricted effects of preexisting semantic associations, 116–18
Retention, 36
Reticular activating system, 200
Retractors, 49
Retraumatization of child in court, 504–5
Retribution, 49
Retrieval capacity, limited, 108–9
Retrieval competition, 169
Retrieval conditions, and children's event memory, 174–75, 177
Retrieval cues, 19
Retrieval of memory
  absence of sufficiently informative cues to guide or permit, 95–97
  arguments supporting delayed recall of trauma, 36
  inaccuracy and inaccessibility in, 93–126
Retrieval plans, subjective, 102–4
Retrieval strengthening, costs of lack of, 108–9
Retroactive interference, 107, 239

Revelation effect, 116
Reworking memory, 207, 285–86
Reworking of traumatic experience, 144
Right cerebral hemisphere, 255
Right frontal lobe infarction, 124
Rights, victim, 425–28
Risk-management principles, clinically based, 480–93, 523
Rituals, in posttraumatic stress disorder, 229
Robust repression, 44
Role switching, 147, 151
Roman Catholic faith, 32
Rorschach Inkblot Test, and self-memory system, 190
Rule of abstinence, 481–83
Rule-outs, 37
Rules of evidence, 521

Sacrifices, ritual, 15
Sadness
  children's event memory and, 175
  neuroanatomy of stress and, 82
Sam Stone scenario, 171–72
Satanic cults, multigenerational, 366–68, 489
Satanic ritual abuse, 14–17, 33–34, 244, 373, 403, 414, 516
Scant reliability of memory, 230
Scars, physical, 15
Scene of abuse, and neuroanatomy of stress, 82
Schemas, 15
  action, 147
  argument for reality of delayed recall of trauma, 48
  memory retrieval and, 120–21
Schizophrenia, 403, 413
School-age children, early organization of memory in, 272–87
School records, 29, 437
"Scientific," legal definition of, 439
"Scientific proof," 437
Screaming during sleep, in posttraumatic stress disorder, 227
Screener function, of court, 470
Screen phenomena, 26
Scripts, 15
Secondary gain for patient, 37

Secondary process, 364
Secondary repression, 147
Second Circuit Court of Appeals, 449
Secrets, well-guarded, 332
Seduction hypothesis, 140
Seduction theory
  psychodynamic therapy and, 333
  reconstruction and, 294–98
Segregated experiences, 324
Seizures, nonepileptic, 37
Selective Reminding Test (SRT)
  neuroanatomy of stress and, 75
  posttraumatic stress disorder and, 238
Selective serotonin reuptake inhibitors
  (SSRIs), 396
Self esteem, low, 145
Self-attitudes, 16
Self-corrections, 122
Self-determination, patient, 484–85
Self-help books, 4
Self-induced trance, 40
Self-involving emotional events, 9
Self-involving events, 5–6
Self-memory system, 189–92, 198–99,
  204, 209–14, 216–17
Self-mutilation, 33, 252, 366–68, 407
Self-protective experiences, weakened ver-
  sions of, 278–79
Semantic associations, 126
  preexisting, 116–18
Semantic context, intrinsic, 97–98
Semantic knowledge, 161
Semantic memory, 103, 105, 108, 252
Semen, 144
Sensitization, stress, 80–81
Sensory cortex, 68
Sensory-perceptual attributes, 126
Serial Digit Learning Test, in posttraumatic
  stress disorder, 239
Sexual abuse, childhood
  child victims in legal system, 496–505
  developmental perspective on, 212–16
  false memories of, 3–20
  neuroanatomical correlates of effects of
    stress on memory, 61–84
  repeated questioning about, 483
  statistics, 517
  validation of in dissociative identity dis-
    order patients, 29–39

Sexual dysfunction, 407
Sexual exploitation by therapist, 27–28
Shahzade v. Gregory, 469, 471
Shame, 51, 69, 277
Shootings, 43
Short stories, 10
Short-term memory, 68
Showing of corroborative fact, 459
Shutting down, 27
Sibling
  abusive, 31, 32
  confirmation of abuse given by, 27, 31–
    32, 34, 36, 320
Single cues, 96
Single-blow trauma, 50, 478
Sisters, corroboration of abuse provided
  by, 27
"Sitting back," 482
Sixth Amendment rights, Constitutional,
  450–51, 522
Skepticism, 14–16
  motivated, 46–47
Slander, 435, 492–93
SLAPP suit, 435
Sleep
  hypnosis and, 350
  integrative developmental model and,
    204–8
  neuroanatomy of stress and, 78
  posttraumatic stress disorder and, 227,
    229, 232
"Sleeping on rights," 448
Slides, 5
"Slow motion," 286
Slutzker trial, Pennsylvania, 451, 470
Smells
  neuroanatomy of stress and, 82
  posttraumatic stress disorder and, 227
"Snake skin," 191
Sniper attack on school playground, 277–
  78, 286
Social demands in false memory creation,
  9, 10, 12, 16–17
Social-motivational model of memory,
  complex, 287
Societal responses to memories of trauma,
  521–24
Sodium amobarbital, 489
Sodium amytal, 4, 490–92, 514

Somatization, 36, 252
Soul murder, 397
Sounds
    neuroanatomy of stress and, 82
    posttraumatic stress disorder and, 227
Source amnesia, 62–63
Source forgetting, 114
Source misattribution, 114
Source monitoring, 125, 163–64, 178–79
Spacing of interviews, 7
"Spacing out," 32, 250–51
Spatial-textual information, 110
Special child abuse prosecution units, 504
Specialized testimony, 438
Specific memories, generic memories vs.,
    119, 120
Splitting defenses, 146, 150, 295, 353,
    362
    integrative developmental model and,
        189–92, 208–9
Spontaneous abreaction, 362
Spontaneous declaration, 505
Spontaneous trance phenomena, 40, 42
Staff burnout, in behavioral management of
    dissociative identity disorder, 366
Staged event, 5
Standard of proof, 428
Standards of care, 523
Startle reflex, 145
    early organization of memory and, 284
    neuroanatomy of stress and, 66, 78
    posttraumatic stress disorder and, 229
State-dependent recall, 82–83
States
    legal rights of trauma victims in, 435–36
    protection of victim rights by, 521
    statute of limitations in, 450–51, 453–
        59, 463–67, 469–70
    victim rights laws passed by, 426–28,
        430–33
State v. Hungerford, 469–71
State v. Mack, 353
State v. Morahan, 469
Statute of limitations, 522
    countervailing policies and meanings of
        statute of limitations challenge, 447–
        54
    emerging assault on repressed memory
        and implications for law, 461–74

filing claim in trauma case, 428
overview, 445–47
pattern of litigation strategies (1986 to
    present), 454–60
Stereotypic response to trauma, 517
Stitches in leg scenario, 9
Stopping therapy, 493
Storage, memory, 153
Stress, neuroanatomical correlates of ef-
    fects of on memory
    brain mechanisms involved in normal
        memory function, 64–68
    brain regions involved in memory, 69–
        73
    effects of stress on normal memories,
        63–64
    extinction, 80
    hormonal responses to, 516
    introduction, 61–62
    modification of normal memories, 62–63
    stress sensitization, 80–81
    stress-induced neuromodulation of
        memory traces, 71–73
    stress-related alterations in brain memory
        systems in patients with stress-related
        psychiatric disorders, 73–81
    working model for neurobiology of
        memory alterations in childhood abuse
        survivors, 81, 82
Stress sensitization, 80–81, 83
Stress trauma, 143
Stria terminalis, 66
Stroop interference
    posttraumatic stress disorder and, 235–
        36, 239
    neuroanatomy of stress and, 67, 79
Structural theory, 301–2
Structured Clinical Interview for DSM-III-R-
    Dissociative Disorders (SCID-D)
    neuroanatomy of stress and, 74
    posttraumatic stress disorder and, 250
Style, 120
Sub-egos, 365
Subcortical structures, 64, 67, 200
Subicular complex, 64–65
Subjective environment, internal, 101–2
Subjective quality of memory awareness,
    disturbances of, 121–22
Substance abuse, 45, 240

Substantia nigra, 66
Suggestibility, 520
    children's event memory and, 173, 177–
        78, 180
    maintaining therapist neutrality and, 486
    preschoolers and, 498
    reconstruction and, 305–11
Suggestion paradigm, 310–11
Suggestions based on probability, 11–12
Suicide attempts, 36–37
Superego, 301
Super memories, 272
Supervision, and maintaining therapist neu-
    trality, 488–89
Support groups, 4
Supportive environment for remembering,
    19
Support persons, 504
Supreme Court
    U.S., 431–32, 434, 450, 467–68
    Washington State, 455–57
Supreme Judicial Court, Massachussetts,
    432–33
Suspecting abuse when no memories are
    present, 407–11
Suspicion to confirmation progression, 11
Sweating, in posttraumatic stress disorder,
    227
Sympathetic nervous system, in post-
    traumatic stress disorder, 240
Symptom clusters, in posttraumatic stress
    disorder, 225–26, 228–29
Symptom relief, 414
Syndrome evidence, 479
Systematic deception, 48

"Taking cognizance," 216
Talking about abuse, as source of memory,
    16
Taste, in posttraumatic stress disorder, 227
Teacher, sexual exploitation by, 34
Tellegen Absorption Scale (TAS), 8
Temper tantrums, 382
Temporal boundary loss, in posttraumatic
    stress disorder, 228
Temporal grouping, 102
Temporal lobe, 69, 76–77, 111–12, 200, 515
Temporal Orientation Test, in posttrau-
    matic stress disorder, 239

Temporal-parietal cortex, 68
Temporal-spatial information, 126
$10 dollar bill scenario, 11
Terminal illness, confession by abusive
    sibling during, 31–32
Termination
    of active retrieval attempts, 105–7
    of therapy, 493
Terror, in posttraumatic stress disorder,
    231
Testifying, effects of on children, 497–
    503
Texas, statute of limitations in, 450
Thalamus, 65–66, 69–70, 78
Therapists
    abusive, 27–28, 31
    boundary-violating, 32
    instigation of false memory creation by,
        3–20
    neutrality of, 477–93
    validation of patient memories by, 411–
        13
Thrashing during sleep, in posttraumatic
    stress disorder, 227
Threats of harm, 51
Three years of age, credibility of memories
    occuring before as suspect, 486
Time-outs, 382
Tip-of-the-tongue awareness, 351
To-be-forgotten materials, 108–9, 110, 115
To-be-remembered materials, 109
Tolling provision, and statute of limitation,
    449–50, 452–53, 457
Tone-footshock pairing paradigm, 67
Topographic theory, 298–302
Tort liability, 524
    child victims in legal system and, 500
    statute of limitations and, 451, 455
Trace alteration, 169
Tracing birth parents, 28, 29
Trail-Making Test
    in posttraumatic stress disorder, 239
"Trance logic," 482
Transference
    formulation of concept, 297
    psychoanalysis and, 148–49, 153
Trauma. *See different aspects and types of
    trauma*
"Traumatic," definition of as term, 142

Traumatic amnesia phenomenon, 248–49, 436
Traumatic Antecedents Questionnaire (self-rating version) (TAQ[S]), in post-traumatic stress disorder, 253
Traumatic history, lack of importance of, 413–16
Traumatic Memory Inventory (TMI), in posttraumatic stress disorder, 253
Traumatic play, 321
Trauma victim, new identity as, 307
Treatment of children, and memories of trauma
    case studies, 380–90
    overview, 378–80
Tricycle scenario, 9
Triggering, 362
Triple cues, 96
Trust, sense of, 145
Truth
    establishing, 520
    historical, 479, 480
    narrative, 479, 480
    psychodynamic therapy and, 333–37
Truth drugs, 13
Twelve-step programs, 32
Tyson v. Tyson, 446, 454–58, 460–63, 465–66

UFOs, 18
Unabsorbed experiences, 324
"Unavailability," 505
Unconditioned stimulus, 66, 72
Unconscious fixed ideas, 251
Unconscious flashbacks, 36
Uncorroborated memories, considering, 403–7
Uncovered material, and psychoanalysis, 155
Unique specification, 95
Unitary phenomenon, memory as, 35
Universal agent, in neurosogenesis, 298
Unsuppressed memory of childhood abuse, 3–4
Urie v. Thompson, 449, 453
U.S. Constitution
    Equal Protection Clause, 450
    Sixth Amendment, 450–51

U.S. Supreme Court, and statute of limitations, 448–50, 467–68

Vague recollections, 36
Validation
    of patient memories by therapist, 411–13
    of recovered memories in dissociative identity disorder patients, 29–39
    of trauma, 305–11
    of truth, 305–11
Valuelessness, sense of, 145–46
Variety of false events and memories, 6–8
Ventromedial prefrontal cortex, 67
Verbal references during nightmare, 227
Verbatim vs. gist, 118–19
Veridical recollection, *xiii–xiv,* 1, 152
Verification of old memories, 19
Vermont, statute of limitations in, 459
Vertical splitting, 325
Vestibulo-orienting reflex (VOR), integrative developmental model and, 193–94
"Victim," bias indicated in use of term, 497
Victims of Child Abuse Laws (VOCAL), 379
Victims of Violent Crime Act, 428
Victory by intimidation, 434
"Video camera" theory of the mind, 514, 516
Videotaped interviews and testimony, 5, 499, 504
Vietnam veterans
    arguments supporting delayed recall of trauma in, 28
    integrative developmental model and, 212
    neuroanatomy of stress in, 74–75, 79
    posttraumatic stress disorder in, 227–36, 238–39, 251, 253
Violence Against Women Act, federal, 426, 428
Visual appearance of perpetrator, 82
Visual association cortex
    neuroanatomy of stress and, 68
    posttraumatic stress disorder and, 255
Visual hallucinations, and neuroanatomy of stress, 77, 79
Visual-spatial pad, 285

Wabimujichagwan, 211

"Wanting to forget," 226

Washington State Supreme Court, and statute of limitations, 455–57

Weakened versions, of self-protective mechanisms in remembering and recounting traumatic experiences, 278–79

"Weapon focussing" phenomenon, 231

Webs, memory, 515

Wechsler Adult Intelligence Scale (WAIS), and posttraumatic stress disorder, 239

Wechsler Adult Intelligence Scale-Revised (WAIS-R),
  neuroanatomy of stress and, 75
  posttraumatic stress disorder and, 237

Wechsler Memory Scale (WMS)
  neuroanatomy of stress and, 75–76
  posttraumatic stress disorder and, 237–38

White v. Illinois, 504–5

Willful misrepresentation, 26

Wisconsin Card Sorting Test, 71, 125

Witch hunts, 440

Witnessed abuse
  by childhood neighbor, 31–32

  by friend, 31–33

Witnesses, child
  jurors' reponses to, 503
  overview, 500
  preparation of for court, 502–3

Wolf Man, 141, 300

Wood v. Carpenter, 448

Word associations
  posttraumatic stress disorder and, 236–37
  neuroanatomy of stress and, 75

Word lists, 10

Word recall, and neuroanatomy of stress and, 77, 80

Working memory, and neuroanatomy of stress, 64–66

"Working through" of sequelae of childhood events, 416

World War II veterans
  neuroanatomy of stress in, 75
  posttraumatic stress disorder in, 237, 249

X-Files, 35

Zealotry, 484